Emergency Cardiac Surgery

Antonios Kourliouros
Editor

Emergency Cardiac Surgery

Springer

Editor
Antonios Kourliouros
Cardiothoracic Surgery
John Radcliffe Hospital
Oxford, UK

ISBN 978-3-032-15786-7 ISBN 978-3-032-15787-4 (eBook)
https://doi.org/10.1007/978-3-032-15787-4

This Springer imprint is published by the registered company Springer Nature Switzerland AG
The registered company address is: Gewerbestrasse 11, 6330 Cham, Switzerland

To my son Massimo Ilias

Contents

Definition and Clinical Relevance of Emergency Cardiac Surgery

Antonios Kourliouros

Abstract While emergency cardiac surgery represents 3–4% of the performed cardiac procedures in terms of acuteness, it accounts for a six fold, at least, increase in operative mortality compared to elective surgery. It stress-tests healthcare systems due to the requirement for increased resources, preparedness, and trained multidisciplinary teams in the core of which lies the modern cardiac surgeon. Strategies for early identification of precarious clinical conditions and support networks for high risk cardiological interventions could mitigate the incidence and improve the outcomes of emergency cardiac surgery. This also applies to cardiothoracic trauma, vascular interventions, and specific vulnerable populations such as those with congenital heart conditions and those awaiting heart transplantation. Emergency cardiac surgery lies in the intersection of these clinical disciplines and has not been examined in detail. It is often underreported in large databases and national audits, risk stratification models lack predictive value and specific training and education is sparse. This introductory chapter aims to better define emergency cardiac surgery and its asymmetric impact on outcomes and resources, and to identify potential strategies for risk management.

Keywords Emergency cardiac surgery · Operative urgency classification · Risk stratification in cardiac surgery · Performance monitoring in cardiac surgery · Risk management in cardiac surgery · Simulation training · Cardiac surgical education and competency · Regional rota for emergency cardiac surgery · Hub-and-spoke networks in cardiac surgery · Healthcare resource utilisation in cardiac surgery

A. Kourliouros (✉)
Cardiothoracic Surgery, John Radcliffe Hospital, Oxford, UK
e-mail: a.kourliouros@gmail.com

A. Kourliouros (ed.), *Emergency Cardiac Surgery*,
https://doi.org/10.1007/978-3-032-15787-4_1

1 Definition of Emergency Cardiac Surgery

International task force groups providing guidelines for cardiac surgical interventions define emergency surgery as one performed within 24 h from when the indication is established (Delgado et al. 2023). Clinical urgency is defined in one of the most widely applied risk prediction models in cardiac surgery, the EuroSCORE II, with emergency surgery taking place before the beginning of the next working day from the time the decision was made to operate (Nashef et al. 2012). This operative urgency definition was reviewed by the Society for Cardiothoracic Surgery in Great Britain and Ireland (SCTS) and revised for the purposes of UK outcome reporting due to potential ambiguity in the one provided by EuroSCORE II; examples of which include who makes the decision to operate, i.e. whether it is unanimous within all members of the surgical team, and at which time point during the patient's hospital admission surgery is performed. For this reason, SCTS have adopted as emergency cardiac surgery those cases operated within 24 h of admission for life-threatening conditions or where clinical deterioration of an inpatient warrants surgical intervention within 24 h (SCTS Annual Report 2019–20 2020). In the same document there is further distinction of salvage surgery wherein rapid clinical deterioration requires expeditious life-saving surgery or requirement of cardiopulmonary resuscitation, commencement of inotropes, and presence of shock prior to conduct of surgery. It is also worth noting that patients on the urgent inpatient pathway (i.e. those admitted as non-electives and that do not require surgery within 24 h) can occasionally cross over to emergency and salvage cases. For the purposes of this book, we have endorsed the SCTS definition for emergency surgery—accepting that the 24h window can still be interpreted differentially—but within the same spirit of acuteness and rapid clinical deterioration.

2 Clinical Relevance

2.1 Impact on Outcomes

Despite an increase in the risk profile of patients undergoing cardiac surgery over the years, mortality rates continue to decrease (Grant et al. 2021). In an analysis of 2022/23 UK data, the unadjusted overall mortality was 2.6% for all cardiac surgery (NACSA Summary Report 2024 n.d.). However, for those patients undergoing emergency cardiac surgery, the mortality rate has been reported at 17.6% (Grant et al. 2013). This represents a sixfold increase in the odds of death, a statistic that is less pronounced in other surgical specialties (Mullen et al. 2017).

Without incorporating the most recent data, an analysis of the UK national cardiac surgical database between 2002 and 2016 has demonstrated a static incidence of emergency surgery accounting for 3.5% of all cases (and approximately 0.5% incidence of salvage procedures) (Grant et al. 2021). One has to appreciate nonetheless, that many emergency cardiac surgical procedures may not be captured or are potentially excluded from national registries and databases, such as surgery for cardiac trauma or complications of cardiovascular interventions; thus their incidence is likely to be systematically underestimated.

2.2 *Impact on Risk Management*

Cardiac surgery has pioneered performance monitoring principles and the implementation of risk prediction modelling in clinical practice. Risk prediction is central to the informed consent of patients, multidisciplinary decision making, and public reporting of outcomes. EuroSCORE (and its current iteration EuroSCORE II), and the Society of Thoracic Surgeons (STS) score are the most commonly applied risk prediction models, both of which possess independent strengths and inherent limitations (Sinha et al. 2021). When tested in a more historic cohort, EuroSCORE II underpredicted emergency surgery mortality in the lower-risk patient cohort (observed mortality at 8.9% vs predicted at 4.4%) and overpredicted it in the higher-risk group (observed mortality 30.4% vs predicted at 39.5%) (Grant et al. 2013). The opposite was identified in an analysis of a broad US database applying the STS score where salvage cases had observed mortality significantly higher than predicted (Chancellor et al. 2020). Such discrepancies expose the methodological limitations of regression-based risk stratification models for rarer pathologies or events, with important repercussions to appropriate patient consent, availability of resources in and out-of-hours, assessment of futility, team dynamics, and transparency.

The public reporting of emergency surgery ceased taking place in the UK to prevent risk-averse behaviour by the surgeons but also due to the aforementioned inability of risk performance tools to provide satisfactory discriminatory capabilities. The effect of this practice on the frequency and outcomes of emergency cardiac surgery has not been studied extensively yet but while there are potential benefits to very high-risk patients, it could also allow for "gaming" through manipulation of operative urgency. Chap. 33 provides a more detailed and critical analysis of risk stratification and performance monitoring in emergency cardiac surgery.

2.3 *Impact on Resources*

In addition to the financial implications of emergency cardiac surgery which are substantially greater than the same procedures being performed electively (Haider et al. 2015), there are also hidden strains posed to healthcare systems. Overnight emergencies could impact the routine conduct of daytime surgery and prolonged intensive care treatments for such patients can also lead to bed blocking, causing an indirect impact on waiting lists and revenue loss. Preparedness for rare events requires additional resources and staff training, a typical example being the provision of mechanical circulatory support (MCS) in the postcardiotomy setting conducted in a unit without routine MCS or cardiac transplant practice (Kourliouros and Tsui 2018). All the above can have both direct and indirect effects on patients waiting for elective cardiac surgery and the viability of healthcare organisations that have to prioritise efficiency whilst maintaining resource-intensive specialist emergency care.

3 Strategies to Mitigate the Risk of Emergency Cardiac Surgery

3.1 Risk Stratification and Standard Operating Procedures

Interventional cardiology procedures often take place in high-risk patient groups or possess an intrinsic technical complexity which can lead to complications that may require emergency cardiac surgery. As we will explore further in the relevant chapters, transcatheter valve implantations, electrophysiology procedures, cardiac device lead extractions, and high-risk coronary percutaneous interventions are associated with rare but potentially catastrophic complications for which cardiac surgical availability is essential. Risk scores have been developed to help with prediction and optimal resource utilisation in interventional procedures. Such examples are the PROGRESS-CTO score for predicting complications including pericardiocentesis and emergency surgery in percutaneous coronary interventions for chronic total occlusions, and the ELECTRa Registry Outcome Score (EROS) in transvenous lead extractions (Simsek et al. 2022; Sidhu et al. 2021) With postoperative bleeding being the most common complication that may lead to emergency re-exploration, risk stratification tools have been developed to predict excessive bleeding following cardiac surgery (Vuylsteke et al. 2011).

Alongside validated risk prediction models, it is paramount that standard operating procedures (SOP) and policies are in place, to ensure that complications can be anticipated and that appropriate resources are in place. An example of such an SOP can be found in Chap. 17 underlying the complex transvenous lead extractions at the Oxford Heart Centre in the UK, where among other provisions, the cardiac surgeon, perfusionist, and operating theatre scrub team are physically present throughout a high-risk procedure. Other local policies such as the Hemostasis Checklist introduced by Papworth Hospital in the UK have led to improved outcomes, including emergency re-exploration for bleeding, and have been adopted by other centres (Ali et al. 2021).

3.2 Simulation Training

The accepted definitions of emergency cardiac surgery often imply "intention" in the surgical decision. Emergency re-sternotomy after cardiac surgery for haemodynamic instability (e.g. bleeding, low cardiac output) or cardiac arrest is originally unintended but with potentially detrimental impact to the patient. It is recognised that cardiac arrest in the intensive care unit can occur in up to 3% of patients with almost half of such arrests managed with emergency re-exploration. Due to great variation in such practices and associated outcomes, the Clinical Guideline Committee of the European Association for Cardio-Thoracic Surgery (EACTS) developed guidelines for cardiac arrest resuscitation following cardiac surgery (Dunning et al. 2009).

It has been demonstrated that high-fidelity training can elicit a stress-response similar to real crisis conditions, which when utilised effectively can improve safety, technical skills, and teamwork spirit in intensive care settings (Kennedy-Metz et al. 2022). The Cardiac Surgery Advanced Life Support Course (CALS) was introduced around the same time to the EACTS guidelines, offering standardised simulation training on emergency chest re-opening in the intensive care setting. Since its implementation the CALS course has been delivered in numerous cardiothoracic units and its protocol endorsed by various specialty groups and societies (Dunning et al. 2006; Karcher et al. 2022). Its basic principles and more advanced concepts in emergency re-exploration following cardiac surgery are presented in Chap. 32. Simulation training for emergency management of cardiac surgical adverse events (in addition to re-exploration) is incorporated in resident and faculty training curricula with very good reception and improvement in technical skills (Mokadam et al. 2017).

3.3 Establishment of Regional Rota for Certain Emergency Conditions

There is evidence of a positive association between volume and outcome in the surgical treatment of many cardiac conditions. This association is more pronounced in rarer pathologies and where specialist expertise is necessary such as congenital cardiac surgery and heart transplantation (Welke et al. 2023; Pettit et al. 2012). With regard to certain types of emergency cardiac surgery and type A aortic dissection repairs in particular, the establishment of a rotational on-call system among hospitals within geographical vicinity of one another has been shown to offer superior outcomes compared to stand alone units (Vaja et al. 2019). As these are often observational analyses and direct causation cannot be established, plausible explanations could be the delivery of surgery by experienced aortic surgeons, familiarity of the operating theatre team with complex repair techniques and perfusion strategies, and standardised postoperative care. In the UK the practice of regional aortic rotas has now been expanded to units with a wider geographic distribution, the focus being the timely and streamlined diagnosis and management of acute aortic syndromes, alongside purpose-specific patient transportation networks (Krasopoulos et al. 2024).

3.4 Hub-and-Spoke Networks

Aside from the aforementioned volume-outcome relationship in emergency surgery for type A aortic dissections, certain cardiothoracic units possess a comparative expertise in the management of critical conditions rendering them more appropriate destinations. Where there is anticipation of postcardiotomy failure or evolving cardiogenic shock in a patient requiring cardiac surgery, provision of MCS could have an important role to play, and it is best delivered in centres with the relevant expertise(Nakata et al. 2023; Banayosy et al. 2019). The establishment of MCS-capable hub centres to support patients in cardiogenic shock (including postcardiotomy ones) presented in spoke hospitals is supported in the guidance produced by the International Society for Heart and Lung Transplantation (Bernhardt et al. 2023). Further evidence also exists in the prevention of infective endocarditis (IE) complications which could lead to emergency cardiac surgery, such as heart failure, by the adoption of a regional IE network (Diab et al. 2021).

The centralisation of trauma services is another initiative seen in the UK and other countries, and management of cardiothoracic trauma in particular has led to changes in practice favouring hub or "major trauma" centres. Indeed, patients having suffered major cardiothoracic trauma and treated exclusively in non-designated trauma centres experienced worse outcomes when compared to those transferred to major trauma centres for their definitive management (Khorsandi et al. 2015).

With an increasing number of percutaneous coronary interventions (PCI) taking place in settings without surgery on site (no-SOS), there has been scepticism with regard to patient safety in the unlikely event of a complication requiring an emergency sternotomy. This consideration will be explored in more detail in Chap. 7; however current data suggest there remains no difference in outcomes between PCI in settings with surgery and in no-SOS. Clinical reasons (such as call to balloon times), patient preference, and financial incentives have driven this increase in PCI in no-SOS centres supported by consensus statements from expert groups (Shamkhani et al. 2024). It has to be noted, however, that very high-risk cases such as chronic total occlusions and unprotected left main stem interventions tend to take place in hub centres, ideally with on-site surgical cover.

3.5 Education

In an era of sub-specialisation with simultaneous expansion of modalities to treat cardiovascular pathologies, it is less likely for the modern cardiac surgeon to obtain adequate exposure to effectively treat all emergency conditions. For instance, a surgeon with mitral interest and predominant practice faced with an acute aortic dissection may not possess the necessary experience for complex aortic repairs. Similarly a principally coronary surgeon with no previous exposure to MCS will not be adequately equipped to manage postcardiotomy failure following coronary artery bypass grafting. Larger cardiac units are likely to have surgeons on site with designated roles, though this is not always the case in smaller units or out-of-hours. The benchmarking of surgical competency in emergencies can be achieved with focused professional development and training from the time of specialisation which extends into the later independent specialist practice (Wang et al. 2011). Sabbaticals, regular exposure to non-dominant sub-specialty practice (e.g. aortic surgeon attending and performing supervised noncomplex mitral repairs alongside a mitral surgeon), and double scrubbing in rarer emergencies (e.g. double valve replacement with reconstruction of the aortomitral curtain—Commando procedure) may play a pivotal role (Doll et al. 2022). Finally, dedicated reading on emergency cardiac surgery, such as the material provided in this book, will allow clinicians to better understand the relevant pathologies and management recommendations and translate them into clinical practice aiming at optimal outcomes for this this high-risk patient population.

4 Conclusions

Emergency cardiac surgery imposes an asymmetric impact on mortality and morbidity, resource utilisation, and systems performance. It is also an area that occasionally lies within the intersection of different specialties and that has not been studied in a comprehensive way, until the production of this specialist book. The authors sought to identify mitigating mechanisms for its occurrence and provide best-practice recommendations for optimal operative management.

References

Ali JM, Gerrard C, Clayton J, Moorjani N (2021) Hemostasis checklist reduces bleeding and blood product consumption after cardiac surgery. Ann Thorac Surg 111. https://doi.org/10.1016/j.athoracsur.2020.07.016

Banayosy AME, Harper MD, Koerner MM, Vanhooser D, Chaffin J, Sasevich M et al (2019) Postcardiotomy cardiogenic shock: initial results of Oklahoma hub-and-spoke model. J Heart Lung Transplant 38. https://doi.org/10.1016/j.healun.2019.01.1095

Bernhardt AM, Copeland H, Deswal A, Gluck J, Givertz MM, Garan AR et al (2023) The International Society for Heart and Lung Transplantation/Heart Failure Society of America Guideline on Acute Mechanical Circulatory Support. J Heart Lung Transplant 42. https://doi.org/10.1016/j.healun.2022.10.028

Chancellor WZ, Mehaffey JH, Beller JP, Krebs ED, Hawkins RB, Yount K et al (2020) Current quality reporting methods are not adequate for salvage cardiac operations. J Thorac Cardiovasc Surg 159. https://doi.org/10.1016/j.jtcvs.2019.01.060

Delgado V, Aimone Marsan N, De Waha S, Bonaros N, Brida M, Burri H et al (2023) ESC guidelines for the management of endocarditis. Eur Heart J 44. https://doi.org/10.1093/eurheartj/ehad193

Diab M, Franz M, Hagel S, Guenther A, Struve A, Kuehn H et al (2021) The impact of establishing a regional infective endocarditis (IE) network on pre-operative IE-related complications and

on post-operative outcome. Eur Heart J 42:ehab724.1721. https://doi.org/10.1093/eurheartj/ehab724.1721
Doll JA, Lata K, Kearney KE (2022) Feedback and the early career proceduralist: how am I doing? J Am Coll Cardiol 79. https://doi.org/10.1016/j.jacc.2021.08.079
Dunning J, Nandi J, Ariffin S, Jerstice J, Danitsch D, Levine A (2006) The Cardiac Surgery Advanced Life Support Course (CALS): delivering significant improvements in emergency cardiothoracic care. Ann Thorac Surg 81. https://doi.org/10.1016/j.athoracsur.2005.12.012
Dunning J, Fabbri A, Kolh PH, Levine A, Lockowandt U, Mackay J et al (2009) Guideline for resuscitation in cardiac arrest after cardiac surgery. Eur J Cardiothorac Surg 36. https://doi.org/10.1016/j.ejcts.2009.01.033
Grant SW, Hickey GL, Dimarakis I, Cooper G, Jenkins DP, Uppal R et al (2013) Performance of the EuroSCORE models in emergency cardiac surgery. Circ Cardiovasc Qual Outcomes 6. https://doi.org/10.1161/CIRCOUTCOMES.111.000018
Grant SW, Kendall S, Goodwin AT, Cooper G, Trivedi U, Page R et al (2021) Trends and outcomes for cardiac surgery in the United Kingdom from 2002 to 2016. JTCVS Open 7. https://doi.org/10.1016/j.xjon.2021.02.001
Haider AH, Obirieze A, Velopulos CG, Richard P, Latif A, Scott VK et al (2015) Incremental cost of emergency versus elective surgery. Ann Surg 262. https://doi.org/10.1097/SLA.0000000000001080
Karcher C, Jurisevic C, Southwood T, McCormack D, Rogers A, Levine A et al (2022) The Australasian ANZSCTS/ANZICS guidelines on cardiothoracic advanced life support (CALS-ANZ). Crit Care Resuscit 24. https://doi.org/10.51893/2022.3.SA3
Kennedy-Metz LR, Barbeito A, Dias RD, Zenati MA (2022) Importance of high-performing teams in the cardiovascular intensive care unit. J Thorac Cardiovasc Surg 163. https://doi.org/10.1016/j.jtcvs.2021.02.098
Khorsandi M, Skouras C, Prasad S, Shah R (2015) Major cardiothoracic trauma: eleven-year review of outcomes in the North West of England. Ann R Coll Surg Engl 97. https://doi.org/10.1308/003588415X14181254789169
Kourliouros A, Tsui S (2018) Veno-arterial extracorporeal membrane oxygenation—a solution for the UK? In: Modi P, Ionescu M (eds) Perspectives in cardiothoracic surgery: the SCTS Ionescu University, vol III. Society for Cardiothoracic Surgery in Great Britain and Ireland, London, pp 126–131
Krasopoulos G, Brooks M, Modi A, Asopa S, Balmforth D et al (2024) NHS England. Supra-regional SOP on the Acute Management of Aortic Dissections. https://pearl.plymouth.ac.uk/cgi/viewcontent.cgi?article=1108&context=more-foh-research. Accessed 25 Dec 2024
Mokadam NA, Fann JI, Hicks GL, Nesbitt JC, Burkhart HM, Conte JV et al (2017) Experience with the cardiac surgery simulation curriculum: results of the resident and faculty survey. Ann Thorac Surg 103. https://doi.org/10.1016/j.athoracsur.2016.06.074
Mullen MG, Michaels AD, Mehaffey HJ, Guidry CA, Turrentine LE, Hedrick TL et al (2017) Risk associated with complications and mortality after urgent surgery vs elective and emergency surgery: implications for defining "quality" and reporting outcomes for urgent surgery. JAMA Surg 152. https://doi.org/10.1001/jamasurg.2017.0918
NACSA Summary Report 2024 (n.d.) National Audit. nacsa-final-report-2022-23
Nakata J, Yamamoto T, Saku K, Ikeda Y, Unoki T, Asai K (2023) Mechanical circulatory support in cardiogenic shock. J Intensive Care 11. https://doi.org/10.1186/s40560-023-00710-2
Nashef SAM, Roques F, Sharples LD, Nilsson J, Smith C, Goldstone AR et al (2012) Euroscore II. Eur J Cardiothorac Surg 41. https://doi.org/10.1093/ejcts/ezs043
Pettit SJ, Jhund PS, Hawkins NM, Gardner RS, Haj-Yahia S, McMurray JJV et al (2012) How small is too small? A systematic review of center volume and outcome after cardiac transplantation. Circ Cardiovasc Qual Outcomes 5. https://doi.org/10.1161/CIRCOUTCOMES.112.966630
SCTS Annual Report 2019–20 (2020) pp 33–34. https://scts.org/_userfiles/pages/files/reports/201920_scts_annual_report_nm_3rd_march_2020.pdf

Shamkhani W, Rashid M, Moledina S, Ludman P, Curzen N, Wijeysundera HC et al (2024) Complex high-risk percutaneous coronary intervention types, trends, and outcomes in nonsurgical centres. Can J Cardiol 40. https://doi.org/10.1016/j.cjca.2024.01.003

Sidhu BS, Ayis S, Gould J, Elliott MK, Mehta V, Kennergren C et al (2021) Risk stratification of patients undergoing transvenous lead extraction with the ELECTRa Registry Outcome Score (EROS): an ESC EHRA EORP European lead extraction ConTRolled ELECTRa registry analysis. Europace 23. https://doi.org/10.1093/europace/euab037

Simsek B, Kostantinis S, Karacsonyi J, Alaswad K, Krestyaninov O, Khelimskii D et al (2022) Predicting periprocedural complications in chronic total occlusion percutaneous coronary intervention: the PROGRESS-CTO complication scores. JACC Cardiovasc Interv 15. https://doi.org/10.1016/j.jcin.2022.06.007

Sinha S, Dimagli A, Dixon L, Gaudino M, Caputo M, Vohra HA et al (2021) Systematic review and meta-analysis of mortality risk prediction models in adult cardiac surgery. Interact Cardiovasc Thorac Surg 33. https://doi.org/10.1093/icvts/ivab151

Vaja R, Talukder S, Norkunas M, Hoffman R, Nienaber C, Pepper J et al (2019) Impact of a streamlined rotational system for the management of acute aortic syndrome: sharing is caring. Eur J Cardiothorac Surg 55. https://doi.org/10.1093/ejcts/ezy386

Vuylsteke A, Pagel C, Gerrard C, Reddy B, Nashef S, Aldam P et al (2011) The Papworth Bleeding Risk Score: a stratification scheme for identifying cardiac surgery patients at risk of excessive early postoperative bleeding. Eur J Cardiothorac Surg 39. https://doi.org/10.1016/j.ejcts.2010.10.003

Wang TT, Ahmed K, Patel VM, Harling L, Jawad M, Darzi A et al (2011) A competency framework in cardiothoracic surgery for training and revalidation—an international comparison. Eur J Cardiothorac Surg 40. https://doi.org/10.1016/j.ejcts.2011.01.018

Welke KF, Karamlou T, O'Brien SM, Dearani JA, Tweddell JS, Kumar SR et al (2023) Contemporary relationship between hospital volume and outcomes in congenital heart surgery. Ann Thorac Surg 116. https://doi.org/10.1016/j.athoracsur.2023.08.006

Management of Acute Aortic Dissection

Benjamin Adams and Luke Holland

Abstract Acute aortic dissection is a total aortic catastrophe which must be managed emergently and preferably by experts in the field within expert centres who are able to manage the patients post operatively. The operating is challenging, even for the most experienced surgeon, and frequently in the night which adds to the difficulties. However, it can be immensely rewarding as a life can be saved and the natural history of such a severe pathology halted in its tracks. This chapter aims to help the reader navigate through the decision making processes involved from referral to discharge home and we hope you find it useful.

Keywords Acute aortic dissection · Aortic dissection classification · Intramural haematoma · Malperfusion syndromes · Cannulation for aortic dissection repair · Ascending aorta replacement · Aortic root surgery · Aortic arch surgery · Bentall procedure · Frozen Elephant Trunk procedure · Cerebral perfusion/methods · Hypothermia

1 Introduction

Acute aortic dissection is a life-threatening emergency that requires prompt recognition, triage, facilitated by computed tomography (CT) imaging and expert management, ideally within a specialist aortic centre.

Without treatment, the classical mortality rate of a 1–2% risk per hour still resonates but was based on historical data from the 1950s, before the improvement of medical therapy, and cardiovascular surgery became routine (Hirst et al. 1958).

Dedication
For my sons and family.

B. Adams (✉) · L. Holland
Barts Heart Centre, St Bartholomew's Hospital, London, UK
e-mail: benjamin.adams6@nhs.net

A. Kourliouros (ed.), *Emergency Cardiac Surgery*,
https://doi.org/10.1007/978-3-032-15787-4_2

However, despite these advances in care, the mortality from acute type A dissection unfortunately remains high with a trend towards single digit survival seemingly elusive worldwide.

In the classic IRAD series, published over 20 years ago now, the mortality rate, even with surgical treatment, was 26% (Hagan et al. 2000). The Society for Cardiothoracic Surgery in Great Britain and Ireland (SCTS) Blue Book data mortality rate was 22.8% in 2008 although dropped to 18.3% in the 6-year period of 2007–2013 (Bridgewater et al. 2008). The German registry GERAADA data similarly was 17% in 2012 (Kruger et al. 2012). The USA type A mortality is also in the region of 17%. It is only the Japanese Registry of Acute Aortic Dissection (JRAD) that have achieved a better published mortality rate of 10.8% after surgical treatment for acute type A aortic dissection (Inoue et al. 2000). In addition, this paper highlights the challenges of managing this condition in the context of preoperative haemodynamic instability, including the need for resuscitation, reduced levels of consciousness, and advanced age, all factors that are associated with increased in-hospital mortality, even when referral to treatment is prompt. This figure of 10.8% is therefore aspirational and cannot be achieved without dedicated teams and pathways and the necessary range of tools in the armamentarium to treat this complex condition.

1.1 Referral Pathways and Regional Dissection Rotas

Bashir et al published in 2016 on the benefits of introduction a dissection rota for repair of type A dissection. In this paper they found a marked benefit in mortality from 30% prior to a dedicated dissection rota, down to 13% after the introduction (Bashir et al. 2016). A subsequent paper by the same group a year later delved deeper and looked at individual surgeons and outcomes. They showed that surgeons with a mean volume of less than four dissections per year had a significantly higher mortality (19.3% vs 12.6%) (Bashir et al. 2017). This has been implemented successfully in many regions across the UK including London and Liverpool.

However, and perhaps rather surprisingly, the UK mortality rate from Type A dissection still remains stuck at 17.7% in the 3-year period from 2016 to 2019. Thus, one could argue that there has essentially been no improvement in the last decade in the UK despite adoption of a regional rotas like London. To investigate this in more detail, NICOR looked at specific outcome measurements across centres in the UK as part of the National Adult Cardiac Surgery Audit (NACSA). Specifically, when units did less than 12 acute type A cases per year, or had less than five surgeons in the unit, or had less than 50% of surgeons performing dissections. In addition, they also looked at units that did less than 4 cases per year by less than two surgeons or each surgeon doing less than two cases per year. The only variable that made a difference, despite the evidence, was when a unit did more than 12 cases per year (16.3% v 19.6%). Thus, volume must be important, but it is the unit experience and pathways that may be more conducive to an outcome relationship.

The acute aortic dissection pathway toolkit was therefore written and published by NHS England in March 2022 with seven key principles and actions to improve care for acute emergency aortic dissection patients (https://jvsgbi.com/wp-content/uploads/2022/08/vol-1-issue-4-s1-s20.pdf).

The toolkit supports the creation of rotas of specialists in regional networks or referring hospitals in a specific geographical area that can deliver emergency care for both type A and B aortic dissection (https://jvsgbi.com/wp-content/uploads/2022/08/vol-1-issue-4-s1-s20.pdf). It also describes the level of governance required to demonstrate improvement in outcomes and reduction in variation. However, it is still cognizant of the fact that eventual agreed models may vary according to the local geography, circumstances, and expertise (https://jvsgbi.com/wp-content/uploads/2022/08/vol-1-issue-4-s1-s20.pdf).

2 Diagnosis and Risk Stratification

In truth, acute aortic dissection is one facet of the acute aortic syndromes (AAS) spectrum reflecting a range of aortic diseases that are all potentially fatal (Bossone et al. 2018). Acute aortic dissections (AADs) represent the most frequently encountered conditions, with an incidence ranging between 3 and 6/100 000 cases a year in western jurisdictions (Fleck et al. 2002; Uchida et al. 2009; Nienaber 2011). Stanford type A dissections account for about 60% of all cases followed by Stanford type B (Rylski et al. 2017), and those involving the arch and distal aorta (defined as non-A non-B [NANB]) occur in about 3–11% of cases (Rylski et al. 2017; Sievers et al. 2020; Urbanski and Wagner 2016).

Campaigns such as Think Aorta have done a lot to advocate for the fact that AAD is a time critical, life-threatening disease and to raise awareness amongst emergency department staff as the first responders and gate keepers. It is humbling to realise that 48% of patients do not even make it to hospital alive with this condition and in those that do, the diagnosis is considered in less than half of patients who arrive in the emergency department with the condition. Furthermore, one-third of patients with AAD are actively treated for a different, incorrect diagnosis. For example, it is not uncommon for a patient to arrive in the operating theatre having been pre-loaded with strong antiplatelet agents as initial management of a suspected but incorrect acute coronary syndrome. This is not withstanding the fact that AAD may present as coronary ischaemia due to malperfusion because of a dynamic dissection flap within the aortic root. Ultimately, a CT aortogram is required for a definitive diagnosis and interpretation of the scan is critical for subsequent treatment algorithms.

Identification of a dissection flap and its location within the aorta is critical to categorising the AAD into a Type A or B dissection as per the Stanford classification. The location of the entry tear on CT can usually be ascertained as a breach in the septum of the aorta and is helpful in planning the likely extent of the surgery required in the context of a Type A dissection. The presence of a pericardial effusion can also be noted and is usually associated with a degree of instability and raises immediate concern of the possibility of contained rupture within the pericardial space.

Of course, this disease is a spectrum as mentioned above, and some patients present with severe pain and have the finding of an intra-mural haematoma (IMH) of the aorta which again can be in the distribution of a Type A or B dissection and therefore generally managed in the same way. IMH is an atypical form of aortic dissection due to a contained haemorrhage into the aortic wall usually from the vasa vasorum and often without an obvious intimal tear.

When approaching a patient with an IMH, it is important to consider the depth of the haematoma with >10 mm in diameter associated with a greater risk of rupture and evolution into a classical dissection flap. In the descending aorta it can sometimes be difficult to distinguish from a mural thrombus in which case the direction of atheromatous calcification displacement can be helpful (Urban et al. 1999). For example, an inwards displacement towards the aortic lumen occurs in IMHs. There may also be an associated so-called ulcer like projection which in reality translates to a localised area of intimal disruption that can progressively enlarge and if so, herald a poor prognosis.

On occasion, an intramural haematoma may be managed conservatively with medical therapy and serial CT imaging. This is reasonable if the patient is free of pain, the IMH is of low volume (<5 mm) and there is no pericardial effusion. However, an increase in the diameter of the IMH or transformation of the appearances of the IMH particularly when a small region of contrast within the haematoma (blood pool) appears, suggests progression and depending on the size and location would generally prompt urgent surgical intervention. Thus, serial CT imaging is critical with this management algorithm.

Both the Stanford and Crawford classifications of aortic dissection evolved before safe surgical techniques for aortic arch replacement were established (Ott et al. 1977). Techniques of deep hypothermia and complete circulatory arrest that were developed in the late 1970s by Cooley et al. (Ott et al. 1977) enabled an increasing number of intimal tears extending into or originating in the arch to be identified and repaired at the same sitting (Ott et al. 1977). In addition, it is now clear that aortic dissection can propagate in both an anterograde and less commonly, in a retrograde fashion. Thus, the description of Non-A, Non-B was coined (Von Segesser et al. 1994) including the therapeutic challenges and conundrums that arise in management of these patients.

3 Cannulation and Planning for the Case

When planning a repair of acute Type A dissection, the principles of surgery to save the patient's life is paramount. These principles essentially are relief of cardiac tamponade, resection of the intrapericardial aorta with reconstruction of the true lumen of the aorta, resection of the entry tear (with inspection of the aortic arch), and restoration of aortic valve function.

A rapid image transfer of the CT aortogram is vital in pre-operative planning and briefing of the team on the expected strategy for aortic cannulation, likely extent of the repair and necessary prosthesis or equipment that is needed. Furthermore, from an anaesthetic perspective, the location of the dissection flap and optimal sites for monitoring of the proximal and distal blood pressure is critical to safe induction of anaesthesia and monitoring of the patient on cardiopulmonary bypass.

Traditionally, the femoral artery was used for arterial cannulation in acute dissection cases as it was felt to be easier to establish full bypass and generally one side was free of a dissection flap. However, there are several disadvantages which mean that this option is much further down the list of preferred arterial cannulation sites in the modern era. Firstly, the inward flow to the body is retrograde and therefore potentially more unpredictable in terms of flow within the true lumen and comes with an inherent higher risk of stroke. Furthermore, if the artery is cannulated directly the arterial supply to the leg may be compromised. If using this technique therefore, a side graft to the artery to allow bidirectional flow would be preferred.

In the case of visceral malperfusion and a dynamic flap which is not perfused anterogradely, it may be necessary to have dual arterial inflow with a cannula proximally and split line with an additional inflow cannula to the femoral artery. Another application of femoral cannulation could be to establish, or be ready to establish, cardiopulmonary bypass (CPB) at the time of induction of anaesthesia in the case of tamponade and instability on transfer or theatre. The femoral vessels can be safely explored under local anaesthesia with the chest prepped and draped ready for example. This can save critical time from the converse situation of the patient arresting at induction with the need for external massage until sternotomy and institution of CPB.

Central cannulation is the current go to strategy for the majority of AAD cases therefore. The easiest technique, probably, to teach is the seldinger cannulation technique. This is feasible if the true lumen is not collapsed in the ascending aorta and is accessible from the front of the aorta after sternotomy. It may be necessary to perform epiaortic ultrasound to help with this decision making and necessitates real time transoesophageal echo (TOE) guidance to confirm the placement of the wire within the true lumen of the descending aorta. A purse string suture is placed at the site of cannulation in the aorta, usually in the distal ascending or proximal arch, of course remembering that the strength of the tissues is in the adventitia and not going deeper. The patient should be fully heparinised before the purse string is placed as there can be troublesome bleeding around the cannula. Usually, this settles sufficiently once on full flow.

Generally, it is not advisable to use the dilators, as it will be very difficult to control the resultant bleeding after each dilation, but to simple place the wire over the needle and make a stab incision into the aorta with the aortic cannula preloaded onto the wire and remembering to remove the "ring" of the cannula if present.

If the true lumen of the aorta looks collapsed and is very narrowed this technique becomes challenging. It is usual to feel a "give" or slight "crunch" as the needle passes through the septum into the true lumen but if the true lumen is compressed and posterior, placement is almost impossible.

Thus, the innominate artery would be the next obvious choice. This does require a stable patient and the time necessary to expose the innominate artery and left common carotid artery. The CT scan is essential here to be sure that the artery is free of a dissection flap and communicates with the true lumen of the aorta. Two tapes are passed around the artery to allow sufficient length of the artery after clamping to facilitate an end to side anastomosis with an 8 mm graft. It is essential to test clamp the artery for a minute or so to be sure that the cerebral saturations/near infra-red spectrometry (NIRS) are stable and implies an intact circle of Willis.

The axillary artery, particularly the right, is an elegant choice for cannulation for AAD but requires around 20–30 min to expose and cannulate. Again, it is far safer to use an end to side anastomosis usually via an 8 mm graft to facilitate a sufficient size of aortic cannula. The arteriotomy should be large enough to allow adequate haemostasis and sufficient flow to achieve full bypass. If a small arteriotomy is performed with resultant narrowing of the inflow, it may be difficult to achieve the necessary required flow and resultant malperfusion. One great advantage to cannulating the right axillary artery during these cases is that at the time of circulatory arrest, the origin of the innominate artery can be clamped, the flow reduced and anterograde cerebral perfusion to be delivered negating the need for extra cannula's into the supra-aortic trunk at the time of circulatory arrest. Reducing instrumentation of these vessels is important in reducing the risk of stroke or neurological dysfunction during surgery of this nature.

The final option is the so called Samurai cannulation, a term first described in Japan by Minatoya in 2003 (Minatoya et al. 2003). However, the description of direct and rapid true lumen aortic cannulation was first described by Borst and then later by Jacob et al. (2007). The technique involves passing several tapes around the distal ascending aorta which requires some practice but is best achieved by dividing the pericardial reflection superiorly underneath the innominate vein and dividing the epicardium between the main pulmonary artery and ascending aorta.

The right atrium is then cannulated after full heparinisation and the patient placed head down in the Trendelenburg position. The cardioplegia line should be ready with a coronary ostia cannula attached and the aortic cannula attached to the arterial line of the bypass circuit. The perfusionist is then asked to "drain the patient" to achieve a systolic blood pressure of 40–50 mmHg. The ascending aorta is then transected and the ensuing 'exsanguination' to be controlled with cardiotomy 'pump' suckers. This should allow visualisation of the true lumen sufficiently that the aortic cannula can be placed within it and the perfusionist asked to "come-up" on the arterial line of the circuit. As the prime turns to bright red of blood, the assistant surgeon ties the tapes around the remaining aortic tissue and around the aortic cannula tightly.

The whole process from controlled hypotension to full flow on CPB usually takes around 90 s or less and provides a good 'adrenal squeeze' for the surgeon! If the heart is fibrillated prior to opening the aorta then there is even more control as the heart does not eject during this period. Once the patient is safely onto bypass, cardioplegia can be delivered directly into each coronary ostia. This technique is particularly useful when the need to go on bypass quickly is necessary and if there is complete rupture on opening of the pericardium then this technique can be lifesaving.

Once safely onto CPB and at full flow with good NIRS readings and no suggestion of malperfusion with acceptable lactate results, the actual operation to repair the dissection can ensue.

4 Cerebral Protection

Protection of the brain particularly during surgery for AAD with the need for circulatory arrest is absolutely critical for the optimum outcome. To complicate matters, a patient presents with a stroke in approximate 6% of cases of AAD according to the IRAD registry. The cause of this is usually therefore acute malperfusion which could be completely reversible with surgery (Hagan et al. 2000). However, this then raises questions on the timing of surgery and particularly if there is a haemorrhagic stroke the question of whether full heparinisation would worsen the neurology further. Patients presenting with stroke in the context of AAD are typically older and exhibit higher rates of hypertension and atherosclerosis. In addition, the presentation differs being less likely to have chest pain and more likely to have syncope and a pulse deficit with shock also being more common. This therefore translates into less favourable outcomes with less surgical management, longer hospital stays, and higher in hospital mortality (30.9% vs 19.3%) (Bossone et al. 2013).

In 1955, Cooley and colleagues used hypothermia to achieve cerebral protection during total replacement of the aortic arch in a 49-year-old patient who had a syphilitic aneurysm involving the arch and descending aorta (Cooley and DeBakey 1955). Surface cooling lowered the patient's temperature to 33 °C, and temporary shunts were placed for blood flow to the carotid arteries and distal aorta. However, the patient had a stroke, attributed to an 8-min occlusion of the right carotid shunt (Gupta et al. 2018).

In 1975, Griepp and colleagues reported the cases of 4 patients who underwent aortic arch replacement with the use of DHCA and cerebral protection during major, complex aortic operations (Griepp et al. 1975). The patients' brain activity and energy demand were minimised while the surgeons were able to excise distal clamp sites, completely view the aortic anatomy in bloodless fields, and perform distal anastomoses without leaving clamp-compromised tissue (Griepp et al. 1975). Despite these advantages, practitioners have continually expressed concerns about the optimal temperature for DHCA and the longest safe interval for repair without risking adverse neurologic sequelae (Gupta et al. 2018). The safe cutoff duration for DHCA was generally considered to be 35–40 min at a temperature of 20 °C, but experience suggests that this interval may be extended beyond this time with the addition of adjuncts such as cerebral perfusion (Gupta et al. 2018; Griepp et al. 1975).

There are several ways to achieve this. The concept for retrograde cerebral perfusion came about in the context of emergency management of cerebral embolism during cardiopulmonary bypass to help "flush" out any air in the cerebral circulation. It will also provide "backwards" perfusion to the brain tissue. Practically, retrograde cerebral perfusion can be achieved by placing a perfusion cannula into the superior vena cavae through a purse string suture and either snaring or clamping the SVC proximal to it. Flow is then begun, usually at between 150 and 450 mls/min to achieve a central venous pressure (CVP) of around 25 mmHg. However, there are concerns with this technique in terms of cerebral oedema and inadequacy of perfusion due to the tendency of the blood to flow to capacitance vessels within the brain. Most studies show the stroke rate with this technique to be very acceptable at between 2.8% and 9.1% (Rimmer et al. 2014; Stein and Elefteriades 2010). However, if there is a pre-operative stroke, the technique should be avoided as there is a higher risk of death of 55% in RCP supported patients as reported by Bavaria and colleagues (2002).

However, in my mind, the only opportunity where I perhaps wouldn't use the generally more favoured technique of anterograde cerebral perfusion (ACP) is if, for example, the implantation of an Ascyrus Medical Dissection Stent (AMDS™) device was not foreseen and if the innominate or right axillary artery had not been cannulated. Once this device is deployed, it is tricky to insert cannula into the open arch as the stent "windows" can obscure the orifice of the supra-aortic trunk somewhat. However, a 10F cannula may be possible to insert if the angulation and alignment is correct.

Generally, ACP allows for reliable and physiological perfusion to the brain, and this corresponds to a safer duration of circulatory arrest to the brain allowing a "brighter" extubation and protection if more extensive surgery in the arch is needed. One of the most stressful aspects of this period is "flying blind", knowing that the risk of stroke is highest during this period, but not certain on how to navigate the interruption of flow to the brain optimal for the individual.

At present, intraoperative monitoring of brain function includes bispectral index (BIS) to ascertain how deeply a patient is asleep during anaesthesia and near infrared spectroscopy (NIRS) to determine the level of oxygen in the blood at the front of the brain. However, neither of these provide a true measure of the blood supply to the brain.

Robotic transcranial doppler (TCD) has recently been developed which provides continuous automated measurement of blood flow in the middle cerebral artery of the brain using ultrasound. This will have several benefits over existing monitoring. Firstly, robotic TCD allows adjustment of the of rate of blood delivered to the brain to ensure adequate flow in the middle cerebral artery. Secondly, flow in both sides of the brain can be visualised and if either is inadequate, the position of the cannulas supplying blood to the brain can be adjusted immediately rather than waiting for a drop in NIRS which can sometimes be difficult to interpret.

Finally, TCD allows small particles of gas or solid material that can shower to the brain during surgery to be detected for the first time. During a trial of TCD in patients undergoing total arch replacement, our group examined how the velocity of blood to the middle cerebral artery (MCA) changed as the patient was cooled. The general physiological response to hypothermia is a reduction in cerebral blood flow. We found that at normothermia, the average velocity in the MCA was between 32 and 34 cm/s but this then dropped by around 40% at the target temperature to on average of 19 cm/s. This corresponded to an average total ACP flow to the brain of

5.9 ml/kg/min. This then translated into zero post-operative strokes, both clinically and radiologically and this data, although as yet unpublished and a small, isolated case series, appears to be continuing in the same very promising trend. The new standardised protocol therefore in our unit for target ACP flow is now 6 ml/kg/min. This is significantly less that the classical 8–10 ml/kg/min target ACP flow that was generally recommended.

In addition, topical ice around the head is generally used to help with cerebral cooling and has been shown, in animal studies at least, to improve neurological outcomes and survival. However, the ice should be removed on rewarming as it may interfere with cerebral vasoregulation and cause cerebral oedema. A cooling cap may offer superior cooling than topical ice in addition and is a necessary addition with the use of robotic TCD.

Pretreatment with intravenous steroids has also been shown to reduce total body oedema and cerebral vascular permeability and was also associated with improved immunohistochemical indices of neuroprotection after hypothermic circulatory arrest (Shum-Tim et al. 2001). It is nice to also note that the EEG is flat on BIS monitoring if available. The use of thiopental may provide some added benefit by lowering oxygen consumption in the brain but the timing of administration is important as if given too early it may replete the cerebral energy state and be detrimental (Al-Hashimi et al. 2013).

5 Proximal Aorta and When to Replace the Root

The proximal aorta will be assessed early after opening the dissected aorta, to firstly identify the position and state of the coronary ostia and to facilitate safe delivery of cardioplegia. The perioperative transoesophageal echo (TOE) would have provided some information on the competency of the aortic valve and if the dissection flap has propagated into the aortic root. Once the heart is arrested, the dissected aorta can be trimmed to the level of the sinotubular junction and retraction sutures placed, usually at the commissures of the valve, to help assess the root.

When I do this, I keep Elefteriades in mind when he stated *that "Certain technical truths regarding the surgical management of acute type A dissection are nearly self-evident. One is that performance of a composite graft replacement on an acutely dissected aorta is a dangerous procedure, best avoided if possible. Mobilization and connection of acutely dissected coronary artery buttons is potentially dangerous and problematic"* (Elefteriades 2002). In addition, on the aortic valve, he states that *"a pertinent physiologic truth is that mild to moderate aortic insufficiency is well tolerated. It is widely known that onset of left ventricular dilatation and heart failure may take many years to become manifest in a general cardiologic patient with aortic insufficiency. Many patients are left with mild to moderate aortic insufficiency after type A dissection repair and do well for many years. This represents a successful outcome, even if further surgical attention is required many years later"* (Elefteriades 2002).

Thus, it follows that a supracoronary tube graft replacement of the ascending aorta is preferred whenever feasible and sensible. The way to do this varies between a Teflon "sandwich" in which two strips of Teflon around 1 cm in width are secured on either side of the aortic wall to reconstruct the layers. A pledgeted suture is then placed at the top of each commissural post to resuspend the aortic valve if the valve is sufficiently competent and free of pathology. A running suture is then used to suture the graft onto the newly constructed aortic wall. Limitations of this, I find, is that on occasion there may be persistent flow into the non-coronary sinus and the appearance of a pseudoaneurysm on post-operative imaging. To negate this a tongue of surgical graft can be placed deep down into the sinus between the layers, possibly with a thin layer of bioglue to help reapproximate the layers.

The neomedia technique is the alternative to the sandwich where Teflon is used between the layers of the aorta this time and has the advantage that the integrity of the intima can be visualised (as it is not hidden by Teflon) and checked for any small tears as the tissue is sutured and corrected with an additional suture.

However, even with the above in mind it is usually immediately apparent if this is going to be possible or not. The modern aortic surgeon should have no qualms about performing a root replacement if there is any doubt. Namely, if the dissection tear clearly goes deep into the aortic sinus, or if the coronary ostia are affected by the tear or if their position is widely abnormal due to a large pre-existing root aneurysm then a root replacement is necessary. Furthermore, if the aortic valve is abnormal in addition to the above reasons, then the decision is clear cut.

In a review of this matter (Munir et al. 2020), we wrote that under certain indications the Bentall is not always the optimum interventional approach for a root replacement, and in some such cases a valve-sparing root replacement (VSRR) can be considered (Harky et al. 2019). The decision to use a mechanical or biological conduit must be balanced for the individual patient and whether lifelong anticoagulation is more appropriate than a higher risk of reoperation.

In a meta-analysis of 9 studies comprising 706 patients treated for ATAAD, VSRR was systematically reviewed as an option for intervention were able to conclude that the use of VSRR in ATAAD provided highly favourable outcomes in the early and late period in comparison to the patients undergoing Bentall procedure (Wu et al. 2019). However, these are results from surgeons who are expect in VSRR and in highly selected patients. In the majority of cases of acute type A dissection, I would not consider VSRR a realistic option. Particularly if the extent of the distal aortic repair is not fully known yet when planning the case.

6 Distal Aorta and When to Replace the Arch

Firstly, an open distal anastomosis, I would say, is essential in the management of acute type A dissection in the modern era. There should not be a fear of doing so as the modern aortic surgeon should be comfortable with the management of the operation to enable this to be performed safely as we described above. Secondly, sewing to a dilated and weakened aortic tissue is dangerous and will lead to either the anastomosis giving away or late rupture. A bevelled hemiarch anastomosis can easily be performed to eliminate a deep tear on the underside of the arch if present. The anastomosis should be performed in the same way as described for the proximal supra-coronary technique, that is, a Teflon sandwich or neo-media technique.

However, there are several situations where this may not be sufficient and replacing the arch, commonly with a frozen elephant trunk (FET) prosthesis is advisable. If the arch is torn, this is usually obvious on the scan and a replacement can be predicted but it is not until the cross clamp is removed and the open arch inspected that this decision can finally be made. In this scenario, the stented portion of the FET offers the theoretical advantage of false lumen decompression, which may lessen bleeding at the collared arch anastomosis (Mariscalco et al. 2019).

Secondly, in cases where there is an arch tear with compression of the true lumen in the distal aorta and radiological evidence or risk of malperfusion, this therapy can dramatically reverse both radiological and clinical malperfusion. However, if leg ischaemia persists even after instituting cardiopulmonary bypass, a femoral–femoral crossover graft becomes essential to restore limb perfusion as proximal tear repair, even with FET, may not re-establish flow and limb reperfusion would then be undertaken too late.

In the presence of clinical malperfusion however, particularly of the gut, operability should be seriously considered as the mortality can be extremely high and a simple life saving approach should invariably be deployed.

One approach could be to implant the AMDS device here, with the benefit of a shorter clamp time and the advantage of the open stent to help expand the compressed true lumen downstream. In the DARTS trial, all patients presented with DeBakey I aortic dissection with evidence of malperfusion in half of patients, albeit small numbers of 8. Despite this, the overall mortality at 30 days was only 6.3% with complete or partial thrombosis and remodelling of the aortic arch occurring in 91.7% of cases (Bozso et al. 2019).

FET can also be used to treat retrograde Type A dissection as the stent is able to bridge the intimal tear in the proximal descending thoracic aorta. However, the sizing of the prosthesis is crucial if this treatment option is chosen as the risk of distal rupture is very real in these cases. This may indeed be a situation where a hybrid approach with TEVAR extension could be the optimum strategy.

Careful review of pre-operative CT imaging is essential in planning of the case when considering a FET (Adams 2023). Analysis of the supra-aortic arch configuration is critical in planning the ideal zone of implantation (Adams 2023). In an acute Type A dissection, zone 2 is preferable with zone 3 being avoided where possible due to the risk of recurrent laryngeal nerve injury and technical difficulties of being so deep in the chest (Adams 2023).

Once the zone of implantation is known and knowing the stent lengths that are available, the surgeon can define the estimated location of the landing zone for the stented portion of the graft (Adams 2023). Generally, this is opposite the left atrium, although may vary, and enables the diameter of the aorta to be measured at this level on axial imaging (Adams 2023). It is useful to ascertain the depth of the left subclavian from the front of the sternum on the sagittal views of the CT scan and the extent of disease in proximity to the artery (Adams 2023). If deemed difficult to mobilise and reimplant from the front of the chest, an extra-anatomical bypass can be performed using an 8 mm graft onto the axillary artery which is accessed with an infraclavicular incison in the deltopectoral groove (Adams 2023). The graft can then be tunnelled between the ribs and brought back into the mediastinum and joined to the main graft (Adams 2023).

In terms of sizing of the stent and in the event of an acute dissection, a true size would be taken (assuming the descending aorta is not dilated) to avoid the risk of implanting a larger stent than needed in acutely dissected tissues with the inherent risk of rupture (Adams 2023). A shorter stent length would generally be preferred in these circumstances to reduce the risk of spinal cord injury (Adams 2023).

7 Post-operative Management

For me the post-operative management begins in the operating theatre with the management of reversal of protamine and blood product administration in an acute type A dissection critical. It is helpful to know the volume of blood returning to the pump via the cardiotomy suckers once off bypass and the vent is removed. Generally, anything up to 100 mls/min would give me confidence that everything is ok surgically. Next the protamine is administered with the aortic graft packed and these are kept in situ for a couple of minutes after the protamine is completed. Next, I prefer Octoplex over fresh frozen plasma (FFP) as the volume required of invariable four units is a risk at this point which I deem unnecessary. It may be necessary to give FFP but this can be done later, perhaps on the ITU and can be TEG guided. The heart has been off bypass for a while now by that stage and can cope better with volume loading if needed. Platelets are the other essential blood product in this early phase of haemostasis management. The packing of the chest needs to be systematic and with some patience and once needle hole bleeding has stopped there should be evidence of clots and a much-improved field to allow general haemostasis of the mediastinum to ensue.

Once on the ITU, if the patient is stable, lactate falling and not bleeding the sedation can be held at the earliest opportunity and proceeded with extubation if appropriate. If a FET has been implanted it is important to keep the mean arterial pressure high to perfuse the spinal cord and fairly high doses of vascoconstrictive agents such as noradrenaline and vasopressin may be necessary. However, this needs to be done sensibly as there is no point in saving the spinal cord if the digits or bowel become ischemic.

An early post-operative CT scan is useful and can be very satisfying to view after what was a challenging case in a critical patient. The scan can reassure that the suture lines are all intact and can ascertain how the repair has impacted the downstream aorta. It may be necessary to have an early endovascular consultation to consider extending a FET with a TEVAR for example if there is still ongoing radiological concern.

Once the patient is recovering on the ward and being prepared for discharge, it is helpful to have the option of enrolling them on an App to allow follow up on a virtual ward. In this way, advice can be given remotely on optimal blood pressure control and symptom checks. An agreed departmental follow-up strategy in terms of CT imaging is also helpful with discussion in aortic MDT's really important in the long term management of these patients.

References

Adams B (2023) Implantation of frozen elephant trunk (FET)—surgical technique. Thoraflex Cardiovasc Diagn Ther 13(3):550–556

Al-Hashimi S, Hamilton M, Arifi AA et al (2013) Thiopental during DHCA in aortic arch surgery: a re-evaluation. Interact Cardiovasc Thorac Surg 17(2):392–397

Bashir M, Markar S, Bilkhu R et al (2016) Repair of type A dissection—benefits of dissection rota. Ann Cardiothorac Surg 5(3):209–215

Bashir M, Mousavizadeh M, Baghai M et al (2017) Acute type A aortic dissection in the United Kingdom: surgeon volume-outcome relation. J Thorac Cardiovasc Surg 154(2):398–406

Bavaria JE, Appoo JJ, Makaroun MS et al (2002) Integrated treatment approach in acute type A dissection. Ann Thorac Surg 74(5):S1848–S1852

Bossone E, Czerny M, Lerakis S et al (2013) Stroke and outcomes in acute type A aortic dissection: findings from IRAD. Circulation 128(11 Suppl 1):S175–S179

Bossone E, LaBounty TM, Eagle KA (2018) Acute aortic syndromes: diagnosis and management, an update. Eur Heart J 39(9):739–749

Bozso SJ, Yousef S, Nagendran J et al (2019) The DARTS trial: Canadian results on hybrid arch repair. J Thorac Cardiovasc Surg 158(2):524–532

Bridgewater B, Gummert JF, Kappetein AP et al (2008) Sixth national adult cardiac surgical database report. Society for Cardiothoracic Surgery in Great Britain and Ireland

Cooley DA, DeBakey ME (1955) Total excision of the aortic arch: a report of two cases. Surg Gynecol Obstet 101(6):667–672

Elefteriades JA (2002) Operation for acute type A dissection. J Thorac Cardiovasc Surg 123(2):199–203

Fleck T, Hutschala D, Czerny M et al (2002) Combined surgical and endovascular treatment of acute aortic dissection type A: preliminary results. Ann Thorac Surg 74(3):761–765

Griepp RB, Stinson EB, Hollingsworth JF, Buehler D (1975) Prosthetic replacement of the aortic arch. J Thorac Cardiovasc Surg 70(6):1051–1063

Gupta P, Harky A, Jahangeer S, Adams B et al (2018) Varying evidence on deep hypothermic circulatory arrest in thoracic aortic aneurysm surgery. Tex Heart Inst J:70–75

Hagan PG, Nienaber CA, Isselbacher EM, Bruckman D, Karavite DJ, Russman PL et al (2000) The International Registry of Acute Aortic Dissection (IRAD): new insights into an old disease. JAMA 283(7):897–903

Harky A, Shaw M, Bashir M (2019) Valve sparing aortic root surgery in acute type A dissection: when and how. J Vis Surg 5:14

Hirst AE Jr, Johns VJ, Kime SW (1958) Dissecting aneurysm of the aorta: a review of 505 cases. Medicine (Baltimore) 37(3):217–279

https://jvsgbi.com/wp-content/uploads/2022/08/vol-1-issue-4-s1-s20.pdf

Inoue Y, Matsuda H, Ogino H et al (2000) Analysis of acute type A aortic dissection in the Japan Registry of Aortic Dissection (JRAD). Ann Thorac Surg 110(3):790–798

Jakob H, Dohle DS, Hamann M et al (2007) Rapid and safe direct cannulation of the true lumen in acute type A aortic dissection. J Thorac Cardiovasc Surg 135(2):244–245

Kruger T, Weigang E, Hoffmann I, Blettner M, Aebert H (2012) Acute aortic dissection type A. Br J Surg 99:1331–1344

Mariscalco G, Debry N, Patel HJ et al (2019) Frozen elephant trunk in type A dissection: rationale and evidence. Semin Thorac Cardiovasc Surg 31(4):686–690

Minatoya K, Ogino H, Matsuda H et al (2003) Ascending aortic cannulation for Stanford type A aortic dissection. J Thorac Cardiovasc Surg 125(4):952–953

Munir W, Ahmed I, Desai N et al (2020) Adding a root replacement in type A dissection: is it worth the risk? J Card Surg 35(7):1575–1580

Nienaber CA (2011) Influence and critique of the INSTEAD Trial. Semin Vasc Surg 24(3):167–171

Ott DA, Cooley DA, Mullins CE (1977) Resection of the aortic arch using DHCA. Circulation 58(Suppl I):I227–I231

Rimmer L, Nawaytou O, Carrel T (2014) History of DHCA in thoracic aortic surgery. Aorta (Stanford) 2(4):183–186

Rylski B, Branchetti E, Bavaria JE et al (2017) Acute non-A non-B aortic dissection: a novel classification. Eur J Cardiothorac Surg 52(6):1111–1117

Shum-Tim D, Goldstein MA, Dagenais F et al (2001) Steroid pretreatment improves cerebral protection during circulatory arrest. Ann Thorac Surg 72(5):1465–1472

Sievers HH, Rylski B, Czerny M et al (2020) Aortic dissection reconsidered. Interact Cardiovasc Thorac Surg 30(3):451–457

Stein L, Elefteriades JA (2010) Protecting the brain during aortic surgery: an update. J Cardiothorac Vasc Anesth 24(2):316–321

Uchida N, Shibamura H, Katayama A et al (2009) Operative strategy for acute type A aortic dissection: ascending aortic or hemiarch vs total arch with FET. Ann Thorac Surg 87(3):773–777

Urban BA, Bluemke DA, Johnson KM et al (1999) Imaging of thoracic aortic disease. Cardiol Clin 17(4):659–682

Urbanski PP, Wagner M (2016) Acute non-A-non-B aortic dissection. Eur J Cardiothorac Surg 49(4):1249–1254

Von Segesser LK, Tkebuchava T, Niederhäuser U et al (1994) Dissection of the descending aorta extending into the ascending aorta. J Thorac Cardiovasc Surg 108(4):755–761

Wu J, Huang Y, Qiu J, Saeed B, Yu C (2019) Is valve-sparing root replacement a safe option in acute type A aortic dissection? A systematic review and meta-analysis. Interact Cardiovasc Thorac Surg 29(5):766–775. https://doi.org/10.1093/icvts/ivz180. PMID: 31365078

Emergency Management of Iatrogenic Injury of the Thoracic Aorta

Constantine N. Antonopoulos, Filippos-Paschalis Rorris, and George Geroulakos

Abstract Iatrogenic injury of the thoracic aorta is a rare but potentially fatal complication, most frequently encountered during spinal, cardiothoracic, or esophageal surgery. Its incidence ranges from 0.01% to 1%, yet the associated mortality remains high, reaching up to 65%. Early recognition is essential, as clinical presentation may be subtle or delayed. Mechanisms include direct vessel laceration, erosion from surgical equipment, or iatrogenic catheter-related trauma. Multimodal imaging, particularly CT angiography, plays a crucial role in diagnosis and management planning. Treatment strategies depend on the site and extent of the lesion and may include open surgical repair, thoracic endovascular aortic repair (TEVAR) or hybrid procedures. Endovascular management has become the preferred approach due to lower morbidity and excellent technical success, even in emergent settings. A high index of suspicion, multidisciplinary coordination, and prompt vascular surgical involvement are key to optimising outcomes.

Keywords Iatrogenic aortic injury · Thoracic aorta · Spinal surgery complication · TEVAR · Endovascular repair · Pedicle screw impingement · Aortic dissection · Vascular injury · Haemothorax · Emergency management · Aortic perforation · Hybrid aortic repair

C. N. Antonopoulos (✉)
1st Department of Vascular Surgery, "Attikon" University Hospital, Athens, Greece

F.-P. Rorris
Department of Pediatric and Congenital Heart Surgery, Onassis Cardiac Surgery Center, Athens, Greece

G. Geroulakos
2nd Department of Vascular Surgery, Mediterraneo Hospital, Athens, Greece

Imperial College London, London, UK
e-mail: g.geroulakos@imperial.ac.uk

A. Kourliouros (ed.), *Emergency Cardiac Surgery*,
https://doi.org/10.1007/978-3-032-15787-4_3

1 Introduction

Iatrogenic injuries of the thoracic aorta are rare and they usually occur after spinal surgery due to the close anatomic relationship of the vertebral bodies to the aorta. Although these injuries are uncommon, with an incidence ranging from 0.01% to 1%, they may be life-threatening, with an overall mortality from 15% to 65% (Giotta Lucifero et al. 2021). The available literature on the true incidence, identification, and overall management of these sporadic injuries during thoracic and lumbar spine procedures is sparse and along with the subtle clinical course in some cases may point to underreporting of the true rate of outcome and complications (Giotta Lucifero et al. 2021).

2 Clinical Presentation

The clinical manifestation may not be readily identifiable, particularly in cases when the lesion is associated with a posterior spinal surgery approach. The patient's presentation and recognition of the vascular damage may be varied by the method of approach, vessel's size, and mechanism of injury. Arterial or venous lacerations can cause immediate haemorrhage (Giotta Lucifero et al. 2021), rapid haematoma, haemodynamic instability (Giotta Lucifero et al. 2021; Kayacı et al. 2019), while absence of femoral pulses, pallor, decrease in limb temperature, abdominal distension, and an abdominal mass can be found when abdominal aorta and iliac vessels are affected (van Zitteren et al. 2013). Other vascular injuries related to progressive damage to the vessel wall by the material used can be manifested lately after the initial procedure and may escape detection for long periods (van Zitteren et al. 2013). These vascular injuries include pseudoaneurysms and or arteriovenous fistulas (Giotta Lucifero et al. 2021; van Zitteren et al. 2013). Adequate intraoperative management, early repair, and a prompt prognosis are essential for the prevention of catastrophic sequelae.

3 Indication for Treatment, Type of Operation, and Spinal Levels

In a recent study (Giotta Lucifero et al. 2021), assessing 261 patients from 56 studies, the authors found that the most common indications for treatment in thoracic or lumbar spinal were spondylolisthesis (34%), degenerative disc disease (24%), disc herniation (16%), scoliosis (11%), fractures (6%), osteomyelitis (4%), pseudarthrosis (3%), and spinal stenosis (2%). An instrumented thoracic or lumbar spinal surgery was performed in the majority of the cases (82%), while in the remaining, a discectomy, corpectomy, or osteophytectomy were involved. The authors found that the most common spinal levels were L4–L5 (12%), L5–S1 (10%), L3–L4 (9%), L2–L3 (8%), and L1–L2 (7%). This comprehensive review found a higher rate of vascular lesions during anterior (59%), compared to the posterior (33%) and lateral approach (8%).

4 Approaches in Thoracic or Lumbar Spinal Surgery: Anterior, Posterior, and Lateral

The anterior approach to the thoracic and lumbar spine includes dissection and mobilisation of thoracic and abdominal vessels, such as the thoracoabdominal aorta, vena cava, iliac vein, and other vessels, in order to approach the anterior surface of the spine. This technique provides with an excellent exposure of the ventral surface of vertebral discs, which offers adequate release to the anterior longitudinal ligament, placement of cages with a wider footprint and possibility of achieving better restoration of lumbar lordosis, resulting in postoperative pain relief and good mechanical stability. However, it increases the possibility for vascular injuries (Giotta Lucifero et al. 2021). A 2% rate for transthoracic anterior approach was reported, mainly due to intercostal and thoracic aorta injuries (Giotta Lucifero et al. 2021).

Posterior approach, on the contrary, does not require exposure and mobilisation of the retroperitoneal vessels, which results in significantly lower risk of vascular complications. Incorrect placement of the screw tip in the proximity to the vessel wall is the mechanism of injury in these cases. However, in posterior non-instrumented operations, manipulation of the disc with curettes or rongeurs may increase the likelihood for vascular injury (Giotta Lucifero et al. 2021). In lateral approach, retroperitoneal trans-psoas or anterior to psoas route is used, providing access to the lumbar vertebral discs. A direct focal laceration of the segmental vessels may be complicate this approach (Giotta Lucifero et al. 2021).

A comprehensive review of aetiology and management for vascular injuries and complications in neurosurgical spine surgery has been published, containing detailed information for anterior screw fixation of the odontoid fracture, anterior cervical spine surgery, posterior C1–2 arthrodesis, posterior cervical spine surgery, anterolateral approach for thoracolumbar spine fracture, posterior thoracic spine surgery, scoliosis surgery, anterior lumbar interbody fusion, lumbar disc arthroplasty, lumbar discectomy, and posterior lumbar spine surgery (Inamasu and Guiot 2006).

5 How to Avoid, When and How to Treat Vascular Injury During Thoracic or Lumbar Spinal Surgery

Understanding of the vascular anatomy and preoperative planning is of paramount importance. The use of preoperative Computed Tomography (CT) and Magnetic Resonance Imaging (MRI) can facilitate in recognising potential surgical difficulties before surgery. Intraoperative CT and the use of CT-based navigation (Kayacı et al. 2019) is also important to prevent the catastrophic consequence of major bleeding (Giotta Lucifero et al. 2021). Biplanar technique and mini-laminotomy may also decrease the rate of vascular injuries (Kayacı et al. 2019). All instruments must be present and working in the operating room, including those which may be needed in case of severe bleeding, such as large bore suckers, topical haemostats, clips, ligature, and vascular sutures. The team should be also prepared to rigorously accommodate a complication and haemodynamic monitoring should be continuously read with blood product readily available.

In cases of aortic perforation, vascular repair followed by screw revision is mandatory. However, there is no consensus regarding the optimal management of aortic impingement by pedicle screw. Some authors have proposed aortic repair with prophylactic Thoracic EndoVascular Aortic Repair (TEVAR) before screw revision, due to high risk of aortic bleeding, while others removed the screw with later or without vascular repair (Kayacı et al. 2019). It is even reported an aortic repair with no screw removal (Zerati et al. 2017). It seems that anterior screws within 5 mm of the aorta should be removed, because the screw tip can cause chronic microtrauma from aortic pulsations, eventually leading to aortic wall thinning and erosion (Kayacı et al. 2019). In cases with less than 5 mm of screw impingement on the aortic wall and no bleeding from the aorta, screw revision without aortic repair may be logical, given that rigorous follow-up would be applied (Kayacı et al. 2019).

Once acute bleeding is suspected, balloon occlusion with resuscitative endovascular balloon occlusion of the aorta (REBOA) might be helpful to control the bleeding and stabilise the patient. Historically, repair of iatrogenic thoracic injuries to the aorta required open surgical thoracotomy with repair of the injured aorta (Carmignani et al. 2013). Primary repair was preferred in cases with aortic wall erosion and pseudoaneurysm, while other repair techniques included patch angioplasty and interposition grafting (Kayacı et al. 2019). However, this approach can lead to a high mortality and morbidity rate and can be complicated with spinal cord ischaemia and respiratory failure (Carmignani et al. 2013) and thus, nowadays, is being used in a limited fashion. Currently, the most frequent repair option in iatrogenic thoracic injuries is TEVAR, as it is less invasive method and can be used with excellent technical success and good outcome for both bleeding and screw impingement on the aortic wall. Usually, the nail that is impinging on the aorta needs to be removed just before the deployment of the endograft, as the continuous friction of the metal on the fabric of the aorta may damage the graft. Although preoperative planning and TEVAR in case of aortic bleeding has helped in reducing mortality and morbidity, iatrogenic thoracic injuries will continue to occur. Emergent consultation with a vascular surgeon should be prompt (Hans et al. 2011).

6 Special Considerations for Anterior, Posterior, and Lateral Approaches in Spinal Surgery

Concerning surgical approaches used in thoracic and lumbar spinal surgery, in anterior approach, injuries can be minimised by pre-emptive intercostal arteries clip ligation, intubation with double lumen endotracheal tube and left lung deflation according to the needs of the procedure, mobilisation of the diaphragm, and removal of the inferior ribs. This approach facilitates an easier exposure of the damaged vessel, bleeding control and direct vessel wall suture repair (Giotta Lucifero et al. 2021). In posterior approach, vascular injuries can be minimised by careful manipulations in cases of both instrumental and non-instrumental surgery. Although rare, the patient has to be turned in supine position and this can be catastrophic in cases of urgent vascular repair. Endovascular techniques, such as stent-graft placement, embolisation, and thrombectomy, in lumbar spine surgery complicated with iliac vessel occlusion can be useful (Giotta Lucifero et al. 2021). In lateral approach, direct pressure and topical haemostatics can be used to control the bleeding. An endovascular repair of the injury can be then applied (van Zitteren et al. 2013), with increasingly and preferably use during the last decade (van Zitteren et al. 2013).

7 Other Anecdotal Types of Iatrogenic Injury of the Thoracic Aorta

Other types include inadvertent puncture of the aortic root (AR) as a complication of transseptal puncture (TSP) requiring urgent pericardiocentesis and surgical repair (Chen et al. 2019) or use of Amplatzer duct occluder (4 × 5 mm) under TEE guidance (Lee et al. 2019). Another rare iatrogenic injury included coronary catheter-related dissection of the aorta, treated with stenting (Núñez-Gil et al. 2015). Interestingly, a patient with a tear between the brachiocephalic trunk and left common carotid artery after percutaneous tracheostomy, managed with sternotomy and direct aortic repair, has been reported (Ulatowski et al. 2020). The authors of another study reported the successful percutaneous treatment of an acute left main coronary occlusion due to iatrogenic dissection extending into the ascending aorta (Unzue et al. 2018). Similarly, in another study, iatrogenic dissection of the right coronary artery and the ascending aorta secondary to percutaneous coronary intervention led to emergency surgery of right coronary artery ostium repair with aortic valvoplasty, ascending aorta replacement and aortic arch descending stent implantation (Yu et al. 2020). Duque Santos et al. have published a case of an unusual rupture of the

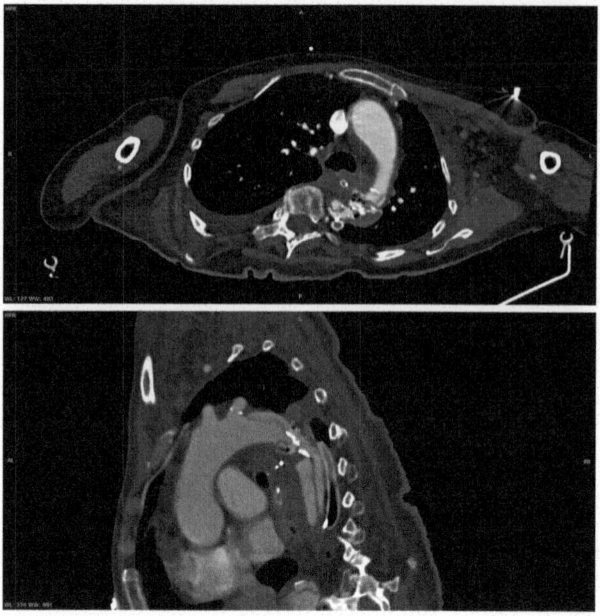

Figs. 1 and 2 CT scan images showing cross-sectional view (top) and sagittal view (bottom) of the thoracic aortic dissection

descending thoracic aorta with massive haemothorax after failed transcatheter valve intervention (TAVI); the valve failed to deploy in the aortic root, migrated in the ascending aorta, and during catheter manipulation to pull it back, the aortic rupture occurred, which was treated with emergency TEVAR (Duque Santos et al. 2018). Injury to the thoracic aorta has also been reported during esophageal surgery for carcinomas, both in thoracotomy (Vrba et al. 2019) and abdominal approaches (Bonavina et al. 2009). Such cases were managed intra-operatively with aortic repair under direct visualisation of the injury.

Out team had also a recent experience with a female, 73-year-old patient who was urgently transferred to our Department after iatrogenic descending thoracic aortic injury, during left upper lobectomy for lung carcinoma (Figs. 1 and 2). The severely injured aorta massively bled during the index operation. Bleeding was controlled by the operating surgeons and the patient was transferred to the Intensive Care Unit (ICU). However, she developed bilateral lower limb ischaemia 2 days later. The postoperative CTA showed antegrade and retrograde aortic dissection and complete thrombosis of the infrarenal segment (Fig. 3). We treated the patient with axillo-bifemoral bypass.

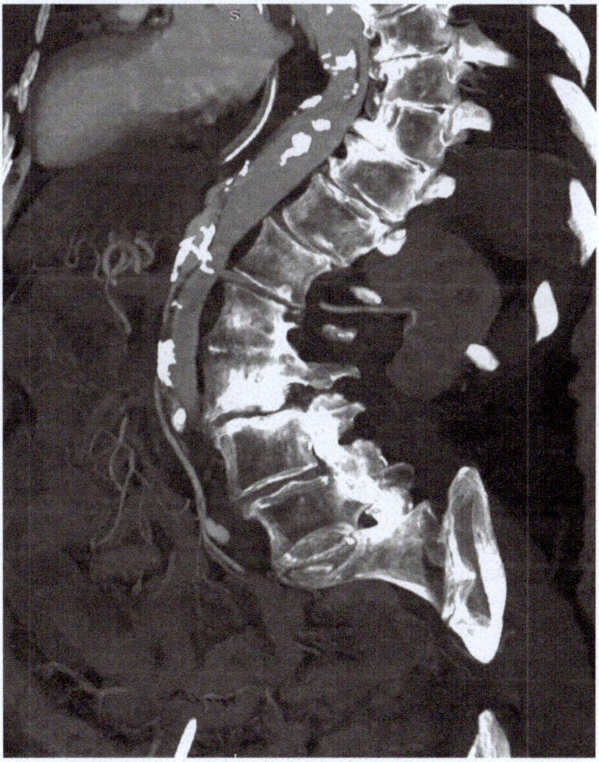

Fig. 3 CT scan image showing a sagittal view of thoracic aortic dissection with complete thrombosis of the infrarenal aortic segment

8 Conclusion

Iatrogenic injury of the thoracic aorta is very rare, but potentially lethal. A high index of suspicion is required to quickly recognise this surgical emergency. Treatment depends on the type and location of the injury.

References

Bonavina L, Bona D, Saino G, Nencioni M (2009) Injury of the thoracic aorta during laparoscopic esophagectomy. Surg Laparosc Endosc Percutan Tech 19(2):e55–e56

Carmignani A, Lentini S, Acri E, Vazzana G, Campello M, Volpe P et al (2013) Combined thoracic endovascular aortic repair and neurosurgical intervention for injury due to posterior spine surgery. J Card Surg 28(2):163–167

Chen H, Fink T, Zhan X, Chen M, Eckardt L, Long D et al (2019) Inadvertent transseptal puncture into the aortic root: the narrow edge between luck and catastrophe in interventional cardiology. Europace 21(7):1106–1115

Duque Santos A, Reyes Valdivia A, Gallo Gonzalez P, Gonzalez Ferrer E, Ocana Guaita J, Gandarias Zuniga C (2018) Descending aorta rupture after transcatheter aortic valve embolization. Ann Vasc Surg 49(312):e1–e4

Giotta Lucifero A, Gragnaniello C, Baldoncini M, Campero A, Savioli G, Tartaglia N et al (2021) Rating the incidence of iatrogenic vascular injuries in thoracic and lumbar spine surgery as regards the approach: a PRISMA-based literature review. Eur Spine J 30(11):3172–3190

Hans S, Shepard A, Reddy P, Rama K, Romano W (2011) Iatrogenic arterial injuries of spine and orthopedic operations. J Vasc Surg 53(2):407–413

Inamasu J, Guiot B (2006) Vascular injury and complication in neurosurgical spine surgery. Acta Neurochir 148(4):375–387

Kayacı S, Cakir T, Dolgun M, Cakir E, Bozok Ş, Temiz C et al (2019) Aortic injury by thoracic pedicle screw. when is aortic repair required? Literature review and three new cases. World Neurosurg 128:216–224

Lee W, Tsai T, Huang C, Wu C (2019) Successful rescue with transcatheter repair for aortic iatrogenic perforation during transseptal puncture. J Interv Card Electrophysiol 55(1):121–123

Núñez-Gil I, Bautista D, Cerrato E, Salinas P, Varbella F, Omedè P et al (2015) Incidence, management, and immediate- and long-term outcomes after iatrogenic aortic dissection during diagnostic or interventional coronary procedures. Circulation 131(24):2114–2119

Ulatowski N, Karolak W, Łoś A, Kołaczkowska M, Siondalski P (2020) Iatrogenic aortic arch injury after unsuccessful percutaneous tracheostomy. J Card Surg 35(3):686–688

Unzue L, Díaz-Antón B, Rodríguez-Rodrigo F, Garcia E (2018) Successful percutaneous treatment of an acute left main coronary occlusion due to iatrogenic dissection extending into the ascending aorta. JACC Cardiovasc Interv 11(18):1897–1899

van Zitteren M, Fan B, Lohle P, de Nie J, de Waal Malefijt J, Vriens P et al (2013) A shift toward endovascular repair for vascular complications in lumbar disc surgery during the last decade. Ann Vasc Surg 27(6):810–819

Vrba R, Neoral C, Aujesky R, Spicka P, Utikal P (2019) Iatrogenic thoracic aortic injury in esophagectomy—a case report and literature review. Rozhl Chir 98(6):256–259

Yu C, He F, Chen H, Hong J, Qian X (2020) Iatrogenic dissection of the right coronary artery and the ascending aorta secondary to percutaneous coronary intervention: a case report. Heart Surg Forum 23(3):E366–E3E9

Zerati A, Leiderman D, Teixeira W, Narazaki D, Cristante A, Wolosker N et al (2017) Endovascular treatment of late aortic erosive lesion by pedicle screw without screw removal: case report and literature review. Ann Vasc Surg 39:285.e17–285.e21

Emergency Surgery for Thoracic Aortic Trauma

M. Yousuf Salmasi, Mohamed Hamady, Thanos Athanasiou, and Alessandro Viviano

Abstract Out of all types of chest trauma, thoracic aortic injury is perhaps the most lethal. Mechanisms of injury can either be penetrating or blunt. The majority of patients do not survive the initial insult, and management of those making it to hospital is quite complex. Surgery used to be the mainstay of in-hospital management, although this has been superseded over the years by endovascular techniques.

In this chapter, we discuss the mechanisms of traumatic aortic injury, early management strategies once transferred to hospital, decision-making for intervention, and predictors of long-term outcome.

Keywords Traumatic aortic injury · Blunt aortic injury · Aortic isthmus · Endovascular stenting · TEVAR

Abbreviations

ATAI	Acute traumatic aortic injury
BTAI	Blunt traumatic aortic injury
CT	Computerised tomography
ICU	Intensive care unit
TEVAR	Thoracic endovascular aortic repair

1 Introduction

Despite advances in diagnosis and management, acute traumatic aortic injury (ATAI) continues to be associated with high rates of morbidity and mortality. The aorta is the largest artery in the body, subject to high systemic pressures, and thus

M. Y. Salmasi (✉) · M. Hamady · T. Athanasiou · A. Viviano
Department of Surgery and Cancer, Imperial College London, London, UK
e-mail: y.salmasi@imperial.ac.uk; alessandro.viviano@nhs.net

A. Kourliouros (ed.), *Emergency Cardiac Surgery*,
https://doi.org/10.1007/978-3-032-15787-4_4

disruption in its integrity can lead to fatal exsanguination and early death, prior to attaining any form of emergency medical attention (Creasy et al. 1997).

Overall, ATAI is relatively rare, with an estimated prevalence of 1–2% in all trauma patients presenting at level 1 or 2 centres (Steenburg and Ravenel 2008). Most incidences of ATAI occur in the setting of motor vehicle collisions; thus, the demographics of patients with ATAI tend to reflect the incidence of such injuries: the majority of ATAI are male subjects falling within ages of 16–50 years. Among patients involved in motor vehicle accidents, ATAI is the second leading cause of death, which is superseded by head injuries.

Both physical and haemodynamic forces have been postulated as mechanisms of aortic injury during a traumatic event (Turney et al. 1976). For patients who survive the initial injury, rapid detection is critical for diagnosis and prognostic outcomes. This also aids in procedural planning, requiring a thorough knowledge of various diagnostic imaging modalities and interventional strategies.

Historically, operative management, while carrying a major procedural burden, was the only way to provide a chance for survival in this highly morbid patient group (Sanborn et al. 1970). However, with the dawn of endovascular stenting more than 20 years ago, this rapidly replaced most surgeries for ATAI. The unique aspect of managing aortic injury is the combined involvement of cardiac, aortovascular surgeons, as well as interventional radiologists. Guidelines from a number of specialist bodies therefore inform best practice and impact patient outcome.

The purpose of this chapter is to provide the reader with a comprehensive overview of traumatic aortic injury. This includes the epidemiology and demographics of ATAI, as well as mechanisms of injury, diagnosis/treatment options for and post-therapeutic follow-up.

2 Mechanisms of Injury

In patients who survive the immediate traumatic incident, studies have shown that the aortic isthmus is the common anatomical site—this represents the region at the insertion of the ligamentum arteriosum, just distal to the left subclavian artery.

Trauma remains the most common cause of death in young adults. Head injury is most prevalent followed by blunt thoracic aortic injury (BTAI), which has been demonstrated by multiple autopsy studies

2.1 Penetrating Traumatic Aortic Injury

Penetrating trauma occurs when the aorta is directly punctured or cut, most commonly due to stab injuries or gunshot wounds. These injuries often cause extensive bleeding, with tissues surrounding the aorta often containing the bleeding, and allowing patients to survive long enough to reach medical attention.

2.2 *Blunt Traumatic Aortic Injury*

Blunt traumatic aortic injury (BTAI) is a more common cause of death compared to penetrating injury. Up to 80% of patients die prior to reaching hospital. Of the remaining survivors of BTAI, in-hospital mortality can be as high as 46% (Teixeira et al. 2011). In these cases, there is invariably high energy blunt trauma with rapid deceleration. Motor vehicle collisions, particularly those with head-on impact, account for 80% of the cases (Schulman et al. 2007; Richens 2003). The remaining 20% of cases can be due to a number of other mechanisms: aircraft injuries, falls from significant height, motorcycle crashes and pedestrian vs motor vehicle accidents (Mouawad et al. 2020).

Most commonly, there are other life-threatening injuries present which complicate management and the risk of poor outcomes. Aortic dissection can occur spontaneously or secondary to blunt trauma (Gammie et al. 1996; Yamasaki et al. 2022).

3 Anatomy and Function of the Thoracic Aorta

According to most recently published aortic guidelines, the aorta is now considered an organ. It serves two main functions in the cardiovascular system: (i) a conduit from the heart to the peripheries and (ii) as a reservoir of blood. The aortic root is subject to the highest mechanical loads from the heart, being the closest in proximity to the left ventricle. The mechanical properties of the thoracic aorta, namely elasticity and tensile strength, arise from its two main constituents: elastin and collagen fibers, respectively. Furthermore, the lamellar structure of the media interspersed with vascular smooth muscle cells anchored within the matrix, provide the aorta with extraordinary tensile strength and make it the toughest vascular tissue in the body. (Humphrey et al. 2015). It is therefore understandable that only the highest impact injuries can lead to disruption of proximal aortic wall integrity (Humphrey and O'Rourke 2015).

4 Mechanistic Principles of BTAI

With rapid deceleration injuries of the thoracic aorta, multiple types of stressors are most likely involved (Gaffey et al. 2020). *Torsion stressors* are created just above the aortic valve by displacement and rotation of the heart at the time of impact. *Hydrostatic forces* are important in creating the so-called waterhammer effect. Pressure waves are created at the time of impact and are propagated through the aorta (Lundevall 1964). When intraluminal pressures exceed 580–2500 mmHg during rapid deceleration impact, ascending aorta and aortic isthmus become prone to injury.

In addition to this, *shearing stressors* occur around the aortic isthmus, which is a stress point between the mobile traverse aorta, and the relatively fixed relatively fixed descending aorta. As such, the aortic arch and descending aorta have a relative difference in deceleration rates (Gaffey et al. 2020). (Feczko et al. 1992). *Bending stressors* occur as the aorta is flexed over the left main pulmonary artery.

In summary, there are three major theories that account for the mechanism of injury, although it is likely that all co-exist in the disruption of aortic integrity:

1. The aortic isthmus is a transition zone from the "mobile" aortic arch to the "fixed" descending aorta—this leads predisposes the aorta to move in opposite vectors during a rapid deceleration and can lead to a tear in the intima (Feczko et al. 1992)
2. Weaker tensile strength at certain "pressure points", such as the isthmus, making it intrinsically more vulnerable to injury
3. A compression point between the sternum anteriorly, and the spine posteriorly, "pinches" the aorta during a deceleration trauma (Crass et al. 1990)

Porcine models identified that traumatic forces cause an initial tear in the intima and media causing a dissection in the first instance. Blood fills the dissection plane which can ultimately penetrate the adventitia causing a pseudoaneurysm and/or free rupture and this process happens over a variable amount of time. Understandably, increased blood pressure and afterload decrease lead to a more rapid onset of rupture from the dissection stage, which explains the need for permissive hypotension and the avoidance of overzealous fluid resuscitation in the acute patient. Rarely, an aortic dissection flap propagates to a distal site as part of the pathological process (Yamasaki et al. 2022).

5 Classification of BTAI

According to the level of disruption in aortic wall integrity, with an increasing level of severity, BTAI can be classified as follows:

- Grade I: Intimal tear, where the aorta's external contour is normal
- Grade II: Intramural haematoma or dissection
- Grade III: Pseudoaneurysm
- Grade IV: Complete rupture of the aortic wall

This classification is vital for two main reasons:

1. Determining the early prognosis of the patient from, and thus guiding the immediate need for blood pressure control
2. Guiding the choice of intervention and its timing, or whether conservative management appropriate

Grade I can be managed conservatively (Class 1 indication), while grade III and grade IV require early intervention (Class 1 indication). Many grade II patients

Table 1 Summary of recommendations from recent ESC/EACTS guidelines (Mazzolai et al. 2024)

Clinical scenario	Recommendation	Class of recommendation
BTAI grade I	Requires non-operative management, including close imaging follow-up	I
BTAI grade II without high-risk features	Should be considered for conservative management and follow-up imaging	IIb
BTAI grade II with high-risk imaging features (see separate table)	Should be considered for TEVAR	IIa
BTAI grade III–IV and suitable anatomy (see stent graft placement section below)	Should be considered for TEVAR	I

should perhaps also undergo early intervention, although most recent AHA guidelines suggest that in the absence of high-risk imaging features (outlined below in the diagnostic section) conservative management can be recommended (class 2b indication) (Table 1).

6 Diagnosing Traumatic Aortic Injury

Symptomatology in traumatic aortic injury may have large variability, ranging from completely asymptomatic to haemorrhagic shock, depending on the severity of the lesion. Not-specific pain can also be a source of confusion. Therefore, it is of paramount importance that physicians exercise a high index of suspicion based on the type of traumatic event and preclinical state of the patient.

Clinicians should follow the primary survey outlined in the stepwise Advanced Trauma Life Support (ATLS) guidelines. Important clinical signs that may raise suspicion of BTAI include active bleeding, pulsating, or expanding haematoma, thrill over a wound, absence of distal pulses or ischaemia of the extremities (pain, pallor, paralysis, hypothermia).

Physical examination may reveal obvious chest wall injuries, subcutaneous emphysema, distended neck veins, tracheal deviation. With detailed examination, suspicion should be raised with absent or muffled heart sounds, a precordial or midscapular murmur, abnormal breath sounds and differential blood pressure between two arms or upper and lower body owing to “pseudocoarctation syndrome”.

6.1 Chest Radiography

Chest radiographs, while useful, have low sensitivity and specificity to reliably diagnose or rule out blunt thoracic aortic injury (Lee et al. 1997). Nevertheless, they are commonly performed during the primary survey. Most commonly, radiographically detectable BTAI demonstrate widening of the mediastinal silhouette to greater than 8 cm or 25% of the total thoracic width. They may also display a loss of aortic contour, rightward deviation of the trachea, and loss of the aortopulmonary window. Other concomitant findings may also be present, including apical capping from blood in the apex, large left pleural effusion (haemothorax), and widening of the paravertebral stripe (Dalldorf et al. 1990). Though these findings are sensitive for aortic injury when present, they are not always specific. In fact, up to 7% of chest radiographs appear normal despite underlying injury (Malhotra et al. 2001).

6.2 Bedside Ultrasonography

Focused assessment with sonography for trauma (FAST) scan ultrasounds are now widely used in emergency care. Free rupture of the aorta can lead to a left haemothorax and pericardial effusion leading to tamponade, both of which can be seen on FAST (Uflacker et al. 1999). However, these findings on bedside ultrasound also have a low sensitivity/specificity and would mean late signs of the disease process if present.

As a result of above mentioned factors, cross-sectional imaging is crucial for definitive diagnosis and should be pursued as early as possible if the patient's presentation displays clinical concern.

7 CT Imaging in BTAI

Computed tomographic angiography (CTA) which has now become by far the imaging modality of choice (Dyer et al. 2000) in BTAI, which has created a major shift in the last few decades. The increased use of CTA has in fact led to a rise in the incidence of BTAI due to its widespread use and excellent sensitivity/specificity in detecting the disrupted integrity of the aortic wall (Fabian et al. 1998). Transoesophageal echocardiography (TOE) is also a good option in the unstable polytrauma patient that cannot be transported to radiology for CTA. An intimal flap, aortic valve regurgitation, an intramural haematoma or signs of a free rupture can be identified and help expedite treatment and medical management where appropriate (Heneghan et al. 2016).

7.1 *Causes of False Positive Results on CT*

A few anatomic conditions can mimic traumatic aortic injury on CT, including:

1. Ductus diverticulum: remnant of ductus arteriosus. On CT, this has smooth obtuse margins contiguous with the wall of aorta and is often calcified.
2. Aortic spindle: a bulge in the proximal descending thoracic aorta just distal to the isthmus, shows a typical smooth contour.
3. Infundibulum: small conical shaped outpouching at the origin of a bronchial or intercostal artery. This may be identified by tracing the related artery to its origin.

Breathing movements or cardiac pulsations may cause motion artefacts, especially in the non-gated images, often creating diagnostic dilemmas, especially at the level of aortic root where this can mimic aortic dissection. Repeating the scan with ECG gating, if available, is an obvious way to mitigate this dilemma (Morgan et al. 2010). Mediastinal haematomas can often aggravate confusion, although traumatic aortic injury may safely be ruled out if the fat planes around the aorta are clear or the haematoma is evidently further away from the aorta.

7.2 *What Are the High Risk Features on Cross-Section Imaging?*

Identifying high-risk imaging features in patients with lower grade traumatic aortic injury is crucial to help determine whether intervention is warranted. According to recently published American Heart Association (AHA) guidelines (Isselbacher et al. 2023), high risk imaging features in BTAI include the following:

- Posterior mediastinal haematoma >10 mm
- Lesion to normal aortic diameter ratio >1.4
- Mediastinal haematoma causing mass effect
- Pseudocoarctation of the aorta
- Large left haemothorax
- Ascending aortic, aortic arch, or great vessel involvement
- Aortic arch haematoma

The presence of above imaging features is indicative of urgent intervention in the context of BTAI. This is particular relevant in stable patients with grades I–II BTAI in whom conservative management could have otherwise been considered.

8 Primary Management of Traumatic Aortic Injury

Blunt thoracic aortic injury requires a high index of suspicion based on mechanism of injury in trauma patients. Patients arriving to the emergency department in relative haemodynamic stability with a recent history of major high-impact blunt trauma to the chest, suspicion of aortic injury should stimulate the In the stable patient arriving to the emergency department,

Traditionally, non-operative management consists of permissive hypotension, negative inotropy and, when needed, supplementation with a vasodilator. These measures aim to minimise shear stress on the vessel through reduction in blood pressure and cardiac contractility. Typical targets include systolic pressures between 100 and 120 mm Hg accompanied by a heart rate between 60 and 90 beats/min (Erbel et al. 2014).

There is a variation in the agent of choice, although esmolol is most favoured due to its rapid onset and short half-life, making it easy to reverse if haemorrhagic and other causes of shock arise (Mosquera et al. 2011). Diltiazem, nitroglycerin, and nitroprusside can also be used in conjunction with, or as an alternative to, esmolol. Pharmacologic control of blood pressure and heart rate dramatically reduce the risk of rupture to <2%. The aim of these therapeutic measures is to prevent lesion progression or rupture.

9 Conservative Management vs Intervention

According to 2011 SVS guidelines (Lee et al. 2011), stable patients require urgent (<24 h) repair, after excluding other serious concomitant non-aortic injuries or immediately after treatment of other injuries.

The decision for conservative versus operative/management of BTAI includes complex and dynamic factors, including:

1. Patient's clinical stability
2. Concomitant injuries
3. Imaging characteristics

Grade 1 BTAIs are likely to resolve and are associated with extremely low aortic-related death (Estrera et al. 2013). Medical management and follow-up imaging to ensure resolution is now shown to be the most appropriate, resulting in virtually no long-term aortic-injury-related fatalities (Estrera et al. 2013). Interestingly, outcomes of grade 1 and 2 injuries were similar between conservative management and TEVAR, including in-hospital and aortic-related death ($P > .05$) (DuBose et al. 2015). High-volume centres reported no differences in aortic-related mortality rates between conservative and operative management of grade 1–2 injuries (Fortuna et al. 2016).

In contrast, grade 3 and 4 BTAIs are at high risk of progression and rupture and should be treated in an urgently. In grade 3 injuries, non-operative management was found to be an independent predictor of all-cause death, independent of additional imaging characteristics (Fortuna et al. 2016). Concomitant injuries and multiple secondary signs are more common in patients with higher grade aortic injuries and should prompt stronger consideration for operative intervention. In particular, Starnes et al found that the presence aortic arch haematoma >15 mm in thickness was predictive of death (Starnes et al. 2012).

Once patients are selected for intervention (i.e. grade 3–4 injuries), optimal timing of intervention remains unclear. A slight delay may confer an advantage by allowing the haematoma to organise and the aortic tissue quality to improve (Isselbacher et al. 2023). In fact, a recent study from the National Trauma Data Bank in the United States found that delayed repair favoured early survival and that early (<24 h) repair had increased odds of death (adjusted OR, 2.39; 95% CI, 1.01–5.67; $P = .047$) (Marcaccio et al. 2018). A multicentre study showed worse adjusted mortality rate with early repair overall (adjusted OR, 7.78; 95% CI, 1.69–35.70; adjusted $P = .008$) although, in subgroup analysis, mortality rate differences only trended towards favouring delayed repair ($P > .05$) (Demetriades et al. 2009).

10 Principles of Surgical Repair in Traumatic Aortic Injury

Since it was successfully introduced in 1959, open surgical repair has been the standard treatment option for BTAI for several decades (Passaro and Pace 1959). This procedure most commonly involves a left thoracotomy, allowing the most convenient exposure to the aortic isthmus. The thoracotomy can be extended, either inferiorly, to gain more exposure of the descending aorta (e.g. for the purpose of shunting/bypassing the aortic injury), or contralaterally (as a clamshell) in the event of other intrathoracic injuries requiring repair. Sternotomy has a role, especially in cases of concomitant cardiac injury and where proximal aortic control is challenging, although this can also be extended to a thoracosternotomy for additional exposure (Mosquera et al. 2013).

Operating in the left pleural space requires single-lung ventilation with anaesthetic adjuncts and expertise to achieve this. Additionally, systemic anticoagulation and aortic cross-clamping are necessary steps prior to incision and repair. It is possible to conduct the procedure without the use of bypass, although the most likely methods used are a left heart bypass, or the use of a Gott shunt, with the aim of diverting blood away from the injured aorta. In cases where shunts are used, aortic cannulation is performed prior to cross clamping (Turney et al. 1976).

10.1 Exposure of the Injured Aorta

It is important to conduct careful blunt and sharp dissection of the surrounding adventitia to identify the phrenic, vagus and recurrent laryngeal nerves, although extensive haematoma formation can make this challenging. Recurrent laryngeal nerve palsy was reported in up to 25% of patients.

Methods to gain proximal control of the aorta have been described, usually at the arch level between the left common carotid and left subclavian arteries, using clamps or circumferential tapes.

Following this, the mediastinal haematoma overlying the rupture is rapidly entered and inspected. If necessary, the clamps can be readjusted to ensure the injured aorta is isolated and to reduce retrograde bleeding from intercostal collateral arteries. The aorta is then opened wide circumferentially over the rupture site and debrided abundantly so that no torn aorta is left behind (Fig. 1).

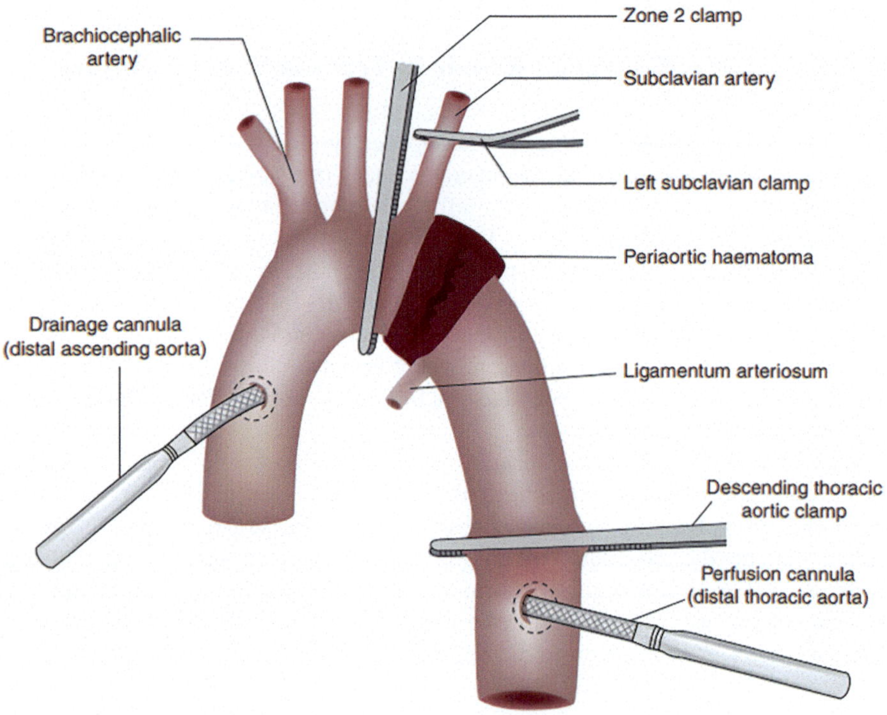

Fig. 1 Principles of vascular clamping during operative repair of traumatic aortic injury at the aortic isthmus

10.2 Aortic Repair

Following debridement, reconstruction usually comprises the use of a short woven Dacron graft using a running 3-0 prolene stitch. Primary repair with the use of graft material is feasible, but only in the case of small primary tears.

Clamps are then released in the following order: (i) distal aorta, (ii) arch (iii) subclavian artery. Decannulation, heparin reversal, and closure of thoracotomy are then the remaining steps to complete the procedure.

10.3 Special Cases: Injury to the Ascending/Arch Aorta

Injuries proximal to the left subclavian artery will require access via a median sternotomy with cardiopulmonary bypass (CPB) and cardioplegic arrest. Patients may also require total circulatory arrest for injuries involving the arch. Full heparinisation is necessary for CPB and bleeding risk in the trauma patient must be considered.

Although open surgery is well-described and has been used in several centres over the last few decades to improve chances of survival, some aspects of open repair may actually exacerbate co-existing injuries sustained. This may result in frequent major postoperative complications and high postoperative mortality.

11 Endovascular Repair for Traumatic Aortic Injury

When TEVAR was licensed for use in 2005, it was almost immediately recognised as a viable alternative to operative aortic repair in the acute trauma setting. Up to 20 year follow-up data now exist for TEVAR in traumatic aortic injury, which show promising results and adequate radiological outcomes in stent graft appearance (Minici et al. 2024).

Society of Vascular Surgeons (SVS) guidelines provide specific considerations when performing TEVAR summarised in Table 2.

Table 2 Clinical considerations during TEVAR according to SVS guidelines 2011 (Lee et al. 2011)

Consideration	Recommendation
Sedation vs anaesthesia	General anaesthesia
Femoral access technique	Open femoral exposure
Systemic heparinisation	Should be done routinely
Heparin dosage	Should be a lower dose than in elective TEVAR
Spinal drainage	Not recommended
Left subclavian artery involvement	Revascularisation of LSA is recommended

11.1 Endovascular Treatment Planning: Vascular Access

Open femoral artery cut down recommended by the SVS guidelines and particular useful to facilitate access to small calibre vessels, or those with significant atherosclerosis. Percutaneous arterial access methods are also possible with reported success rates (Azizzadeh et al. 2014). Alternatively, if the iliofemoral vessels are especially small, diseased, or in spasm, open retroperitoneal exposure can be performed, allowing for direct cannulation of the common iliac artery or via a Dacron conduit. Pelvic or lower extremity fixation devices may also pose challenges during vascular access and need to be considered in operative planning.

11.2 Endovascular Treatment Planning: Stent Placement

There are vital anatomic criteria that need to be assessed in order to confirm suitability of TEVAR in BTAI. For TEVAR to be possible, a healthy 2 cm of aorta at the proximal and distal landing zones is crucial. A proximal landing zone diameter of less than or equal to 42 mm appropriate access vessels is also important. In addition, there should be minimal aortic calcification, tortuosity, or thrombus, especially at the anticipated landing zones. When such criteria are not met, then operative intervention may need to be considered.

11.3 Hybrid Options During TEVAR

Patients with more proximal injuries may require supra-aortic debranching (Uchida et al. 2019). Revascularisation of the left subclavian artery is recommended in SVS guidelines and is especially required in cases of left vertebral dominance or if clinical signs of arterial insufficiency arise. If arm ischaemia occurs, it can be treated non-urgently with a left carotid-subclavian bypass or subclavian-to-carotid transposition. Despite this, in general, coverage of the left subclavian artery by TEVAR is usually well-tolerated and not a major cause of poor outcome. It is also worth noting, that spinal cord ischaemia risk increases with left subclavian coverage, especially when in combination with extended thoracic aortic coverage (Lee et al. 2011).

Analysis of US registry data in 2019 since the inception of TEVAR found that the endovascular approach significantly reduced mortality and ICU stay (Scalea et al. 2019). The study evaluated the national experience of BTAI management over a decade, during which TEVAR was introduced. During this period, the use of surgical repair declined significantly, while the use of TEVAR increased. Even after adjusting for the overall incidence of BTAI and change in study population over time, the relative rate of TEVAR use continued to rise. Furthermore, mortality associated with TEVAR was significantly lower when compared with matched patients undergoing surgical repair (Scalea et al. 2019).

12 Complications Following Intervention in Traumatic Aortic Injury

Both endovascular and operative intervention are associated with major adverse events. Open repair has been associated with high complication rates: namely mortality (28%) and paraplegia (16%) (Lee et al. 2011). Surgical access to the aortic arch is itself traumatic and increases the risk of bleeding, infection, and extended post-operative critical care (Cowley et al. 1990).

12.1 Complications Specific to TEVAR

Endovascular repair has certainly decreased the rate of the aforementioned complications, although it has also introduced new challenges related to stent complications, including endoleaks, endograft collapse, or inadequate stent coverage of aortic injury. In severe circumstances, these require urgent correction and most can be managed with additional endovascular intervention and further stent graft deployment. Rarely, open surgical correction may be required (Brown et al. 2021).

Type 1 endoleaks are the most common complication, whereby the deployed stent does not adequately seal at its edge with the vessel wall (reported incidence of 15% (Neschis et al. 2009)). Milder endoleaks can be followed up with interval imaging over time and many spontaneously resolve (Minici et al. 2024).

Endograft infection is a rare but severe complication, and may lead to formation of mycotic aneurysms and/or sepsis with multisystem organ dysfunction (Heyer et al. 2009). If conservative antibiotic treatment is unable to treat the infection, open repair with stent extraction and replacement with a new may be required (Orton et al. 2000).

13 Predictors of Long-Term Outcome After BTAI

Midterm outcomes after open and endovascular repair for BTAI are good for patients who survive to discharge from hospital. Earlier series reported endovascular complications (namely endoleaks) of up to 14% (Demetriades et al. 2008). However, more recent series report early occurrences of endograft malposition and endoleak to be as low as 2% and 3% respectively (de Mestral et al. 2013). Once a few months pass from the initial insult, midterm data suggest a low incidence of endoleak, stent migration, or reintervention after both open and endovascular repairs (mean period of 52–60 months) (Jacob-Brassard et al. 2019).

Longer term comparative data which compares open vs endovascular repair are limited. The SVS clinical practice guidelines for traumatic thoracic aortic injury (Lee et al. 2011) suggest that follow-up after TEVAR could be decreased to every 2–5 years in the absence of abnormalities on follow-up imaging (i.e. stent graft migration, endoleak). Despite this, there are no published guidelines available outlining postoperative surveillance strategies after open or endovascular aortic repair for blunt aortic injury.

A recent systemic review of non-operative management of blunt thoracic aortic injuries showed injury progression in 7.6% of patients on surveillance imaging despite having low aortic-related event rates (follow-up, 1 day to 118 months) (Jacob-Brassard et al. 2019).

For patients managed non-operatively (BTAI grade 1–2), injury healing or improvement was observed in 34% of patients (period of follow up: 1 day to 10 years). Injury progression, with or without intervention, occur in 0.68% of patients with grade 1–2 BTAI. In published series of blunt aortic injury, patients with disease progression on repeat imaging all undergo repair (de Mestral et al. 2013) (Fig. 2).

13.1 Timing to Repair

SVS and, more recently, ESC/EACTS guidelines (Mazzolai et al. 2024) suggest early repair, within 24 h, is recommended for those patients with grade >2 injuries. Despite this, the literature in fact shows a paradox in outcome for those who have delayed repair: the lag time between aortic injury and intervention with open or endovascular procedures correlated with improved survival. That is, patients who survived longer after their injury up to the time of treatment had better outcomes regardless of procedure (Hemmila et al. 2004). However, other studies, while confirming improved outcome after interventional delay, delayed repair was also associated with longer hospital stay and increased risks of complications (Holmes et al. 2002). In contrast, studies using both endovascular and open repair, failed to show a difference in mortality (early repair 4/21 [19%], delayed repair 2/48 [4.2%], $P = \text{NS}$)—repair times ranging from 8 h to 3.4 months (Pacini et al. 2005).

14 Comparison of Outcomes TEVAR vs Open Repair

The latest AHA guidelines now suggest as a class 1 recommendation, that with favourable anatomy, TEVAR is preferred over open repair (Isselbacher et al. 2023).

Many published studies in the literature comparing endovascular versus open repair have important limitations. Since this patient category are the subject of

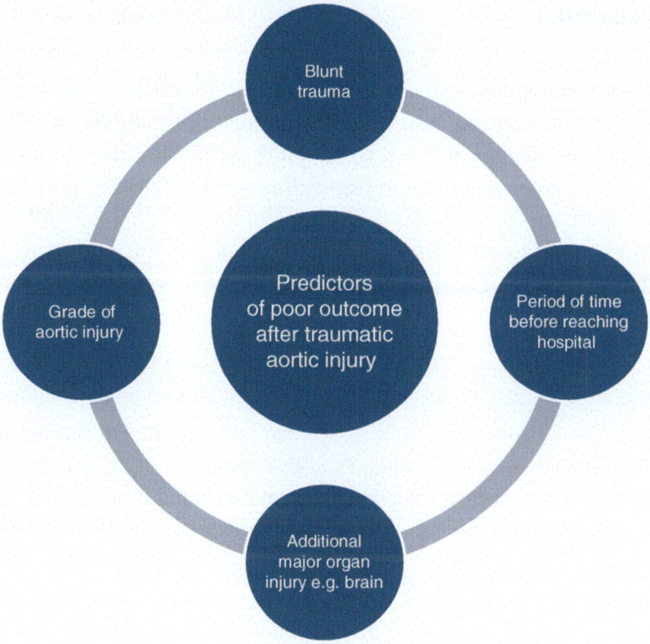

Fig. 2 Diagram summarising the factors influencing poor outcomes following traumatic aortic injury

major trauma, injury patterns and coexisting injuries are grossly varied. Therefore, when comparing outcomes, it is unclear whether underlying aortic pathology or other non-aortic injuries, rather than the procedure itself, are what is ultimately affecting survival.

To date, no randomised controlled trials on the choice of intervention in traumatic aortic injury exist. The most widely reported meta-analysis on the subject (Murad et al. 2011) suggests more favourable outcomes following TEVAR in a number of key domains. When meta-analysing 27 non-randomised studies, the mortality rate was significantly lower in patients who underwent endovascular repair, followed by open repair and non-operative management (9%, 19%, and 46%, respectively; $P < .01$). Open repair was also associated with increased risk of graft infection and systemic infections. The risk of spinal cord ischaemia and renal failure were also higher in open repair compared with TEVAR (9% vs 3% $P = .01$ for SCI and 8% vs 5% $P = .01$ for ESRD). Despite this, there was no significant difference in stroke incidence between TEVAR and open repair (Von Oppell et al. 1994).

15 Conclusion

In summary, high-impact thoracic trauma resulting in aortic injury requires timely management and intervention. Although the majority of patients suffering this life-threatening condition do not make it to hospital, rapid assessment and intervention can potentially save lives and prevent impending aortic rupture. Endovascular repair has replaced open surgical modes of treatment in most cases, although trauma centres should be able to perform open repair given the polytraumatic injuries that these patients often present with.

References

Azizzadeh A, Ray HM, Dubose JJ, Charlton-Ouw KM, Miller CC, Coogan SM, Safi HJ, Estrera AL (2014) Outcomes of endovascular repair for patients with blunt traumatic aortic injury. J Trauma Acute Care Surg 76(2):510–516. https://doi.org/10.1097/TA.0b013e3182aafe8c

Brown SR, Still SA, Eudailey KW, Beck AW, Gunn AJ (2021) Acute traumatic injury of the aorta: presentation, diagnosis, and treatment. Ann Transl Med 9(14):1193

Cowley RA, Turney SZ, Hankins JR, Rodriguez A, Attar S, Shankar BS (1990) Rupture of thoracic aorta caused by blunt trauma. J Thorac Cardiovasc Surg 100(5):652–661. https://doi.org/10.1016/S0022-5223(19)35462-5

Crass JR, Cohen AM, Motta AO, Tomashefski JF, Wiesen EJ (1990) A proposed new mechanism of traumatic aortic rupture: the osseous pinch. Radiology 176(3):645–649. https://doi.org/10.1148/radiology.176.3.2389022

Creasy JD, Chiles C, Routh WD, Dyer RB (1997) Overview of traumatic injury of the thoracic aorta. RadioGraphics 17(1):27–45. https://doi.org/10.1148/radiographics.17.1.9017797

Dalldorf P, McCarthy M, Tarver R, Mail J, Broadie T, Solotkin K, Yaw PB (1990) Traumatic rupture of the aorta. Indications for aortography. Am Surg 56(8):500–503

de Mestral C, Dueck A, Sharma SS, Haas B, Gomez D, Hsiao M, Hill A, Nathens AB (2013) Evolution of the incidence, management, and mortality of blunt thoracic aortic injury: a population-based analysis. J Am Coll Surg 216(6):1110–1115. https://doi.org/10.1016/j.jamcollsurg.2013.01.005

Demetriades D, Velmahos GC, Scalea TM, Jurkovich GJ, Karmy-Jones R, Teixeira PG, Hemmila MR, O'Connor JV, McKenney MO, Moore FO, London J, Singh MJ, Lineen E, Spaniolas K, Keel M, Sugrue M, Wahl WL, Hill J, Wall MJ et al (2008) Operative repair or endovascular stent graft in blunt traumatic thoracic aortic injuries: results of an American Association for the Surgery of Trauma Multicenter Study. J Trauma Injury Infect Crit Care 64(3):561–571. https://doi.org/10.1097/TA.0b013e3181641bb3

Demetriades D, Velmahos GC, Scalea TM, Jurkovich GJ, Karmy-Jones R, Teixeira PG, Hemmila MR, O'Connor JV, McKenney MO, Moore FO, London J, Singh MJ, Spaniolas K, Keel M, Sugrue M, Wahl WL, Hill J, Wall MJ, Moore EE et al (2009) Blunt traumatic thoracic aortic injuries: early or delayed repair—results of an American Association for the Surgery of Trauma Prospective Study. J Trauma Injury Infect Crit Care 66(4):967–973. https://doi.org/10.1097/TA.0b013e31817dc483

DuBose JJ, Leake SS, Brenner M, Pasley J, O'Callaghan T, Luo-Owen X, Trust MD, Mooney J, Zhao FZ, Azizzadeh A (2015) Contemporary management and outcomes of blunt thoracic aortic injury. J Trauma Acute Care Surg 78(2):360–369. https://doi.org/10.1097/TA.0000000000000521

Dyer DS, Moore EE, Ilke DN, McIntyre RC, Bernstein SM, Durham JD, Mestek MF, Heinig MJ, Russ PD, Symonds DL, Honigman B, Kumpe DA, Roe EJ, Eule J (2000) Thoracic aortic injury: how predictive is mechanism and is chest computed tomography a reliable screening tool? A prospective study of 1,561 patients. J Trauma Injury Infect Crit Care 48(4):673–683. https://doi.org/10.1097/00005373-200004000-00015

Erbel R, Aboyans V, Boileau C, Bossone E, Di Bartolomeo R, Eggebrecht H, Evangelista A, Falk V, Frank H, Gaemperli O, Grabenwöger M, Haverich A, Iung B, Manolis AJ, Meijboom F, Nienaber CA, Roffi M, Rousseau H, Sechtem U et al (2014) 2014 ESC Guidelines on the diagnosis and treatment of aortic diseases: document covering acute and chronic aortic diseases of the thoracic and abdominal aorta of the adult. The Task Force for the Diagnosis and Treatment of Aortic Diseases of the European. Eur Heart J 35(41):2873–2926. https://doi.org/10.1093/eurheartj/ehu281

Estrera AL, Miller CC, Guajardo-Salinas G, Coogan S, Charlton-Ouw K, Safi HJ, Azizzadeh A (2013) Update on blunt thoracic aortic injury: fifteen-year single-institution experience. J Thorac Cardiovasc Surg 145(3):S154–S158. https://doi.org/10.1016/j.jtcvs.2012.11.074

Fabian TC, Davis KA, Gavant ML, Croce MA, Melton SM, Patton JH, Haan CK, Weiman DS, Pate JW (1998) Prospective study of blunt aortic injury. Ann Surg 227(5):666–677. https://doi.org/10.1097/00000658-199805000-00007

Feczko JD, Lynch L, Pless JE, Clark MA, McClain J, Hawley DA (1992) An autopsy case review of 142 nonpenetrating (BLUNT) injuries of the aorta. J Trauma Injury Infect Crit Care 33(6):846–849. https://doi.org/10.1097/00005373-199212000-00009

Fortuna GR, Perlick A, DuBose JJ, Leake SS, Charlton-Ouw KM, Miller CC, Estrera AL, Azizzadeh A (2016) Injury grade is a predictor of aortic-related death among patients with blunt thoracic aortic injury. J Vasc Surg 63(5):1225–1231. https://doi.org/10.1016/j.jvs.2015.11.046

Gaffey AC, Zhang J, Saka E, Quatromoni JG, Glaser J, Kim P, Szeto W, Kalapatapu V (2020) Natural history of nonoperative management of grade II blunt thoracic aortic injury. Ann Vasc Surg 65:124–129. https://doi.org/10.1016/j.avsg.2019.10.084

Gammie JS, Katz WE, Swanson ER, Peitzman AB (1996) Acute aortic dissection after blunt chest trauma. J Trauma Injury Infect Crit Care 40(1):126–127. https://doi.org/10.1097/00005373-199601000-00025

Hemmila MR, Arbabi S, Rowe SA, Brandt M-M, Wang SC, Taheri PA, Wahl WL (2004) Delayed repair for blunt thoracic aortic injury: is it really equivalent to early repair? J Trauma Injury Infect Crit Care 56(1):13–23. https://doi.org/10.1097/01.TA.0000108634.15989.07

Heneghan RE, Aarabi S, Quiroga E, Gunn ML, Singh N, Starnes BW (2016) Call for a new classification system and treatment strategy in blunt aortic injury. J Vasc Surg 64(1):171–176. https://doi.org/10.1016/j.jvs.2016.02.047

Heyer KS, Modi P, Morasch MD, Matsumura JS, Kibbe MR, Pearce WH, Resnick SA, Eskandari MK (2009) Secondary infections of thoracic and abdominal aortic endografts. J Vasc Interv Radiol 20(2):173–179. https://doi.org/10.1016/j.jvir.2008.10.032

Holmes JH, Bloch RD, Hall RA, Carter YM, Karmy-Jones RC (2002) Natural history of traumatic rupture of the thoracic aorta managed nonoperatively: a longitudinal analysis. Ann Thorac Surg 73(4):1149–1154. https://doi.org/10.1016/S0003-4975(01)03585-8

Humphrey JD, O'Rourke SL (2015) An introduction to biomechanics: solids and fluids, analysis and design, 2nd edn. Springer, New York. https://doi.org/10.1007/978-1-4939-2623-7

Humphrey JD, Schwartz MA, Tellides G, Milewicz DM (2015) Role of mechanotransduction in vascular biology: focus on thoracic aortic aneurysms and dissections. Circ Res 116(8):1448–1461. https://doi.org/10.1161/CIRCRESAHA.114.304936

Isselbacher EM, Preventza O, Hamilton Black J, Augoustides JG, Beck AW, Bolen MA, Braverman AC, Bray BE, Brown-Zimmerman MM, Chen EP, Collins TJ, DeAnda A, Fanola CL, Girardi LN, Hicks CW, Hui DS, Schuyler Jones W, Kalahasti V, Kim KM et al (2023) 2022 ACC/AHA guideline for the diagnosis and management of aortic disease. J Thorac Cardiovasc Surg 166(5):e182–e331. https://doi.org/10.1016/j.jtcvs.2023.04.023

Jacob-Brassard J, Salata K, Kayssi A, Hussain MA, Forbes TL, Al-Omran M, de Mestral C (2019) A systematic review of nonoperative management in blunt thoracic aortic injury. J Vasc Surg 70(5):1675–1681.e6. https://doi.org/10.1016/j.jvs.2019.02.023

Lee J, Harris JH, Duke JH, Williams JS (1997) Noncorrelation between thoracic skeletal injuries and acute traumatic aortic tear. J Trauma Injury Infect Crit Care 43(3):400–404. https://doi.org/10.1097/00005373-199709000-00002

Lee WA, Matsumura JS, Mitchell RS, Farber MA, Greenberg RK, Azizzadeh A, Murad MH, Fairman RM (2011) Endovascular repair of traumatic thoracic aortic injury: clinical practice guidelines of the Society for Vascular Surgery. J Vasc Surg 53(1):187–192. https://doi.org/10.1016/j.jvs.2010.08.027

Lundevall J (1964) The mechanism of traumatic rupture of the aorta. Acta Pathol Microbiol Scand 62(1):34–46. https://doi.org/10.1111/apm.1964.62.1.34

Malhotra AK, Fabian TC, Croce MA, Weiman DS, Gavant ML, Pate JW (2001) Minimal aortic injury: a lesion associated with advancing diagnostic techniques. J Trauma Acute Care Surg 51(6):1042–1048. https://doi.org/10.1097/00005373-200112000-00003

Marcaccio CL, Dumas RP, Huang Y, Yang W, Wang GJ, Holena DN (2018) Delayed endovascular aortic repair is associated with reduced in-hospital mortality in patients with blunt thoracic aortic injury. J Vasc Surg 68(1):64–73. https://doi.org/10.1016/j.jvs.2017.10.084

Mazzolai L, Teixido-Tura G, Lanzi S, Boc V, Bossone E, Brodmann M, Bura-Rivière A, De Backer J, Deglise S, Della Corte A, Heiss C, Kałużna-Oleksy M, Kurpas D, McEniery CM, Mirault T, Pasquet AA, Pitcher A, Schaubroeck HAI, Schlager O et al (2024) 2024 ESC guidelines for the management of peripheral arterial and aortic diseases. Eur Heart J 45(36):3538–3700. https://doi.org/10.1093/eurheartj/ehae179

Minici R, Serra R, Ierardi AM, Petullà M, Bracale UM, Carrafiello G, Laganà D (2024) Thoracic endovascular repair for blunt traumatic thoracic aortic injury: long-term results. Vascular 32(1):5–18. https://doi.org/10.1177/17085381221127740

Morgan TA, Steenburg SD, Siegel EL, Mirvis SE (2010) Acute traumatic aortic injuries: post-therapy multidetector CT findings. RadioGraphics 30(4):851–867. https://doi.org/10.1148/rg.303105009

Mosquera VX, Marini M, Lopez-Perez JM, Muñiz-Garcia J, Herrera JM, Cao I, Cuenca JJ (2011) Role of conservative management in traumatic aortic injury: comparison of long-term results of conservative, surgical, and endovascular treatment. J Thorac Cardiovasc Surg 142(3):614–621. https://doi.org/10.1016/j.jtcvs.2010.10.044

Mosquera VX, Marini M, Muñiz J, Gulias D, Asorey-Veiga V, Adrio-Nazar B, Herrera JM, Pradas-Montilla G, Cuenca JJ (2013) Blunt traumatic aortic injuries of the ascending aorta and aortic arch: a clinical multicentre study. Injury 44(9):1191–1197. https://doi.org/10.1016/j.injury.2012.12.011

Mouawad NJ, Paulisin J, Hofmeister S, Thomas MB (2020) Blunt thoracic aortic injury—concepts and management. J Cardiothorac Surg 15(1):62. https://doi.org/10.1186/s13019-020-01101-6

Murad MH, Rizvi AZ, Malgor R, Carey J, Alkatib AA, Erwin PJ, Lee WA, Fairman RM (2011) Comparative effectiveness of the treatments for thoracic aortic transaction. J Vasc Surg 53(1):193–199.e21. https://doi.org/10.1016/j.jvs.2010.08.028

Neschis DG, Moainie S, Flinn WR, Scalea TM, Bartlett ST, Griffith BP (2009) Endograft repair of traumatic aortic injury—a technique in evolution. Ann Surg 250(3):377–382. https://doi.org/10.1097/SLA.0b013e3181b3b5c9

Orton DF, LeVeen RF, Saigh JA, Culp WC, Fidler JL, Lynch TJ, Goertzen TC, McCowan TC (2000) Aortic prosthetic graft infections: radiologic manifestations and implications for management. RadioGraphics 20(4):977–993. https://doi.org/10.1148/radiographics.20.4.g00jl12977

Pacini D, Angeli E, Fattori R, Lovato L, Rocchi G, Di Marco L, Bergonzini M, Grillone G, Di Bartolomeo R (2005) Traumatic rupture of the thoracic aorta: ten years of delayed management. J Thorac Cardiovasc Surg 129(4):880–884. https://doi.org/10.1016/j.jtcvs.2004.10.012

Passaro E, Pace WG (1959) Traumatic rupture of the aorta. Surgery 46(4):787–791

Richens D (2003) Rupture of the aorta following road traffic accidents in the United Kingdom 1992–1999. The results of the co-operative crash injury study. Eur J Cardiothorac Surg 23(2):143–148. https://doi.org/10.1016/S1010-7940(02)00720-0

Sanborn JC, Heitzman ER, Markarian B (1970) Traumatic rupture of the thoracic aorta. Radiology 95(2):293–298. https://doi.org/10.1148/95.2.293

Scalea TM, Feliciano DV, DuBose JJ, Ottochian M, O'Connor JV, Morrison JJ (2019) Blunt thoracic aortic injury: endovascular repair is now the standard. J Am Coll Surg 228(4):605–610. https://doi.org/10.1016/j.jamcollsurg.2018.12.022

Schulman CI, Carvajal D, Lopez PP, Soffer D, Habib F, Augenstein J (2007) Incidence and crash mechanisms of aortic injury during the past decade. J Trauma Injury Infect Crit Care 62(3):664–667. https://doi.org/10.1097/TA.0b013e318031b58c

Starnes BW, Lundgren RS, Gunn M, Quade S, Hatsukami TS, Tran NT, Mokadam N, Aldea G (2012) A new classification scheme for treating blunt aortic injury. J Vasc Surg 55(1):47–54. https://doi.org/10.1016/j.jvs.2011.07.073

Steenburg SD, Ravenel JG (2008) Acute traumatic thoracic aortic injuries: experience with 64-MDCT. Am J Roentgenol 191(5):1564–1569. https://doi.org/10.2214/AJR.07.3349

Teixeira PGR, Inaba K, Barmparas G, Georgiou C, Toms C, Noguchi TT, Rogers C, Sathyavagiswaran L, Demetriades D (2011) Blunt thoracic aortic injuries: an autopsy study. J Trauma Injury Infect Crit Care 70(1):197–202. https://doi.org/10.1097/TA.0b013e3181df68b3

Turney SZ, Attar S, Ayella R, Cowley RA, McLaughlin J (1976) Traumatic rupture of the aorta. J Thorac Cardiovasc Surg 72(5):727–734. https://doi.org/10.1016/S0022-5223(19)39620-5

Uchida K, Nishimura T, Yamamoto H, Mizobata Y (2019) Efficacy and safety of TEVAR with debranching technique for blunt traumatic aortic injury in patients with severe multiple trauma. Eur J Trauma Emerg Surg 45(6):959–964. https://doi.org/10.1007/s00068-019-01123-3

Uflacker R, Horn J, Phillips G, Selby JB (1999) Intravascular sonography in the assessment of traumatic injury of the thoracic aorta. Am J Roentgenol 173(3):665–670. https://doi.org/10.2214/ajr.173.3.10470899

Von Oppell UO, Dunne TT, De Groot MK, Zilla P (1994) Traumatic aortic rupture: twenty-year metaanalysis of mortality and risk of paraplegia. Ann Thorac Surg 58(2):585–593. https://doi.org/10.1016/0003-4975(94)92270-5

Yamasaki G, Sugimoto M, Kondo T, Takahashi M, Morichika M, Kuse A, Nakagawa K, Ueno Y, Asano M (2022) Blunt traumatic aortic dissection death by falling: an autopsy case report. Forensic Sci Med Pathol 19(3):388–392. https://doi.org/10.1007/s12024-022-00527-9

Revascularisation Strategy for Acute Coronary Syndrome with Unstable Symptoms in Surgical Pattern Disease

Jason Leo Walsh, Jean-Luc Duval, Giovanni Luigi De Maria, and Priya Sastry

Abstract Coronary specialists (cardiology and surgical) are often faced with patients with acute coronary syndrome (ACS) and surgical pattern coronary disease and a spectrum of stability and risk. These patients fall into a watershed zone of evidence between the impulse to revascularise quickly with PCI (percutaneous coronary intervention) for the acute ischaemia, but durably with CABG (coronary artery bypass grafting) surgery for the long-term outcome. Initial targeted PCI can incur delays in performing safe durable CABG as stents "bed in" with dual antiplatelets. Equally some patients may be too unstable and the heart too irritable to withstand surgery. Such patients therefore require a tailored approach accounting for multiple factors including coronary anatomy and lesion characteristics, comorbid conditions, institutional expertise and facilities, patient preferences, haemodynamic stability, and symptoms. This chapter aims to discuss and inform the reader about current evidence and rationale for the various approaches (conservative, PCI, CABG, and hybrid techniques).

As the choice of best strategy in ACS with surgical pattern coronary disease is often complex involving several interacting variables, decisions should be guided by multidisciplinary heart team discussion. Here we discuss revascularisation approaches and the factors to consider when selecting an optimal revascularisation strategy in this complex patient group.

Keywords Acute coronary syndrome · Cardiogenic shock · Percutaneous coronary intervention · Coronary artery bypass grafting · Multivessel disease · Left main stem disease · Heart team · Hybrid revascularisation

---

J. L. Walsh · J.-L. Duval · G. L. De Maria (✉) · P. Sastry
John Radcliffe Hospital, Oxford, UK
e-mail: GiovanniLuigi.DeMaria@ouh.nhs.uk; Priya.Sastry@ouh.nhs.uk

A. Kourliouros (ed.), *Emergency Cardiac Surgery*,
https://doi.org/10.1007/978-3-032-15787-4_5

1 Introduction

A true coronary emergency requiring emergency surgical revascularisation is thankfully rare and usually results from iatrogenic injury or other PCI complications, or when a planned surgical case has become acutely unstable and ischemic. These scenarios will be covered in more detail in forthcoming sections. In this chapter, the focus will be on the clinical challenge of deciding the optimal approach to revascularisation in NSTEMI and UA (NSTE-ACS) in the presence of unstable symptoms and a surgical pattern of coronary disease. We will describe and discuss the main strategies for coronary revascularisation and symptom management in such patients, outlining the major factors that need to be considered when deciding which approach to take (Box 1). Finally, we discuss the importance of the role of the heart team in individualising the approach to managing this complex group of patients.

Box 1 Key Factor Guiding the Revascularisation Approach

- *Coronary anatomy and lesion characteristics* (consider tortuosity, calcification, long segments of disease, number of lesions, location of lesions)
- *Symptoms* (persistent ischemic symptoms should prompt consideration of urgent revascularisation)
- *Co-morbidities* (does the patient have: diabetes, heart failure, previous cardiac surgery, frailty, CKD, COPD, PVD, cancer or concurrent valvular disease?)
- *Institutional expertise and facilities* (does the centre offer complex PCI? Is CABG available on-site? Is urgent PCI available 24/7? Is there a cardiac intensive care on-site? Could a hybrid procedure be offered?)
- *Patient choice* (the patient should be informed on the revascularisation options, the risks and benefits of each and involved in shared decision-making)
- *Haemodynamic stability* (haemodynamically unstable patients (with cardiogenic shock) should undergo urgent revascularisation)

2 Definitions

Acute coronary syndrome (ACS) comprises both acute myocardial infarction (AMI) and unstable angina (UA). AMI is acute myocardial injury (evidenced by an elevated troponin level that is rising and/or falling) combined with at least one clinical marker of acute myocardial ischaemia, either anginal symptoms, new ischemic ECG changes or imaging evidence of new loss of myocardial viability (e.g. a new regional wall motion abnormality on echocardiography) (Thygesen et al. 2018). UA is defined as myocardial ischaemia, with unstable ischemic symptoms, without myocardial injury (no troponin rise). Unstable ischemic symptoms can refer to prolonged angina at rest, new onset severe angina and angina that is becoming progressively more frequent and/or longer in duration and/or more easily precipitated (Byrne et al. 2023).

The most common pathophysiological cause of AMI is atherothrombotic coronary disease. AMI can be further sub-divided into STEMI and NSTEMI (Byrne et al. 2023). STEMI typically correlates with an acutely occluded or sub-totally occluded coronary artery and is almost invariably initially treated with primary percutaneous coronary intervention (pPCI) or fibrinolysis when pPCI is not available within 120 minutes. On the other hand, NSTEMI and UA can be treated either by percutaneous coronary intervention (PCI), coronary artery bypass grafting (CABG) or pharmacological management alone (conservative management). When NSTEMI or UA are suspected and myocardial injury has not yet been confirmed (troponin results are pending), the condition is referred to as non-ST-elevation ACS (NSTE-ACS).

Surgical pattern coronary disease refers to lesion patterns that are typically expected to be treated more effectively with CABG than PCI. Surgical pattern disease is generally held to mean multivessel disease involving the left main stem (LMS) or left anterior descending artery (LAD). Isolated LMS lesions used to be considered de facto surgical disease, but no longer. In the generality of these cases, graft durability is anticipated to be better than stent durability and single-setting complete revascularisation can often be achieved while technical considerations may require staged PCI therapy. Complex lesions (e.g. long, tortuous, heavily calcified, chronic occlusions or major bifurcation involvement) increase the risk of PCI and thus can (though not always) favour surgery and there are other patient factors (e.g. diabetes, impaired left ventricular function, other cardiac disease such as aortic stenosis) that also favour a surgical strategy.

3 Revascularisation Strategies in ACS with Surgical Pattern Disease

The main strategies for revascularisation in surgical pattern disease are PCI, CABG, or hybrid revascularisation. PCI involves obtaining access to the coronary arteries (traditionally via the radial or femoral artery) with the use of specialised catheters, then using a range of equipment including coronary catheters, wires, balloons, and stents to mechanically improve patency and flow within the coronary arteries. CABG is a surgical approach, where vessels are harvested from the patient (traditionally an internal mammary artery, radial artery or saphenous vein) and then grafted onto the coronary arteries with the distal end of the graft anastomosed distal to the stenosis or occlusion. Traditionally CABG was always performed via median sternotomy with use of the cardiopulmonary bypass machine. However advances in surgical technology have created the options of minimally invasive incisions and off-pump surgery, which will be explored in greater detail later in this section. Hybrid coronary revascularisation (HCR) combines PCI and CABG, commonly utilising minimally invasive incisions to graft the LAD and either concomitantly or stepwise treating the remaining diseased vessels with PCI.

3.1 Coronary Artery Bypass Grafting Versus Percutaneous Coronary Intervention in ACS?

The landmark trials PRECOMBAT (Premier of Randomized Comparison of Bypass Surgery versus Angioplasty Using Sirolimus-Eluting Stent in Patients with Left Main Coronary Artery Disease), BEST (The Randomized Comparison of Coronary Artery Bypass Surgery and Everolimus-Eluting Stent Implantation in the Treatment of Patients with Multivessel Coronary Artery Disease), and SYNTAX (The Synergy Between Percutaneous Coronary Intervention with Taxus and Cardiac Surgery) provide robust evidence for the superiority of CABG over PCI in surgical pattern coronary disease for reducing major adverse cardiac and cerebrovascular events (MACCE) (Park et al. 2011, 2015; Serruys et al. 2009). However a closer look at these three trials shows that most of the patients recruited had stable coronary disease. Only 2.2% of the patients included in SYNTAX, BEST, and PRECOMBAT presented with NSTEMI (Chang et al. 2017). No randomised controlled trial (RCT) exists comparing CABG to PCI specifically in the context of NSTE-ACS.

Studies and meta-analyses have demonstrated benefits of rapid revascularisation with PCI in patients with NSTEMI/UA (Milosevic et al. 2016; Li et al. 2017). However only a small proportion of the patients in these trials had surgical pattern disease. Current ESC guidance suggests risk stratifying NSTE-ACS patients into very high-, high, and non-high risk based on clinical parameters. For very high-risk patients, with features such as cardiogenic shock and ongoing chest pain refractory to medical treatment, it suggests treating them similarly to a STEMI with immediate PCI (Byrne et al. 2023).

An additional consideration is that PCI technology and techniques are rapidly advancing and this may influence strategies in the future. These advancements include: intravascular imaging, improved stent technology, coronary physiology guidance and new calcium modification technology, such as intravascular lithotripsy. For example, SYNTAX II demonstrated significantly better MACCE outcomes with modern PCI versus conventional PCI with durable results up to 5 years of follow-up. "State of the art" PCI proved also to offer comparable outcomes to CABG in an exploratory analysis (Escaned et al. 2017; Banning et al. 2022). Trials comparing modern PCI to CABG in traditional surgical pattern coronary disease are awaited (Fremes et al. 2023). It is to be noted though, that immediate (salvage) PCI can complicate future CABG and in scenarios where hybrid strategies might be useful, the decision for immediate PCI should take place with an impromptu heart team MDT.

Patients with acute coronary syndrome, surgical pattern coronary disease and unstable symptoms fall into a no-man's land of sparse evidence. CABG is known to be more durable in multivessel disease but rapid revascularisation, with minimal stress to the heart and patient's physiology, is clearly of benefit in acute ischaemia, particularly when there is ongoing cardiogenic shock and refractory angina. This emphasises the importance of careful case-by-case decision-making in this context.

3.2 Indications for Emergent CABG

While the role of surgical revascularisation for emergency reperfusion in ACS has changed considerably over the past 50 years, it remains an important treatment option in the management of these patients. Approximately, 5–10% of NSTEMI patients require CABG (Ranasinghe et al. 2011); however the majority of these can be operated on non-emergently. The timing of non-emergent CABG should be determined on an individual basis as there is an absence of robust evidence to inform optimal timing. Non-randomised data suggests a mortality benefit if CABG can be delayed 3–7 days post-MI; however this fails to differentiate between NSTEMI and STEMI and creates bias as higher-risk patients were more likely to be treated more rapidly (Weiss et al. 2008).

Current guidelines recommend emergent surgery in NSTEMI for patients with "ongoing ischaemia or haemodynamic instability with an indication for CABG". The ambiguity of this recommendation can be ascribed to the aforementioned paucity of randomised data on PCI versus CABG in the context of ACS. Despite this, non-randomised studies seem to support the conjecture that the indications for CABG in ACS are similar to those for stable angina (i.e. severe multivessel and/or left main-stem disease). A 2021 Surgical Myocardial Infarction report from Germany (Thielmann et al. 2021) recognised three common ACS scenarios in which emergent CABG remains a vital intervention: (1) ongoing ischaemia and large areas of jeopardised myocardium where PCI is not feasible due to technical or anatomical reasons; or (2) following successful PCI of the culprit lesion with further indication for CABG; or (3) where PCI was incomplete, insufficient, or failed.

When the decision is made to proceed with emergent CABG, it is widely recognised in the literature that there are worsened mortality and other post-operative outcomes. In-hospital mortality rates following emergent CABG have been reported ranging between 6% and 15%; with a significant increase in mortality in the cohorts of patients being operated on within 24 h of PCI or following failed PCI (Thielmann et al. 2021; Khaladj et al. 2013; Christiansen and Autschbach 2010; Sezai et al. 2012; Shahian et al. 2009; Schumer et al. 2016; Yang et al. 2005). In addition to worsened mortality outcomes, emergent CABG is also associated with more frequent and severe post-operative sequalae, including MACCE, re-operation for bleeding and renal failure, as well as considerably longer mechanical ventilation, intensive-care unit and overall in-hospital stays (Christiansen and Autschbach 2010; Schumer et al. 2016).

Given the established risk of emergent CABG, careful patient selection is crucial to improving outcomes. Preoperative variables such as age, female sex, hyperlipidaemia, peripheral vascular disease, reduced left ventricular ejection fraction, prior cardiopulmonary resuscitation, and cardiogenic shock have been reported as independent predictors for in-hospital mortality and MACCE (Thielmann et al. 2021). Many of these are encompassed within risk stratification systems such as EuroSCORE II, which while accurate in predicting post-operative death, do not alone reliably preclude patients from consideration of emergent CABG and neglect other significant determinates such as recent/failed PCI or very poor coronary targets.

Emergent CABG is indicated in a small and select cohort of patients presenting with ACS, however is associated with a disproportionately high rate of adverse sequelae and death. There is a general lack of evidence to inform guidelines, and decision-making in these often time-critical scenarios is reliant on local expertise and experience of the heart team. Understanding of the available data is therefore essential to eventually improving outcomes for these patients.

3.3 Operative Considerations in Emergent CABG

Anaesthetic and Pre-operative Considerations

In the case of emergent CABG, the imperative has to be to rest the heart, i.e. get on bypass quickly and effectively. Induction of anaesthesia can result in catastrophic hypotension or cardiac arrest and there should be a clear plan established at the WHO team briefing regarding escalation in such an event. The need for external defibrillator pads prior to induction should be agreed with the theatre team. Surgical and perfusion teams should be present and prepared to respond to any deterioration. These patients may also have received loading doses of anti-platelet medications at presentation, and the urgency to get on cardiopulmonary bypass (CPB) must be balanced against meticulous haemostasis, as the heart may not tolerate poly-transfusion as the third insult after ischaemia and CPB. Pre-emptive strategies such as whole blood Thromboelastograph Platelet Mapping to guide transfusion and the use of antifibrinolytic agents (aprotinin or tranexamic acid) may aid operative haemostasis, reduce the quantity of blood products transfused and decrease the incidence of post-operative bleeding.

Surgical Strategy

Surgical coronary revascularisation has advanced significantly in the last 30 years and the best surgical strategy for CABG, regardless of urgency, remains debated. In addition to conventional cardiopulmonary bypass and cardioplegic arrest (on-pump CABG (ONCAB)), there has been the emergence of off-pump (OPCAB), on-pump beating heart (OnBHCAB) and minimally invasive direct (MIDCAB) CABG. A detailed examination of traditional on-pump versus more modern approaches to CABG is beyond the scope of this chapter; however, it is important to appreciate the relative merits and limitations of the various approaches and how these interplay in the context of ACS.

The key theoretical benefit of the more modern approaches (whether OPCAB, OnBHCAB or MIDCAB) in ACS is broadly derived from two separate processes. Firstly, keeping the heart beating preserves coronary flow, hence reducing global myocardial ischemic injury, avoiding reperfusion injury and reducing myocardial oedema in the already stressed heart. In traditional on pump surgery, the surgeon must rely on diligent ventricular decompression, maintenance of diastolic arrest and cooling for myocardial protection. Secondly, in the case of OPCAB/off-pump MIDCAB, the local and systemic insults of CPB and cardioplegic arrest, such as aortic manipulation and cross clamping, haemodilution and hypothermia can be avoided. ACS can induce a pro-inflammatory state, and while there is a theoretical benefit in the avoidance of CPB so as to not worsen this, the relationship remains unclear. The trade-off to avoiding these deleterious effects of ONCAB with off-pump surgery is that the heart—which is already impaired—must continue to fully support the circulation, and when, for example, it is positioned for circumflex territory there is typically a degree of mitral/tricuspid insufficiency that may not be tolerated. In the scenario of an initially "unhappy" ventricle with concern that the heart will not separate from bypass because of the quality of the revascularisation (poor targets), then OnBHCAB may represent a suitable compromise; however there is no evidence to support this. Another major drawback of these novel techniques is their more technically demanding nature, which may lead to longer operative times in the context of time-critical ACS, incomplete revascularisation or dubious long-term patency of grafts.

Despite the theoretical advantages of avoiding CPB and diastolic arrest, there is lack of consensus in the literature regarding the overall benefit of on- versus off-pump CABG, particularly in the lesser-studied context of ACS. There is however a body of work supporting the use of off-pump CABG in a sub-group of high-risk patients (cardiogenic shock, poor ventricular function or ongoing myocardial ischaemia) to confer both short- and long-term mortality benefits (Hwang et al. 2022; Rastan et al. 2006; Stamou et al. 2005; Locker et al. 2000). On the other hand, there is an established high mortality and morbidity associated with the intraoperative conversion from off-pump to on-pump surgery (Patel et al. 2004; Jin et al. 2005; Reeves et al. 2006). As such, this highlights the fact that there is no singular correct approach to emergent CABG for ACS, and that the choice of surgical strategy should be made weighing patient presentation, institutional expertise and infrastructure.

Choice of Conduits

There is a well-established hierarchy in the longevity of conduits for CABG. The in situ left internal mammary artery (LIMA) anastomosed to the LAD is considered the "gold-standard" of surgical coronary revascularisation, with patency reaching 95% at 20 years. Other arterial conduits (RIMA, radial artery) have demonstrated better mid- and long-term outcomes than saphenous vein grafts (Zeff et al. 1988; Goldman et al. 2004; Ahmed and Yandrapalli 2023). The choice of conduit in elective CABG is determined considering a constellation of patient and technical factors, and similarly in emergent cases this choice should not differ within most circumstances. Several studies have confirmed that there is no increased mortality or complication rate if the internal mammary artery is used in emergent scenarios, as compared to saphenous vein grafts (Zapolanski et al. 1991, 1995; Bonacchi et al. 2006; Caes and Van Nooten 1994). Despite this, it is important to recognise possible rationale for deviation from the standard of elective CABG in the emergent situation. Saphenous veins can be harvested rapidly and concurrently to chest opening, whereas internal mammary artery harvest is relatively slower, more technically challenging with CPB pipes in situ and the mammary bed can end up a significant source of bleeding in the anticoagulated patient. Furthermore, there is a theoretical risk to arterial grafts by means of vasospasm in the context high-dose vasoactive medications which may be necessitated in the post-operative period following emergent surgery for ACS.

3.4 Hybrid Revascularisation

The idea of hybrid coronary revascularisation (HCR) was underpinned by the well-established durability and prognostic value of the LIMA-LAD graft. This promoted innovation, whereby the LIMA can be grafted to the LAD via a mini-thoracotomy (even robot-assisted) followed by PCI for the remaining lesions. This buys the benefits of the LIMA-LAD graft without incurring the "expenses" of a sternotomy and cardiopulmonary bypass associated morbidity.

Li et al. compared hybrid revascularisation with MIDCAB to off-pump CABG (with median sternotomy), finding a lower rate of perioperative transfusion, less new-onset atrial fibrillation, a shorter time on mechanical ventilation and a shorter length of stay in hospital with MIDCAB (Li et al. 2021). However, this benefit is demonstrated in the context of elective surgery for stable disease. In the context of an acutely ischemic heart with recent high-dose antiplatelets on board, the results are unlikely to be quite so clearly in favour of a hybrid approach, certainly while the technique is in its infancy. Furthermore, HCR obligates well-established infrastructure and experienced surgical, cardiology, anaesthetic and technical teams, which can generate logistical challenges in the context of ACS.

In the scenario of surgical pattern ACS with unstable refractory symptoms and bystander LAD disease, it could be considered that the culprit (non-LAD) vessel be treated with PCI, to maximise the benefits of rapid revascularisation in the context of refractory ischaemia. Subsequently, the LAD could be treated with less invasive LIMA-LAD bypass, particularly if the bystander LAD disease is complex. However, the risks of operating with dual antiplatelets on board for stent patency are significantly higher than without and thus, surgery to the bystander disease would generally be deferred for 3–6 months with conventional stents. New stent technologies with thinner struts or resorbable polymers are facilitating shorter regimens (1 month) of dual antiplatelet therapies after PCI (Hong et al. 2021), but these may not be available to all centres and thus such an approach needs to be discussed up-front between surgeon and cardiologist. Currently, no randomised trials have demonstrated non-inferiority or superiority of HCR over traditional CABG in terms of long-term durability and outcomes, only limited observational comparisons exist (Hannan et al. 2020). Heart team discussion should guide which patients may benefit from HCR in centres with the appropriate expertise.

3.5 *No Revascularisation—Conservative Management*

Conservative management in ACS refers to the avoidance of invasive revascularisation strategies such as PCI and CABG, opting (either provisionally or definitively) for pharmacological and other supportive treatments. Pharmacological treatment of ACS, particularly with aspirin, P2Y12 inhibitors, anti-coagulants and statins, undoubtedly improves patient outcomes (ISIS-2 1988; Yusuf et al. 2001; Eikelboom et al. 2000; Schwartz 2001). Rarely does the risk of these therapies outweigh the benefits and they are therefore given to virtually all ACS patients, irrespective of their revascularisation status. Revascularisation offers large incremental survival benefits in addition to medical therapy, particularly in ACS with ongoing ischaemia (Puymirat et al. 2012; de Winter and Tijssen 2012). The RITA-3 trial (Randomized Intervention Trial of unstable Angina) randomised NSTE-ACS patients to either early revascularisation (PCI or CABG) or initial pharmacological management only with revascularisation reserved for patients with refractory or recurrent ischaemia. A significant reduction in the combined endpoint of death, non-fatal myocardial infarction, or refractory angina was seen in patients with early revascularisation compared to a conservative strategy (Fox et al. 2002). Therefore, in contemporary practice, only a small sub-group of ACS patients should be considered for conservative management. Typically these are patients with significant objections to intervention, other prognosis-limiting comorbidities, extremely unfavourable metabolic status or coronary anatomy completely unamenable to intervention. In a few cases, an initial conservative approach can be taken to allow a period of stability for normalisation of metabolic status prior to definitive revascularisation with CABG or PCI; however there is no evidence for this. As always, heart team discussion should be central in guiding when conservative management should be employed, whether as a temporising measure or definitively.

4 Case Studies

Case 1

An 81-year-old gentleman presented to the emergency department with a prolonged episode of central chest pain. He was functionally independent and walked several miles regularly. His ECG showed anterolateral T-wave inversion, and his troponin was elevated. He was loaded with aspirin and ticagrelor and transferred to the cardiology ward. He had a further episode of chest pain at rest, which resolved with sublingual nitrate. On examination he had an ejection systolic murmur. Echocardiogram showed a normal left ventricular function and thickened calcified aortic valve leaflets with mild aortic stenosis. An invasive angiogram was performed (Fig. 1), showing severe heavily calcific proximal left main stem stenosis, severe heavily calcified proximal LAD stenosis and critical heavily calcified proximal right coronary artery (RCA) stenosis with poor antegrade flow. The findings were

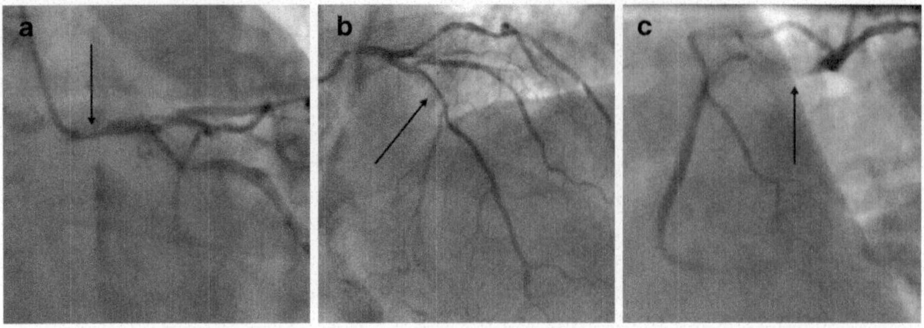

Fig. 1 Coronary angiogram showing (**a**) severe calcific proximal left main stem stenosis, (**b**) severe calcific proximal left anterior descending artery stenosis and (**c**) critical calcific proximal right coronary artery stenosis resulting in poor flow into the distal vessel

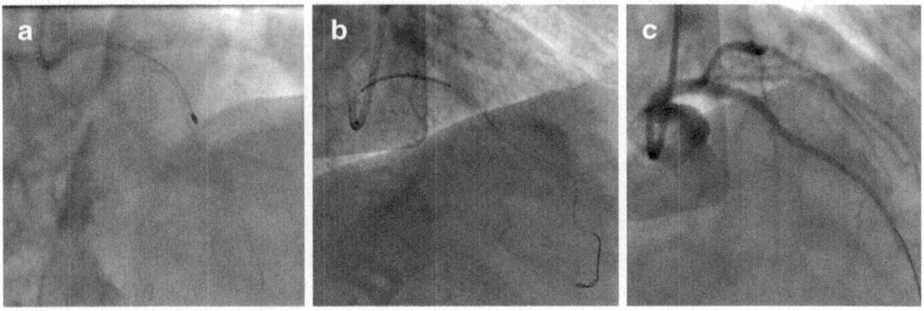

Fig. 2 Complex percutaneous coronary intervention which included (**a**) rotational atherectomy to modify coronary calcium, (**b**) deployment of two overlapping drug eluting stents into the left main stem and proximal left anterior descending artery. (**c**) A good angiographic result was achieved with good expansion of the left main stem and left anterior descending artery

explained to the patient, the benefits and limitations of both PCI and CABG were explained and the patient was told his case would be discussed in an expert meeting. The patient expressed a preference for PCI if feasible.

The patients SYNTAX score was calculated as 33 (high, favouring CABG); his SYNTAX II score estimated a 6.9% 4-year mortality with PCI and a 16.2% 4-year mortality with CABG (favouring PCI); his EUROSCORE II predicted a 2.48% risk of perioperative mortality with CABG.

His case was for discussion in the heart team meeting the following day, and he was started on a nitrate infusion overnight due to chest pain recurrence. Several factors including the patient's age, ongoing symptoms, and preference weighted the decision towards PCI. Local complex PCI operators were confident that heavily calcific disease could be well-managed with PCI using rotational atherectomy +/− intravascular lithotripsy. Heart team consensus was that PCI should be performed as an inpatient.

The patient proceeded to intravascular imaging guided, rotational atherectomy assisted PCI to the left main stem into the LAD with two drug = eluting stents (Fig. 2).

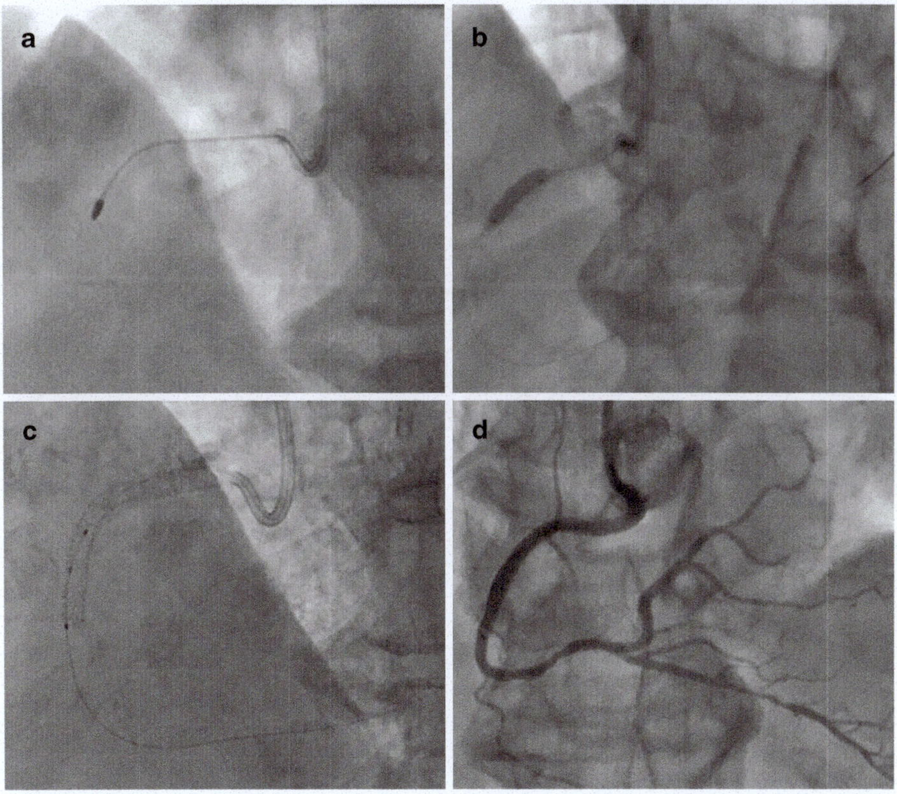

Fig. 3 Complex percutaneous coronary intervention which included (**a**) rotational atherectomy to the proximal and mid right coronary artery and (**b**) intravascular lithotripsy to modify coronary calcification. (**c**) Stent deployment with one long drug eluting stent from the ostium to mid vessel. (**d**) A good angiographic result was achieved, with flow restored to the distal vessel

A staged intravascular imaging guided procedure was performed two days later to the RCA. The calcific lesions were prepared with rotational atherectomy and intravascular lithotripsy. A single drug-eluting stent was deployed (Fig. 3).

The patient was discharged the following day. At 12-month follow-up, the patient was symptom-free and completing all his usual activities of daily living.

Case 2

A normally fit and active 42-year-old gentleman, with no other medical history besides well-controlled type 2 diabetes presented to the emergency department of a district general hospital. He reported a month's history of progressive exertional angina, but developed central crushing chest pain at rest leading to presentation. A 12-lead ECG demonstrated anterolateral T-wave inversion and his initial troponin I resulted at 500 ng/L; he was thus transferred to the cardiology department at a tertiary centre for ongoing management. On arrival, he underwent invasive coronary angiography which revealed critical diffuse three-vessel disease (Fig. 4). Following

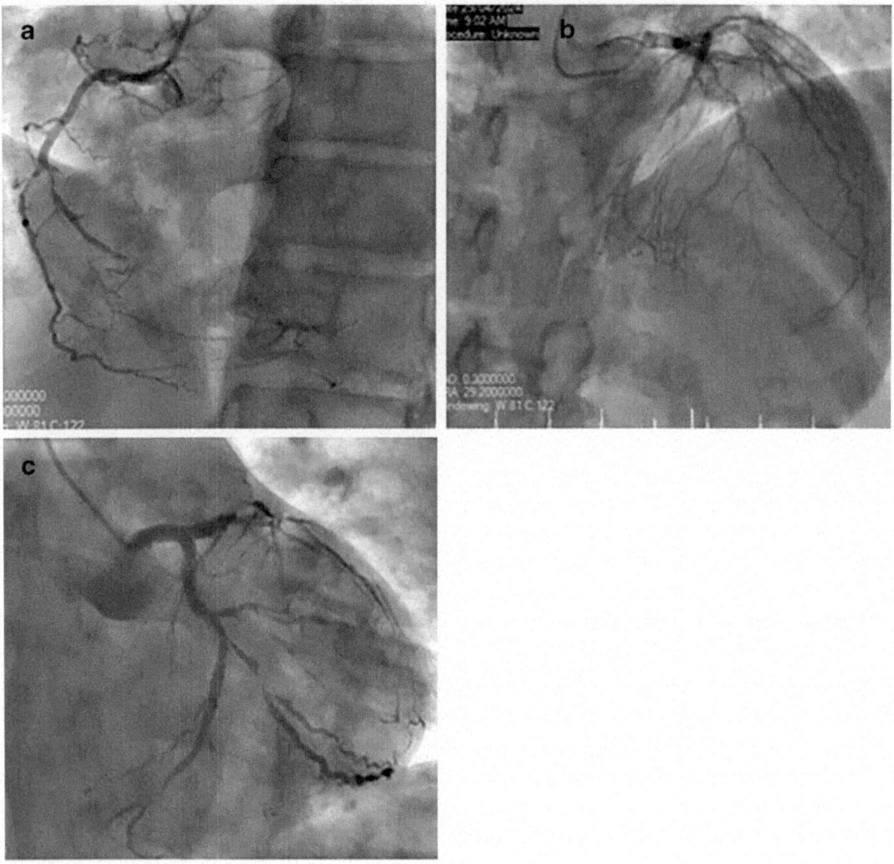

Fig. 4 Coronary angiogram showing (**a**) co-dominant RCA with sub-total occlusion distally, (**b**) Sub-totally occluded LAD from the mid vessel with retrograde filling from the RCA and (**c**) co-dominant LCx, with severe disease in distal segment and OM. Technically graftable targets

angiography, he had ongoing chest pain at rest, with no dynamic ECG changes but an interval increase in troponin I to 1279 ng/L. He was given loading doses of aspirin and ticagrelor, sub-lingual, then intravenous nitrates with no cessation of chest pain. Echocardiogram demonstrated preserved left ventricular function with regional wall-motion abnormalities.

The patients SYNTAX score was calculated as 26 (intermediate); his SYNTAX II score estimated a 2.6% 4-year mortality with PCI and a 1.0% 4-year mortality with CABG; his EUROSCORE II predicted a 1.62% risk of perioperative mortality with CABG. An impromptu heart team MDT rationalised that given his age, diabetes, surgical pattern of disease and ongoing symptoms, emergent CABG would be the most appropriate management for revascularisation, and the patient consented to proceed with surgery.

Emergent CABG was performed on cardiopulomonary bypass with complete cardioplegic arrest (cumulative CPB time—99 min, cumulative cross clamp time—40 min). The left internal mammary artery, radial artery (endoscopic harvest), and one length of saphenous vein (endoscopic harvest) were utilised as conduits. Three grafts were constructed: left internal mammary artery to the left anterior descending, radial artery to the second obtuse marginal branch and saphenous vein to the right-originating posterior descending branch. The patient separated from bypass easily on low-dose milrinone and noradrenaline and was transferred to critical care in a stable condition.

On post-operative day 1, he was started on dual antiplatelet therapy. He was noted to be hypotensive and tachycardic, and transoesophageal echocardiography on critical care revealed a very large left-sided haemothorax resulting in tension physiology. The decision was made to return to theatre for re-exploration and washout, where a 2 L left-sided pleural collection was evacuated, but no active bleeding point identified; with the bleeding being attributed to generalised coagulopathy. Between both theatre visits he received a total of 13 units of packed red cells, 14 units of fresh frozen plasma and 2 pools of platelets. He returned to critical care in a stable condition and was stepped down to ward-based care on post-operative day 4. He had an otherwise uneventful recovery and was discharged home on post-operative day 7.

He was reviewed in surgical follow-up clinic at 2-months post-op. He was regularly walking more than 2 miles daily with no recurrence of shortness of breath or angina. His sternal wound had fully healed, and he was fit to return to work and his other normal daily activities. He was discharged from surgical follow-up and remains under the ongoing care of his local cardiology team.

5 Conclusions

There is no one-size fits all strategy to revascularisation in ACS with "surgical pattern" coronary disease. Generally, patients that are unstable with ongoing ischemic symptoms despite medical management and/or haemodynamic instability should be offered immediate PCI; however, if PCI is contraindicated, emergent CABG should be considered to achieve revascularisation.

Factors such as coronary anatomy, lesion complexity, patient co-morbidities, patient preferences, and institutional experience should be carefully considered in deciding the optimal revascularisation strategy in these cases.

While more definitive evidence is awaited, the expertise of the heart team, comprising of cardiologists, cardiothoracic surgeons and other specialists, should determine revascularisation strategies through systematic discussions. This aims to ensure the revascularisation strategy chosen is optimal for each individual patient's circumstances, ultimately aiming to optimise outcomes and quality-of-life.

References

Ahmed I, Yandrapalli S (2023) Internal mammary artery bypass. StatPearls [Internet]. StatPearls Publishing, Treasure Island. Available from: https://www.ncbi.nlm.nih.gov/books/NBK560835/

Banning AP et al (2022) Five-year outcomes after state-of-the-art percutaneous coronary revascularization in patients with *de novo* three-vessel disease: final results of the SYNTAX II study. Eur Heart J 43:1307–1316

Bonacchi M et al (2006) Urgent/emergent surgical revascularization in unstable angina: influence of different type of conduits. J Cardiovasc Surg 47:201–210

Byrne RA et al (2023) 2023 ESC Guidelines for the management of acute coronary syndromes. Eur Heart J 44:3720–3826

Caes FL, Van Nooten GJ (1994) Use of internal mammary artery for emergency grafting after failed coronary angioplasty. Ann Thorac Surg 57:1295–1299

Chang M et al (2017) Comparison of outcome of coronary artery bypass grafting versus drug-eluting stent implantation for non–ST-elevation acute coronary syndrome. Am J Cardiol 120:380–386

Christiansen S, Autschbach R (2010) Results and treatment strategy for patients undergoing emergent coronary artery bypass grafting. Ann Thorac Cardiovasc Surg 16:168–173

de Winter RJ, Tijssen JGP (2012) Non–ST-segment elevation myocardial infarction. JACC Cardiovasc Interv 5:903–905

Eikelboom JW et al (2000) Unfractionated heparin and low-molecular-weight heparin in acute coronary syndrome without ST elevation: a meta-analysis. Lancet 355:1936–1942

Escaned J et al (2017) Clinical outcomes of state-of-the-art percutaneous coronary revascularization in patients with de novo three vessel disease: 1-year results of the SYNTAX II study. Eur Heart J 38:3124–3134

Fox K et al (2002) Interventional versus conservative treatment for patients with unstable angina or non-ST-elevation myocardial infarction: the British Heart Foundation RITA 3 randomised trial. Lancet 360:743–751

Fremes SE et al (2023) STICH3C: rationale and study protocol. Circ Cardiovasc Interv 16

Goldman S et al (2004) Long-term patency of saphenous vein and left internal mammary artery grafts after coronary artery bypass surgery. J Am Coll Cardiol 44:2149–2156

Hannan EL et al (2020) Hybrid coronary revascularization versus conventional coronary artery bypass surgery. Circ Cardiovasc Interv 13

Hong S-J et al (2021) 1-month dual-antiplatelet therapy followed by aspirin monotherapy after polymer-free drug-coated stent implantation. JACC Cardiovasc Interv 14:1801–1811

Hwang B, Williams ML, Tian DH, Yan TD, Misfeld M (2022) Coronary artery bypass surgery for acute coronary syndrome: a network meta-analysis of on-pump cardioplegic arrest, off-pump, and on-pump beating heart strategies. J Card Surg 37:5290–5299

ISIS-2 (Second International Study of Infarct Survival) Collaborative Group (1988) Randomised trial of intravenous streptokinase, oral aspirin, both, or neither among 17,187 cases of suspected acute myocardial infarction: ISIS-2. ISIS-2 (Second International Study of Infarct Survival) Collaborative Group. Lancet 2:349–360

Jin R, Hiratzka LF, Grunkemeier GL, Krause A, Page US (2005) Aborted off-pump coronary artery bypass patients have much worse outcomes than on-pump or successful off-pump patients. Circulation 112

Khaladj N et al (2013) Immediate surgical coronary revascularisation in patients presenting with acute myocardial infarction. J Cardiothorac Surg 8:167

Li Y et al (2017) Immediate/early vs. Delayed invasive strategy for patients with non-ST-segment elevation acute coronary syndromes: a systematic review and meta-analysis. Front Physiol 8

Li D et al (2021) One-stop hybrid coronary revascularization versus off-pump coronary artery bypass grafting in patients with multivessel coronary artery disease. Front Cardiovasc Med 8

Locker C et al (2000) Emergency myocardial revascularization for acute myocardial infarction: survival benefits of avoiding cardiopulmonary bypass. Eur J Cardiothorac Surg 17:234–238

Milosevic A et al (2016) Immediate versus delayed invasive intervention for non-STEMI patients. JACC Cardiovasc Interv 9:541–549
Park S-J et al (2011) Randomized trial of stents versus bypass surgery for left main coronary artery disease. N Engl J Med 364:1718–1727
Park S-J et al (2015) Trial of Everolimus-Eluting stents or bypass surgery for coronary disease. N Engl J Med 372:1204–1212
Patel NC, Patel NU, Loulmet DF, McCabe JC, Subramanian VA (2004) Emergency conversion to cardiopulmonary bypass during attempted off-pump revascularization results in increased morbidity and mortality. J Thorac Cardiovasc Surg 128:655–661
Puymirat E et al (2012) Use of invasive strategy in non–ST-segment elevation myocardial infarction is a major determinant of improved long-term survival. JACC Cardiovasc Interv 5:893–902
Ranasinghe I et al (2011) Risk stratification in the setting of non-ST elevation acute coronary syndromes 1999-2007. Am J Cardiol 108:617–624
Rastan AJ et al (2006) Emergency coronary artery bypass graft surgery for acute coronary syndrome. Circulation 114
Reeves BC, Ascione R, Caputo M, Angelini GD (2006) Morbidity and mortality following acute conversion from off-pump to on-pump coronary surgery. Eur J Cardiothorac Surg 29:941–947
Schumer EM et al (2016) Emergency coronary artery bypass grafting: indications and outcomes from 2003 through 2013. Tex Heart Inst J 43:214–219
Schwartz GG (2001) Effects of atorvastatin on early recurrent ischemic events in acute coronary syndromes. The MIRACL study: a randomized controlled trial. JAMA 285:1711
Serruys PW et al (2009) Percutaneous coronary intervention versus coronary-artery bypass grafting for severe coronary artery disease. N Engl J Med 360:961–972
Sezai A et al (2012) Results of emergency coronary artery bypass grafting for acute myocardial infarction: importance of intraoperative and postoperative cardiac medical therapy. Ann Thorac Cardiovasc Surg 18:338–346
Shahian DM et al (2009) The Society of Thoracic Surgeons 2008 cardiac surgery risk models: part 1—coronary artery bypass grafting surgery. Ann Thorac Surg 88:S2–S22
Stamou SC et al (2005) Coronary revascularization without cardiopulmonary bypass versus the conventional approach in high-risk patients. Ann Thorac Surg 79:552–557
Thielmann M et al (2021) Coronary artery bypass graft surgery in patients with acute coronary syndromes after primary percutaneous coronary intervention: a current report from the north-rhine westphalia surgical myocardial infarction registry. J Am Heart Assoc 10
Thygesen K et al (2018) Fourth universal definition of myocardial infarction (2018). Circulation 138
Weiss ES, Chang DD, Joyce DL, Nwakanma LU, Yuh DD (2008) Optimal timing of coronary artery bypass after acute myocardial infarction: a review of California discharge data. J Thorac Cardiovasc Surg 135:503–511.e3
Yang EH et al (2005) Emergency coronary artery bypass surgery for percutaneous coronary interventions. J Am Coll Cardiol 46:2004–2009
Yusuf S et al (2001) Effects of clopidogrel in addition to aspirin in patients with acute coronary syndromes without ST-segment elevation. N Engl J Med 345:494–502
Zapolanski A et al (1991) Emergency coronary artery bypass surgery following failed balloon angioplasty: role of the internal mammary artery graft. J Card Surg 6:439–448
Zapolanski A et al (1995) Arterial conduits in emergency coronary artery surgery. J Card Surg 10:32–39
Zeff RH et al (1988) Internal mammary artery versus saphenous vein graft to the left anterior descending coronary artery: prospective randomized study with 10-year follow-up. Ann Thorac Surg 45:533–536

Surgical Revascularisation for Acute ST Elevation Myocardial Infarction Unsuitable for Percutaneous Intervention

Dimitrios Angouras and Grigorios Karamasis

Abstract While primary percutaneous coronary intervention (PCI) remains the gold-standard reperfusion therapy for ST-elevation myocardial infarction (STEMI), a subset of patients is unsuitable for PCI because of anatomical, technical, or clinical constraints. This chapter examines the evolving role of emergency coronary artery bypass grafting (CABG) in STEMI, tracing its progression from a primary reperfusion approach to a selective treatment reserved for high-risk cases. Contemporary registry data indicate that surgery is now performed mainly in the most critically ill patients—those with cardiogenic shock, failed PCI, mechanical complications, or complex coronary anatomy. The timing of surgery is discussed, with evidence suggesting increased risk with early (<24 h) CABG, but also recognising that unnecessary delay may be harmful in unstable patients. Perioperative considerations, including conduit selection, off-pump surgery and myocardial protection strategies, mechanical circulatory support, and antiplatelet management, are critically reviewed. Although CABG cannot rival PCI's speed in achieving reperfusion, it remains indispensable in carefully selected cases, underscoring the importance of multidisciplinary decision-making and institutional expertise to optimise outcomes in this challenging patient group.

Keywords ST-elevation myocardial infarction (STEMI) · Coronary artery bypass grafting (CABG) · Percutaneous coronary intervention (PCI) · Cardiogenic shock · Mechanical complications · Surgical timing · Myocardial protection · Mechanical circulatory support · Antiplatelet therapy · Emergency revascularisation

---

D. Angouras
Department of Cardiac Surgery, Attikon University Hospital, Medical School, National and Kapodistrian University of Athens, Athens, Greece

G. Karamasis (✉)
Department of Cardiology, Attikon University Hospital, Medical School, National and Kapodistrian University of Athens, Athens, Greece

A. Kourliouros (ed.), *Emergency Cardiac Surgery*,
https://doi.org/10.1007/978-3-032-15787-4_6

1 Introduction

In patients with acute ST-elevation myocardial infarction (STEMI), the primary goal is the rapid restoration of epicardial flow in the culprit vessel and the reperfusion of the affected myocardium. Timely reperfusion is critical, as the duration of ischaemia is directly correlated with the extent of myocardial necrosis and the likelihood of adverse clinical outcomes (Cannon et al. 2000; Fu et al. 2001). Current guidelines recommend primary percutaneous coronary intervention (PCI) as the preferred reperfusion strategy, emphasising that PCI-mediated reperfusion should be achieved within 120 min of STEMI diagnosis (Lawton et al. 2022; Byrne et al. 2023). For patients who initially present at PCI-capable hospitals, the time from diagnosis to reperfusion—referred to as door-to-wire crossing time—should be under 60 min. In cases where primary PCI cannot be performed within 120 min, immediate thrombolysis followed by prompt transfer to a PCI centre is advised (Lawton et al. 2022; Byrne et al. 2023).

Given the time-sensitive nature of STEMI treatment, coronary artery bypass grafting (CABG) plays a limited role, primarily due to practical and logistical challenges. Moreover, robust evidence supporting CABG as a primary treatment for acute STEMI is lacking, as it has not been evaluated in major randomised controlled trials (RCTs). As a result, the use of CABG has diminished with the widespread adoption of primary PCI. Data from a nationwide registry in the United States show that CABG utilisation in STEMI patients declined from 8.3% in 2007 to 5.4% in 2014, with 45.8% of patients undergoing CABG alone, 38.7% receiving CABG after PCI, and 8.2% undergoing CABG following thrombolysis (Pi et al. 2017). Nevertheless, emergency CABG remains a viable option in specific clinical scenarios for the management of acute STEMI.

2 Historical Perspectives and Contemporary Outcomes of CABG in STEMI Treatment

During the late 1970s and 1980s, CABG emerged as a leading revascularisation option for acute myocardial infarction (AMI). DeWood et al. reported a 2.0% hospital mortality rate among 701 patients with transmural AMI who underwent surgical reperfusion within 6 h of symptom onset (DeWood et al. 1983). Similarly, Flameng et al. found no mortality among haemodynamically stable patients with evolving AMI when surgical reperfusion occurred within an average of 3 h from symptom onset (Flameng et al. 1987). A 1988 randomised trial, the only one published to date, demonstrated that surgical myocardial reperfusion was both safe and effective in treating evolving transmural AMI, significantly reducing early (2.9%) and late (0%) mortality rates compared to those of conventional medical treatment (8.8% and 11.7%, respectively), excluding thrombolysis and PCI (Koshal et al. 1988). However, the advent and widespread adoption of primary PCI, with its ability to rapidly restore blood flow, has dramatically altered our perspective since then.

Time constraints of myocardial reperfusion challenge the ability of CABG to act as a first-line treatment for STEMI. Issues with resource availability and the inherently time-consuming nature of the procedure significantly limit its potential to achieve infarct-related artery (IRA) reperfusion within the ideal timeframe and save sufficient myocardium to impact prognosis (Byrne et al. 2023). Additionally, emergency surgical revascularisation may exacerbate ischaemia-reperfusion injury, not only due to prolonged flow deprivation but also because of potential further myocardial damage caused by cardiopulmonary bypass (CPB) and cardioplegic arrest (Vinten-Johansen and Thourani 2000; Buja 2023). Furthermore, surgery, with or without CPB, is likely to intensify the acute systemic inflammatory response associated with STEMI (Anzai et al. 1997; Fransen et al. 1998; Lee et al. 2003; Lang et al. 2022).

These factors may partly explain the higher mortality rates observed with emergency CABG for STEMI compared to primary PCI. In countries with well-established PCI programs, primary PCI consistently demonstrates an average hospital mortality rate of approximately 5% (Alkhouli et al. 2020; Thrane et al. 2023). In contrast, Creswell et al. reported a 9.1% mortality rate for surgical procedures performed within 6 h and 8.3% for those conducted between 6 h and 2 days after AMI (Creswell et al. 1995). Similarly, Weiss et al. documented an 8.2% mortality rate for CABG performed on day 0 (Weiss et al. 2008). More recent data from Axelsson et al. over the past decade indicate hospital mortality rates of 13% for emergency CABG and 41% for salvage procedures (Axelsson et al. 2016). Data from the North Rhine Westphalia surgical myocardial infarction (NRW-SMI) registry in Germany further revealed substantial mortality (12.6%) and major adverse cardio-cerebral events (MACCE) (28.5%) associated with CABG for STEMI (Liakopoulos et al. 2020).

However, these figures do not necessarily imply that CABG is inferior to PCI or that its outcomes have worsened over time. Because no RCTs have directly compared PCI with surgical revascularisation in patients with acute coronary syndromes (ACS), interpreting observational data requires caution, especially given the differences in patient populations. The seemingly higher CABG mortality rates compared to the 1980s primarily reflect differences in patient selection rather than the procedure itself. Early CABG studies mainly included patients with one- or two-vessel disease and minimal comorbidity. In contrast, contemporary emergency CABG for STEMI is typically reserved for patients with cardiogenic shock (CS), mechanical complications, or situations where primary PCI is unfeasible, incomplete, insufficient, or has failed. These scenarios often involve critically ill patients with ongoing ischaemia, extensive myocardial jeopardy, a high atherosclerotic burden, and poor coronary targets (Byrne et al. 2023). Data from the NRW-SMI registry show that hospital mortality for STEMI patients undergoing CABG without prior PCI was 11.8%, rising to 12.3% when PCI was performed more than 24 h before CABG, 15.8% when PCI was performed within 24 h before CABG, and 21.1% in cases of failed PCI ($P < 0.05$). Prior PCI (OR 1.25; $P = 0.039$) and failed PCI (OR 1.88, $P = 0.001$) were identified as independent predictors for the combined endpoint of hospital mortality and MACCE (Thielmann et al. 2021).

Given the severity of the clinical status and comorbidities of patients referred for surgery, current outcomes are indeed commendable. An analysis of 11,485 patients from the Acute Coronary Syndrome Israeli Survey (2000–2010) revealed that those referred for early surgery (5% of the total cohort) exhibited higher-risk characteristics and a more frequent use for mechanical ventilation and intra-aortic balloon pump (IABP) support (all $p < 0.01$). Nevertheless, mortality rates following CABG were comparable to those observed with PCI or medical treatment (11.4% vs. 10.2%; $P = 0.40$) (Klempfner et al. 2018). Data from the Japan AMI Registry, collected retrospectively during the current PCI era (2011–2016), offer additional insights (Tomura et al. 2024). Among 19,428 STEMI patients, 2.3% underwent CABG, while 90.0% underwent primary PCI. Although all-cause mortality was significantly higher in the CABG group compared to those who did not undergo surgery (15.9% vs. 7.3%, $P < 0.001$), CABG patients had a greater incidence of heart failure, CS, diabetes, and left main or multivessel disease. After multivariable analysis, CABG was associated with lower all-cause mortality (adjusted OR = 0.43, 95% CI 0.26–0.72).

In summary, primary PCI remains the preferred treatment for STEMI due to its promptness and well-established benefits. Although earlier studies suggested favourable outcomes for emergency surgical revascularisation in STEMI, recent evidence associates it with higher mortality rates. This discrepancy likely arises from patient selection bias, as those now referred for early CABG are typically critically ill with poor prognoses. For those high-risk STEMI patients, CABG remains a valuable therapeutic option.

3 Clinical Scenarios for Emergency CABG

Emergency CABG for acute STEMI should be considered in the following clinical scenarios (Lawton et al. 2022; Byrne et al. 2023):

1. In STEMI patients who develop mechanical complications (i.e. ventricular septal defect, acute mitral regurgitation due to papillary muscle rupture, or left ventricle free wall rupture). Emergency cardiac surgery in this clinical scenario is discussed in detail in Chapter "Emergency Surgery for Mechanical Complications of Myocardial Infarction."
2. In patients with STEMI complicated by cardiogenic shock, when PCI is not feasible. In this case, CABG should be considered regardless of the time elapsed since symptom onset (Lawton et al. 2022; Byrne et al. 2023).
3. In STEMI patients when PCI is either not feasible or unsuccessful. In contemporary practice, primary PCI successfully restores epicardial vessel patency in >95% of the cases (Keeley et al. 2003; De Waha et al. 2017). When anatomical or technical factors (e.g. uncrossable lesions, extreme tortuosity, iatrogenic coro-

nary dissection) prevent percutaneous antegrade blood flow restoration, emergency CABG can serve as an effective reperfusion strategy. However, emergency surgical revascularisation following failed primary PCI should be reserved for cases with ongoing ischaemia or a large area of myocardium at risk (Lawton et al. 2022; Byrne et al. 2023). Additionally, if myocardial perfusion fails despite a patent epicardial vessel due to unsuccessful microvascular reperfusion (i.e. no-reflow), surgical revascularisation offers no benefit (Lawton et al. 2022).

In contemporary practice, the primary goal during the initial revascularisation procedure is to restore flow in the IRA. Therefore, complex multivessel disease in the context of STEMI does not mandate treatment with emergency CABG if primary PCI of the culprit vessel is feasible. However, since complete revascularisation post-STEMI is recommended based on strong clinical evidence (Reddy et al. 2024), a staged CABG procedure following primary PCI may be appropriate for selected patients with multivessel disease (Besola et al. 2024). Extensive discussion for such a strategy is beyond the scope of this chapter.

4 Timing of Surgical Revascularisation

Determining the ideal timing of surgery in STEMI patients may be challenging and requires close collaboration between interventional cardiologists and cardiac surgeons. Factors to consider include clinical acuity, ongoing ischaemia, extent of jeopardised myocardium, and operability. The latter involves assessing operative risk, technical feasibility, logistical issues, and potential futility.

Some patients may be too high-risk for surgery due to substantial comorbidities, particularly when combined with advanced age or limited life expectancy. Patients who have experienced cardiac arrest/intubation are deemed inoperable if they present with irreversible neurological injury or multi-organ failure (Krishnan et al. 2018). Conversely, operable patients with STEMI-related CS or electrical instability and unfeasible or unsuccessful PCI of the IRA represent true surgical emergencies despite reported high operative mortality rates, ranging from 24% to 62% (Liakopoulos et al. 2019; Thielmann et al. 2021; Grothusen et al. 2022; Liu et al. 2024). This recommendation is classified as I/B in current European ACS guidelines (Byrne et al. 2023).

In stable patients, the optimal timing for surgery remains debatable. Substantial evidence indicates that early surgery is associated with a higher mortality risk (Creswell et al. 1995; Lee et al. 2003; Voisine et al. 2006; Weiss et al. 2008; Abd-Alaal et al. 2010; Assmann et al. 2012; Liakopoulos et al. 2019; Bernard et al. 2023). A meta-analysis of 100,048 STEMI and NSTEMI patients showed hospital mortality rates of 7.7% for early CABG (within 1 or 2 days) versus 3.0% for late CABG (Chen and Liu 2014). The mortality OR for early surgery was 3.76 ($P = 0.000$) for the entire cohort and 5.28 ($P = 0.000$) for the STEMI subgroup. A dose-response analysis demonstrated a significant correlation between mortality and CABG timing, prompting the authors to advise against early CABG, especially within the first 2 weeks post-AMI (Chen and Liu 2014). A subsequent meta-analysis of 19 studies and 113,984 patients (including STEMI, NSTEMI, and an undefined STEMI/NSTEMI category) reaffirmed these findings (Lang et al. 2022). Early CABG (within 24 h) had significantly higher hospital mortality rates compared to delayed surgery (>24 h), both in the STEMI subgroup (OR 2.62) and the undefined STEMI/NSTEMI subgroup (OR 3.88). The authors concluded that CABG should be deferred until at least 24 h after STEMI onset whenever feasible (Lang et al. 2022). Similarly, in their meta-analysis involving 137,373 patients with AMI, Weigel et al. showed an average mortality rate after CABG of 12.7% when the procedure was performed within 6 h of AMI, 10.9% when performed within 6–24 h, 9.8% within 1 day, 3.0% any time after 1 day, 5.9% within 7 days, and 2.7% when CABG was performed any time after 7 days of AMI. However, a significant risk of bias due to patient selection and confounding, as well as considerable heterogeneity in mortality rates within subgroups, was detected in this meta-analysis (Weigel et al. 2022).

It appears that the increased mortality linked to early surgery reflects the higher clinical acuity of these patients rather than a direct etiological association with surgical timing. In a retrospective analysis of 2058 STEMI and NSTEMI patients who underwent early versus late (<24 vs. ≥24 h) isolated CABG, the operative mortality rate was significantly higher in the <24 h cohort (7.19% vs. 3.79%; $P = .01$) (Bianco et al. 2021). Nonetheless, the early group had a higher prevalence of previous PCI, CS (24.7% vs. 3.3%), and IABP use. After adjusting for baseline characteristics, the mortality difference disappeared (4.15% vs. 4.58%; $P = .62$). Interestingly, in the subgroup of 390 STEMI patients, risk-adjusted analysis revealed a numerical—but not statistically significant—increase in operative mortality in the late surgery group (4.0% vs. 8.4%; $P = 0.17$). Similarly, in some series of STEMI patients who underwent early vs. late CABG (<24 vs. ≥24 h or <12 h vs. 12–72 h vs. >72 h), the timing of surgery did not significantly impact early or long-term survival (Khan et al. 2015; Kang et al. 2023).

In this context, it is inadvisable to delay surgery for clinically stable patients with an extensive myocardial area at risk. Prolonged delays could result in ischaemia recurrence (reported in 19% of cases) or preoperative low cardiac output, both associated with approximately tripled operative mortality (Grieshaber et al. 2017; Bernard et al. 2023). This consideration also applies to cases where successful primary PCI on the IRA has been performed, but the patient has complex multivessel and/or left main disease. In such situations, complete surgical revascularisation during the index hospitalisation may be suggested by the Heart Team based on the patient's comorbidities and disease complexity, following the principles of myocardial revascularisation management in non-ACS cases (Head et al. 2018; Sabatine et al. 2021; Byrne et al. 2023; Besola et al. 2024). STEMI and NSTEMI patients with multivessel disease appear to be better served by a single-setting complete versus staged complete revascularisation strategy. A recent meta-analysis showed the former offering the greatest reductions in cardiovascular events (Maqsood et al. 2024).

Discrepancies in the medical literature regarding the optimal timing of CABG after STEMI may stem not only from patient heterogeneity and differing definitions of early versus late surgery but also from variations in the effectiveness of local teams and therapeutic strategies (Biancari et al. 2015). In this context, exercising clinical judgement is crucial. During decision-making, it is essential to assess each patient's unique clinical characteristics while also considering the availability of local resources and expertise.

5 Perioperative Strategies and Surgical Considerations

While most centres adhere to institutionally established or preferred therapeutic approaches, the overall management of STEMI patients undergoing surgical revascularisation may vary based on each patient's specific needs.

5.1 Mechanical Circulatory Support

In patients with CS, mechanical circulatory support (MCS) should be considered. The IABP is the most accessible and commonly used haemodynamic support device. It offers haemodynamic benefits through afterload reduction and enhanced coronary and peripheral perfusion, coupled with ease of implantation and management, as well as a favourable safety profile. However, the IABP-SHOCK II trial did not show a reduction in 30-day or 12-month all-cause mortality when IABP was used in CS patients following AMI (Thiele et al. 2012; Thiele et al. 2013). Consequently, current guidelines discourage routine IABP use in ACS patients with CS who do not present mechanical complications (class III/B recommendation) (Byrne et al. 2023). It is important to underline, however, that in the IABP-SHOCK II trial, only 1.0% of the 600 patients underwent immediate CABG, and an additional 2.5% had surgery after initial PCI (Thiele et al. 2012). Thus, the trial results have limited relevance to the surgical population. While the modest effects of IABP on cardiac output are unlikely to reduce mortality in the late phases of CS with systemic inflammation-induced inappropriate vasodilation (Geppert et al. 2006; Dettling et al. 2024), counterpulsation may be beneficial during the initial phases of compensatory vasoconstriction as the patient approaches surgery. Preoperative IABP use in high-risk CABG patients has consistently been shown to reduce mortality, morbidity, and the length of ICU and hospital stay (Deppe et al. 2017). Therefore, we continue to support its use in the surgical STEMI population with CS. If IABP is insufficient to achieve meaningful haemodynamic and metabolic improvement, circulatory support can be escalated to veno-arterial extracorporeal membrane oxygenation (VA-ECMO), with IABP serving as an adjunct device for left ventricular unloading. Although the ECMO-CS trial did not show significant improvement in clinical outcomes for 122 patients (51% with STEMI) with rapidly deteriorating or severe CS (Ostadal et al. 2023), the trial's validity is questionable due to limited statistical power and methodological issues, including a high (39%) crossover rate to VA-ECMO in the conservative arm. Conversely, a recent network meta-analysis involving 48,749 CS patients found that the ECMO-IABP configuration was associated with reduced mortality (network OR 0.54, 95% CI 0.33–0.86), while other MCS devices, including ECMO, IABP, microaxial ventricular assist device (mVAD), ECMO-mVAD, centrifugal VAD, and mVAD-IABP, did not demonstrate similar benefits (Low et al. 2024). Escalation to ECMO-IABP can be performed preoperatively or postoperatively as needed. For further details on MCS in perioperative CS, refer to Chapter "Mechanical Circulatory Support in Perioperative Cardiogenic Shock".

5.2 *Conduit Selection*

In patients with STEMI, the urgency of revascularisation often influences the choice and utilisation of CABG conduits. For stable patients, graft selection need not differ from elective cases. However, in haemodynamically or electrically unstable patients, prolonged conduit harvesting poses challenges occasionally leading to total venous graft-based CABG. In a recent prospective multicentre registry involving 618 STEMI patients who underwent CABG, the left internal thoracic artery (LITA) was employed in only 78.9% of those presenting with CS, compared to 92.2% among those without CS (Liakopoulos et al. 2019). A second arterial graft (RITA or radial artery) was rarely utilised (in 3.7% and 9.3% of the patients, respectively).

We advocate for the routine harvest and utilisation of the LITA in all patients. Not only does LITA grafting offer undeniable medium- and long-term survival benefits (Cameron et al. 1995; Karthik et al. 2004), but compelling evidence also associates it with significantly reduced hospital mortality (Leavitt et al. 2001; Locker et al. 2003). In their analysis of 21,873 consecutive, first-time CABG procedures, Leavitt et al. reported an adjusted OR for hospital mortality (LITA versus no LITA) of 0.40 ($P < 0.001$). Remarkably, even urgent or emergency surgery patients benefited from LITA use (OR = 0.36 for urgent patients; OR = 0.30 for emergency patients; $P < 0.001$). Furthermore, after developing five mortality risk groups using multivariate analysis, Leavitt et al. consistently demonstrated a protective effect of LITA grafting on perioperative mortality. In the highest-risk group (predicted mortality risk ≥10.0%), the relative risk (RR) was 0.59, with a risk difference of −9.61% (13.82% mortality for LITA versus 23.43% without LITA), representing the most substantial difference across all groups. In unstable patients, the LITA can be safely harvested under CPB. During harvesting, CPB (a) maintains systemic organ perfusion, (b) decompresses the heart, significantly reducing myocardial oxygen demands (Allen et al. 1986), and (c) eliminates the need for catecholamine administration, further improving the oxygen demand-supply balance and mitigating the direct toxic effects of catecholamines on the myocardium (Kumar et al. 2021).

5.3 *Cardiopulmonary Bypass and Myocardial Protection Strategies*

Conventional on-pump CABG with cardioplegic arrest is the predominant surgical technique for treating STEMI patients in Western countries (Liakopoulos et al. 2020). Both crystalloid HTK (Custodiol®) solution and blood cardioplegia with antegrade or retrograde administration can be used (Rastan et al. 2006; Liakopoulos et al. 2020). The optimal temperature of blood cardioplegic solution remains debated. While cold cardioplegia minimises myocardial oxygen demand by lowering basal metabolic rate, it has been criticised for impairing enzymatic activity and disrupting metabolic processes (Whittaker et al. 2021). Conversely, warm blood cardioplegia provides a metabolically balanced environment, stabilising cell membranes and enhancing substrate, oxygen, and ATP utilisation. For cases of STEMI-related CS, warm induction cardioplegia with glutamate-enriched blood followed by cold cardioplegia has been suggested to resuscitate energy- and substrate-depleted myocardium (Rosenkranz et al. 1983). We favour induction with warm resuscitative cardioplegia for emergency STEMI surgery due to its theoretical advantages, although this is not unequivocally proven (Asai et al. 1995). However, cold blood cardioplegia remains our primary protection strategy. Warm cardioplegia is less attractive because of impaired visualisation of distal anastomoses, higher hyperkalemia risk, increased crystalloid and alpha-agonist use to maintain perfusion pressures, and greater reported endothelial injury and rates of neurological complications (Whittaker et al. 2021). Furthermore, data from the NRW-SMI registry indicated that warm blood cardioplegia is an independent predictor of MACCE in STEMI patients, including those with CS (Liakopoulos et al. 2019).

While CPB remains the standard approach for surgical revascularisation, some surgeons advocate for off-pump CABG (OPCABG), even in emergencies. In addition to its other theoretical advantages, OPCABG, in the context of AMI, purportedly prevents further global myocardial ischaemia and reduces ischaemia-reperfusion injury (Emerson et al. 2015). Multiple studies have demonstrated OPCABG's safety and effectiveness in this setting (Locker et al. 2003; Rastan et al. 2006; Fattouch et al. 2009; Ben-Gal et al. 2011; Kawamoto et al. 2018), though its superiority is debated. In the only relevant RCT involving 128 STEMI patients, Fattouch et al. found OPCABG reduced early mortality and morbidity compared to the conventional procedure (Fattouch et al. 2009). Interestingly, their findings showed improved outcomes in patients undergoing off-pump surgery within 6 h of symptom onset and in those with CS, despite other experts advocating OPCABG in carefully selected patients with stable haemodynamics (Kerendi et al. 2005). In a study of 251 AMI patients, Locker et al. also found significantly lower early mortality in off-pump compared to on-pump CABG, but only for those who underwent surgery within the first 48 h (4.3% vs. 16.5%, $P = 0.044$) (Locker et al. 2003). However, late reinterventions were more frequent (6.5% vs. 0.8%; $P = 0.028$).

Other studies did not show improved early outcomes for off-pump surgery, regardless of revascularisation timing, but confirmed higher unplanned reintervention rates (Ben-Gal et al. 2011; Liakopoulos et al. 2019; Bernard et al. 2023). A meta-analysis of 3001 ACS patients who underwent CABG found comparable mortality between the two strategies at 30 days and mid-term follow-up but noted that OPCABG was associated with significantly lower completeness of revascularisation (Harling et al. 2013). These findings highlight a highly debated shortcoming of off-pump surgery, namely incomplete revascularisation and inferior graft patency rates. In the study of Locker et al., OPCABG was associated with fewer grafts per patient (1.75 vs. 3.04; $P < 0.001$), lower circumflex marginal grafting (11.5% vs. 90%; $P < 0.001$), and reduced use of ITA grafts (82% vs. 92%; $P = 0.033$) (Locker et al. 2003). These factors likely impact long-term outcomes.

Incomplete revascularisation is mainly due to intractable haemodynamic instability. Upward retraction of the heart, particularly during circumflex branch grafting, can be challenging in unstable STEMI patients, even for experienced teams. Beating-heart on-pump CABG (BH-CABG) may act as a compromise, preventing additional global myocardial ischaemia while offering the benefits of a decompressed heart and haemodynamic stability provided by CPB. However, BH-CABG also entails the adverse effects of CPB, the technical challenges of heart motion, blood flow at the anastomosis site, and the potential risk of regional myocardial ischaemia. A network meta-analysis of 11,841 ACS patients who underwent OPCABG, BH-CABG, or arrested-heart on-pump CABG demonstrated comparable 30-day mortality across ACS, but a significant mortality benefit for OPCABG in AMI patients (OR 0.28, 95% CI 0.07–0.83) (Hwang et al. 2022). Moderate heterogeneity in the on-pump CABG and OPCABG comparison ($I^2 = 48.9\%$) suggests differences in team expertise and familiarity with the OPCABG technique as factors for successful outcomes.

Overall, on-pump surgery using a single ITA and additional venous grafting is still considered by most surgeons the safest strategy for higher-risk patients (Liakopoulos et al. 2020). Among the 2432 ACS patients in the NRW-SMI registry, 92% underwent on-pump arrested-heart CABG, with only 6% undergoing OPCABG and 2% BH-CABG (Liakopoulos et al. 2020). The percentages were similar in the STEMI subgroup, except for BH-CABG, which was slightly more frequent in STEMI patients with CS compared to those without CS (6.6% vs. 1.6%; $P = 0.002$) (Liakopoulos et al. 2019).

5.4 Bleeding Risk Considerations and Antiplatelet Management

Most STEMI patients (56% in the NRW-SMI registry) receive dual antiplatelet therapy (DAPT), preferably with a potent P2Y12 inhibitor (prasugrel or ticagrelor), or clopidogrel if these are unavailable, intolerable, or contraindicated (Liakopoulos et al. 2020; Byrne et al. 2023). The preoperative use of potent antiplatelet drugs increases postoperative bleeding, transfusion requirements, and reoperation rate after CABG (Kremke et al. 2013; Cao et al. 2014; Hansson et al. 2016; Rohman et al. 2020). Consequently, European guidelines recommend considering the postponement of non-emergent cardiac surgery for at least 3 days after discontinuing ticagrelor, 5 days after clopidogrel, and 7 days after prasugrel (recommendation IIa/B) (Neumann et al. 2019). However, if emergency surgery is indicated, it should not be postponed due to antiplatelet treatment exposure, as the imminent hazards, including death, far outweigh the risks of bleeding complications (Neumann et al. 2019).

While some meta-analytic data suggest a significantly greater incidence of mortality for those undergoing CABG while on clopidogrel (Biancari et al. 2012; Cao et al. 2014; Siller-Matula et al. 2017), this association has not been consistently confirmed (Nijjer et al. 2011; Kremke et al. 2013). In the NRW-SMI registry, DAPT was not found to be an independent predictor for hospital mortality or MACCE (Liakopoulos et al. 2020).

Compared to clopidogrel, ticagrelor offers advantageous features and a more favourable bleeding profile due to its short half-life and reversible receptor binding, which allows for a more rapid recovery of platelet function (Hansson et al. 2016). In a subgroup analysis of the PLATO trial involving 1261 ACS patients who underwent CABG, ticagrelor was associated with a comparable risk of CABG-related major bleeding to clopidogrel when withheld for only 24–72 h before surgery, as opposed to 5 days for clopidogrel (Held et al. 2011). Similarly, an analysis of propensity score-matched ACS patients from the E-CABG registry demonstrated that, if discontinued more than 24 h before surgery, ticagrelor is associated with a similar degree of bleeding compared to aspirin alone, although with a higher rate of platelet transfusion (Gherli et al. 2016).

Unlike ticagrelor, prasugrel is a potent antiplatelet drug with a long half-life. Prasugrel is recommended for P2Y12 receptor inhibitor-naïve patients undergoing PCI (recommendation I/B) (Byrne et al. 2023). However, this recommendation may be problematic if primary PCI becomes unfeasible or fails. It is primarily based on the ISAR-REACT 5 trial, which showed that among STEMI/NSTEMI patients, the incidence of death, MI, or stroke at 1 year was significantly lower in those who received prasugrel compared to those who received ticagrelor (Schüpke et al. 2019). However, the validity of this study for CABG patients is limited, as only 2.1% of randomised patients underwent surgical revascularisation. Interestingly, the 1-year hazard ratio (HR) of the primary endpoint in the pre-specified CABG subgroup numerically, but not significantly, favoured ticagrelor (HR 0.66, 95% CI 0.19–2.30).

For emergency surgery where discontinuation of ticagrelor is not feasible, two novel approaches are under clinical investigation to reduce or eliminate circulating drug levels by exploiting its reversible binding to the P2Y12 receptor. The first approach employs a device with adsorbent polymer micro-beads, effective in removing low molecular weight substances from the blood. This device (CytoSorb® 300 mL; CytoSorbent Europe GmbH), initially used to adsorb cytokines in severe inflammatory conditions such as sepsis, is incorporated into the CPB circuit and has shown efficacy in adsorbing ticagrelor and DOACs (Ling et al. 2022). Initial clinical reports are promising (Javanbakht et al. 2020; Cohen et al. 2023; Schmoeckel et al.

2024), as is our limited experience. However, high-quality RCTs are needed to draw definitive conclusions about the clinical benefit. The Safe and Timely Antithrombotic Removal–Ticagrelor (STAR-T) trial is currently in progress in the USA (Gibson et al. 2022). The second approach involves intravenous administration of bentracimab, a recombinant human monoclonal antibody that binds ticagrelor and its major active metabolite with high affinity. An interim analysis of an ongoing multicentre, single-arm, open-label trial demonstrated that bentracimab provides immediate and sustained reversal of ticagrelor's antiplatelet effects, achieving haemostasis in over 90% of cases (Bhatt et al. 2022). However, 5.3% of patients experienced thrombotic events, including MI with graft occlusion, raising serious safety concerns for emergency CABG.

6 Conclusions

While primary PCI remains the gold standard for the treatment of acute STEMI, emergency cardiac surgery is indispensable in select clinical scenarios. Although only a small subset of patients requires surgical intervention, it is essential that surgical teams involved in acute MI management are well-versed in the specific surgical considerations and key perioperative strategies.

References

Abd-Alaal MM, Alsabban MA, Abbas OA, Alshaer AA, Al-Saddique A, Fouda M (2010) Timing of revascularization after acute myocardial infarction. Asian Cardiovasc Thorac Ann 18:118–121. https://doi.org/10.1177/0218492310361001

Alkhouli M, Alqahtani F, Kalra A, Gafoor S, Alhajji M, Alreshidan M, Holmes DR, Lerman A (2020) Trends in characteristics and outcomes of patients undergoing coronary revascularization in the United States, 2003–2016. JAMA Netw Open 3

Allen BS, Rosenkranz ER, Buckberg GD (1986) STUDIES OF CONTROLLED REPERFUSION AFTER ISCHEMIA: VII. High oxygen requirements of dyskinetic cardiac muscle. J Thorac Cardiovasc Surg 92:543–552. https://doi.org/10.1016/S0022-5223(19)36505-5

Anzai T, Yoshikawa T, Shiraki H, Asakura Y, Akaishi M, Mitamura H, Ogawa S (1997) C-reactive protein as a predictor of infarct expansion and cardiac rupture after a first Q-wave acute myocardial infarction. Circulation 96:778–784. https://doi.org/10.1161/01.CIR.96.3.778/ASSET/9DE399D4-1EFE-43BA-B878-932850130FA5/ASSETS/GRAPHIC/HC1570703003.JPEG

Asai T, Grossi EA, Iii ML, Parish MA, Baumann FG, Spencer FC, Colvin SB, Galloway AC, York N (1995) Resuscitative retrograde blood cardioplegia: are amino acids or continuous warm techniques necessary?

Assmann A, Boeken U, Akhyari P, Lichtenberg A (2012) Appropriate timing of coronary artery bypass grafting after acute myocardial infarction. Thorac Cardiovasc Surg 60:446–451. https://doi.org/10.1055/S-0032-1304542

Axelsson TA, Mennander A, Malmberg M, Gunn J, Jeppsson A, Gudbjartsson T (2016) Is emergency and salvage coronary artery bypass grafting justified? The Nordic Emergency/Salvage coronary artery bypass grafting study. Eur J Cardiothorac Surg 49:1451–1456. https://doi.org/10.1093/ejcts/ezv388

Ben-Gal Y, Stone GW, Smith CR, Williams MR, Weisz G, Stewart AS, Takayama H, Genereux P, Argenziano M (2011) On-pump versus off-pump surgical revascularization in patients with acute coronary syndromes: analysis from the Acute Catheterization and Urgent Intervention Triage Strategy trial. J Thorac Cardiovasc Surg 142:e33–e39. https://doi.org/10.1016/j.jtcvs.2011.03.022

Bernard C, Morgant MC, Jazayeri A, Perrin T, Malapert G, Jazayeri S, Bernard A, Bouchot O (2023) Optimal timing of coronary artery bypass grafting in haemodynamically stable patients after myocardial infarction. Biomedicine 979:11. https://doi.org/10.3390/BIOMEDICINES11030979

Besola L, Colli A, De Caterina R (2024) Coronary bypass surgery for multivessel disease after percutaneous coronary intervention in acute coronary syndromes: why, for whom, how early? Eur Heart J. https://doi.org/10.1093/EURHEARTJ/EHAE413

Bhatt DL, Pollack CV, Mazer CD, Angiolillo DJ, Steg PG, James SK, Weitz JI, Ramnath R, Arnold SE, Mays MC, Umstead BR, White B, Hickey LL, Jennings LK, Curry BJ, Lee JS, Verma S (2022) Bentracimab for ticagrelor reversal in patients undergoing urgent surgery. NEJM Evid 1. https://doi.org/10.1056/evidoa2100047

Biancari F, Airaksinen KEJ, Lip GYH (2012) Benefits and risks of using clopidogrel before coronary artery bypass surgery: Systematic review and meta-analysis of randomized trials and observational studies. J Thorac Cardiovasc Surg 143. https://doi.org/10.1016/j.jtcvs.2011.01.069

Biancari F, Onorati F, Rubino AS, Mosorin MA, Juvonen T, Ahmed N, Faggian G, Mariani C, Mignosa C, Cottini M, Beghi C, Mariscalco G (2015) Outcome of emergency coronary artery bypass grafting. J Cardiothorac Vasc Anesth 29:275–282. https://doi.org/10.1053/j.jvca.2014.10.019

Bianco V, Kilic A, Gleason TG, Aranda-Michel E, Wang Y, Navid F, Sultan I (2021) Timing of coronary artery bypass grafting after acute myocardial infarction may not influence mortality and readmissions. J Thorac Cardiovasc Surg 161:2056–2064.e4. https://doi.org/10.1016/j.jtcvs.2019.11.061

Buja LM (2023) Pathobiology of myocardial ischemia and reperfusion injury: models, modes, molecular mechanisms, modulation, and clinical applications. Cardiol Rev 31:252–264

Byrne RA, Rossello X, Coughlan JJ, Barbato E, Berry C, Chieffo A, Claeys MJ, Dan GA, Dweck MR, Galbraith M, Gilard M, Hinterbuchner L, Jankowska EA, Jüni P, Kimura T, Kunadian V, Leosdottir M, Lorusso R, Pedretti RFE, Rigopoulos AG, Gimenez MR, Thiele H, Vranckx P, Wassmann S, Wenger NK, Ibanez B (2023) 2023 ESC Guidelines for the management of acute coronary syndromes. Eur Heart J 44:3720–3826. https://doi.org/10.1093/eurheartj/ehad191

Cameron AAC, Green GE, Brogno DA, Thornton J (1995) Internal thoracic artery grafts: 20-year clinical follow-up. J Am Coll Cardiol 25:188–192. https://doi.org/10.1016/0735-1097(94)00332-K

Cannon CP, Gibson CM, Lambrew CT, Shoultz DA, Levy D, French WJ, Gore JM, Weaver WD, Rogers WJ, Tiefenbrunn AJ (2000) Relationship of symptom-onset-to-balloon time and door-to-balloon time with mortality in patients undergoing angioplasty for acute myocardial infarction. JAMA 283:2941–2947. https://doi.org/10.1001/JAMA.283.22.2941

Cao C, Indraratna P, Ang SC, Manganas C, Park J, Bannon PG, Yan TD (2014) Should clopidogrel be discontinued before coronary artery bypass grafting for patients with acute coronary syndrome? A systematic review and meta-analysis. J Thorac Cardiovasc Surg 148:3092–3098. https://doi.org/10.1016/j.jtcvs.2014.04.054

Chen HL, Liu K (2014) Timing of coronary artery bypass graft surgery for acute myocardial infarction patients: a meta-analysis. Int J Cardiol 177:53–56. https://doi.org/10.1016/j.ijcard.2014.09.127

Cohen BG, Chingcuanco F, Zhang J, Reid NM, Lee V, Hong J, Deliargyris EN, Padula WV (2023) Cost-effectiveness and budget impact of a novel antithrombotic drug removal system to reduce bleeding risk in patients on preoperative ticagrelor undergoing cardiac surgery. Am J Cardiovasc Drugs 23:429–440. https://doi.org/10.1007/s40256-023-00587-4

Creswell LL, Moulton MJ, Cox JL, Rosenbloom M (1995) Revascularization after acute myocardial infarction

De Waha S, Patel MR, Granger CB, Ohman EM, Maehara A, Eitel I, Ben-Yehuda O, Jenkins P, Thiele H, Stone GW (2017) Relationship between microvascular obstruction and adverse events following primary percutaneous coronary intervention for ST-segment elevation myocardial infarction: an individual patient data pooled analysis from seven randomized trials. Eur Heart J 38:3502–3510. https://doi.org/10.1093/EURHEARTJ/EHX414

Deppe AC, Weber C, Liakopoulos OJ, Zeriouh M, Slottosch I, Scherner M, Kuhn EW, Choi YH, Wahlers T (2017) Preoperative intra-aortic balloon pump use in high-risk patients prior to coronary artery bypass graft surgery decreases the risk for morbidity and mortality-a meta-analysis of 9,212 patients. J Card Surg 32:177–185. https://doi.org/10.1111/JOCS.13114

Dettling A, Weimann J, Sundermeyer J, Beer BN, Besch L, Becher PM, Brunner FJ, Kluge S, Kirchhof P, Blankenberg S, Westermann D, Schrage B (2024) Association of systemic inflammation with shock severity, 30-day mortality, and therapy response in patients with cardiogenic shock. Clin Res Cardiol 113:324–335. https://doi.org/10.1007/s00392-023-02336-8

DeWood MA, Spores J, Berg Jr R, Kendall RW, Grunwald RP, Selinger SL, Hensley GR, Sutherland KI, Sheilds JP (1983) Acute myocardial infarction: a decade of experience with surgical reperfusion in 701 patients. Circulation. https://pubmed.ncbi.nlm.nih.gov/6872200/. Accessed 11 July 2024

Emerson DA, Conor Þ, Hynes F, Greenberg MD, Trachiotis GD (2015) Coronary artery bypass grafting during acute coronary syndrome outcomes and comparison of off-pump to conventional coronary artery bypass grafting at a Veteran Affairs Hospital

Fattouch K, Guccione F, Dioguardi P, Sampognaro R, Corrado E, Caruso M, Ruvolo G (2009) Off-pump versus on-pump myocardial revascularization in patients with ST-segment elevation myocardial infarction: a randomized trial. J Thorac Cardiovasc Surg 137:650–657. https://doi.org/10.1016/j.jtcvs.2008.11.033

Flameng W, Sergeant P, Vanhaecke J, Suy R (1987) Emergency coronary bypass grafting for evolving myocardial infarction. Effects on infarct size and left ventricular function. J Thorac Cardiovasc Surg 94:124–131. https://doi.org/10.1016/s0022-5223(19)36327-5

Fransen E, Maessen J, Dentener M, Senden N, Geskes G, Buurman W (1998) Systemic inflammation present in patients undergoing CABG without extracorporeal circulation. Chest 113:1290–1295. https://doi.org/10.1378/chest.113.5.1290

Fu Y, Goodman S, Chang WC, Van De Werf F, Granger CB, Armstrong PW (2001) Time to treatment influences the impact of ST-segment resolution on one-year prognosis: insights from the assessment of the safety and efficacy of a new thrombolytic (ASSENT-2) trial. Circulation 104:2653–2659. https://doi.org/10.1161/HC4701.099731

Geppert A, Dorninger A, Delle-Karth G, Zorn G, Heinz G, Huber K (2006) Plasma concentrations of interleukin-6, organ failure, vasopressor support, and successful coronary revascularization in predicting 30-day mortality of patients with cardiogenic shock complicating acute myocardial infarction. Crit Care Med 34:2035–2042. https://doi.org/10.1097/01.CCM.0000228919.33620.D9

Gherli R, Mariscalco G, Dalén M, Onorati F, Perrotti A, Chocron S, Verhoye JP, Gulbins H, Reichart D, Svenarud P, Faggian G, Santarpino G, Fischlein T, Maselli D, Dominici C, Musumeci F, Rubino AS, Mignosa C, De Feo M, Bancone C, Gatti G, Maschietto L, Santini F, Nicolini F, Gherli T, Zanobini M, Kinnunen EM, Ruggieri VG, Rosato S, Biancari F (2016) Safety of preoperative use of ticagrelor with or without aspirin compared with aspirin alone in patients with acute coronary syndromes undergoing coronary artery bypass grafting. JAMA Cardiol 1:921–928. https://doi.org/10.1001/JAMACARDIO.2016.3028

Gibson CM, Mack MJ, Lee VT, Schneider DJ, Sellke FW, Ohman EM, Thourani VH, Doros G, Kroger H, Cutlip DE, Deliargyris EN (2022) Rationale and design of the safe and timely antithrombotic removal—ticagrelor (STAR-T) trial: a prospective, multi-center, double-blind, randomized controlled trial evaluating reductions in postoperative bleeding with intraoperative removal of ticagrelor by the drugsorbTM-ATR device in patients undergoing cardiothoracic surgery within 48 hours from last ticagrelor dose. Am Heart J 245:19–28. https://doi.org/10.1016/j.ahj.2021.10.188

Grieshaber P, Roth P, Oster L, Schneider TM, Görlach G, Nieman B, Böning A (2017) Is delayed surgical revascularization in acute myocardial infarction useful or dangerous? New insights into an old problem. Interact Cardiovasc Thorac Surg 25:772–779. https://doi.org/10.1093/icvts/ivx188

Grothusen C, Friedrich C, Ulbricht U, Meinert J, Attmann T, Huenges K, Borzikowsky C, Haneya A, Schoettler J, Cremer J (2022) Coronary artery bypass grafting in patients with acute myocardial infarction and cardiogenic shock. Rev Cardiovasc Med 23. https://doi.org/10.31083/J.RCM2307237

Hansson EC, Jidéus L, Åberg B, Bjursten H, Dreifaldt M, Holmgren A, Ivert T, Nozohoor S, Barbu M, Svedjeholm R, Jeppsson A (2016) Coronary artery bypass grafting-related bleeding complications in patients treated with ticagrelor or clopidogrel: a nationwide study. Eur Heart J 37:189–197. https://doi.org/10.1093/EURHEARTJ/EHV381

Harling L, Moscarelli M, Kidher E, Fattouch K, Ashrafian H, Athanasiou T (2013) The effect of off-pump coronary artery bypass on mortality after acute coronary syndrome: a meta-analysis. Int J Cardiol 169:339–348. https://doi.org/10.1016/J.IJCARD.2013.09.003

Head SJ, Milojevic M, Daemen J, Ahn JM, Boersma E, Christiansen EH, Domanski MJ, Farkouh ME, Flather M, Fuster V, Hlatky MA, Holm NR, Hueb WA, Kamalesh M, Kim YH, Mäkikallio T, Mohr FW, Papageorgiou G, Park SJ, Rodriguez AE, Sabik JF, Stables RH, Stone GW, Serruys PW, Kappetein AP (2018) Mortality after coronary artery bypass grafting versus percutaneous coronary intervention with stenting for coronary artery disease: a pooled analysis of individual patient data. Lancet 391:939–948. https://doi.org/10.1016/S0140-6736(18)30423-9

Held C, Senblad N, Bassand JP, Becker RC, Cannon CP, Claeys MJ, Harrington RA, Horrow J, Husted S, James SK, Mahaffey KW, Nicolau JC, Scirica BM, Storey RF, Vintila M, Ycas J, Wallentin L (2011) Ticagrelor versus clopidogrel in patients with acute coronary syndromes undergoing coronary artery bypass surgery: results from the PLATO (platelet inhibition and patient outcomes) trial. J Am Coll Cardiol 57:672–684. https://doi.org/10.1016/j.jacc.2010.10.029

Hwang B, Williams ML, Tian DH, Yan TD, Misfeld M (2022) Coronary artery bypass surgery for acute coronary syndrome: a network meta-analysis of on-pump cardioplegic arrest, off-pump, and on-pump beating heart strategies. J Card Surg 37:5290–5299

Javanbakht M, Trevor M, Rezaei Hemami M, Rahimi K, Branagan-Harris M, Degener F, Adam D, Preissing F, Scheier J, Cook SF, Mortensen E (2020) Ticagrelor removal by CytoSorb® in patients requiring emergent or urgent cardiac surgery: a UK-based cost-utility analysis. Pharmacoecon Open 4:307–319. https://doi.org/10.1007/s41669-019-00183-w

Kang J, Marin-Cuartas M, Auerswald L, Deo SV, Borger M, Davierwala P, Verevkin A (2023) Does timing of coronary artery bypass grafting after ST-elevation myocardial infarction impact early- and long-term outcomes? Thorac Cardiovasc Surg. https://doi.org/10.1055/S-0044-1787851

Karthik S, Srinivasan AK, Grayson AD, Jackson M, Mediratta NK (2004) Left internal mammary artery to the left anterior descending artery: effect on morbidity and mortality and reasons for non-usage. Ann Thorac Surg 78:142–148. https://doi.org/10.1016/J.ATHORACSUR.2004.02.025

Kawamoto S, Miyata H, Motomura N, Tanemoto K, Takamoto S, Saiki Y (2018) Surgical outcomes of isolated coronary artery bypass grafting for acute coronary syndrome: based on the Japan adult cardiovascular surgery database. Circ J 82:123–130. https://doi.org/10.1253/circj.CJ-17-0561

Keeley EC, Boura JA, Grines CL (2003) Primary angioplasty versus intravenous thrombolytic therapy for acute myocardial infarction: a quantitative review of 23 randomised trials. Lancet 361:13–20. https://doi.org/10.1016/S0140-6736(03)12113-7

Kerendi F, Puskas JD, Craver JM, Cooper WA, Jones EL, Lattouf OM, Vega JD, Guyton RA (2005) Emergency coronary artery bypass grafting can be performed safely without cardiopulmonary bypass in selected patients. Ann Thorac Surg 79:801–806. https://doi.org/10.1016/j.athoracsur.2004.08.010

Khan AN, Sabbagh S, Ittaman S, Abrich V, Narayan A, Austin B, Rezkalla SH (2015) Outcome of early revascularization surgery in patients with ST-elevation myocardial infarction. J Interv Cardiol 28:14–23. https://doi.org/10.1111/joic.12177

Klempfner R, Barac YD, Younis A, Kopel E, Younis A, Ronen G, Maor E, Arbel Y, Rott D, Goldenberg I, Aravot D (2018) Early referral to coronary artery bypass grafting following acute coronary syndrome, trends and outcomes from the Acute Coronary Syndrome Israeli Survey (ACSIS) 2000–2010. Heart Lung Circ 27:175–182. https://doi.org/10.1016/j.hlc.2017.01.017

Koshal A, Beanlands DS, Davies RA, Nair RC, Keon W J (1988) Urgent surgical reperfusion in acute evolving myocardial infarction. A randomized controlled study—PubMed. Circulation 78(3 Pt 2). https://pubmed.ncbi.nlm.nih.gov/3044642/. Accessed 3 July 2024

Kremke M, Tang M, Bak M, Kristensen KL, Hindsholm K, Andreasen JJ, Hjortdal V, Jakobsen CJ (2013) Antiplatelet therapy at the time of coronary artery bypass grafting: a multicentre cohort study. Eur J Cardiothorac Surg 44. https://doi.org/10.1093/ejcts/ezt230

Krishnan U, Brejt JA, Schulman-Marcus J, Swaminathan RV, Feldman DN, Goyal P, Wong SC, Minutello RM, Bergman G, Singh H, Kim LK (2018) Temporal trends in the clinical acuity of patients with ST-segment elevation myocardial infarction. Am J Med 131:100.e9–100.e20. https://doi.org/10.1016/J.AMJMED.2017.06.040

Kumar A, Pappachan JM, Fernandez CJ (2021) Catecholamine-induced cardiomyopathy: an endocrinologist's perspective. Rev Cardiovasc Med 22:1215–1228

Lang Q, Qin C, Meng W (2022) Appropriate timing of coronary artery bypass graft surgery for acute myocardial infarction patients: a meta-analysis. Front Cardiovasc Med 9

Lawton JS, Tamis-Holland JE, Bangalore S, Bates ER, Beckie TM, Bischoff JM, Bittl JA, Cohen MG, DiMaio JM, Don CW, Fremes SE, Gaudino MF, Goldberger ZD, Grant MC, Jaswal JB, Kurlansky PA, Mehran R, Metkus TS, Nnacheta LC, Rao SV, Sellke FW, Sharma G, Yong CM, Zwischenberger BA (2022) 2021 ACC/AHA/SCAI Guideline for Coronary Artery Revascularization: a report of the American College of Cardiology/American Heart Association Joint Committee on Clinical Practice Guidelines. J Am Coll Cardiol 79:e21–e129. https://doi.org/10.1016/J.JACC.2021.09.006

Leavitt BJ, O'Connor GT, Olmstead EM, Morton JR, Maloney CT, Dacey LJ, Hernandez F, Lahey SJ (2001) Use of the internal mammary artery graft and in-hospital mortality and other adverse outcomes associated with coronary artery bypass surgery. Circulation 103:507–512. https://doi.org/10.1161/01.CIR.103.4.507

Lee DC, Oz MC, Weinberg AD, Ting W, Guyton R (2003) Appropriate timing of surgical intervention after transmural acute myocardial infarction. J Thorac Cardiovasc Surg 125:115–120. https://doi.org/10.1067/mtc.2003.75

Liakopoulos OJ, Schlachtenberger G, Wendt D, Choi YH, Slottosch I, Welp H, Schiller W, Martens S, Welz A, Neuhäuser M, Jakob H, Wahlers T, Thielmann M (2019) Early clinical outcomes of surgical myocardial revascularization for acute coronary syndromes complicated by cardiogenic shock: a report from the North-Rhine-Westphalia surgical myocardial infarction registry. J Am Heart Assoc 8. https://doi.org/10.1161/JAHA.119.012049/SUPPL_FILE/JAH34068-SUP-0001-SUPINFO.PDF

Liakopoulos OJ, Slottosch I, Wendt D, Welp H, Schiller W, Martens S, Choi YH, Welz A, Pisarenko J, Neuhäuser M, Jakob H, Ruhparwar A, Wahlers T, Thielmann M (2020) Surgical revascularization for acute coronary syndromes: a report from the North Rhine-Westphalia surgical myocardial infarction registry. Eur J Cardiothorac Surg 58:1137–1144. https://doi.org/10.1093/EJCTS/EZAA260

Ling CNY, Umakumar K, Moss L, Stock UA, Raja SG, de Waal EEC, Marczin N (2022) Cytosorb® haemoadsorption: a potential game changer for patients needing myocardial surgical revascularisation. Vessel Plus 5

Liu SS, Wang J, Tan HQ, Yang YM, Zhu J (2024) Cardiac arrest and cardiogenic shock complicating ST-segment elevation myocardial infarction in China: a retrospective multicenter study. Heliyon 10. https://doi.org/10.1016/j.heliyon.2024.e34070

Locker C, Mohr R, Paz Y, Kramer A, Lev-Ran O, Pevni D, Shapira I (2003) Myocardial revascularization for acute myocardial infarction: benefits and drawbacks of avoiding cardiopulmonary bypass

Low CJW, Ling RR, Lau MPXL, Liu NSH, Tan M, Tan CS, Lim SL, Rochwerg B, Combes A, Brodie D, Shekar K, Price S, MacLaren G, Ramanathan K (2024) Mechanical circulatory support for cardiogenic shock: a network meta-analysis of randomized controlled trials and propensity score-matched studies. Intensive Care Med 50:209–221

Maqsood MH, Tamis-Holland JE, Rao SV, Stone GW, Bangalore S (2024) Culprit-only revascularization, single-setting complete revascularization, and staged complete revascularization in acute myocardial infarction: insights from a mixed treatment comparison meta-analysis of randomized trials. Circ Cardiovasc Interv 17. https://doi.org/10.1161/CIRCINTERVENTIONS.123.013737

Neumann FJ, Sousa-Uva M, Ahlsson A, Alfonso F, Banning AP, Benedetto U, Byrne RA, Collet JP, Falk V, Head SJ, Jüni P, Kastrati A, Koller A, Kristensen SD, Niebauer J, Richter DJ, Seferovic PM, Sibbing D, Stefanini GG, Windecker S, Yadav R, Zembala MO, Wijns W, Glineur D, Aboyans V, Achenbach S, Agewall S, Andreotti F, Barbato E, Baumbach A, Brophy J, Bueno H, Calvert PA, Capodanno D, Davierwala PM, Delgado V, Dudek D, Freemantle N, Funck-Brentano C, Gaemperli O, Gielen S, Gilard M, Gorenek B, Haasenritter J, Haude M, Ibanez B, Iung B, Jeppsson A, Katritsis D, Knuuti J, Kolh P, Leite-Moreira A, Lund LH, Maisano F, Mehilli J, Metzler B, Montalescot G, Pagano D, Petronio AS, Piepoli MF, Popescu BA, Sádaba R, Shlyakhto E, Silber S, Simpson IA, Sparv D, Tavilla G, Thiele H, Tousek P, Van Belle E, Vranckx P, Witkowski A, Zamorano JL, Roffi M (2019) 2018 ESC/EACTS Guidelines on myocardial revascularization. Eur Heart J 40:87–165

Nijjer SS, Watson G, Athanasiou T, Malik IS (2011) Safety of clopidogrel being continued until the time of coronary artery bypass grafting in patients with acute coronary syndrome: a meta-analysis of 34 studies. Eur Heart J 32:2970–2988. https://doi.org/10.1093/eurheartj/ehr151

Ostadal P, Rokyta R, Karasek J, Kruger A, Vondrakova D, Janotka M, Naar J, Smalcova J, Hubatova M, Hromadka M, Volovar S, Seyfrydova M, Jarkovsky J, Svoboda M, Linhart A, Belohlavek J (2023) Extracorporeal membrane oxygenation in the therapy of cardiogenic shock: results of the ECMO-CS randomized clinical trial. Circulation 147:454–464. https://doi.org/10.1161/CIRCULATIONAHA.122.062949/SUPPL_FILE/SUPPLEMENTAL

Pi Y, Roe MT, Holmes DN, Chiswell K, Garvey JL, Fonarow GC, De Lemos JA, Garratt KN, Xian Y (2017) Utilization, characteristics, and in-hospital outcomes of coronary artery bypass grafting in patients with ST-segment-elevation myocardial infarction: results from the national cardiovascular data registry acute coronary treatment and intervention outcomes network registry-get with the guidelines. Circ Cardiovasc Qual Outcomes 10. https://doi.org/10.1161/CIRCOUTCOMES.116.003490

Rastan AJ, Eckenstein JI, Hentschel B, Funkat AK, Gummert JF, Doll N, Walther T, Falk V, Mohr FW (2006) Emergency coronary artery bypass graft surgery for acute coronary syndrome: beating heart versus conventional cardioplegic cardiac arrest strategies. Circulation 114. https://doi.org/10.1161/CIRCULATIONAHA.105.001545

Reddy RK, Howard JP, Jamil Y, Madhavan MV, Nanna MG, Lansky AJ, Leon MB, Ahmad Y (2024) Percutaneous coronary revascularization strategies after myocardial infarction: a systematic review and network meta-analysis. J Am Coll Cardiol 84:276–294. https://doi.org/10.1016/J.JACC.2024.04.051

Rohman MS, Purnamasari Y, Ilmawan M, Mahdi BA, Tamara F, Mahendra AI, Mazen M, Heriansyah T, Yamin M, Pikir BS, Fajar JK (2020) Comparison of major bleeding in patients with acute coronary syndrome that underwent coronary artery bypass grafting treated with clopidogrel or ticagrelor: a systematic review and meta-analysis. F1000Res 9:99. https://doi.org/10.12688/f1000research.21925.1

Rosenkranz ER, Buckberg GD, Laks H, Mulder DG, Calif A (1983) Warm induction of cardioplegia with glutamate-enriched blood in coronary patients with cardiogenic shock who are dependent on inotropic drugs and intra-aortic balloon support

Sabatine MS, Bergmark BA, Murphy SA, O'Gara PT, Smith PK, Serruys PW, Kappetein AP, Park SJ, Park DW, Christiansen EH, Holm NR, Nielsen PH, Stone GW, Sabik JF, Braunwald E (2021) Percutaneous coronary intervention with drug-eluting stents versus coronary artery bypass grafting in left main coronary artery disease: an individual patient data meta-analysis. Lancet 398:2247–2257. https://doi.org/10.1016/S0140-6736(21)02334-5

Schmoeckel M, Thielmann M, Hassan K, Geidel S, Schmitto J, Meyer AL, Vitanova K, Liebold A, Marczin N, Bernardi MH, Tandler R, Lindstedt S, Matejic-Spasic M, Wendt D, Deliargyris EN, Storey RF (2024) Intraoperative haemoadsorption for antithrombotic drug removal during cardiac surgery: initial report of the international safe and timely antithrombotic removal (STAR) registry. J Thromb Thrombolysis. https://doi.org/10.1007/s11239-024-02996-x

Schüpke S, Neumann F-J, Menichelli M, Mayer K, Bernlochner I, Wöhrle J, Richardt G, Liebetrau C, Witzenbichler B, Antoniucci D, Akin I, Bott-Flügel L, Fischer M, Landmesser U, Katus HA, Sibbing D, Seyfarth M, Janisch M, Boncompagni D, Hilz R, Rottbauer W, Okrojek R, Möllmann H, Hochholzer W, Migliorini A, Cassese S, Mollo P, Xhepa E, Kufner S, Strehle A, Leggewie S, Allali A, Ndrepepa G, Schühlen H, Angiolillo DJ, Hamm CW, Hapfelmeier A, Tölg R, Trenk D, Schunkert H, Laugwitz K-L, Kastrati A (2019) Ticagrelor or prasugrel in patients with acute coronary syndromes. N Engl J Med 381:1524–1534. https://doi.org/10.1056/nejmoa1908973

Siller-Matula JM, Petre A, Delle-Karth G, Huber K, Ay C, Lordkipanidzé M, De Caterina R, Kolh P, Mahla E, Gersh BJ (2017) Impact of preoperative use of P2Y12 receptor inhibitors on clinical outcomes in cardiac and non-cardiac surgery: a systematic review and meta-analysis. Eur Heart J Acute Cardiovasc Care 6:753–770

Thiele H, Zeymer U, Neumann F-J, Ferenc M, Olbrich H-G, Hausleiter J, Richardt G, Hennersdorf M, Empen K, Fuernau G, Desch S, Eitel I, Hambrecht R, Fuhrmann J, Böhm M, Ebelt H, Schneider S, Schuler G, Werdan K (2012) Intraaortic balloon support for myocardial infarction with cardiogenic shock. N Engl J Med 367:1287–1296. https://doi.org/10.1056/nejmoa1208410

Thiele H, Zeymer U, Neumann FJ, Ferenc M, Olbrich HG, Hausleiter J, De Waha A, Richardt G, Hennersdorf M, Empen K, Fuernau G, Desch S, Eitel I, Hambrecht R, Lauer B, Böhm M, Ebelt H, Schneider S, Werdan K, Schuler G (2013) Intra-aortic balloon counterpulsation in acute myocardial infarction complicated by cardiogenic shock (IABP-SHOCK II): Fi nal 12 month results of a randomised, open-label trial. Lancet 382:1638–1645. https://doi.org/10.1016/S0140-6736(13)61783-3

Thielmann M, Wendt D, Slottosch I, Welp H, Schiller W, Tsagakis K, Schmack B, Weymann A, Martens S, Neuhäuser M, Wahlers T, Choi YH, Ruhparwar A, Liakopoulos OJ (2021) Coronary artery bypass graft surgery in patients with acute coronary syndromes after primary percutaneous coronary intervention: a current report from the north-rhine westphalia surgical myocardial infarction registry. J Am Heart Assoc 10. https://doi.org/10.1161/JAHA.121.021182

Thrane PG, Olesen KKW, Thim T, Gyldenkerne C, Mortensen MB, Kristensen SD, Maeng M (2023) Mortality trends after primary percutaneous coronary intervention for ST-segment elevation myocardial infarction. J Am Coll Cardiol 82:999–1010. https://doi.org/10.1016/j.jacc.2023.06.025

Tomura N, Honda S, Takegami M, Nishihira K, Kojima S, Takayama M, Yasuda S (2024) Characteristics and in-hospital outcomes of patients who underwent coronary artery bypass grafting during hospitalization for ST-segment elevation or non-ST-segment elevation myocardial infarction. Ann Thorac Cardiovasc Surg 30. https://doi.org/10.5761/atcs.oa.23-00016

Vinten-Johansen J, Thourani VH (2000) Myocardial protection: an overview. Journal of Extra-Corporeal Technology. American Society of Extra-Corporeal Technology, In, pp 38–48

Voisine P, Mathieu P, Doyle D, Perron J, Baillot R, Raymond G, Métras J, Dagenais F (2006) Influence of time elapsed between myocardial infarction and coronary artery bypass grafting surgery on operative mortality. Eur J Cardiothorac Surg:319–323

Weigel F, Nudy M, Krakowski G, Ahmed M, Foy A (2022) Meta-analysis of nonrandomized studies to assess the optimal timing of coronary artery bypass grafting after acute myocardial infarction. Am J Cardiol 164:44–51. https://doi.org/10.1016/j.amjcard.2021.10.033

Weiss ES, Chang DD, Joyce DL, Nwakanma LU, Yuh DD (2008) Optimal timing of coronary artery bypass after acute myocardial infarction: a review of California discharge data. J Thorac Cardiovasc Surg 135:503–511.e3. https://doi.org/10.1016/j.jtcvs.2007.10.042

Whittaker A, Aboughdir M, Mahbub S, Ahmed A, Harky A (2021) Myocardial protection in cardiac surgery: how limited are the options? A comprehensive literature review. Perfusion (United Kingdom) 36:338–351

Management of Complications During Percutaneous Coronary Interventions

Randal J. B. Low, Gianluca Lucchese, and Antonis N. Pavlidis

Abstract Percutaneous coronary intervention (PCI) has revolutionised the management of coronary artery disease. Advances in equipment and technique have led to a steady increase in both the volume and complexity of PCIs performed. Fortunately, complications remain rare, and most can be managed effectively through percutaneous means. However, in the subset of patients where percutaneous strategies are unsuccessful, emergency cardiac surgery remains the final bailout option. The unpredictable nature of PCI complications and the lack of standardised management algorithms underscores the need for cardiothoracic surgeons to be familiar with both the technical aspects of PCI-related events and their percutaneous treatment options. This chapter provides a comprehensive overview of major PCI complications that may necessitate emergency cardiac surgery, including coronary perforation, coronary dissection, iatrogenic aortic dissection, and equipment entrapment and loss. For each, we review the epidemiology, pathophysiology, classification, clinical sequelae, prognosis, and available percutaneous management strategies. Emphasis is placed on considerations relevant to surgical planning and intervention. A thorough understanding of these rare but potentially life-threatening complications is essential for interventional cardiologists, cardiothoracic surgeons, and the entire heart team to ensure optimal patient outcomes during the acute phase of care.

Keywords Percutaneous coronary intervention (PCI) · PCI complications · Coronary perforation · Coronary dissection · Iatrogenic aortic dissection · Pericardial effusion · Tamponade · PCI equipment entrapment · PCI without surgery on-site (no SOS)

R. J. B. Low (✉)
St Thomas' Hospital, London, UK

Woodlands Health, Singapore, Singapore

G. Lucchese · A. N. Pavlidis
St Thomas' Hospital, London, UK
e-mail: gianluca.lucchese@gstt.nhs.uk; antonis.pavlidis@gstt.nhs.uk

A. Kourliouros (ed.), *Emergency Cardiac Surgery*,
https://doi.org/10.1007/978-3-032-15787-4_7

1 Introduction

Percutaneous coronary intervention (PCI) is currently performed for various clinical indications, with the strongest evidence for the management of acute coronary syndromes (ACS) and relief of refractory angina.

PCI complications are thankfully rare, and most can be effectively managed percutaneously. However, when these measures fail, emergency cardiac surgery remains the final bailout option. Due to their low incidence, data guiding optimal management strategies are limited. Moreover, complications vary widely in presentation depending on the nature of the procedure, necessitating a highly individualised approach to management. Such individualisation requires a thorough understanding of the tools and techniques commonly employed during PCI. Accordingly, this chapter is written from the perspective of an interventional cardiologist and aims to provide a technical appraisal of common PCI complications, including percutaneous salvage manoeuvres that would have been typically attempted before referral to the cardiothoracic surgeon.

In the following sections, we address specific PCI complications, namely:

1. Coronary perforation
2. Coronary dissection
3. Iatrogenic aortic dissection
4. Equipment entrapment and loss

Finally, we also dedicate a section to discuss the evidence and recommendations for PCI in centres without on-site surgical support.

2 The Incidence and Impact of Percutaneous Coronary Intervention Complications Requiring Emergency Cardiac Surgery

In the United Kingdom (UK), approximately 100,000 PCIs are performed annually across 119 centres, with a gradual increase both in the volume of PCI cases and the number of PCI centres over the years. Additionally, advances in equipment, technique, and experience have empowered operators to tackle cases with higher complexity. Currently, unprotected left main (LM) intervention represents 4.5% of all PCIs, while chronic total occlusion (CTO) PCI accounts for 11.0% of elective cases (British Cardiovascular Intervention Society (BCIS) 2022).

Despite increasing procedural complexity, the incidence of PCI-related adverse events has fortunately remained low. An analysis of the *British Cardiovascular Intervention Society (BCIS)* database of PCIs performed between 2007 and 2014 reported an emergency cardiac surgery rate of just 0.07%, with a

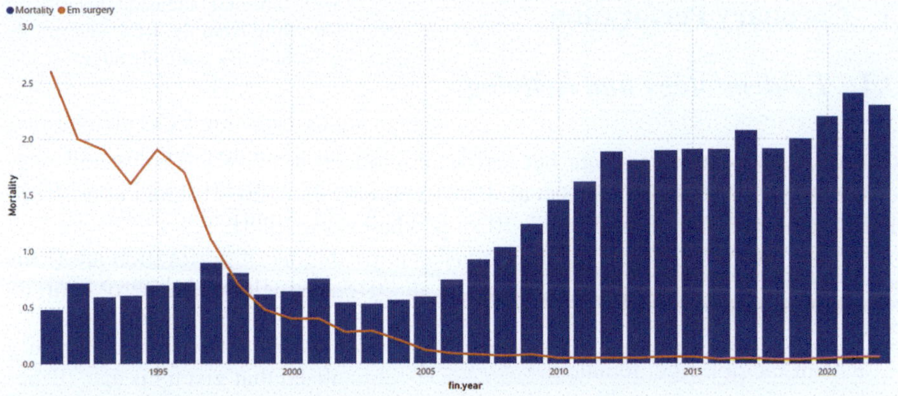

Fig. 1 Trends in PCI-related mortality and need for emergency cardiac surgery in the UK in recent years. (Reproduced with permission from the *BCIS National Audit for Adult Interventional Procedures* for 2022–23 activity (British Cardiovascular Intervention Society (BCIS) 2022))

modest decline from 0.09% in 2007 to 0.06% in 2014. Unsurprisingly, such patients had increased odds of 30-day mortality, in-hospital major adverse cardiac and cerebrovascular events (MACCE), and longer average hospital stays. The most common complications requiring surgical intervention were, in decreasing order, aortic dissection, coronary dissection, coronary perforation, and cardiac tamponade (Kwok et al. 2020). Encouragingly, a more recent analysis from the same database revealed that the need for emergency cardiac surgery has not increased over the last decade (Fig. 1) (British Cardiovascular Intervention Society (BCIS) 2022).

Many PCI complications can be managed conservatively or percutaneously, thus only patients with the most severe complications are referred for urgent cardiac surgery. It should also be noted that the lack of an opportunity for pre-operative evaluation and optimisation constitutes a considerable anaesthetic risk on top of the inherent surgical risks. Predictably, outcomes following emergency surgical intervention are poor, with perioperative mortality reported as high as 20.8%. Long-term prognosis is also guarded, with 5-year and 10-year survival rates of 63.9% and 49.6%, respectively. The strongest predictors of long-term mortality include a critical perioperative state and coronary artery occlusion during PCI, suggesting that mortality is largely driven by cardiogenic shock and end-organ hypoperfusion. Notably, when patients who die within the first 30 days are excluded, long-term survival among hospital survivors improves significantly (Verevkin et al. 2018). Therefore, despite poor peri-operative outcomes, the substantial resource investment in urgent cardiac surgery is justified, as patients who can be supported through the acute phase still have a favourable prognosis.

3 Coronary Perforation

3.1 Epidemiology and Aetiology

Coronary perforation is a rare but serious complication of PCI. The overall incidence is low at 0.3–0.5% (Ellis et al. 1994; Shimony et al. 2011; Bauer et al. 2015; Kinnaird et al. 2016; Nairooz et al. 2020; Mikhail et al. 2022).

Across multiple studies, the most consistent predictors of perforation are (Ellis et al. 1994; Shimony et al. 2011; Bauer et al. 2015; Kinnaird et al. 2016; Nairooz et al. 2020; Mikhail et al. 2022):

- Patient factors: Age, female
- Lesion factors: Complex lesions (American College of Cardiology type C lesions, LM PCI, saphenous venous graft (SVG) PCI), prior coronary artery bypass graft (CABG) surgery, CTO PCI
- Procedural factors: Use of atheroablative devices (e.g. rotational atherectomy)

3.2 Classification

Coronary perforations are classified in two ways: according to location and severity. These have important implications on treatment strategy.

3.2.1 Classification by Location

Coronary perforations occur in three main locations:

1. Proximal or large vessel
2. Distal or branch vessel
3. Collaterals vessel (septal or epicardial)

Large vessel perforations are most commonly caused by balloon or stent oversizing, particularly when inflated at high pressures. However, they may also occur with appropriately sized balloons in vessels with reduced compliance, particularly in those with heavy calcification. Distal vessel perforations are almost always the result of inadvertent guidewire tip migration, especially with use of aggressive wires with high tip load or hydrophilic coatings. Collateral vessel perforations, typically encountered during retrograde crossing techniques, present a unique challenge in CTO PCI.

3.2.2 Classification by Severity

A classification of coronary perforations based on angiographic severity was proposed by Ellis et al. in 1994 (Table 1) (Ellis et al. 1994). This system remains widely used today due to its ease of use and validated ability to predict patient morbidity

Table 1 The Ellis classification of coronary perforation by severity (Ellis et al. 1994)

Type I	Extraluminal crater without extravasation
Type II	Pericardial or myocardial blush without contrast jet extravasation
Type III	Extravasation though frank (≥1 mm) perforation
Type III - Cavity spilling (CS)	Perforation into an anatomic cavity chamber, coronary sinus, etc.

and mortality. Types I through III represent a progressive increase in angiographic severity, corresponding with exponential rises in clinical complications. Type III-cavity spilling (CS) perforations refer to a small subset in which the perforation leaks into another anatomic chamber, most commonly the ventricles or coronary sinus. Paradoxically, these patients exhibit symptoms of a new shunt but rarely develop pericardial effusion, and the condition is generally well tolerated.

3.3 *Clinical Sequelae*

When coronary perforation occurs, blood typically extravasates into the pericardial space. The risk of developing cardiac tamponade is related to the rate of fluid accumulation and compliance of the pericardium. Unlike chronic effusions, where the pericardium has been given ample time to accommodate the slow increase in pericardial volume, acute effusions are poorly tolerated. A large, rapidly accumulating pericardial effusion increases intrapericardial pressures and compromises diastolic filling, particularly of the right heart chambers which normally function within a low-pressure system. Once this exceeds the distending pressures of the right heart, critical cardiac compression ensues, resulting in tamponade. Recognition of this pathophysiology (the “last drop” phenomenon) is important as blood pressure can fall precipitously rather than gradually, catching operators off guard. By the same principle, the initial release of even a small amount of fluid during pericardiocentesis produces significant decompression and rapid haemodynamic improvement.

3.4 *Percutaneous Management*

Sudden chest pain during intervention or unexplained haemodynamic compromise should prompt immediate angiographic assessment to evaluate for coronary perforation. If confirmed, prompt measures must be taken to minimise further coronary extravasation and stabilise haemodynamics. These interventions serve as temporising measures, providing a critical window for determining the most appropriate definitive treatment.

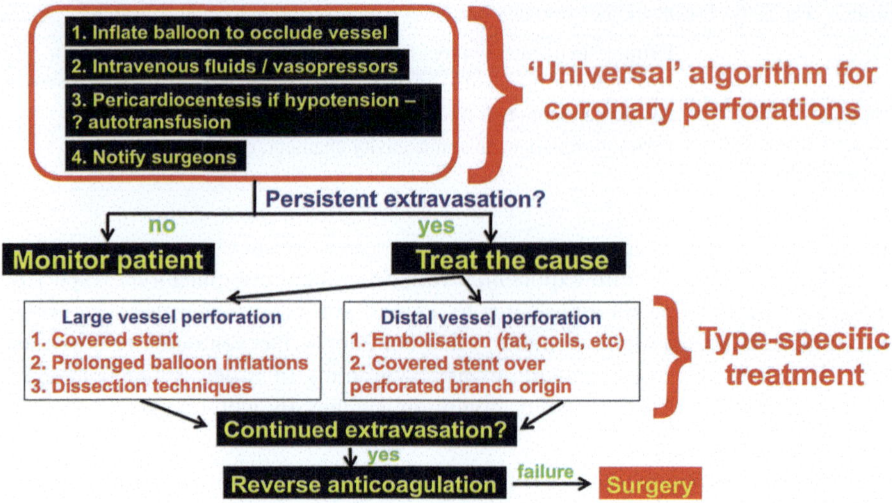

Fig. 2 Coronary perforation management algorithm. (Reproduced from Karacsonyi et al. 2021. Licensed under CC-BY 4.0 at https://creativecommons.org/licenses/by/4.0/. No changes were made to the original image)

Typical management algorithms follow a two-step approach (Fig. 2): first, a series of immediate manoeuvres aimed at stabilising the patient, applicable to all cases of perforation; second, a targeted management strategy based on the location and severity of the perforation (Karacsonyi et al. 2021).

3.4.1 Immediate Management Strategies

Step 1. Immediate balloon occlusion

A balloon, sized to the vessel of interest, is positioned proximal to or at the site of perforation and inflated at low pressures to limit further coronary extravasation. A repeat angiogram should be performed to confirm successful sealing, after which the balloon is left inflated for a prolonged duration (up to 15 min), while proceeding to the subsequent steps in this algorithm.

In cases of small perforations (e.g. Ellis type I), balloon occlusion alone may be sufficient to achieve haemostasis. Prolonging the duration of inflation increases the likelihood of success, but this must be carefully balanced against the risk of myocardial ischaemia from extended vessel occlusion.

Step 2. Management of pericardial effusion and cardiac tamponade

Once coronary extravasation has been temporarily controlled, the next step is to perform an urgent on-table transthoracic echocardiogram (TTE) to assess for the presence and size of any pericardial effusion. Small effusions can be monitored with serial echocardiograms, but there should be a low threshold to perform pericardiocentesis in cases of large or expanding effusions.

Special consideration should be given to patients with a history of CABG, as pre-existing pericardial adhesions can result in loculated effusions that may be difficult or even impossible to drain using standard percutaneous approaches. These patients may require advanced imaging-guided approaches (e.g. CT-guided drainage) or surgical drainage.

Step 3. Haemodynamic optimisation

While the above manoeuvres are being performed, concurrent pharmacotherapy should be initiated to stabilise the patient. This may include aggressive intravenous fluid resuscitation (which augments diastolic filling and can delay the onset of tamponade), inotropic support with vasopressors, and adjunctive agents such as atropine for bradycardia.

Step 4. Reversal of anticoagulation

The decision to reverse anticoagulation involves balancing potential risks and benefits. In patients with freshly implanted stents, there is a theoretical increased risk of acute stent thrombosis. However, in cases of large perforations or incomplete haemostasis, the risk of developing cardiac tamponade often outweighs the thrombotic risk, justifying reversal. Unfractionated heparin is the most commonly used anticoagulant during PCI, and reversal can be achieved with protamine, aiming for an activated clotting time (ACT) of less than 150 s.

Other antithrombotic drugs, such as glycoprotein IIb/IIIa inhibitors, should be discontinued immediately to minimise further bleeding risk.

3.4.2 Specific Management Strategies

The previously described classifications of coronary perforations (by location and severity) play a central role in determining the definitive management strategy.

Main vessel perforations require a decisive and structured management approach, including serial angiographic assessments to monitor for worsening extravasation, and a low threshold for escalation of intervention. Ellis type I perforations are essentially contained and generally do not require active intervention beyond close monitoring. Ellis type II perforations are often managed initially with prolonged balloon inflation, which is frequently sufficient as definitive treatment.

Ellis type III perforations can rapidly lead to cardiac tamponade and circulatory collapse. Placement of a covered stent is the most effective treatment strategy (Briguori et al. 2000). Early generations of covered stents featured a polytetrafluoroethylene (PTFE) membrane layer sandwiched between two stents. While this design effectively created a non-porous barrier, they were often bulky and challenging to deliver, particularly in tortuous or heavily calcified vessels. Significant advancements have since been made, with newer-generation covered stents

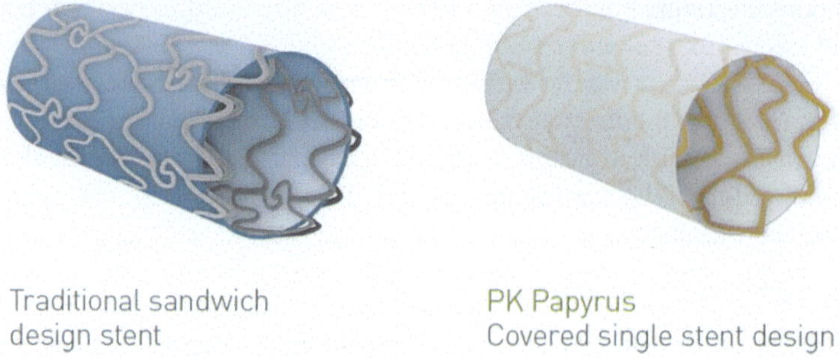

Fig. 3 Comparison of traditional and contemporary covered stent designs. (Reproduced with permission from Biotronik Pte Ltd)

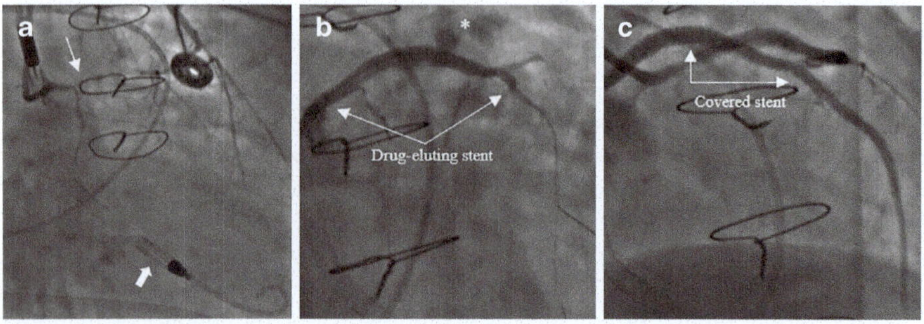

Fig. 4 Case of Ellis type II coronary perforation treated with a covered stent. (**a**) High-risk PCI to ostial left anterior descending (LAD) CTO (thin arrow), supported by an Impella device (thick arrow). (**b**) This was successfully crossed and stented with a drug-eluting stent (DES). Ellis type II perforation occurred after post-dilation (asterisk). (**c**) Successful treatment with a covered stent, with no extravasation at the end of PCI

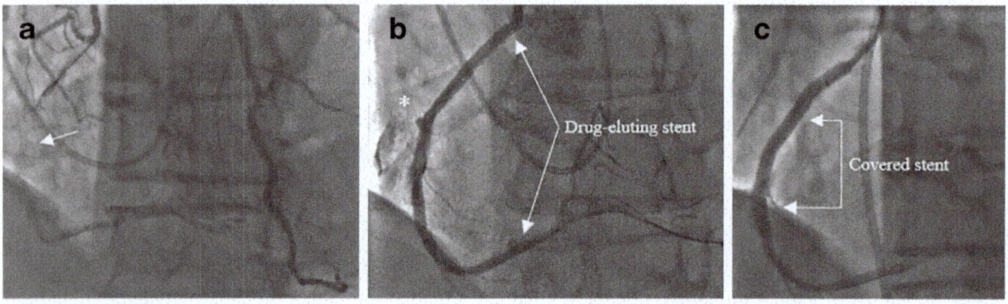

Fig. 5 Case of Ellis type III coronary perforation treated with a covered stent. (**a**) Elective PCI of mid right coronary artery (RCA) CTO (arrow). (**b**) This was successfully crossed with a subintimal technique and stented with a conventional DES. Ellis types III perforation occurred after post-dilation within the subintimal space (asterisk). (**c**) Successful treatment with a covered stent, with no extravasation at the end of PCI

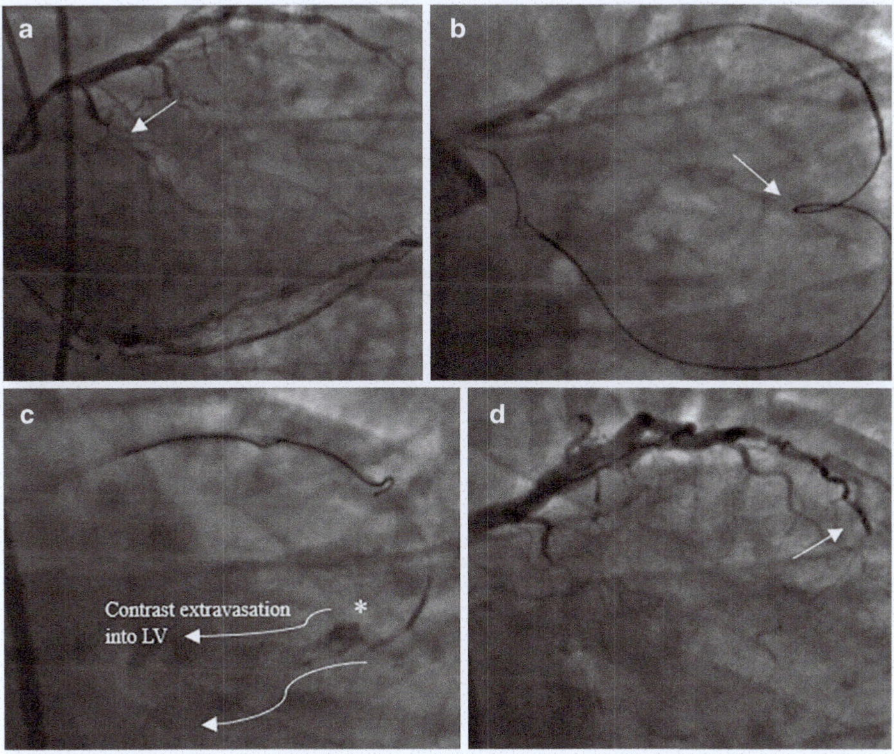

Fig. 6 Case of Ellis type III-CS perforation into the left ventricle, treated with coils. (**a**) Elective PCI to proximal left circumflex (LCx) CTO (arrow). (**b**) This was performed with a retrograde approach via an epicardial collateral from the LAD, with a very tortuous course mid-vessel (arrow). (**c**) Microcatheter-induced injury led to Ellis type III-CS perforation (asterisk) with rapid clearance of contrast outlining the left ventricle (arrows). (**d**) Perforation persisted despite prolonged balloon occlusion, thus this was treated with coils (arrow). The patient was asymptomatic

adopting a single-layer design, thereby improving deliverability and clinical safety (Figs. 3, 4, and 5).

Ellis type III-CS perforations are relatively benign and can often be managed expectantly. In cases of persistent leakage, operators may choose to pursue definitive treatment (Fig. 6).

Distal vessel and side branch perforations typically permit repeated prolonged balloon inflations, as ischaemia is rarely a concern in these territories. If this fails, distal vessels may be embolised using a variety of materials, most commonly coils (Aslam et al. 2000) (Fig. 7).

Other reported materials include clotted autologous blood (Hadjimiltiades et al. 1998), gelfoam (Dixon et al. 2000), harvested subcutaneous fat (George et al. 2015), and thrombin (Fischell et al. 2003). Alternatively, a perforated side branch can be sealed by deploying a covered stent across the main vessel; however, this approach

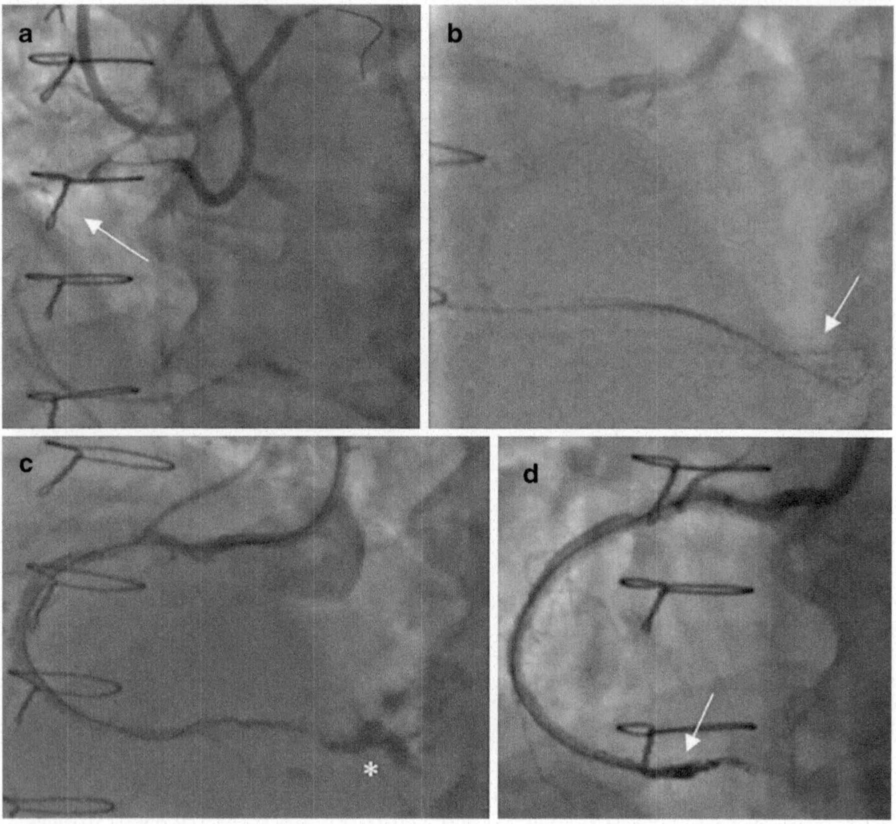

Fig. 7 Case of distal wire perforation treated with coils. (**a**) Elective PCI to mid RCA CTO (arrow). (**b**) A guidewire was advanced in a knuckle to the distal vessel, as part of an antegrade subintimal dissection technique. (**c**) This led to distal vessel perforation (asterisk). While most guidewire tip perforations are small and self-limiting, in this case the wire knuckle caused a large perforation and a more definitive treatment was indicated. (**d**) This was successfully treated with coils, with no extravasation at the end of PCI (arrow)

results in obligatory ischaemia in the territory supplied by the entire occluded side branch.

Collateral vessel perforations typically occur during retrograde CTO PCI and are caused by trauma from equipment such as guidewires and microcatheters. Epicardial collateral perforations can rapidly lead to cardiac tamponade and require prompt recognition, as successful sealing necessitates occlusion of both the antegrade and retrograde blood supplies (Boukhris et al. 2015).

In contrast, septal collateral perforations are generally well tolerated because blood extravasates into the interventricular septum rather than the pericardial space, resulting in a lower risk of tamponade. Consequently, septal collaterals are preferred over epicardial collaterals for retrograde access. Most septal perforations are clinically benign and managed conservatively. However, rare cases of septal haematoma

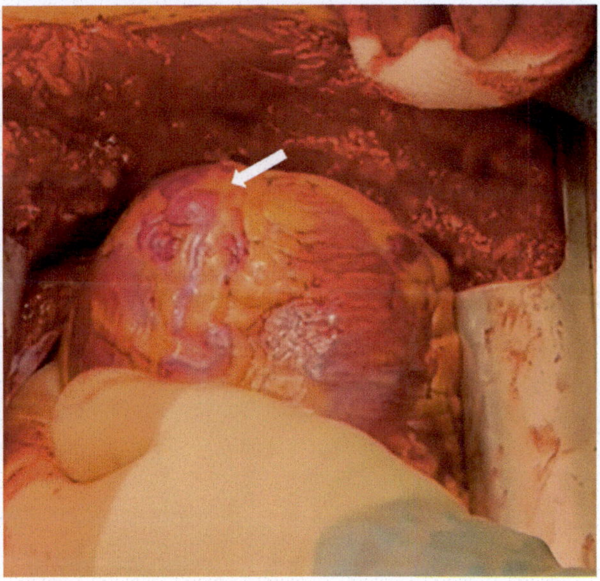

Fig. 8 Case of Ellis type III perforation of the distal LAD requiring surgical intervention. This was repaired off-pump with a sutureless patch-and-glue technique (arrow)

and infarction have been reported, and occlusion should be considered if extravasation persists (Lin et al. 2006).

While most coronary perforations can be managed percutaneously, urgent cardiac surgery is still required in 3–17% of cases when percutaneous strategies fail (Figs. 8 and 9) (Kinnaird et al. 2016; Mikhail et al. 2022; Ang and Tan 2013).

3.5 *Prognosis*

Coronary perforation is strongly associated with an increased risk in adverse outcomes, including in-hospital major adverse cardiovascular events (MACE), 30-day and 1-year mortality, cardiac tamponade, in-hospital bleeding, and longer length of hospital stay. Overall mortality has been shown to increase five-fold (Bauer et al. 2015; Kinnaird et al. 2016).

The rate of adverse events increases with perforation severity in a non-linear fashion. The incidence of myocardial infarction, cardiac tamponade, and death for Ellis type I perforations was reported as 0%, 8%, and 0%, respectively; this rose to 14%, 13%, and 0% for type II, and 50%, 63%, and 19% for type III perforations (Ellis et al. 1994). Type III perforations, in particular, are associated with significantly higher rates of long-term MACE (Al-Lamee et al. 2011), with effects persisting well beyond hospital discharge. However, this may reflect the more vulnerable patient profile rather than being a direct consequence of the perforation itself.

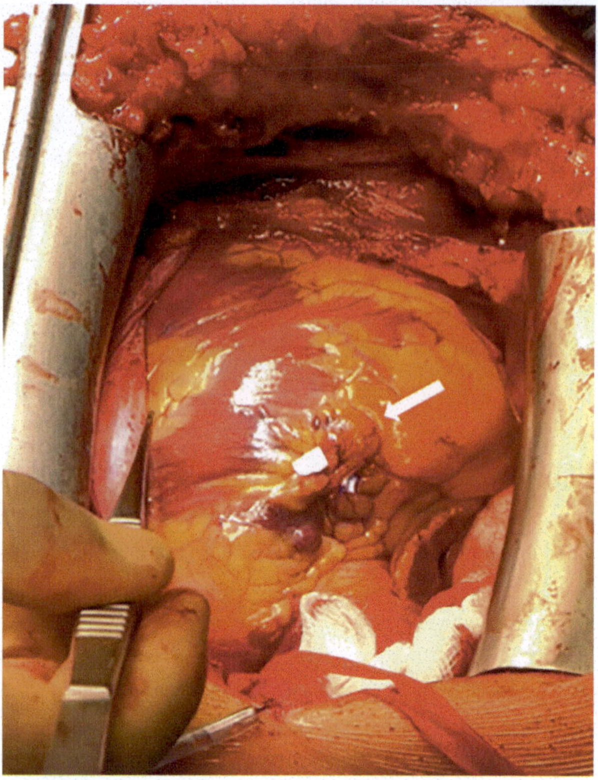

Fig. 9 Case of Ellis type III perforation of the RCA requiring surgical intervention. This was repaired off-pump by approximating the epicardial fat with pledgeted stitches onto the perforation, sealing the leak without occluding the vessel (arrow)

3.6 Summary

Coronary perforation is a rare but serious complication of PCI. Although overall incidence is low, it carries a high risk of both in-hospital and long-term morbidity and mortality. Acute deterioration is typically due to cardiac tamponade and myocardial infarction. A well-structured management algorithm is crucial for prompt vessel occlusion and definitive sealing of the perforation.

4 Coronary Dissection

4.1 Epidemiology and Aetiology

Coronary dissection is the most common major complication of PCI, with a reported incidence of ~30% in the early balloon angioplasty era. With marked improvements in PCI technique, equipment, and pharmacotherapy, this has substantially reduced to ~1.4% in the contemporary era (Huber et al. 1991; Page et al. 2023).

The true incidence of coronary dissection is likely grossly underestimated. In a post-mortem study by Hoshino et al., angiographic dissection was identified in 47%

of cases, but histological analysis revealed intimal disruption in 100% and medial involvement in 65%. Only when dissections extended to more than one-fourth of the vessel circumference were they angiographically evident (Hoshino et al. 1987). These findings suggest that coronary dissection is virtually ubiquitous during PCI and may represent an obligatory consequence of balloon angioplasty, rather than a true "complication".

Iatrogenic coronary dissection results from several mechanisms during PCI. In a large contemporary series, the most common causes identified were guidewire advancement (30%), stenting (22%), balloon angioplasty (20%), and guide catheter engagement (18%) (Page et al. 2023).

Guidewire-induced dissection occurs with inadvertent wiring into the subintimal space, particularly when aggressive guidewires (e.g. polymer-jacketed wires with high tip load) are used to cross challenging lesions. These dissections tend to be localised and easily managed if recognised early. In some cases, notably in CTO interventions, subintimal wiring may even be intentional.

Dissections post-stenting typically occur at the proximal or distal stent edges, at the transition between the rigid stent platform and the immediate adjacent native vessel wall. Contributing factors include high pressure stent deployment, or stent edges landing in diseased segments with significant plaque burden ("unhealthy landing zones").

Balloon angioplasty as part of the pre-dilation process frequently leads to dissections, particularly if specific devices (e.g. scoring or cutting balloons, atherectomy devices) are used. This is generally benign as long as coronary flow remains uncompromised, and may even be desirable as part of optimal plaque modification prior to stenting. However, on rare occasions, high-pressure inflation can cause balloon rupture, leading to extensive flow-limiting dissections or even coronary perforation.

Guide catheter-induced dissections, while least common, deserve special attention. These often result from mechanical trauma at the coronary ostium due to catheter tip manipulation or "deep-seating", frequently compounded by forceful contrast injections exerting high hydraulic pressure to a focal point within the vessel. The incidence has been reported to be ~0.09–1.1% (Hiraide et al. 2018; Ramasamy et al. 2020). The right coronary artery (RCA) is more frequently affected than the LM, likely due to its smaller calibre and greater anatomical variability, including anomalous origins. Guide catheters are more likely to induce injury compared to diagnostic catheters, primarily due to their stiffer tips and more aggressive manipulation to achieve co-axial alignment and support at the aortic cusp. Notably, catheter-induced dissections tend to be extensive, with up to two-thirds being high-grade and flow-limiting (Ramasamy et al. 2020).

4.2 *Classification*

Coronary dissection is diagnosed by the presence of multiple radiolucent lumens on angiography. The *National Heart, Lung and Blood Institute (NHLBI)* classification, which categorises dissections according to angiographic morphology and flow, is widely adopted due to its ease of use (Fig. 10) (Geeslin et al. 2025).

TYPE A	Radiolucent area within the coronary lumen.	
TYPE B	Parallel tracts or double lumen separated by radiolucent area.	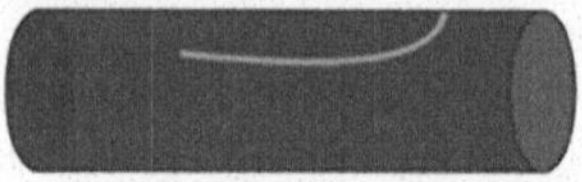
TYPE C	Contrast outside the coronary lumen.	
TYPE D	Spiral luminal filling defect.	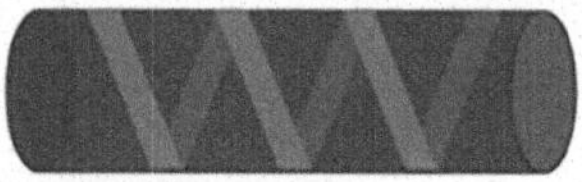
TYPE E	Persistent filling defect.	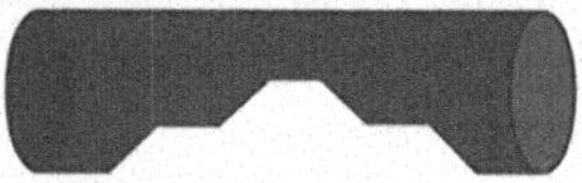
TYPE F	Total occlusion without antegrade flow.	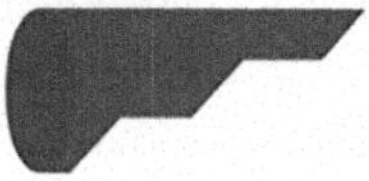

Fig. 10 The *National Heart, Lung and Blood Institute (NHLBI)* classification for coronary dissections. (Reproduced from Geeslin et al. 2025. Licensed under CC-BY 4.0 at https://creativecommons.org/licenses/by/4.0/. No changes were made to the original image)

4.3 Clinical Sequelae

The immediate clinical impact of coronary dissection is driven by myocardial ischaemia, the severity of which depends on two key factors: the degree of coronary flow impairment and the location of the dissection. Flow may be preserved, partially reduced, or completely obstructed. Proximal dissections compromise a larger myocardial territory and can rapidly precipitate malignant arrhythmias or cardiogenic shock. This risk is further amplified in patients with poor coronary reserve, such as those with multi-vessel disease or when the dissection involves a donor vessel in CTO PCI.

Huber et al. demonstrated a strong correlation between the NHLBI dissection classification and clinical outcomes. Type A and B dissections showed comparable rates of procedural success, morbidity, and mortality to cases without dissection, suggesting they are generally benign. In contrast, types C to F were associated with significantly worse outcomes, including abrupt vessel closure (31%), emergency

CABG (37%), MI (13%), and the need for repeat PCI (24%). Overall clinical success in this group was markedly lower, at just 38% (Huber et al. 1991).

Even after technically successful PCI, coronary dissection carries an increased risk of late vessel closure. Though less concerning in the era of drug-eluting stents (DES), this risk remains relevant when the dissection extends beyond the treated segment. While initial data suggested that dissections did not increase the risk of long-term restenosis (Matthews et al. 1988), subsequent studies demonstrated a significant association between coronary dissection and MACE. Even in the absence of abrupt vessel closure at the time of PCI, delayed ischemic complications (ischemic chest pain, MI, need for CABG, death) occurred in 9% of patients during prospective follow-up. Post-hoc geometric and videodensitometric analysis identified several key predictors of adverse outcomes, in decreasing order of significance: dissection length, post-PCI residual stenosis, post-PCI vessel area, and the presence of extra-luminal contrast (Black et al. 1989). These findings underscore that, while many dissections are benign, a distinct subset of patients remains at elevated risk of late ischemic events.

Of greater relevance to contemporary practice is the occurrence of stent edge dissections. Many of these are not apparent on angiography and are best detected using intravascular imaging, with optical coherence tomography (OCT) being the modality of choice due to its superior resolution. Management may be conservative or involve deployment of an overlapping stent to seal the dissection. OCT-defined "major" dissections (≥60° of the vessel circumference and/or extending ≥3 mm in length) warrant stenting (Ali et al. 2023).

4.4 Percutaneous Management

Many iatrogenic coronary dissections are potentially preventable with meticulous PCI technique. Catheter selection should take into account the size and anatomical characteristics of the target vessel to ensure appropriate shape, alignment, and support. Co-axial alignment of the catheter tip with the coronary ostium is essential, and pressure waveforms should be closely monitored for signs of damping prior to contrast injection. Lesion wiring should begin with workhorse wires, escalating only when necessary. Balloon angioplasty must be performed using appropriately sized balloons, with high-pressure inflations reserved only for un-dilatable lesions.

Once coronary dissection occurs, the immediate priority is to maintain coronary flow. Localised, non–flow-limiting dissections (NHLBI types A and B) are typically benign and may be managed conservatively. In contrast, more extensive dissections with extra-luminal contrast staining, particularly those that are flow-limiting (types C–F), generally require stenting. A typical management algorithm is outlined below (Fig. 11) (Doll et al. 2020).

If there is current guidewire access to the distal true lumen, percutaneous management is generally straightforward. Balloon inflation at the dissection site usually restores flow by "tagging up" the dissection flap and compressing any associated

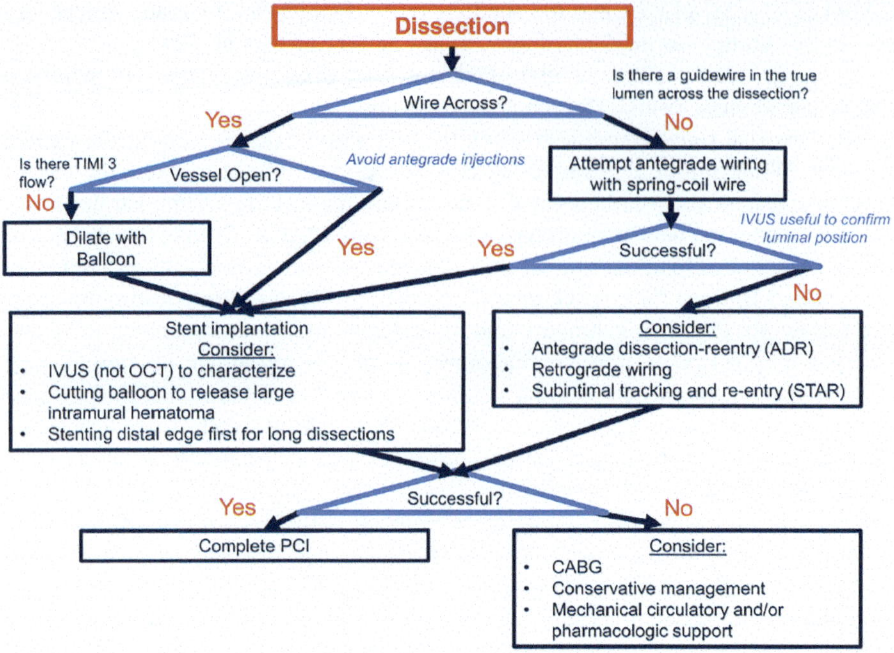

Fig. 11 Coronary dissection management algorithm. (Reproduced with permission from Doll et al. 2020)

intramural haematoma. In some cases, prolonged balloon inflation alone may suffice. Repeated antegrade contrast injections should be avoided, as they risk extending the dissection plane. Intravascular imaging, particularly intravascular ultrasound (IVUS) when available, is invaluable for delineating the entry point and length of the dissection. Because stenting can potentially compress any intramural haematoma and propagate the dissection, it is recommended to deploy a sufficiently long stent, ensuring generous coverage both proximal and distal to the dissected segment (Fig. 12).

If there is no access to the distal true lumen, percutaneous management becomes challenging. The critical step is to successfully navigate a guidewire across the dissected segment into the distal true lumen. This is particularly difficult in catheter-induced ostial dissections, where the dissection flap tends to deflect the guidewire tip, and the catheter often biases towards the dissection entry point. In such cases, using a spring-coil wire with a low tip load is recommended. Additionally, changing to a guiding catheter with a different shape may help re-orientate the catheter tip and guidewire away from the false lumen. If the guidewire reaches the distal vessel but there is uncertainty regarding its true luminal position, IVUS is once again invaluable for confirmation. Thereafter, stenting proceeds as usual. If wiring the true lumen remains impossible, specialised dissection and re-entry techniques, commonly used in CTO PCI, can be

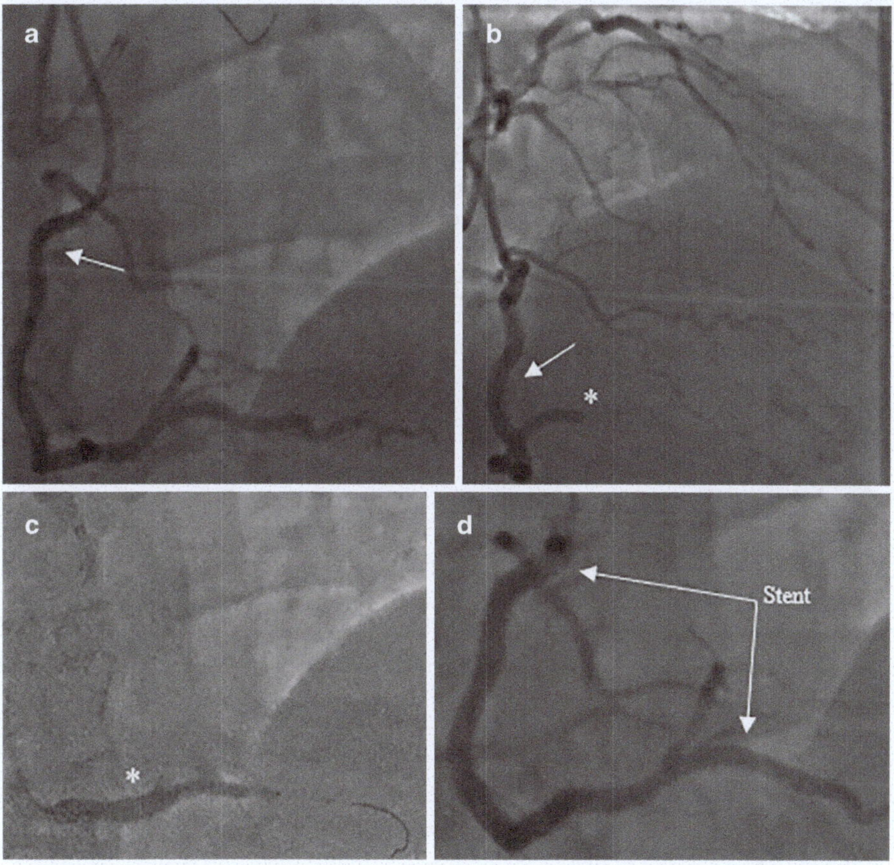

Fig. 12 Case of catheter-induced coronary dissection treated with stenting. (**a**) Elective PCI to LAD CTO. An Amplatz-left (AL) guiding catheter was used to engage the RCA for retrograde angiogram. The catheter tip was "deep-seated" into the proximal vessel but was deemed to be co-axial (arrow at catheter tip). (**b**) Subsequent angiograms led to catheter-induced dissection at the proximal RCA, appreciated as a radiolucent "double lumen" (arrow), with lengthy antegrade extension into the distal RCA (asterisk). A guidewire was immediately advanced past the dissected segment into distal true lumen. (**c**) Persistent contrast staining at the distal RCA despite no further antegrade contrast injections (asterisk). (**d**) This was successfully treated with a long segment of stents from ostial to distal vessel (arrows)

employed to re-enter the true lumen from a subintimal position. However, these techniques require significant expertise and time, and are rarely practical in urgent settings.

If percutaneous strategies fail and there is ongoing evidence of ischaemia, arrhythmia, or cardiogenic shock, emergency CABG may be necessary. This is rare in contemporary practice, with available data showing that 70–80% of dissections are successfully treated with stenting, and only 2–6% require emergency CABG (Page et al. 2023; Ramasamy et al. 2020; Tarbiat and Safarpoor 2015).

4.5 *Prognosis*

The invention of stents has dramatically reduced the adverse outcomes of coronary dissections by lowering the rate of vessel closure (Serruys et al. 1994; Fischman et al. 1994). However, patients who sustain coronary dissection remain at increased risk of in-hospital adverse events, regardless of whether coronary flow was impaired post-PCI (Hiraide et al. 2018). Some postulate that this may result from residual ischemic injury sustained during the event, while others propose that insult to the coronary microcirculation also plays a role. Significant in-hospital major adverse cardiovascular events (MACE) occur in up to 23% of patients, with long-term follow-up showing mortality rates as high as 20% and target lesion revascularisation (TLR) in 11.3%.

4.6 *Summary*

Coronary dissection is the most common PCI-related complication. Intimal dissection resulting from balloon angioplasty should be viewed as an expected consequence rather than a true complication. The NHLBI classification is a valuable tool that predicts clinical outcomes and guides management. Localised, non-flow limiting dissections (types A–B) can typically be managed conservatively, whereas extensive or flow-limiting dissections (types C–F) generally require stenting. Stenting is a highly effective treatment that has dramatically improved outcomes compared to the pre-stent era.

Interestingly, the growing success of drug-coated balloons (DCBs) as definitive treatment in PCI has led to increased confidence in the conservative management of coronary dissections. This trend is likely to continue, and routine stenting may no longer be the universal approach in future. Nonetheless, emergency CABG is rarely required for the management of coronary dissection.

5 Iatrogenic Aortic Dissection

5.1 *Epidemiology and Aetiology*

Iatrogenic aortic dissection is a rare but dramatic complication of PCI. The reported incidence is very low at 0.01–0.06% (Dunning et al. 2000; Núñez-Gil et al. 2015; Leontyev et al. 2012). In large registries evaluating patients undergoing surgery for acute type A aortic dissection from both spontaneous and iatrogenic causes, iatrogenic dissections (from any type of surgery) accounted for 2.6–5% of all cases. Of these, 1.3–2.2% were specifically attributed to coronary catheterisation, either from diagnostic angiography or PCI (Hagan et al. 2000; Rylski et al. 2013; Biancari et al. 2022).

Most PCI-related iatrogenic aortic dissections originate as coronary dissections, typically near or at the coronary ostium. While some dissections remain localised or propagate anterogradely into the distal coronary vessel, others can extend unpredictably in a retrograde fashion into the aortic root and, in severe cases, even beyond the aortic arch. The most common cause is catheter-induced trauma (see earlier section on *coronary dissection*), though there are other mechanisms including subintimal guidewire entry or balloon dilation of ostial lesions. Notably, during PCI of ostial CTO lesions, a retrograde subintimal approach may lead guidewires to track within the subintimal plane towards the aorto-ostial junction and ultimately exit into the ascending aorta.

Predictably, risk factors for iatrogenic aortic dissection overlap significantly with those for guide catheter-induced coronary dissection, given their shared pathogenesis. The RCA is most commonly involved, and guide catheters are more frequently implicated than diagnostic catheters, particularly the Amplatz Left (AL) catheter. Among all predictors, the most consistent is emergency PCI for acute MI (Dunning et al. 2000; Núñez-Gil et al. 2015). This likely reflects a combination of contributing factors: procedural urgency leading to operator haste, a higher-risk patient population with prevalent vascular comorbidities, and the presence of acutely ruptured plaques, particularly at or near the coronary ostia. Histological examination of resected aortic specimens further supports this, revealing frequent associations with pre-existing aortic pathology, including extensive atherosclerosis, cystic medial necrosis, penetrating atherosclerotic ulcers, and inflammatory aortitis (Leontyev et al. 2012).

5.2 *Classification*

Traditional classification systems for spontaneous aortic dissection (Stanford classification, DeBakey classification), which are based on involvement of the ascending aorta, are not well suited for iatrogenic aortic dissections since these typically originate at the aortic cusp and extend retrogradely towards the ascending aorta, rather than following patterns characteristic of spontaneous dissections.

To address this, Dunning et al. proposed a dedicated classification system for PCI-related iatrogenic aortic dissections based on the extent of aortic root involvement (Fig. 14) (Dunning et al. 2000). This system has practical value in guiding treatment decisions and has been shown to correlate with clinical outcomes (Table 2).

Table 2 The Dunning classification of iatrogenic aortic dissection

Proposed classification	Extent of aortic involvement in the dissection
Class I	Involving the ipsilateral cusp
Class II	Involving cusp and extending up the aorta less than 40 mm
Class III	Involving cusp and extending up the aorta greater than 40 mm

Reproduced with permission from Dunning et al. 2000

5.3 *Clinical Sequelae*

Aortic dissection, whether spontaneous or iatrogenic, can lead to coronary and systemic hypoperfusion. Coronary involvement results in myocardial infarction, while extension into the systemic circulation may cause stroke, limb ischaemia, or renal failure. However, there are two key distinctions between iatrogenic and spontaneous dissections in terms of their presentation. First, iatrogenic dissections tend to be localised as the inciting trauma is focal, and they less commonly extend to the supra-aortic, abdominal, or iliac vessels. Second, iatrogenic dissections almost invariably originate at the coronary ostia or aortic cusps, whereas spontaneous dissections often begin within the aortic wall itself. Consequently, iatrogenic dissections are more likely to cause coronary malperfusion and less likely to result in systemic complications such as renal or limb ischaemia.

Because of these differences, patients undergoing surgical repair for iatrogenic aortic dissections are often managed with a more limited surgical approach than those with spontaneous dissections. They are less likely to require complex aortic surgery (e.g. supra-coronary ascending aorta replacement, aortic arch surgery, complex aortic root reconstruction), but more frequently require concomitant CABG (Rylski et al. 2013).

5.4 *Percutaneous Management*

Most cases of iatrogenic aortic dissection can be managed conservatively or percutaneously, with only a small proportion requiring urgent cardiac surgery. Conservative management is reasonable for localised dissections in haemodynamically stable patients, provided facilities with close monitoring are available.

However, if there is evidence of compromised coronary flow or significant extension into the ascending aorta with risk of further propagation, percutaneous intervention is warranted. In such cases, stenting the dissection entry point, typically at the coronary ostium, can effectively seal the dissection flap and prevent retrograde extension into the aorta. Operators are cautioned against repeated contrast injections, as these may exacerbate the dissection. Intravascular imaging is immensely helpful in achieving precise stent placement and ensuring complete ostial coverage (Fig. 13).

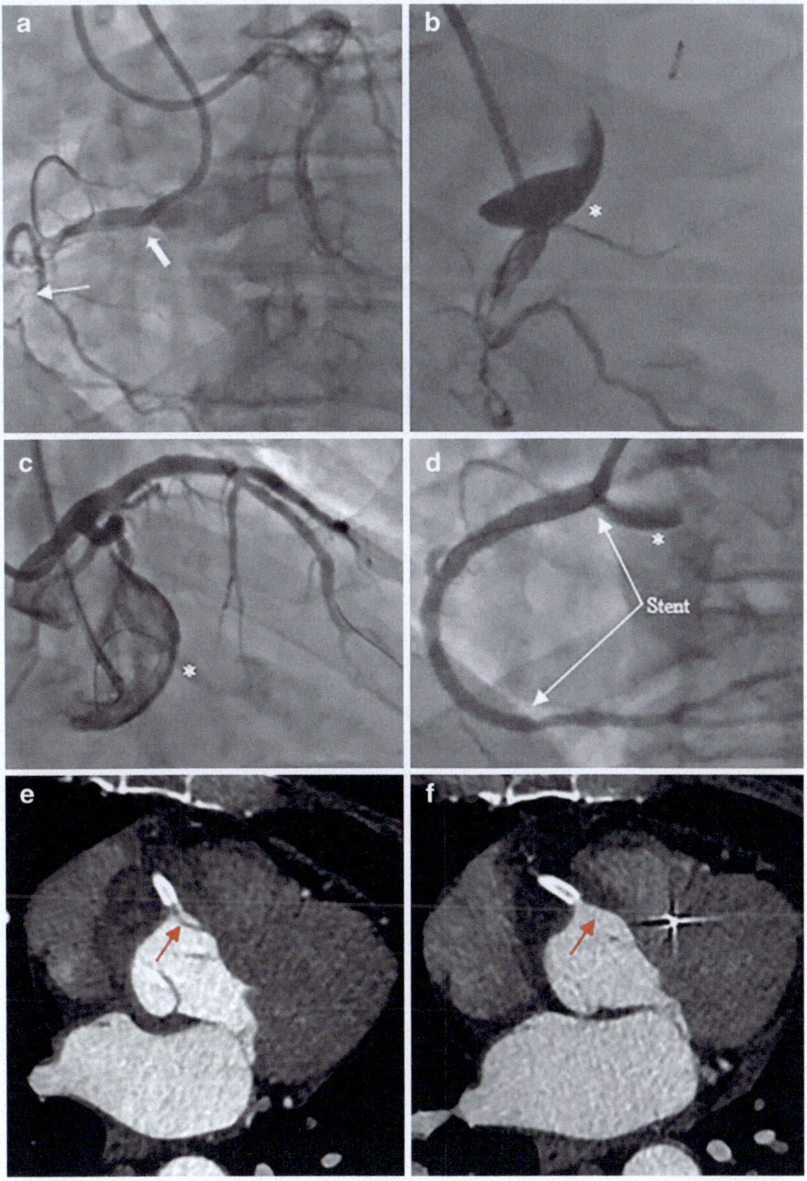

Fig. 13 Case of guider-induced iatrogenic aortic dissection. (**a**) Elective PCI to mid RCA CTO (thin arrow). The RCA ostium was engaged with an AL-1 guider, with its tip pointing inferiorly against the vessel wall (thick arrow). (**b**) Subsequent angiogram resulted in ostial dissection which extended to the right coronary cusp (asterisk). (**c**) No further antegrade injections was done and the rest of the PCI was guided by intracoronary imaging. Persistent contrast staining of the right coronary cusp was evident throughout the procedure (asterisk). (**d**) Successful PCI of the RCA, with a drug-eluting stent (DES) adequately covering the RCA ostium. Final angiogram showed only limited staining of the coronary cusp (asterisk). The procedure was well-tolerated. (**e**) Immediate post-PCI CT aortogram showed the dissection flap involving the right coronary cusp (arrow), with no extension into the ascending aorta. (**f**) A repeat CT aortogram on day 5 post-PCI demonstrated complete resolution, with no residual dissection flap (arrow). The patient was discharged uneventfully

All patients, whether managed conservatively or percutaneously, should be closely monitored in a high-dependency or intensive care setting. Early TTE is essential to assess for pericardial effusion and evaluate aortic valve integrity. A CT aortogram is recommended to establish a baseline should clinical deterioration occur.

A minority of patients may require urgent cardiac surgery. These include cases where stenting cannot be performed (e.g. guidewire access into the distal true lumen is not possible) or when stenting fails to adequately seal the dissection flap. This is particularly warranted if there is ongoing myocardial ischaemia from impaired coronary flow, haemodynamic instability, or acute aortic regurgitation.

Retrospective application of the Dunning classification to published case series suggests that class I and II dissections can be managed conservatively or with PCI, whereas class III dissections often require surgical intervention (Dunning et al. 2000). Registry data on iatrogenic aortic dissection during coronary procedures show that 48.6% of cases were treated conservatively, 47.3% with stenting, and only 4% required cardiac surgery (Núñez-Gil et al. 2015).

5.5 *Prognosis*

Patients with limited dissections generally have favourable outcomes. However, those requiring surgery for PCI-related iatrogenic aortic dissection represent a high-risk cohort, with reported early post-operative mortality rates of up to 50%. Thirty-day mortality has been shown to be comparable to that of spontaneous aortic dissection. Multivariate analyses have identified coronary malperfusion, pre-operative cardiopulmonary resuscitation, and prolonged cardiopulmonary bypass (CPB) time as the strongest predictors of 30-day mortality (Leontyev et al. 2012; Rylski et al. 2013).

On the other hand, among patients who survive the peri-operative period, late adverse events are rare and long-term prognosis is generally favourable (Núñez-Gil et al. 2015; Leontyev et al. 2012; Biancari et al. 2022). This suggests that the elevated risk is largely attributable to the acute iatrogenic insult itself, and that definitive surgical repair effectively corrects the underlying pathology.

5.6 *Summary*

Among all PCI-related complications, iatrogenic aortic dissection is one of the rarest but also among the most severe. It typically results from trauma to the coronary ostium by an aggressive guiding catheter, creating a dissection flap that propagates retrogradely into the ascending aorta. Angiographic assessment of severity is based on the extent of aortic involvement. Most cases with localised dissections can be managed conservatively or with stenting at the coronary ostium to seal the entry point. However, a minority of patients who cannot be treated percutaneously, or who experience clinical deterioration despite stenting, will require urgent surgical intervention. This subset carries a guarded prognosis due to high peri-operative mortality. Nonetheless, patients who survive the initial insult often have a favourable long-term outcome.

6 Equipment Entrapment and Loss

6.1 *Overview*

Equipment entrapment or loss is a particularly challenging complication that may arise during PCI. This includes the entrapment or fracture of guidewires, balloon catheters, microcatheters, stents, and specialised devices such as atherectomy burrs. The overall incidence is estimated to be 0.22–0.55% (Hartzler et al. 1987; Iturbe et al. 2012).

Equipment entrapment can lead to fracture and loss, particularly when forceful attempts are made to free the trapped component. Depending on the size and location of the retained fragment, coronary flow obstruction may result in ischaemia and thrombosis. Conversely, equipment loss poses the risk of distal embolisation into the distal coronary or systemic circulation, with stroke being a major concern if emboli reach cerebral vessels. Generally, equipment retention is more likely to necessitate emergency surgery, whereas device loss can often be managed conservatively or via percutaneous retrieval (Iturbe et al. 2012).

With advancements in PCI technology, operators now have access to an expanding array of specialised tools. However, when addressing device-related complications, the specific procedural context must be carefully considered in formulating a treatment strategy. Consequently, there is no universal "one-size-fits-all" approach. Some proposed algorithms tailored to different scenarios are illustrated below (Fig. 14) (Doll et al. 2020). As with all other complications, emergency cardiac surgery remains the ultimate bailout option if percutaneous interventions are unsuccessful.

6.2 *Stent Entrapment and Loss*

Coronary stents are the most commonly entrapped or embolised devices during PCI, occurring in ~0.3% of cases (Brilakis et al. 2005; Colkesen et al. 2007). Over the past few decades, this incidence has steadily declined, likely due to improvements in stent crimping technology by manufacturers (Alomar et al. 2013).

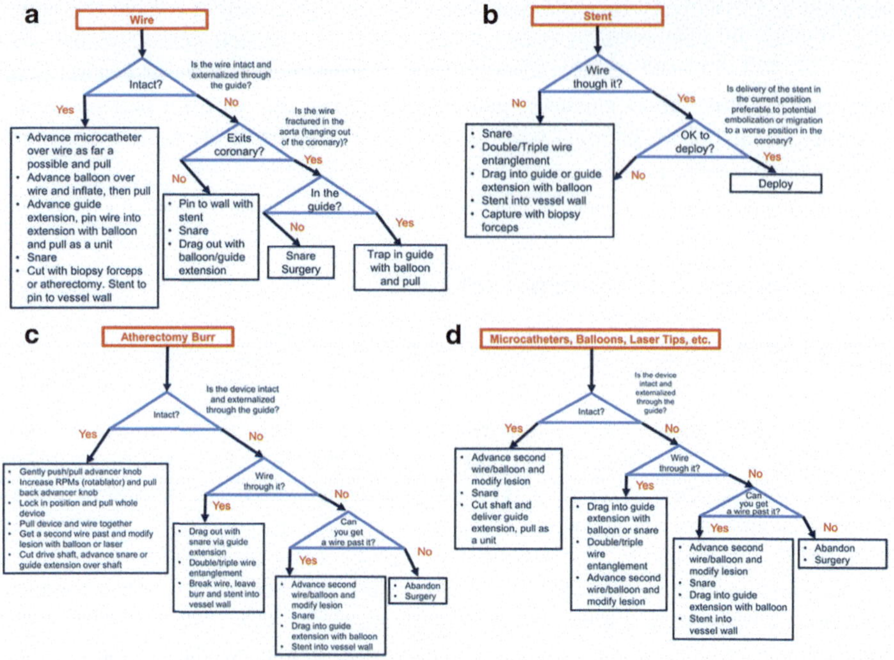

Fig. 14 Management algorithm of various scenarios of equipment entrapment and loss. (Reproduced with permission from Doll et al. 2020)

Stents may become entrapped within lesions, particularly in heavily calcified vessels or when vessel pre-dilation is inadequate. Forceful withdrawal in such cases can cause the stent to dislodge from the balloon to which it is crimped. Significant vessel angulation and severe calcification are key predictors of this complication (Brilakis et al. 2005; Colkesen et al. 2007; Kozman et al. 2001).

The primary consideration in managing an entrapped stent is its location, which determines whether an attempt at retrieval is justified. This decision must be carefully weighed against the risk of uncontrolled stent migration to a less favourable position during the retrieval attempt. Another key factor is the availability of guidewire access through the stent, without which interventional options are significantly more limited (Fig. 14, column B).

If the current location of the stent is unacceptable (e.g. LM artery, cerebral vessel), retrieval is generally warranted. Several techniques can be employed for this purpose. If guidewire access is present, a common initial approach involves advancing a small balloon through the stent, inflating it, and then withdrawing both the balloon and stent together into the guiding catheter as a single unit (Fig. 15). If guidewire access is not available, snaring the stent is the most frequently used strategy, with various commercial snares available for this purpose. Alternatively, multiple guidewires can be advanced alongside the stent and twisted repeatedly in an attempt to entangle and retrieve the stent (the "guidewire twirling" technique).

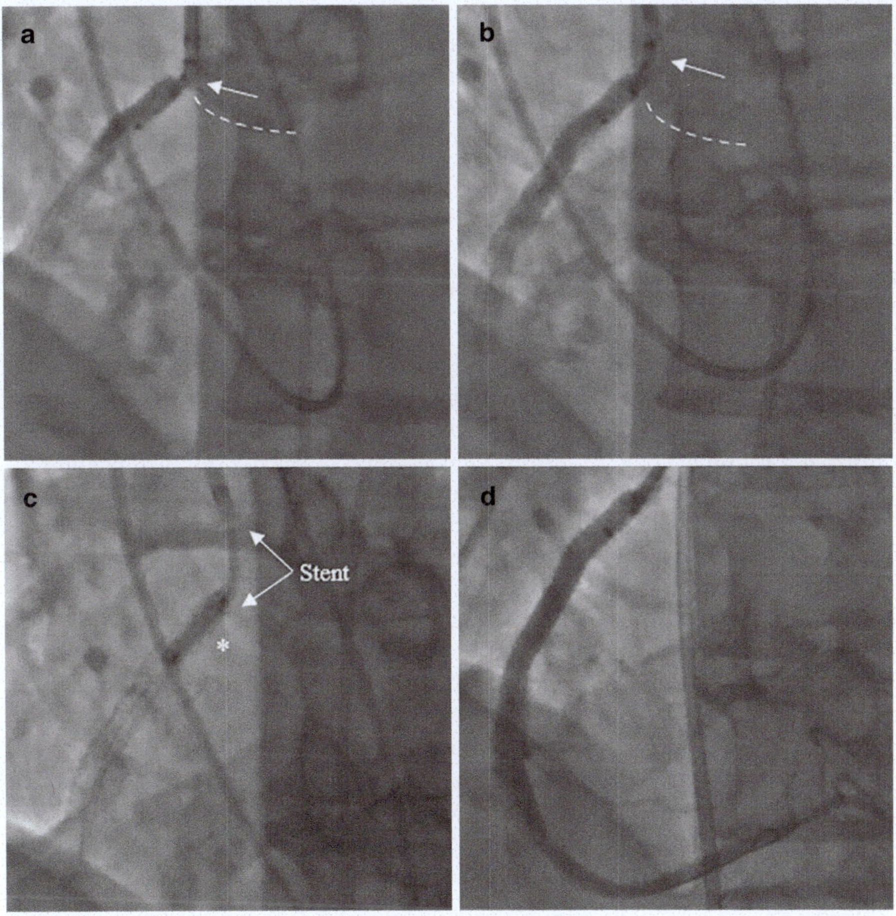

Fig. 15 Case of stent mis-deployment with successful retrieval. (**a**) Positioning a stent at the ostial RCA with the stent proximal marker (arrow) aligned with the aorto-ostial junction (dashed line). (**b**) Stent inadvertently "slipped" proximally during deployment. The stent balloon was immediately deflated upon detection of stent migration, resulting in a partially inflated stent protruding into the aorta. (**c**) A small balloon was advanced distal to the stent and inflated (asterisk), trapping the stent on the guidewire and allowing its withdrawal out of the vessel into the guiding catheter. (**d**) A new stent was successfully deployed at the originally intended position

If the current stent location is acceptable and guidewire access is maintained, the safest approach is to advance a balloon within the stent and deploy it in-situ. If there is no guidewire access, a balloon can be introduced alongside the stent and inflated to "crush" the stent against the vessel wall, typically followed by deployment of another stent to fully cover the crushed material. A meta-analysis on stent loss reported successful retrieval in 66% of cases, deployment in 12%, and crushing in 3% (Alomar et al. 2013).

Stent loss is associated with MACE in 19% of cases, with this increased risk extending beyond the acute hospitalisation period. Stent embolisation within the coronary circulation is linked to poor long-term outcomes, including significantly higher rates of MI, urgent CABG, repeat PCI, and death. In contrast, stent embolisation into the systemic circulation appears to have minimal clinical sequelae (Alomar et al. 2013; Kozman et al. 2001).

6.3 Guidewire Entrapment and Fracture

Interventional cardiologists have access to an extensive range of guidewires, each intended for different tasks. Workhorse wires are designed to be soft and atraumatic, whereas others feature stiff tips with high tip loads to enhance penetrative force—particularly useful in complex lesions such as CTOs or heavily calcified plaques. In these settings, aggressive manipulation can deform the wire, either through interaction with the lesion or intentional knuckling. This loss of wire integrity increases the risk of entrapment, especially if the wire begins to unravel. Entrapment can also occur during bifurcation stenting when a side branch wire is "trapped" after stenting across the main vessel—a widely accepted technique. During retrieval, the wire may rarely catch on stent struts and prevent removal. In all the above scenarios, forceful withdrawal can lead to wire tip fracture, emphasising the need for careful handling.

Entrapped guidewire fragments can serve as a nidus for thrombus formation, raising concerns of late vessel thrombosis and MI. Loss of the wire tip also carries the risk of distal embolisation, potentially affecting distal coronary territories leading to MI, or systemic embolisation resulting in stroke.

Percutaneous management depends on whether the guidewire remains intact (i.e. entrapped but not fractured) (Fig. 14, column A). If the wire is still intact, operators should resist the temptation to apply forceful traction, as this often results in tip fracture—a far more complex scenario. Instead, advancing a microcatheter or a small balloon to the site of entrapment and inflating it is often effective in releasing the wire. If this approach fails, a guide extension catheter can be advanced over the wire as close to the entrapped segment as possible. A balloon is then inflated alongside the wire within the guide extension catheter to "trap" it, facilitating the entire assembly to be withdrawn as a unit. This technique allows traction to be applied more distally, as close to the point of entrapment as possible, and is generally more effective than pulling from outside the body. Even if wire fracture occurs during this manoeuvre, it is more likely to happen distally within the coronary circulation. In contrast, uncontrolled pulling from outside the body may result in mid-wire fracture, leaving a long segment protruding into the aorta—an especially undesirable outcome.

Once a guidewire has fractured, the location of the retained fragment becomes a key determinant in guiding further management. If a substantial length of the wire extends from the coronary artery into the aorta, retrieval is generally advised. This

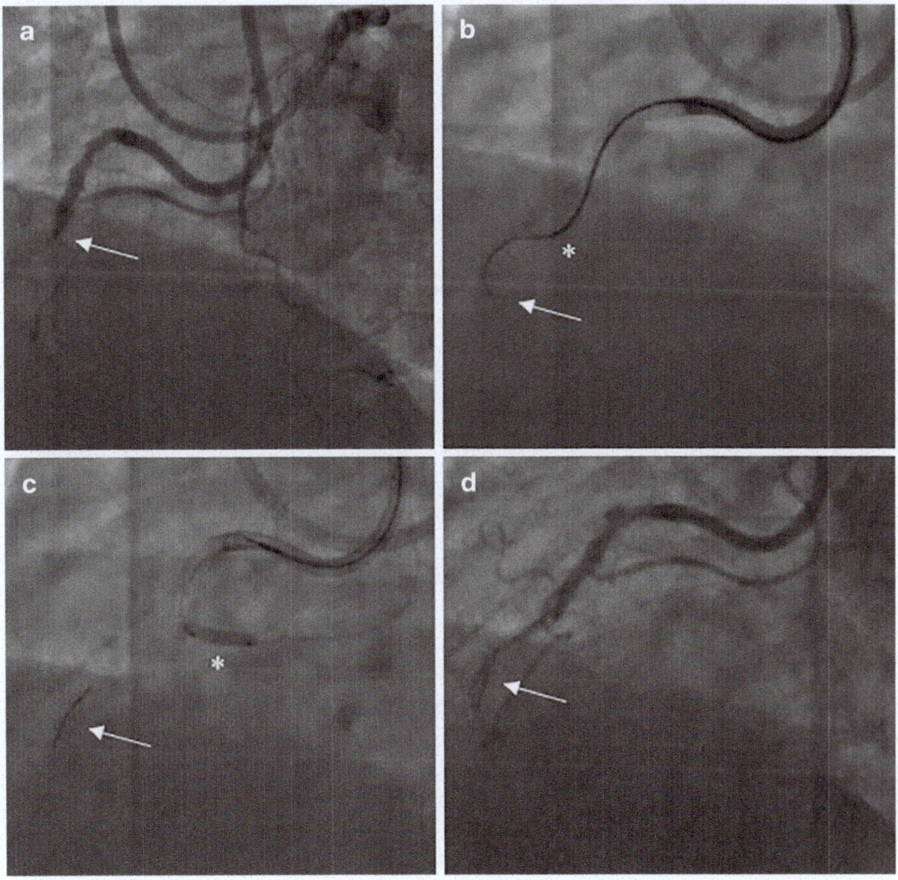

Fig. 16 Case of guidewire fracture managed conservatively. (**a**) Elective PCI to mid RCA CTO (arrow). (**b**) A stiff guidewire (Gaia Third, Asahi Intecc, Japan) was used to attempt antegrade crossing of the highly calcified CTO segment. A microcatheter (asterisk) was used for increased support. (**c**) Further support was provided by anchoring a small balloon in a side branch ("anchoring balloon" technique) (asterisk). Aggressive manipulation of the guidewire resulting in tip fracture (arrow). (**d**) As the fractured wire tip was firmly embedded in a calcified CTO lesion (arrow) with minimal risk of migration, no attempt was made at retrieval. The procedure was completed with balloon dilation in the subintimal space as an "investment" procedure

can be achieved using a snare. Failure to retrieve such a fragment should prompt consideration of emergency cardiac surgery, given the long-term risks of thrombus formation and stroke (Danek et al. 2016). Conversely, small fragments retained in non-critical coronary territories are often best left untreated (Fig. 16). These may embolise distally into side branches or small vessels, where they are unlikely to cause clinically significant harm. When feasible—particularly if the fragment lies within the target lesion—stenting over the wire can anchor it in place, preventing future migration and reducing the risk of thrombosis.

6.4 Microcatheter or Balloon Entrapment and Fracture

Microcatheters are particularly prone to entrapment when subjected to aggressive manipulation, especially torqueable designs intended to "drill" through complex lesions. Excessive rotation can compromise the structural integrity of these devices, leading to tip fracture. Similarly, balloon entrapment can occur when they are forcefully advanced into severely stenosed lesions. Another scenario involves balloon rupture during inflation, where the splayed remnants become lodged within the lesion. In rare cases, balloons may fail to deflate, complicating retrieval.

Entrapped microcatheters or balloons can be retrieved using several techniques. One commonly employed method involves advancing a "trapping" balloon and inflating it within the guiding catheter near its tip. This anchors the entrapped device, allowing the entire system to be withdrawn as a single unit (Kaier et al. 2022). This approach helps concentrate traction distally, enabling more controlled force application. If unsuccessful, a guide extension catheter can be advanced to the site of entrapment, after which counter-traction (by simultaneously pushing the guide extension catheter while pulling on the entrapped device) can focused tension and facilitate release. Alternatively, the device may be retrieved using a snare.

Fractured microcatheter tips or balloon fragments are generally managed similarly to guidewire fractures. If the fragment is located in a critical coronary segment (e.g. LM artery), retrieval using a snare should be attempted. However, in most cases, these fragments embolise to distal or non-critical vessels, where they can often be left untreated without significant clinical consequence. As with guidewire fragments, stenting over the retained material is a viable option, particularly if it lies within the planned treatment segment (Fig. 17).

Failure of balloon deflation ("indeflatable balloon") is very rare but serious complication, as the inflated balloon obstructs coronary flow and can rapidly lead to myocardial ischaemia. This is usually related to indeflator malfunction or kinking of the balloon catheter shaft, which creates a "one-way valve" (i.e. the balloon can be inflated further but not deflated). If due to an indeflator malfunction, it is resolved by simply replacing the indeflator. However, shaft kinking presents a far more challenging scenario. Unless the balloon is significantly undersized relative to the vessel, retrieval in the inflated state is usually not possible. In such cases, only a limited number of high-risk options remain. The first recommended step is to intentionally rupture the balloon by inflating it to very high pressures. This may allow for subsequent removal but carries a substantial risk of vessel perforation. Alternatively, mechanical puncture of the balloon can be attempted using a stiff guidewire or a modified guide extension catheter (with the tip cut to create a sharp edge). These techniques are technically challenging and risky, as directing force precisely towards the balloon is difficult; instead, there is tendency for the stiff guidewire to "slip" off the balloon surface and perforate the coronary artery.

If all percutaneous methods fail, emergency cardiac surgery becomes the definitive solution.

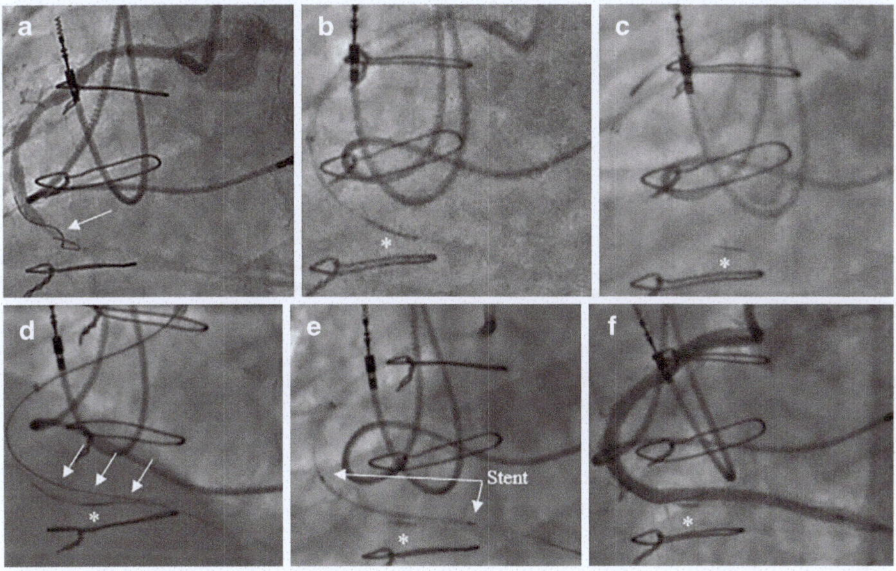

Fig. 17 Case of microcatheter tip fracture with subsequent stenting over the fragment. (**a**) Elective PCI to distal RCA CTO (arrow). (**b**) A microcatheter (asterisk at microcatheter tip) was used to increase support for antegrade wiring. (**c**) Aggressive manipulation of the microcatheter within the calcified lesion led to microcatheter tip fracture, with the radio-opaque tip fragment embedded within the CTO segment (asterisk). (**d**) A separate guidewire was advanced within the subintimal space and successfully crossed into distal vessel ("antegrade dissection and reentry" technique) (arrows). (**e**) The lesion was stented (arrows) across the fractured microcatheter tip (asterisk). (**f**) Final result with the microcatheter tip (asterisk) firmly "trapped" behind stent

6.5 Atherectomy Burr Entrapment

Coronary calcification remains a major challenge in contemporary PCI. Heavily calcified lesions respond poorly to conventional balloon angioplasty, even at high inflation pressures. Moreover, balloon behaviour in these settings is unpredictable; high-pressure inflations may result in asymmetric balloon expansion ("dog-boning"), increasing the risk of coronary dissection or perforation. Inadequate lesion modification often leads to stent under-expansion, which has important long-term consequences including accelerated in-stent restenosis. Atherectomy devices aim to "debulk" calcific plaque and modify lesion morphology, thereby facilitating more effective and safer lesion preparation prior to stent implantation. The main types of atherectomy used in contemporary practice include rotational atherectomy, orbital atherectomy, and excimer laser coronary angioplasty.

The Rotablator system (Boston Scientific, USA) comprises a console, advancer, burr, and a dedicated guidewire (the RotaWire) (Fig. 18). The burr is elliptical in shape, with its distal half coated in microscopic diamond crystals. Burr sizes range 1.25–2.5 mm in diameter, with the 1.25 mm and 1.5 mm burrs most commonly used in clinical practice. The burr, connected to the advancer via

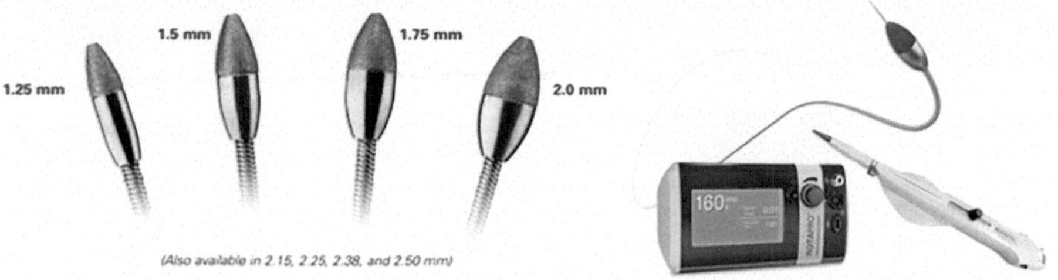

Fig. 18 The Rotablator system for rotational atherectomy (Boston Scientific, USA). (Reproduced with permission from Boston Scientific)

a driveshaft, is mounted onto the RotaWire and advanced to the target lesion. When rotated at high speeds, typically between 150,000 and 200,000 revolutions per minute (rpm), the diamond-coated surface ablates calcific plaque, enhancing lesion crossing and debulking.

The Diamondback 360 Precision Orbital Atherectomy System (OAS) (Abbott, USA) is a similar device designed for calcium modification. While it shares many features with rotational atherectomy, its key distinguishing mechanism is the eccentrically mounted, diamond-coated crown, which orbits rather than rotates within the vessel lumen. Between the two, rotational atherectomy remains more widely used in most regions of the world.

The frequency of atherectomy use varies widely between centres, owing to differences in operator expertise, case complexity, and equipment availability. In recent years, the growing adoption of intravascular lithotripsy (IVL) as an alternative for calcium modification has contributed to a modest decline in atherectomy use (British Cardiovascular Intervention Society (BCIS) 2022). Atherectomy is associated with a higher risk of procedural complications (including no-reflow, coronary spasm, distal embolisation, dissection, and perforation) and should be reserved for select cases. Data from the large national Japan PCI (J-PCI) registry reported that rotational atherectomy was performed in 3.2% of all PCI. The composite rate of major in-hospital complications (death, cardiac tamponade, and emergency surgery) was 1.3%, comprising in-hospital death (0.6%), cardiac tamponade (0.64%), and emergent surgery (0.18%) Sakakura et al. (2016). Notably, centres with higher atherectomy volumes experienced significantly lower complication rates, highlighting the importance of both institutional experience and operator proficiency.

Burr entrapment is a unique complication of rotational atherectomy that merits specific consideration. It occurs when the rotating burr, propelled by high-speed momentum, dives into a heavily calcified stenotic lesion but abruptly decelerates upon encountering resistance, and is left embedded within the plaque. Withdrawal becomes difficult due to both the loss of rotational momentum and the burr's structural design—only the distal (leading) edge is coated with diamond crystals, while the proximal half remains uncoated, with no ability to ablate retrogradely during retraction. This is known as the "Kokesi" phenomenon (Kaneda et al. 2000). Although uncommon, with a reported incidence of 0.4% (Sakakura et al. 2012), prevention is critical. Meticulous technique—including gentle burr advancement with brief lesion contact (the "pecking" motion) and keeping each ablation run short (<15 s)—reduces the risk of entrapment.

Once burr entrapment occurs, coronary flow may be compromised, necessitating immediate intervention (Fig. 14, column C). In some cases, restarting the burr—either at a higher rotational speed or using reduced-speed "Dynaglide" mode—may help regain momentum and enable withdrawal. However, the burr is often too firmly embedded within heavily calcified segments for this strategy to be effective.

The next practical step is to attempt manual retraction by locking the advancer knob and applying steady traction to the entire system. Importantly, excessive force should be avoided, as it increases the risk of vessel injury or driveshaft fracture, which could result in complete burr detachment within the coronary artery.

Several additional bailout techniques have been reported with varying success. One technique describes obtaining a second vascular access and introducing a separate guiding catheter to wire alongside the entrapped burr, followed by balloon advancement and dilation adjacent to the lesion to dislodge the burr (Sakara et al. 2011). Another method involves cutting the driveshaft and advancing a guide extension catheter to the burr to allow controlled counter-traction, which may facilitate retrieval (Chiang and Liu 2017). Alternatively, snaring can be attempted in the same manner as described in the above sections (Chiang and Liu 2017). Finally, emergency cardiac surgery may be required if all else fails (Fig. 19) (Sulimov et al. 2013).

6.6 *Summary*

Equipment entrapment and loss during PCI is a rare but serious complication, with stents being the most commonly involved devices. Management is particularly challenging due to the wide variety of equipment used in PCI and the diverse clinical scenarios in which entrapment or loss can occur. Device entrapment may lead to rapid coronary obstruction and myocardial ischaemia, while device loss carries the risk of embolisation to other coronary territories or the systemic circulation, with stroke being a major concern.

Various percutaneous management strategies have been described in case reports and small case series, with current practice largely informed by anecdotal experience rather than robust evidence. Clinical judgement remains essential in determining whether retrieval should be attempted, as some cases may be more appropriately managed conservatively.

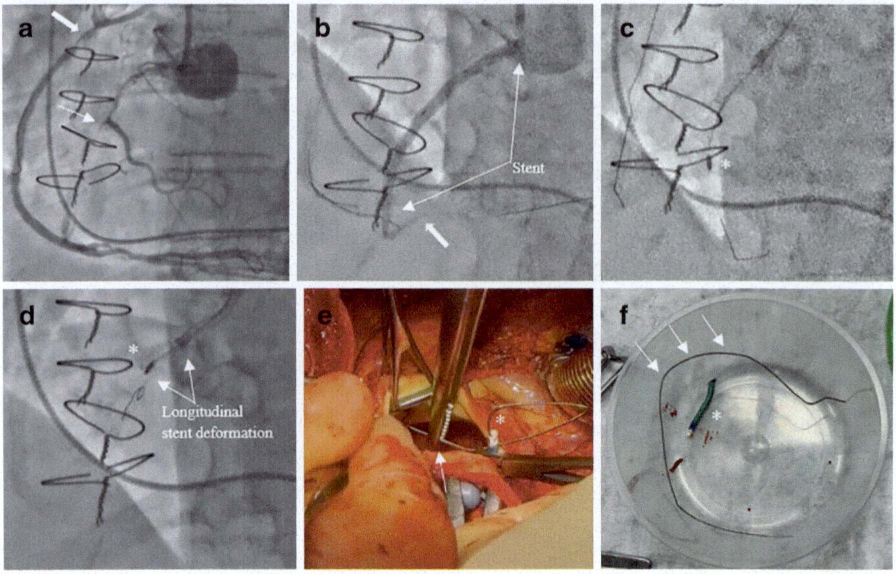

Fig. 19 Case of entrapped rotational atherectomy burr requiring urgent cardiac surgery. (**a**) Elective PCI to native mid RCA CTO (thin arrow). This patient had previous CABG with known critical occlusion of the SVG-RCA (thick arrow). (**b**) Successful stenting of the ostial-distal native RCA (thin arrows). Subsequent angiogram showed poor outflow due to a more distal lesion at the distal RCA (thick arrow). (**c**) The lesion was uncrossable despite the use of small balloons with guide extension catheter support. Decision was made to perform rotational atherectomy. A 1.25 mm burr (asterisk) was advanced past the freshly implanted stents to the distal RCA lesion. (**d**) The burr encountered significant deceleration within the distal RCA lesion and stalled. During retraction, the burr caught onto stent struts, leading to longitudinal stent deformation (LSD) with resultant significant shortening of the stent (thin arrows). The burr was entrapped within a mesh of stent at the proximal RCA (asterisk) and could not be removed despite multiple percutaneous strategies. (**e**) The patient was transferred to the operating theatre for emergency cardiac surgery. After exposing the ascending aorta, the driveshaft (arrow) and guiding catheter distal fragment (asterisk) were located. Despite direct manual traction, the burr could not be extracted. The driveshaft was cut as distally as possible, leaving the burr in-situ within the ostial RCA but with no components extending into the ascending aorta. (**f**) Extracted fragments of the driveshaft (arrows) and guiding catheter tip (asterisk) shown

7 Percutaneous Coronary Interventions in Centres Without On-Site Surgical Support

Once deemed below the standard of care, PCI in centres without surgery on-site (no-SOS) has become routine in many parts of the world. In the UK, only 39% of PCI centres currently have access to on-site cardiothoracic surgical support (British Cardiovascular Intervention Society (BCIS) 2022). This proportion has steadily declined over the past decade, likely reflecting both the increase of PCI-capable centres and the concurrent centralisation of cardiothoracic surgical services into fewer tertiary institutions.

The safety and efficacy of PCI performed in no-SOS centres have been consistently supported by large randomised trials and registry data. The *Cardiovascular Patient Outcomes Research Team Non-Primary PCI (CPORT-E)* trial (2012) demonstrated that PCI performed in no-SOS centres was non-inferior to those with on-site surgery with respect to 6-week mortality and 9-month MACE (death, myocardial infarction, or target-vessel revascularisation) (Aversano et al. 2012). These findings were affirmed by the *Randomized Trial to Compare Percutaneous Coronary Intervention between Massachusetts Hospital with Cardiac Surgery On-Site and Community Hospitals without Cardiac Surgery On-Site (MASS COMM*) trial (2013), which similarly showed that PCI in Massachusetts hospitals with no-SOS was non-inferior to surgical centres, with similar 30-day and 1-year clinical outcomes (death, myocardial infarction, repeat revascularisation, or stroke) (Jacobs et al. 2013).

Notably, the two landmark randomised controlled trials above excluded primary PCI and high-risk PCI (both trials excluded patients with low left ventricular ejection fraction and PCI of unprotected LM coronary artery). However, data from large registries and meta-analyses supports the safety of performing these procedures in no-SOS settings. Analysis from the *Swedish Coronary Angiography and Angioplasty Registry (SCAAR)* found no significant differences in PCI outcomes (30-day mortality, 1-year mortality, stroke, and emergency CABG) between hospitals with and without on-site surgical backup; this finding applied to both elective and primary PCIs (Carlsson et al. 2007). Additionally, a large meta-analysis including 124,074 primary PCI and 914,288 elective PCI cases showed that both cohorts performed in no-SOS centres were not associated with higher rates of in-hospital mortality or emergency CABG compared to centres with on-site surgery (Singh et al. 2011). Primary PCI remains the gold-standard treatment for STEMI, with outcomes strongly linked to call-to-balloon (CTB) and door-to-balloon (DTB) times. Among the 70 PCI centres in the UK providing primary PCI today, only 56% of STEMI patients meet the target CTB time of <150 min. This rate drops dramatically to 39.5% for patients requiring inter-hospital transfer from non-PPCI capable centres, meaning only about one-third of transferred patients achieve the target CTB times (British Cardiovascular Intervention Society (BCIS) 2022). Thus, the success and safety of primary PCI programs in no-SOS settings is a robust argument for expanding such services within the healthcare system.

Recent data from the BCIS registry indicate a steady increase in the proportion of complex high-risk percutaneous coronary intervention (CHiP) cases performed at no-SOS hospitals (12.5% in 2006 to 42% in 2017). Despite this rise, MACCE (in-hospital death, major bleeding, and major cardiovascular or cerebral events) odds were similar between hospitals with and without on-site surgical support. Interestingly, no-SOS centres demonstrated significantly lower mortality and major bleeding rates; however, this finding may reflect patient selection bias, as operators likely refer cases with the highest risk to centres with on-site surgical backup (Shamkhani et al. 2024).

In recognition of evolving practice and outcomes data, the *SCAI expert consensus statement on percutaneous coronary intervention without on-site surgical backup* document was revised in 2023. Compared to the 2014 edition, the updated document endorses a significantly broader range of cases as safe to perform in no-SOS centres (Grines et al. 2023).

Together, these developments reflect a growing consensus that, with appropriate patient selection and institutional protocols, PCI can be safely and effectively performed in no-SOS centres, ultimately facilitating broader access to timely coronary intervention.

8 Conclusion

PCI is a common procedure performed in both acute and elective settings. Although the total volume and complexity of PCI cases have increased over time, the incidence of PCI-related complications and the need for emergency cardiac surgery has remained low, with no evidence of an upward trend. Common complications include coronary perforation, coronary dissection, iatrogenic aortic dissection, and equipment entrapment or loss.

PCI-related complications are particularly challenging to manage due to their acute nature, clinical heterogeneity, and the lack of universal management guidelines. Nonetheless, the collective anecdotal experience within the interventional cardiology community suggests that most of these cases can be successfully managed percutaneously. Various algorithms have been proposed to guide operators through the diverse scenarios that may arise.

Many PCI centres now operate without on-site surgical backup, a model that has proven to be both safe and cost-effective, provided that a clear evacuation protocol is in place to enable timely transfer to a surgical facility when necessary.

Emergency cardiac surgery is seldom required, typically being reserved for cases where percutaneous measures fail and the patient is rapidly deteriorating. This subgroup represents the cohort at the highest risk, often associated with significant peri-operative morbidity and mortality. However, patients who recover from the acute phase generally experience favourable long-term outcomes.

References

Ali ZA, Landmesser U, Maehara A, ILUMIEN IV Investigators (2023) Optical coherence tomography-guided versus angiography-guided PCI. N Engl J Med 389(16):1466–1476

Al-Lamee R, Ielasi A, Latib A et al (2011) Incidence, predictors, management, immediate and long term outcomes following grade III coronary perforations. J Am Coll Cardiol 4:87–95

Alomar ME, Michael TT, Patel VG et al (2013) Stent loss and retrieval during percutaneous coronary interventions: a systematic review and meta-analysis. J Invasive Cardiol 25:637–641

Ang CY, Tan WCJ (2013) Coronary perforation complicating percutaneous coronary intervention – a case illustration and review. ASEAN Heart J 21(2):3
Aslam MS, Messersmith RN, Gilbert J, Lakier JB (2000) Successful management of coronary artery perforation with helical platinum microcoil embolization. Catheter Cardiovasc Interv 51(3):320–322
Aversano T, Lemmon CC, Liu L, Atlantic CPORT Investigators (2012) Outcomes of PCI at hospitals with or without on-site cardiac surgery. N Engl J Med 366:1792–1802
Bauer T, Boeder N, Nef HM et al (2015) Fate of patients with coronary perforation complicating percutaneous coronary intervention (from the Euro Heart Survey Percutaneous Coronary Intervention Registry). Am J Cardiol 116:1363–1367
Biancari F, Pettinari M, Mariscalco G (2022) Outcome after surgery for iatrogenic acute type A aortic dissection. J Clin Med 11(22):6729
Black AJ, Namay DL, Niederman AL et al (1989) Tear or dissection after coronary angioplasty: morphologic correlates of an ischemic complication. Circulation 79:1035–1042
Boukhris M, Tomasello SD, Azzarelli S et al (2015) Coronary perforation with tamponade successfully managed by retrograde and antegrade coil embolization. J Saudi Heart Assoc 27:216–221
Briguori C, Nishida T, Anzuini A et al (2000) Emergency polytetrafluoroethylene-covered stent implantation to treat coronary ruptures. Circulation 102:3028–3031
Brilakis ES, Best PJM, Elesber AA et al (2005) Incidence, retrieval methods, and outcomes of stent loss during percutaneous coronary intervention. Catheter Cardiovasc Interv 65:333–340
British Cardiovascular Intervention Society (BCIS) national audit for adult interventional procedures for 2022–23 activity. Available on BCIS official website at https://www.bcis.org.uk
Carlsson J, James SN, Stahle E et al (2007) Outcome of percutaneous coronary intervention in hospitals with and without on-site cardiac surgery standby. Heart 93:335–338
Chiang CH, Liu SC (2017) Successful retrieval of an entrapped rotablator burr by using a guideliner guiding catheter and a snare. Acta Cardiol Sin 33:96–98
Colkesen AY, Baltali M, Acil T et al (2007) Coronary and systemic stent embolization during percutaneous coronary interventions: a single center experience. Int Heart J 48:129–136
Danek BA, Karatasakis A, Brilakis ES (2016) Consequences and treatment of guidewire entrapment and fracture during percutaneous coronary intervention. Cardiovasc Revasc Med 17:129–133
Dixon SR, Webster MW, Ormiston JA, Wattie WJ, Hammett CJ (2000) Gelfoam embolization of a distal coronary artery guidewire perforation. Catheter Cardiovasc Interv 49(2):214–217
Doll JA, Hira RS, Kearney KE et al (2020) Management of percutaneous coronary intervention complications. Circ Cardiovasc Interv 13:e008962
Dunning DW, Kahn JK, Hawkins ET et al (2000) Iatrogenic coronary artery dissections extending into and involving the aortic root. Catheter Cardiovasc Interv 51:387–393
Ellis SG, Ajluni S, Arnold AZ et al (1994) Increased coronary perforation in the new device era. Incidence, classification, management, and outcome. Circulation 90:2725–2730
Fischell TA, Korban EH, Lauer MA (2003) Successful treatment of distal coronary guidewire-induced perforation with balloon catheter delivery of intracoronary thrombin. Catheter Cardiovasc Interv 58(3):370–374
Fischman DL, Leon MB, Baim DS (1994) Stent restenosis study investigators. A randomized comparison of coronary-stent placement and balloon angioplasty in the treatment of coronary artery disease. N Engl J Med 331:496–501
Geeslin D, Addington M, Trotman D et al (2025) Beyond the incision: understanding catheter induced coronary artery dissection. Curr Treat Options Cardio Med 27:31
George S, Cotton J, Wrigley B (2015) Guidewire-Induced coronary perforation successfully treated with subcutaneous fat embolisation: a simple technique available to all. Catheter Cardiovasc Interv 86(7):1186–1188
Grines CL, Box LC, Mamas MA et al (2023) SCAI expert consensus statement on percutaneous coronary intervention without on-site surgical backup. JACC Cardiovasc Interv 16:847–860
Hadjimiltiades S, Paraskevaides S, Kazinakis G, Louridas G (1998) Coronary vessel perforation during balloon angioplasty: a case report. Catheter Cardiovasc Diagn 45(4):417–420

Hagan PG, Nienaber CA, Isselbacher EM et al (2000) The International Registry of Acute Aortic Dissection (IRAD). JAMA 283(7):897

Hartzler GO, Rutherford BD, McConahay DR (1987) Retained percutaneous transluminal coronary angioplasty equipment components and their management. Am J Cardiol 60:1260–1264

Hiraide T, Sawano M, Shiraishi Y et al (2018) Impact of catheter-induced iatrogenic coronary artery dissection with or without postprocedural flow impairment: a report from a Japanese multicenter percutaneous coronary intervention registry. PLoS One 13:e0204333

Hoshino T, Yoshida H, Takayama S et al (1987) Significance of intimal tears in the mechanism of luminal enlargement in percutaneous transluminal coronary angioplasty: correlation of histologic and angiographic findings in postmortem human hearts. Am Heart J 114:503–510

Huber MS, Mooney JF, Madison J et al (1991) Use of a morphologic classification to predict clinical outcome after dissection from coronary angioplasty. Am J Cardiol 68:467–471

Iturbe JM, Abdel-Karim AR, Papayannis A et al (2012) Frequency, treatment, and consequences of device loss and entrapment in contemporary percutaneous coronary interventions. J Invasive Cardiol 24:215–221

Jacobs AK, Normand SL, Massaro JM, MASS COMM Investigators et al (2013) Nonemergency PCI at hospitals with or without on-site cardiac surgery. N Engl J Med 368:1498–1508

Kaier TE, Kalogeropoulos AS, Pavlidis AN (2022) Use of trapping techniques and a GooseNeck snare to retrieve a fractured balloon catheter. J Invasive Cardiol 34(8):E640–E641

Kaneda H, Saito S, Hosokawa G et al (2000) Trapped rotablator: Kokesi phenomenon. Catheter Cardiovasc Interv 49:82–84

Karacsonyi J, Vemmou E, Nikolakopoulos ID et al (2021) Complications of chronic total occlusion percutaneous coronary intervention. Neth Hear J 29(1):60–67

Kinnaird T, Kwok CS, Kontopantelis E et al (2016) Incidence, determinants and outcomes of coronary perforation during percutaneous coronary intervention in the United Kingdom between 2006 and 2013. An analysis of 527121 cases from the British Cardiovascular Intervention Society Database. Circ Cardiovasc Interv 9:e003449

Kozman H, Wiseman AH, Cook JR (2001) Long-term outcome following coronary stent embolization or misdeployment. Am J Cardiol 88:630–634

Kwok CS, Sirker A, Nolan J et al (2020) A national evaluation of emergency cardiac surgery after percutaneous coronary intervention and postsurgical patient outcomes. Am J Cardiol 130:24–29

Leontyev S, Borger MA, Legare JF, Merk D, Hahn J, Seeburger J et al (2012) Iatrogenic type A aortic dissection during cardiac procedures: early and late outcome in 48 patients. Eur J Cardiothorac Surg 41:641–646

Lin TH, Wu DK, Su HM et al (2006) Septum hematoma: a complication of retrograde wiring in chronic total occlusion. Int J Cardiol 113:e64–e66

Matthews BJ, Ewels CJ, Kent KM (1988) Coronary dissection: a predictor of restenosis? Am Heart J 115(3):547–554

Mikhail P, Howden N, Monjur M et al (2022) Coronary perforation incidence, outcomes and temporal trends (COPIT): a systematic review and meta-analysis. Open Heart 9:e002076

Nairooz R, Parzynski CS, Curtis JP et al (2020) Contemporary trends, predictors and outcomes of perforation during percutaneous coronary intervention (from the NCDR Cath PCI registry). Am J Cardiol 130:37–45

Núñez-Gil IJ, Bautista D, Cerrato E et al (2015) Incidence, management, and immediate-and long-term outcomes after iatrogenic aortic dissection during diagnostic or interventional coronary procedures. Circulation 131:2114–2119

Page E, Kostantinis S, Karacsonyi J et al (2023) Outcomes of coronary artery dissection during percutaneous coronary intervention. J Invasive Cardiol 35(7):E341–E354

Ramasamy A, Bajaj R, Jones DA et al (2020) Iatrogenic catheter-induced ostial coronary artery dissections: prevalence, management, and mortality form a cohort of 55,968 patients over years. Catheter Cardiovasc Interv

Rylski B, Hoffmann I, Beyersdorf F et al (2013) Iatrogenic acute aortic dissection type A: insight from the German Registry for Acute Aortic Dissection Type A (GERAADA). Eur J Cardiothorac Surg 44:353–359

Sakakura K, Ako J, Wada H et al (2012) Comparison of frequency of complications with on-label versus off-label use of rotational atherectomy. Am J Cardiol 110:498–501

Sakakura K, Inohara T, Kohsaka S et al (2016) Incidence and determinants of complications in rotational atherectomy: insights from the National clinical data (J-PCI-Registry). Circ Cardiovasc Interv 9:e004278

Sakara K, Ako J, Momomura SI (2011) Successful removal of an entrapped rotablation burr by extracting drive shift sheath followed by balloon dilatation. Catheter Cardiovasc Interv 78:567–570

Serruys PW, de Jaegere P, Kiemeneij F et al (1994) A comparison of balloon-expandable-stent implantation with balloon angioplasty in patients with coronary artery disease. BENESTENT study group. N Engl J Med 331:489–495

Shamkhani W, Rashid M, Moledina S et al (2024) Complex high-risk percutaneous coronary intervention types, trends, and outcomes in nonsurgical centres. Can J Cardiol 40:1237–1246

Shimony A, Joseph L, Mottillo S et al (2011) Coronary artery perforation during percutaneous coronary intervention: a systematic review and meta-analysis. Can J Cardiol 27:843–850

Singh M, Holmes DR, Dehmer GJ et al (2011) Percutaneous coronary intervention at centers with and without on-site surgery: a meta-analysis. JAMA 306:2487–2494

Sulimov DS, Abdel-Wahab M, Toelg R et al (2013) Stuck rotablator: the nightmare of rotational atherectomy. EuroIntervention 9:251–258

Tarbiat M, Safarpoor G (2015) Emergency coronary artery bypass graft surgery for iatrogenic left main coronary artery dissection. J Tehran Heart Cent 10(4):215–218

Verevkin A, von Aspern K, Leontyev S et al (2018) Early and long-term outcomes in patients undergoing cardiac surgery following iatrogenic injuries during percutaneous coronary intervention. J Am Heart Assoc 7:e010940

Surgery for Coronary Pathologies Leading to Spontaneous Dissection or Rupture

Maria Comanici and Shahzad G. Raja

Abstract Spontaneous coronary artery dissection (SCAD) and coronary artery rupture (CAR) are rare yet important causes of myocardial infarction with significant morbidity and mortality. Despite the serious nature of these pathologies, the exact incidence rates of SCAD and CAR remain difficult to determine due to underdiagnosis and misclassification. Evolution of imaging techniques and increasing clinical awareness have led to improved detection rates. The pace of attainment of knowledge acquisition has been rapid, but ongoing challenges include accurately diagnosing these pathologies and improving outcomes. Both these conditions cause physical and psychosocial distress. Management strategies for these two critical conditions vary. SCAD often starts with conservative medical therapy, while severe cases may require surgical intervention such as coronary artery bypass grafting. CAR generally warrants immediate surgical repair due to its acute nature. The prognosis and outcomes for SCAD and CAR patients are impacted by a variety of factors, including underlying conditions, management strategies, and patient characteristics. Long-term follow-up studies indicate that while many patients can have favourable outcomes, the risk of recurrence and complications remains considerable. Identifying and managing risk factors is pivotal for improving long-term prognosis. Long-term management focuses on recurrence prevention and management of symptoms through medical therapy, cardiac rehabilitation, and psychological support, with regular follow-up and imaging.

Keywords Spontaneous coronary artery dissection (SCAD) · Coronary artery rupture (CAR) · SCAD classification · Fibromuscular dysplasia · Genetics · Myocardial infarction · Pregnancy-associated

---

M. Comanici · S. G. Raja (✉)
Department of Cardiac Surgery, Harefield Hospital, London, UK
e-mail: shahzad.raja1@nhs.net

A. Kourliouros (ed.), *Emergency Cardiac Surgery*,
https://doi.org/10.1007/978-3-032-15787-4_8

1 Introduction

Coronary pathologies leading to spontaneous dissection or rupture represent a significant, though relatively uncommon, subset of cardiovascular conditions that pose serious risks to affected individuals and demand thorough understanding and precise management. These conditions, while less prevalent than other forms of coronary artery disease (CAD), have garnered increasing attention due to their potentially fatal outcomes and the unique challenges they present in clinical practice.

Spontaneous coronary artery dissection (SCAD) and coronary artery rupture (CAR) are characterised by a sudden compromise of the coronary artery wall, leading to myocardial ischaemia and infarction (Adlam et al. 2018). SCAD involves a tear within the coronary artery wall, causing the formation of a false lumen and impeding normal blood flow. This condition has been increasingly recognised as a major cause of acute coronary syndrome (ACS), especially in populations typically not considered at high risk for coronary artery disease, such as younger women without traditional risk factors. Studies indicate that SCAD may account for up to 4% of ACS cases overall and as much as 35% of ACS in women under the age of 50 (Tweet et al. 2012).

In terms of incidence, various studies have sought to elucidate the prevalence of SCAD within different populations. The Canadian SCAD cohort study, one of the largest of its kind, reported that SCAD constituted nearly 24% of ACS cases in women under 60 years of age (Saw et al. 2014). Similarly, data from the Mayo Clinic SCAD registry indicated that SCAD was the underlying cause in 1.7% of all ACS cases, highlighting its significance as an aetiological factor in myocardial infarction among younger patients (Tweet et al. 2012). The increasing recognition of SCAD is partly attributable to advancements in imaging technologies, such as intravascular ultrasound (IVUS) and optical coherence tomography (OCT), which have enhanced diagnostic accuracy and enabled better identification of SCAD cases (Saw et al. 2022).

Coronary artery rupture, although less common than SCAD, is a catastrophic event often associated with high mortality rates. The precise incidence of CAR is challenging to determine due to its rarity and the often fatal nature of the condition, which can result in underreporting. CAR frequently results from the rupture of an atherosclerotic plaque but can also be induced by trauma or iatrogenic causes, such as complications arising from percutaneous coronary interventions (PCI). Limited epidemiological data suggest that CAR is an infrequent but severe complication of coronary interventions, with incidence rates varying widely depending on the population and study context (Longobardi et al. 2017).

Despite the critical nature of these pathologies, the exact incidence rates of SCAD and CAR remain challenging to pinpoint due to underdiagnosis and misclassification. Advancements in imaging techniques and growing clinical awareness have led to improved detection rates. For instance, the use of IVUS and OCT has enhanced the ability to diagnose SCAD accurately, leading to better patient outcomes (Saw et al. 2016b).

Despite the critical nature of these conditions, randomised controlled trials (RCTs) specifically addressing SCAD and CAR are scarce. Most of the existing literature comprises observational studies, case series, and registry data. The rarity and acute presentation of these conditions pose significant challenges to conducting large-scale RCTs. However, some efforts have been made to consolidate data from multiple centres to better understand the clinical characteristics and outcomes associated with SCAD and CAR. For instance, the European Society of Cardiology has established position papers and expert consensus documents to guide the management of SCAD, drawing from pooled data and expert opinion (Adlam et al. 2018).

Coronary pathologies leading to spontaneous dissection or rupture, while relatively rare, represent critical conditions that require prompt recognition and appropriate management. Understanding the incidence, risk factors, and associated conditions is essential for improving diagnosis and treatment outcomes. This chapter aims to provide a comprehensive exploration of these pathologies, offering insights into their complex nature and the latest advancements in their management.

2 Aetiology and Pathogenesis

SCAD, marked by a spontaneous tear in the coronary artery wall, primarily affects younger women and is linked to genetic predispositions, hormonal changes, and connective tissue disorders. CAR, often resulting from trauma or atherosclerotic plaque rupture, impacts older adults with pre-existing coronary artery disease. Both conditions are associated with genetic and syndromic abnormalities. Understanding these genetic predispositions, associated conditions, and pathophysiological mechanisms is essential for developing effective diagnostic and therapeutic strategies.

SCAD is increasingly recognised as having a genetic component, particularly given its occurrence in younger individuals and its association with specific genetic disorders. Genetic predispositions to SCAD often involve mutations affecting the extracellular matrix and vascular integrity.

Approximately 90% of SCAD patients are women (Adlam et al. 2018). SCAD predominantly affects women, especially those during pregnancy, indicating the role for female sex hormones in its pathophysiology. Although the exact mechanisms are not yet fully understood, it is believed that these hormonal influences may impact vascular connective tissue or the vessel microvasculature. This topic will be discussed in more detail later in the text.

Peripartum cases consist approximately 10% of the total number of SCAD (Adlam et al. 2018). Reports of SCAD during pregnancy and the peripartum period have been documented as early as the fifth week of pregnancy (Codsi et al. 2016), although most occurrences are noted in the third trimester. SCAD also presents in the early (less than 6 weeks), late (6 weeks to 12 months), and very late postpartum periods (12–24 months), with the highest incidence observed in the early postpartum phase (Appleby et al. 2009). Anecdotal evidence suggests that late postpartum SCAD might be associated with breastfeeding (Codsi et al. 2016).

SCAD has been associated with various predisposing arteriopathies, with fibromuscular dysplasia (FMD) being the most frequently associated with SCAD. FMD is a non-atherosclerotic, non-inflammatory condition affecting arterial walls, predominantly seen in middle-aged women with minimal cardiovascular risk factors. This disease can cause stenosis, dissections, and aneurysms in medium-sized arteries, including renal, cervico-cephalic, and visceral arteries (Olin et al. 2014).

Genetic factors are also thought to play a significant role in its development. Variants in genes related to connective tissue and smooth muscle cell function, such as PHACTR1, have been implicated in both FMD and SCAD (Kadian-Dodov et al. 2016). Inherited connective tissue disorders, such as Marfan syndrome, Ehlers-Danlos syndrome, and Loeys-Dietz syndrome, significantly increase the risk of SCAD. These conditions are caused by mutations in genes encoding for extracellular matrix proteins, such as fibrillin-1 (FBN1) in Marfan syndrome and collagen type III (COL3A1) in Ehlers-Danlos syndrome, which compromise vascular integrity and elasticity (Elendu et al. 2023). Mutations in genes associated with thoracic aortic diseases, such as TGFBR1, TGFBR2, SMAD3, and ACTA2, also predispose individuals to SCAD. These genes are involved in the transforming growth factor-beta (TGF-β) signalling pathway, which is crucial for maintaining vascular homeostasis (Yagyu et al. 2023).

The pathophysiological mechanisms underlying SCAD include an intimal tear or spontaneous haemorrhage within the vasa vasorum, leading to the formation of an intramural haematoma. This haematoma creates a false lumen, which compresses the true lumen, restricting blood flow and causing ischaemia (Saw et al. 2017). Hormonal changes, particularly during pregnancy and the postpartum period, are significant risk factors for SCAD. Oestrogen and progesterone can induce structural changes in the arterial walls, including increased proteolytic activity and decreased collagen content, which weaken the vessel wall and predispose it to dissection (Tweet et al. 2017). Pregnancy-associated SCAD accounts for 5–10% of all SCAD cases (Tweet et al. 2017). Inflammatory processes and immune responses contribute to the development of SCAD. Systemic inflammatory diseases such as SLE and rheumatoid arthritis can lead to chronic vascular inflammation, resulting in endothelial damage and increased susceptibility to dissection (Adlam et al. 2018).

In contrast, coronary artery rupture (CAR) involves the rupture of the coronary artery, often due to trauma or the rupture of an atherosclerotic plaque. The buildup of plaques within the arterial walls can cause them to become rigid and prone to rupture under stress. Plaque rupture is the most common cause of CAR, particularly in older adults with significant coronary artery disease (Libby 2021). High-impact trauma, such as from motor vehicle accidents or falls, is a significant cause of CAR. The mechanical forces exerted on the chest can cause laceration or rupture of the coronary arteries, especially in individuals with pre-existing vascular conditions (Abu-Hmeidan et al. 2016). Invasive cardiovascular procedures, such as PCI, can cause mechanical injury to the coronary arteries, leading to CAR. The risk is heightened in patients with pre-existing atherosclerosis, where the arterial walls are already compromised. Procedural complications, such as guidewire perforation or balloon over-inflation, can precipitate arterial rupture (Nagalli and Hajouli 2020).

The genetic underpinnings of CAR are less well understood than those of SCAD, primarily due to its rarity and often acute presentation. However, certain genetic factors that affect vascular integrity and response to injury may contribute to its development. It is most frequently observed in older adults with pre-existing coronary artery disease. Genetic factors influencing the development of atherosclerosis, such as polymorphisms in the APOE, LDLR, and PCSK9 genes, can predispose individuals to plaque rupture and subsequent CAR. These genes affect lipid metabolism and arterial wall stability (Libby 2021). Inherited connective tissue disorders can also predispose individuals to CAR, with compromised structural integrity of the arterial walls making them more susceptible to rupture under stress or trauma.

The genetic predispositions and associated conditions for SCAD and CAR are detailed in Tables 1 and 2, respectively.

The pathophysiological mechanisms underlying CAR include plaque rupture and thrombosis, mechanical forces and trauma, and iatrogenic injury. Plaque rupture exposes the lipid-rich core and necrotic material to the bloodstream, triggering thrombus formation. The sudden increase in intraluminal pressure can cause the arterial wall to rupture, leading to haemopericardium and cardiac tamponade (Libby 2021). In cases of traumatic CAR, mechanical forces exerted on the chest can cause direct injury to the coronary arteries. The right coronary artery is particularly susceptible due to its anatomical position. Trauma-induced CAR often results in rapid haemodynamic deterioration and requires immediate intervention (Nagalli and Hajouli 2020). The pathophysiological mechanisms for SCAD and CAR are listed in Table 3.

Table 1 Genetic predispositions for SCAD and CAR

Condition	Genetic factors
SCAD	PHACTR1, FBN1, COL3A1, TGFBR1, TGFBR2, SMAD3, ACTA2
CAR	APOE, LDLR, PCSK9, FBN1, COL3A1

Table 2 Associated conditions for SCAD and CAR

Condition	Associated conditions
SCAD	Fibromuscular dysplasia, hormonal influences, connective tissue disorders, systemic inflammatory diseases
CAR	Atherosclerosis, trauma, iatrogenic causes

Table 3 Pathophysiological mechanisms for SCAD and CAR

Condition	Pathophysiological mechanisms
SCAD	Intimal tear and haematoma formation, hormonal influences, inflammation and immune response
CAR	Plaque rupture and thrombosis, mechanical forces and trauma, iatrogenic injury

3 Clinical Presentation

SCAD and CAR present distinct clinical challenges, characterised by unique presentations and specific risk factors, leading to missed or delayed diagnosis. Maintaining a high level of suspicion in typical patients, along with a thorough understanding of the various forms of SCAD and CAR, is crucial for reducing missed or delayed diagnoses.

SCAD is an important and underrecognised cause of ACS, particularly in younger women without traditional cardiovascular risk factors. The clinical presentation of SCAD can vary widely, but it often mimics other forms of ACS and is associated with positive biomarkers of myocardial necrosis.

Patients with SCAD typically present with symptoms that are similar to those of ACS:

- Chest Pain: The most common symptom of SCAD, often described as severe and sudden in onset. It can be persistent or intermittent and may radiate to the neck, back, or arms.
- Shortness of Breath: Frequently reported by patients, resulting from myocardial ischaemia and reduced cardiac output.
- Nausea and Vomiting: Particularly prevalent in cases involving extensive myocardial infarction. These symptoms can be mistaken for gastrointestinal issues, leading to delayed diagnosis.
- Diaphoresis: A common autonomic response to myocardial ischaemia, often accompanying chest pain.
- Palpitations: Occasionally reported, these can indicate arrhythmias associated with SCAD.
- Dizziness or Syncope: Less common but can occur, particularly if there is significant haemodynamic compromise.
- Fatigue: Some patients report unexplained fatigue or general malaise prior to the acute event.

SCAD predominantly affects women aged 30–50 years and is often associated with specific risk factors and conditions, including:

- Hormonal Influences: Pregnancy and the postpartum period are significant risk factors.
- FMD: A common associated condition.
- Connective Tissue Disorders: Such as Marfan syndrome and Ehlers-Danlos syndrome.
- Systemic Inflammatory Diseases: Including systemic lupus erythematosus (SLE) and rheumatoid arthritis.

CAR, though less common than SCAD, is a catastrophic event often associated with high mortality rates. The clinical presentation of CAR can be sudden and severe, requiring immediate medical intervention.

The clinical presentation of CAR includes:

Table 4 Clinical features of SCAD and CAR

Common symptoms	SCAD	CAR
Chest pain	Severe, sudden onset, may radiate to neck, back, arms	Sudden, intense, tearing sensation
Shortness of breath	Due to myocardial ischaemia and reduced cardiac output	Resulting from impaired cardiac function
Nausea and vomiting	Common in extensive myocardial infarction	Less common, more typical of haemodynamic instability
Sweating (Diaphoresis)	Autonomic response to myocardial ischaemia	Autonomic response, particularly with chest pain
Palpitations	Occasionally reported, indicating possible arrhythmias	Often indicative of severe haemodynamic instability
Dizziness or Syncope	Less common, can indicate significant haemodynamic compromise	Common, indicating severe haemodynamic instability or arrhythmias
Fatigue	Unexplained fatigue or malaise prior to acute event	Rare, acute presentation dominates

- Severe Chest Pain: Typically sudden in onset and described as intense and tearing. The pain may radiate to the back, abdomen, or shoulders.
- Haemodynamic Instability: Manifesting as hypotension, tachycardia, or even bradycardia if there is significant cardiac compromise.
- Rapid Progression to Shock: Due to massive haemorrhage into the pericardium (haemopericardium) leading to cardiac tamponade. Symptoms include jugular venous distension, muffled heart sounds, and pulsus paradoxus.
- Dyspnoea: Resulting from impaired cardiac function and tamponade physiology.
- Syncope: Often indicative of severe haemodynamic instability or arrhythmias.

CAR is most commonly associated with atherosclerosis and trauma, but can also result from iatrogenic causes such as complications from PCI. The key risk factors and associated conditions include:

- Atherosclerosis: The most common underlying cause.
- Trauma: High-impact injuries from accidents or falls.
- Iatrogenic Causes: Complications from invasive cardiovascular procedures.

The clinical features of SCAD and CAR are summarised and compared in Table 4.

4 Diagnostic Approaches

Diagnosing SCAD and CAR requires a high index of suspicion and a comprehensive understanding of their clinical presentations. The diagnostic process involves a combination of clinical evaluation, imaging techniques, and sometimes laboratory tests.

SCAD is a challenging diagnosis due to its variability in presentation and the fact that it often occurs in patients without traditional risk factors for coronary artery disease and there are no currently identified specific blood biomarkers for SCAD. Coronary angiography represents the principal tool for the diagnosis of SCAD in clinical practice. Early and accurate diagnosis is crucial for effective management and improved outcomes.

The initial step in diagnosing SCAD involves a thorough clinical evaluation, including a detailed patient history and physical examination.

Key aspects include:

- Patient History: Focus on the onset, duration, and nature of chest pain, associated symptoms such as shortness of breath, nausea, vomiting, and any recent physical or emotional stress. A history of connective tissue disorders, fibromuscular dysplasia, or recent pregnancy should raise suspicion for SCAD (Saw, Mancini, & Humphries, 2014).
- Physical Examination: Look for signs of myocardial ischaemia, such as diaphoresis, pallor, and tachycardia. Auscultation may reveal murmurs or signs of heart failure in advanced cases.

Electrocardiography (ECG) is a frontline diagnostic tool in evaluating chest pain. In SCAD, ECG findings may include:

- ST-Segment Elevation: Indicative of acute myocardial infarction, seen in approximately 20–30% of SCAD cases (Tweet et al. 2012).
- T-Wave Inversion: Common in the leads corresponding to the affected coronary artery.
- Non-specific ST-T Changes: These can complicate the differentiation from other causes of ACS.

Measurement of cardiac biomarkers, such as troponins, helps to confirm myocardial injury. Elevated troponin levels are common in SCAD, reflecting the extent of myocardial ischaemia or infarction (Saw et al. 2014).

Coronary angiography is the gold standard for diagnosing SCAD. It provides detailed visualisation of the coronary arteries, revealing characteristic findings such as:

- "Pearl and String" Appearance: Alternating segments of narrowed and dilated arteries.
- Multiple Radiolucent Lumens: Indicating the presence of a false lumen (Saw et al. 2017).

The most commonly used angiographic classification of SCAD has been adapted from Saw et al. According to the Saw classification (Saw et al. 2016a), Type 1 SCAD is characterised by the classic angiographic radiolucent "flap" and linear double lumen, often associated with contrast hold-up. This type occurs in 29–48% of cases. However, these features are absent in the more common Type 2 pattern, which is seen in 52–67% of cases. Type 2 SCAD is identified by a long, diffuse, and smooth stenosis predominantly located in mid-to-distal segments. This type is

Table 5 Angiographic classification of SCAD

SCAD type	Features	Occurrence (%)	Additional details
Type 1	Radiolucent "flap", linear double lumen, contrast hold-up	29–48	Classic appearance
Type 2	Long, diffuse, smooth stenosis	52–67	Predominantly mid-to-distal segments
Type 2a	Normal calibre distal vessel	N/A	Subtype of Type 2
Type 2b	Stenosis extends to vessel's end	N/A	Subtype of Type 2
Type 3	Mimics focal atherosclerotic stenosis, requires intracoronary imaging	0–3.9	Diagnostic challenge
Type 4	Total occlusion, usually of distal vessel	N/A	Diagnosis often during intervention

further divided into Type 2a, where there is a return to a normal calibre distal vessel, and Type 2b, where the stenosis extends to the end of the vessel. Intermediate appearances between Type 1 and 2 are also observed. These intermediate types exhibit a typical Type 2 pattern but with a short segment of dual lumen or contrast hold-up, indicating a localised fenestration between the true and false lumen. Type 3 SCAD, which is angiographically indistinguishable from focal atherosclerotic stenosis, requires diagnostic confirmation by intracoronary imaging and accounts for a small minority of cases (0–3.9%). Finally, Type 4 SCAD is described as a total occlusion, usually of a distal vessel. Diagnosing Type 4 can be particularly challenging and is often established during coronary intervention once coronary flow is re-established or inferred by subsequent vessel healing and the exclusion of an embolic cause. The detailed classification of SCAD types is summarised in Table 5.

IVUS and OCT are intravascular imaging techniques that provide high-resolution images of the coronary artery wall, helping to confirm the diagnosis of SCAD and assess its extent. IVUS is particularly useful for visualising the arterial wall and identifying a false lumen, helping to determine the extent of dissection and the presence of intramural haematomas (Saw et al. 2017). On the other hand, OCT offers even higher resolution images than IVUS, allowing for detailed visualisation of the dissection flap, false lumen, and intimal tears (Saw et al. 2017). Most SCAD cases can be diagnosed angiographically, and conservative management is often feasible, avoiding unnecessary coronary instrumentation. However, when diagnostic uncertainty exists or when guiding coronary intervention is necessary, careful intracoronary imaging with IVUS or OCT becomes invaluable and appears safe. SCAD frequently affects more distal coronary segments, which may limit complete imaging of the false lumen. In some series, only a portion of affected cases could be fully imaged along their entire length, though imaging shorter proximal segments often suffices for diagnosis.

IVUS provides tomographic images of the vessel wall and coronary lumen, differentiating atherosclerotic plaques from SCAD. It excels in demonstrating true and false lumens and false lumen thrombosis. Its advantages include no need for blood clearance and superior depth penetration, visualising the entire vessel wall,

Table 6 Diagnostic tools for SCAD

Diagnostic tool	Key features and findings
Clinical evaluation	Patient history, physical examination
Electrocardiography	ST-segment elevation, T-wave inversion, non-specific ST-T changes
Cardiac biomarkers	Elevated troponin levels
Coronary angiography	"Pearl and string" appearance, multiple radiolucent lumens
Intravascular ultrasound	Visualisation of arterial wall, false lumen
Optical coherence tomography	High-resolution images of dissection flap, false lumen

including thrombus. However, IVUS's poor spatial resolution can limit the identification of small structures such as the intimal-medial membrane and localised fenestrations connecting true and false lumens.

OCT offers higher spatial resolution, providing detailed images of SCAD, but requires blood clearance with high-pressure contrast injection, which carries a risk of extending the false lumen. Despite this, careful use of OCT in SCAD cases has been shown to be safe. OCT excels in characterising the true lumen, associated thrombus, false lumen dimensions, and connections between true and false lumens. It is also valuable in guiding revascularisation, ensuring the guidewire is in the true lumen to avoid serious complications.

Computed Tomography Coronary Angiography (CTCA) offers a non-invasive option for assessing acute chest pain and suspected SCAD cases, particularly beneficial for patients with a low atherosclerotic risk profile. However, due to its lower spatial resolution, it may not be ideal for accurately assessing mid-to-distal coronary territories. While CTCA is not currently the primary diagnostic tool for SCAD, it may have a role in follow-up assessments.

The diagnostic tools for SCAD, along with their key features and findings, are summarised in Table 6.

Multi-vessel SCAD refers to the occurrence of simultaneous dissections in multiple arteries without continuity, distinguishing it from recurrent SCAD or a single dissection extending into different coronary territories. This condition is well-documented, with a reported prevalence of 5–13% in larger series (Adlam et al. 2018). Thus, careful angiographic assessment of seemingly unaffected vessels during initial angiography is strongly recommended.

CAR is a medical emergency requiring rapid diagnosis and intervention. The diagnostic approach focuses on identifying the site and extent of rupture, assessing haemodynamic stability, and planning urgent management.

A thorough clinical evaluation is the first step in diagnosing CAR:

- *Patient History*: Obtain a history of trauma, recent invasive cardiac procedures, or known coronary artery disease. Symptoms such as sudden, severe chest pain, syncope, or signs of shock should prompt immediate investigation.
- *Physical Examination*: Look for signs of haemodynamic instability, such as hypotension, tachycardia, distended neck veins, and muffled heart sounds. These findings may indicate cardiac tamponade due to haemopericardium.

Table 7 Diagnostic tools for CAR

Diagnostic tool	Key features and findings
Clinical evaluation	Patient history, physical examination
Electrocardiography	ST-segment changes, arrhythmias
Cardiac biomarkers	Elevated troponin levels
Coronary angiography	Extravasation of contrast media
Echocardiography	Pericardial effusion, signs of cardiac tamponade
Computed tomography (CT)	Detailed coronary artery imaging, rupture location

ECG may reveal:

- *ST-Segment Changes*: Similar to those seen in acute myocardial infarction.
- *Arrhythmias*: Such as ventricular fibrillation or tachycardia, particularly if there is significant myocardial injury.

Elevated cardiac biomarkers, such as troponins, are common in CAR and reflect myocardial injury. However, their role is secondary to imaging in acute settings.

Coronary angiography is critical for identifying the site of rupture and guiding therapeutic interventions:

- *Extravasation of Contrast Media*: Indicates the presence of a coronary artery rupture (Nagalli and Hajouli 2020).

Echocardiography is a key diagnostic tool for assessing haemodynamic status and detecting complications:

- *Pericardial Effusion*: Presence of fluid in the pericardial space, suggesting haemopericardium.
- *Signs of Cardiac Tamponade*: Such as diastolic collapse of the right atrium or ventricle.

CT scans provide detailed images of the coronary arteries and can help identify the site and extent of the rupture, as well as associated complications:

- *Detailed Coronary Artery Imaging*: Helps in planning surgical or interventional repair (Libby 2021).

The diagnostic tools for CAR, along with their key features and findings, are listed in Table 7.

5 Management Strategies

The management of SCAD and coronary artery rupture CAR is multifaceted, involving a range of conservative, interventional, and surgical strategies. The approach to each patient must be individualised, considering the specific characteristics of the dissection or rupture, the patient's clinical stability, and underlying risk factors. The European Society of Cardiology (ESC) provides detailed recommendations for managing these conditions, emphasising a careful, patient-centred approach.

Conservative management is often the first line of treatment for SCAD, especially for patients who are haemodynamically stable without ongoing myocardial ischaemia. The ESC recommends this approach when dissections do not significantly compromise blood flow in the coronary arteries and in the absence of high-risk features such as left main coronary artery involvement or multi-vessel disease (Adlam et al. 2018). The cornerstone of conservative management includes medical therapy, close monitoring, and lifestyle modifications. Medical therapy typically involves antiplatelet agents, beta-blockers, and sometimes angiotensin-converting enzyme (ACE) inhibitors or angiotensin receptor blockers (ARBs) to manage hypertension and reduce myocardial oxygen demand (Tweet et al. 2012). Regular follow-up with repeat imaging is crucial to monitor the healing of the dissection, while patients are advised to avoid extreme physical or emotional stress and adhere to heart-healthy lifestyle changes (Adlam et al. 2018).

There is substantial evidence suggesting that most SCAD cases will stabilise and heal over time with conservative management (Saw et al. 2014). Revascularisation in SCAD patients is challenging due to the disrupted and fragile coronary vessel wall, often resulting in poorer outcomes compared to atherosclerotic coronary disease. Consequently, conservative management is generally preferred in haemodynamically stable patients with maintained distal flow in the culprit coronary artery and no ongoing ischaemia (Adlam et al. 2018). Studies report varying healing rates, with a significant number of cases showing complete resolution upon follow-up angiography (Saw et al. 2014; Tweet et al. 2012; Adlam et al. 2018). However, a small percentage of conservatively managed patients may require subsequent revascularisation, typically early during follow-up.

Conservative management of CAR is less common due to the acute and often life-threatening nature of the condition. However, in selected cases where the rupture is contained and haemodynamic stability is achieved, initial conservative measures may include the administration of antiplatelet agents and beta-blockers to stabilise the patient and reduce the risk of further rupture (Libby 2021). Intensive monitoring in a critical care setting with repeat imaging is essential to assess the integrity of the coronary artery.

Surgical intervention for SCAD is generally reserved for cases where conservative management is not feasible or fails, and where there is ongoing ischaemia or haemodynamic instability. Specific indications for surgery include left main coronary artery involvement due to the high risk of extensive myocardial ischaemia, ongoing ischaemia despite optimal medical therapy, and patients who cannot be stabilised medically (Adlam et al. 2018). Coronary artery bypass grafting (CABG) is often preferred in cases of extensive dissection or when PCI is not feasible. CABG can restore blood flow by bypassing the dissected segment, and in some instances, direct surgical repair is performed to directly address the dissection, although this is less common due to the technical challenges involved (Saw et al. 2014).

For CAR, surgical intervention is typically required due to the acute nature of the condition and the need to prevent further complications. Indications for surgery include ongoing haemorrhage, uncontrolled bleeding or haemopericardium causing cardiac tamponade, and persistent instability despite initial medical therapy (Nagalli and Hajouli 2020). Surgical techniques for CAR primarily involve CABG to bypass the ruptured segment and restore blood flow. Direct surgical repair, which involves suturing the ruptured segment or placing a patch to seal the rupture, is another approach, though it is technically demanding and requires specialised expertise.

PCI is generally reserved for SCAD patients with ongoing ischaemia or haemodynamic instability who are not candidates for conservative management. The ESC emphasises careful consideration before proceeding with PCI due to the risk of exacerbating the dissection (Adlam et al. 2018). Key techniques include stenting and balloon angioplasty. Stenting involves the placement of a stent to cover the dissection and restore vessel integrity, with drug-eluting stents (DES) often preferred to reduce the risk of restenosis (Saw et al. 2014). Balloon angioplasty is used selectively to improve blood flow before stenting, though care must be taken to avoid extending the dissection (Saw et al. 2017).

For CAR, PCI techniques focus on stabilising the patient and preventing further rupture. Stenting involves the placement of a covered stent to seal the rupture and restore vessel integrity, while balloon angioplasty can be used to tamponade the bleeding vessel temporarily before definitive stent placement (Nagalli and Hajouli 2020).

Advanced PCI techniques such as cutting-balloon angioplasty and bioresorbable scaffolds represent innovative approaches in specific scenarios. Cutting-balloon angioplasty uses a balloon with small blades to create controlled incisions in the plaque before dilation, which can be particularly useful in resistant lesions or in-stent restenosis. In SCAD, this technique is rarely used due to the risk of extending the dissection but may be considered in select cases with localised and resistant stenosis (Saw et al. 2017). In CAR, cutting-balloon angioplasty is not typically used due to the acute nature of the rupture and the need for immediate vessel sealing.

Bioresorbable scaffolds (BRS) are temporary stents that provide mechanical support to the vessel while gradually being absorbed by the body, aiming to reduce long-term complications associated with permanent stents. In SCAD, BRS can provide temporary support while allowing the vessel to heal naturally, reducing the risk of late stent thrombosis and restenosis (Saw et al. 2017). However, their use in CAR is limited due to the urgent need for durable and immediate vessel support.

Surgical management of SCAD and CAR is complex and requires a detailed understanding of the anatomical and pathophysiological aspects of these conditions. For SCAD, CABG is the preferred surgical technique, particularly in cases involving the left main coronary artery or when extensive dissection precludes PCI. The procedure involves grafting a new blood vessel to bypass the dissected artery, thus restoring normal blood flow to the myocardium. In some cases, direct surgical repair of the dissected artery may be attempted, although this is less common due to the technical difficulties and potential for further dissection.

For CAR, surgical management is often emergent and involves a combination of techniques to control bleeding, restore coronary blood flow, and repair the ruptured artery. CABG is frequently employed to bypass the damaged segment of the artery. Additionally, direct surgical repair, which may involve suturing the rupture or placing a patch over the defect, is critical in stabilising the patient. The choice of technique depends on the location and extent of the rupture, the patient's haemodynamic status, and the availability of surgical expertise.

Table 8 Indications and techniques for PCI in SCAD and CAR

Condition	Indications for PCI	Key techniques
SCAD	Ongoing ischaemia, haemodynamic instability	Stenting, balloon angioplasty
CAR	Haemodynamic instability, failed conservative management	Covered stenting, balloon angioplasty

Table 9 Advanced PCI techniques for SCAD and CAR

Technique	Application in SCAD	Application in CAR
Cutting-balloon angioplasty	Rarely used, select resistant stenosis	Not typically used
Bioresorbable scaffolds	Temporary support, reduces late complications	Limited use, need for immediate support

Table 10 Surgical management strategies for SCAD and CAR

Condition	Surgical techniques	Indications for surgery	Description
SCAD	Coronary Artery Bypass Grafting (CABG)	Left main coronary artery involvement Ongoing ischaemia despite medical therapy Haemodynamic instability	Preferred for extensive dissection or when PCI is not feasible; restores blood flow by bypassing the dissected segment
	Direct surgical repair	When CABG is not suitable Isolated cases	Less common due to technical challenges; involves direct repair of the dissection
CAR	CABG	Ongoing haemorrhage Uncontrolled bleeding Haemopericardium causing cardiac tamponade Persistent instability despite initial medical therapy	Frequently employed to bypass the ruptured segment and restore blood flow
	Direct surgical repair	Suitable case Location and extent of rupture	Involves suturing the ruptured segment or placing a patch to seal the rupture; technically demanding and requires specialised expertise

A comprehensive management strategy for SCAD and CAR involves a multidisciplinary team approach, integrating cardiologists, cardiac surgeons, interventional radiologists, and critical care specialists. This collaborative approach ensures that all aspects of the patient's condition are addressed, from initial diagnosis and stabilisation to definitive treatment and long-term follow-up (Adlam et al. 2018).

The indications and techniques for PCI in SCAD and CAR are tabulated in Table 8, while advanced PCI techniques for both conditions are outlined in Table 9. The surgical management strategies for SCAD and CAR, including indications and techniques, are detailed in Table 10.

6 Long-Term Management and Follow-Up

Effective long-term management and follow-up are crucial for patients who have experienced SCAD or CAR. The aim is to prevent recurrence, manage symptoms, and improve overall quality of life.

Long-term medical therapy is a cornerstone in the management of both SCAD and CAR patients. For SCAD, antiplatelet therapy, such as aspirin, is commonly prescribed to prevent thrombotic complications. The ESC recommends lifelong aspirin therapy for SCAD patients to reduce the risk of subsequent cardiovascular events (Adlam et al. 2018). Beta-blockers are also frequently used in SCAD patients, especially those with a history of hypertension or left ventricular dysfunction. Beta-blockers help to reduce myocardial oxygen demand, control blood pressure, and prevent arrhythmias. ACE inhibitors or angiotensin receptor blockers (ARBs) may be added for patients with left ventricular dysfunction or persistent hypertension (Tweet et al. 2012).

For CAR, long-term medical therapy also includes antiplatelet agents and beta-blockers. The use of dual antiplatelet therapy (DAPT) with aspirin and a P2Y12 inhibitor may be indicated for patients who have undergone stent placement during initial treatment. Beta-blockers are particularly important in preventing stress on the coronary arteries and reducing the risk of recurrent rupture (Libby 2021). Additionally, managing underlying risk factors such as hypertension, hyperlipidaemia, and diabetes is critical for both SCAD and CAR patients to prevent further cardiovascular events.

Cardiac rehabilitation plays a vital role in the recovery and long-term management of SCAD and CAR patients. Comprehensive cardiac rehabilitation programs typically include supervised exercise training, education on heart-healthy living, and counselling to reduce stress and improve mental health. Exercise training is tailored to the individual's fitness level and clinical status, aiming to improve cardiovascular endurance, strength, and overall physical function (Saw et al. 2014). Education sessions cover topics such as diet, weight management, smoking cessation, and medication adherence. These programs are designed to empower patients with the knowledge and skills needed to make lasting lifestyle changes that benefit their cardiovascular health.

Psychological support is an often underemphasised but critical component of long-term management for SCAD and CAR patients. The emotional impact of experiencing a life-threatening cardiac event can be profound, leading to anxiety, depression, and post-traumatic stress disorder (PTSD). Psychological support can include individual counselling, support groups, and stress management techniques. Cognitive-behavioural therapy (CBT) has been shown to be particularly effective in helping patients cope with anxiety and depression related to their cardiac condition (Adlam et al. 2018). Support groups provide a platform for patients to share their experiences and receive encouragement from others who have undergone similar experiences. Additionally, stress management techniques such as mindfulness, meditation, and relaxation exercises can help patients manage anxiety and reduce the risk of recurrent cardiac events (Saw et al. 2017).

In the long-term follow-up of SCAD and CAR patients, regular medical check-ups and imaging studies are essential to monitor the status of the coronary arteries and assess for any signs of recurrence. Echocardiography, stress tests, and coronary computed tomography angiography (CTA) can be used to evaluate cardiac function and detect any new dissections or aneurysms (Tweet et al. 2012). Blood pressure and lipid levels should be regularly monitored and managed according to current guidelines to reduce cardiovascular risk.

Family members and caregivers also play a crucial role in the long-term management of SCAD and CAR patients. Educating them about the patient's condition, treatment plan, and signs of potential complications can help in early detection and prompt management of any issues that arise. Family support can also provide emotional stability and encouragement for patients, which is essential for their psychological well-being and adherence to treatment regimens.

The long-term management of SCAD and CAR patients involves a multidisciplinary approach that includes medical therapy, cardiac rehabilitation, psychological support, and regular follow-up. Lifelong aspirin therapy, beta-blockers, and management of cardiovascular risk factors are key components of medical therapy. Cardiac rehabilitation programs aid in physical recovery and lifestyle modification, while psychological support addresses the emotional impact of these conditions. Regular monitoring and family support further enhance the overall management strategy, aiming to improve the quality of life and reduce the risk of recurrence for these patients.

7 Prognosis and Outcomes

Understanding the prognosis and long-term outcomes for patients who have experienced SCAD or CAR is essential for guiding management and counselling patients.

The prognosis for SCAD patients has been a subject of increasing study, with various long-term follow-up studies providing valuable insights. Research indicates that while SCAD can have a favourable short-term outcome, there is a significant risk of recurrence and long-term cardiovascular complications. In a large cohort study conducted by Tweet et al. (2012), the 5-year survival rate for SCAD patients was found to be over 90%, highlighting the generally positive long-term outlook. However, the same study reported a recurrence rate of approximately 17% within 3 years, emphasising the need for ongoing vigilance and follow-up.

The risk factors for SCAD recurrence have been extensively studied to better stratify patients and tailor follow-up strategies. Key risk factors include a history FMD, hormonal changes such as those occurring during pregnancy or menopause, and genetic predispositions such as connective tissue disorders. McGrath-Cadell et al. (2016) identified that patients with FMD are at a higher risk for recurrent SCAD, suggesting that these individuals may benefit from more frequent and intensive follow-up. Similarly, Tweet et al. (2012) found that women who experienced

SCAD during the peripartum period were more likely to have recurrent events, underscoring the impact of hormonal fluctuations on arterial integrity.

For CAR, the long-term prognosis can be more variable due to the acute and often severe nature of the initial event. Studies on long-term outcomes are less common, but available data suggest that patients who survive the acute phase can have a reasonably good long-term prognosis if managed appropriately to prevent further events and improve overall outcomes. Recurrence rates and risk factors for CAR are less well defined compared to SCAD, partly due to the rarity and acute presentation of CAR. However, studies suggest that underlying atherosclerosis, hypertension, and previous coronary interventions are significant risk factors for recurrence. Patients with extensive coronary artery disease are particularly vulnerable to further ruptures, indicating the need for aggressive management of atherosclerotic risk factors.

Future research directions for both SCAD and CAR focus on improving our understanding of the pathophysiological mechanisms, identifying genetic markers for predisposition, and developing more effective management strategies. The establishment of international registries and collaborative research networks is also crucial for advancing our knowledge of these conditions. The Canadian SCAD Study (Saw et al. 2014) and the European Position Paper on SCAD (Adlam et al. 2018) both emphasise the need for large-scale, multicentre studies to gather more comprehensive data on long-term outcomes and recurrence rates.

The prognosis and outcomes for SCAD and CAR patients are influenced by a variety of factors, including underlying conditions, management strategies, and patient characteristics. Long-term follow-up studies indicate that while many patients can have favourable outcomes, the risk of recurrence and complications remains significant. Identifying and managing risk factors is crucial for improving long-term prognosis. Future research will likely focus on genetic and molecular mechanisms, as well as optimising treatment protocols to enhance patient outcomes.

8 Conclusion

SCAD and CAR are complex cardiovascular conditions influenced by genetic factors, systemic conditions, and specific pathophysiological mechanisms. Accurate diagnosis is essential, involving clinical evaluation, ECG, biomarkers, and advanced imaging like coronary angiography, IVUS, and OCT. Management strategies vary: SCAD often starts with conservative medical therapy, while severe cases may require surgical intervention such as CABG. CAR generally necessitates immediate surgical repair due to its acute nature.

Long-term management aims to prevent recurrence and manage symptoms through medical therapy, cardiac rehabilitation, and psychological support, with regular follow-up and imaging. SCAD patients generally have a favourable prognosis, though recurrence is possible, especially in those with fibromuscular dysplasia or hormonal factors. CAR survivors can have good outcomes but remain at risk for complications.

Despite significant progress in the clinical characterisation of SCAD through international efforts to register, assess, and follow up with patients, the pathophysiology remains poorly understood, and there is no specific disease-modifying therapy despite a significant recurrence risk. Current international efforts are concentrated on building large, prospectively recruited multicentre cohorts, phenotyped with advanced imaging for pathophysiological (including genetic) and clinical studies. Prospective studies, including ultimately randomised trials, are needed to evaluate the best medical therapies (such as the role and duration of antiplatelet therapy, the use of beta-blockers, and other secondary prevention drugs), as well as the optimal coronary intervention strategies.

Funding No funds, grants, or other support was received.

References

Abu-Hmeidan JH, Arrowaili AI, Yousef RS et al (2016) Coronary artery rupture in blunt thoracic trauma: a case report and review of literature. J Cardiothorac Surg 11:1–6

Adlam D, Alfonso F, Maas A, Vrints C (2018) European Society of Cardiology, acute cardiovascular care association, SCAD study group: a position paper on spontaneous coronary artery dissection. Eur Heart J 39:3353–3368

Appleby CE, Barolet A, Ing D et al (2009) Contemporary management of pregnancy-related coronary artery dissection: a single-centre experience and literature review. Exp Clin Cardiol 14:e8

Codsi E, Tweet MS, Rose CH et al (2016) Spontaneous coronary artery dissection in pregnancy: what every obstetrician should know. Obstet Gynecol 128:731–738

Elendu C, Amaechi DC, Elendu TC et al (2023) Comprehensive review of aortic aneurysms, dissections, and cardiovascular complications in connective tissue disorders. Medicine 102:e36499

Kadian-Dodov D, Gornik HL, Gu X et al (2016) Dissection and aneurysm in patients with fibromuscular dysplasia: findings from the US Registry for FMD. J Am Coll Cardiol 68:176–185

Libby P (2021) The changing landscape of atherosclerosis. Nature 592:524–533

Longobardi A, Iesu S, Baldi C et al (2017) Spontaneous coronary artery rupture presenting as an acute coronary syndrome evolved in pseudoaneurysm and cardiac tamponade: case report and literature review. Eur Heart J Acute Cardiovasc Care 6:666–669

McGrath-Cadell L, McKenzie P, Emmanuel S et al (2016) Outcomes of patients with spontaneous coronary artery dissection. Open Heart 3:e000491

Nagalli S, Hajouli S (2020) Coronary artery perforation

Olin JW, Gornik HL, Bacharach JM et al (2014) Fibromuscular dysplasia: state of the science and critical unanswered questions: a scientific statement from the American Heart Association. Circulation 129:1048–1078

Saw J, Aymong E, Sedlak T et al (2014) Spontaneous coronary artery dissection: association with predisposing arteriopathies and precipitating stressors and cardiovascular outcomes. Circ Cardiovasc Interv 7:645–655

Saw J, Humphries K, Aymong E et al (2017) Spontaneous coronary artery dissection: clinical outcomes and risk of recurrence. J Am Coll Cardiol 70:1148–1158

Saw J, Mancini GBJ, Humphries K et al (2016a) Angiographic appearance of spontaneous coronary artery dissection with intramural hematoma proven on intracoronary imaging. Catheter Cardiovasc Interv 87:E54–E61

Saw J, Mancini GBJ, Humphries KH (2016b) Contemporary review on spontaneous coronary artery dissection. J Am Coll Cardiol 68:297–312

Saw J, Starovoytov A, Aymong E et al (2022) Canadian spontaneous coronary artery dissection cohort study: 3-year outcomes. J Am Coll Cardiol 80:1585–1597

Tweet MS, Hayes SN, Codsi E et al (2017) Spontaneous coronary artery dissection associated with pregnancy. J Am Coll Cardiol 70:426–435

Tweet MS, Hayes SN, Pitta SR et al (2012) Clinical features, management, and prognosis of spontaneous coronary artery dissection. Circulation 126:579–588

Yagyu T, Noguchi T, Asano Y et al (2023) Association between genetic diagnosis and clinical outcomes in patients with heritable thoracic aortic disease. J Am Heart Assoc 12:e028625

Emergency Aortic Valve Replacement

Vinci Naruka, Derek Brinster, and Omar A. Jarral

Abstract Emergency aortic valve replacement (AVR) is a critical intervention for life-threatening conditions for patients with haemodynamic instability, acute heart failure, or cardiogenic shock that cannot be managed medically. Emergency AVR has significantly higher risks than elective procedures due to instability of patients and limited preoperative optimisation. This chapter will explore emergency AVR in the context of three major clinical indications: infective endocarditis, critical aortic stenosis, and severe acute aortic regurgitation. It explores indications, preoperative planning, surgical techniques, and outcomes, emphasising the importance of multidisciplinary management for improving procedural success and survival of critically ill patients.

Keywords Emergency cardiac surgery · Infective endocarditis · Aortic valve replacement · Balloon aortic valvuloplasty · Transcatheter aortic valve replacement (TAVR) · Critical aortic stenosis · Decompensated aortic stenosis · Prosthetic valve thrombosis · Acute aortic regurgitation · Annular rupture · TAVR explantation · TAVR migration

1 Introduction

Emergency aortic valve replacement (AVR) is a critical surgical intervention undertaken in life-threatening situations where failure to replace the aortic valve within 24 h of diagnosis would lead to imminent death or irreversible organ damage.

V. Naruka (✉)
St Bartholomew's Hospital, Barts Heart Centre, London, UK
e-mail: vinci.naruka@nhs.net

D. Brinster · O. A. Jarral
Lenox Hill Hospital, Northwell Cardiovascular Institute, New York, NY, USA
e-mail: dbrinster@northwell.edu; ojarral@northwell.edu

A. Kourliouros (ed.), *Emergency Cardiac Surgery*,
https://doi.org/10.1007/978-3-032-15787-4_9

Acute decompensation and the rapid progression of the aortic valve disease would present with haemodynamic instability, severe heart failure or cardiogenic shock, which cannot be managed by medical therapy alone.

Emergency AVR outcomes differ significantly from elective procedures, primarily due to the critical state of patients presenting at the time of surgery. The risk of complications, including early mortality and prolonged hospital stays, is markedly higher in emergency settings. Despite advancements in surgical techniques and perioperative care, the urgency of the procedure often limits the ability to optimise the patient's condition beforehand or investigate thoroughly the aetiology of the decompensation, which contributes to the increased procedural risk. Nevertheless, with appropriate surgical strategies and multidisciplinary management, favourable outcomes can still be achieved in selected patients, particularly when intervention is performed promptly.

Given the inherent challenges in conducting randomised clinical trials for emergency scenarios, for some of the cases, clear guidelines for managing critical cases requiring emergency AVR are often limited. Much of the current recommendations are derived from observational studies and expertise of specialised centres. Consequently, decision-making in these emergencies often relies on clinical judgement and the experience of multidisciplinary teams rather than standardised protocols.

This chapter will explore emergency AVR in the context of three major clinical indications: infective endocarditis (IE), critical aortic stenosis, and severe acute aortic regurgitation (AR). Each of these conditions represents a distinct pathophysiological challenge, requiring a tailored approach to surgical intervention, which is crucial to understand for optimising surgical outcomes.

Infective endocarditis often involves destruction of the valve and surrounding tissue, increasing the complexity of valve replacement and the risk of postoperative complications. Critical aortic stenosis is characterised by an abrupt narrowing of the valve orifice and thus diminished cardiac output, resulting from prosthetic valve thrombosis or from a sudden decompensation of the aortic stenosis manifesting as acute heart failure or life-threatening cardiogenic shock. Severe acute AR resulting from acute aortic dissection or from iatrogenic complications from catheter-based cardiac interventions leads to rapid volume overload of the left ventricle, precipitating into acute heart failure.

This chapter aims to provide a detailed dive into emergency AVR, focusing on the clinical indications for intervention, preoperative planning, surgical techniques, and outcomes associated with each of these critical conditions. By analysing the latest evidence and exploring key considerations in the management of patients undergoing emergency aortic valve replacement, this chapter will offer valuable insights for clinicians managing these complex and high-risk cases.

2 Acute Endocarditis

Infective endocarditis (IE) is a fatal disease from microorganisms colonising the valvular structures of the heart and manifesting with a wide variety of symptoms. Infective endocarditis of the aortic valve require prompt recognition and intervention should not be delayed especially when meeting criteria for emergency surgery. The in-hospital mortality for IE is 15–20%, rising to 40% at 1-year (Otto et al. 2021).

Infective endocarditis patients require a multidisciplinary team approach (Endocarditis Team) which includes infectious disease specialists, cardiologists, cardiac surgeons, radiologist, and other specialists like neurology and nephrology when required.

2.1 Indications

EACTS/ESC infective endocarditis guidelines (2023) define emergency surgery as within 24 h of diagnosis, while urgent as within 3–5 days and non-urgent as within the same hospital admission (Delgado et al. 2023). The complex decision making for timing and whether a high risk patient should be offered an operation should be determined after a detailed discussion with the experienced Endocarditis Team.

There are three main reasons for undergoing surgery in acute IE: heart failure, uncontrolled infection, and prevention of septic embolisation. A significant proportion of surgical intervention for IE are performed on an urgent basis.

Emergency aortic valve surgery for native or prosthetic valve IE is only recommended (Class I) for patients presenting with heart failure including from severe acute regurgitation, obstruction, fistula causing refractory pulmonary oedema, or cardiogenic shock (Anguera et al. 2005; Nadji et al. 2009; Pericàs et al. 2021). Surgery for PVE follows the general principles and indications as of the native valve endocarditis (Delgado et al. 2023).

Patients with IE complicated by heart failure frequently present with reduced left ventricular ejection fraction, larger vegetations size, perivalvular abscesses, pseudoaneurysms, and leaflet rupture or perforation causing new severe valvular regurgitation (Kiefer et al. 2011; Mir et al. 2022). Cardiogenic shock can be the primary presentation in up to 5% of cases (Pericàs et al. 2021).

Heart failure presentation in the context of IE is independently associated with poor in-hospital and 1-year survival, and surgery is the only treatment to improve such survival (Kiefer et al. 2011; Pericàs et al. 2021; Bohbot et al. 2022). Emergency surgery may be indicated in patients with IE presenting with heart failure with NYHA IV and new onset of elevated filling pressures, pulmonary hypertension, and/or pericardial effusions irrespective of infection status or length of antibiotic treatment (Habib et al. 2010).

A more detailed presentation of the indications, timing, and preoperative planning in infective endocarditis is available in Chapter "Emergency Surgery for Infective Endocarditis".

2.2 Operative Considerations

The principle objectives of IE surgery are to prevent additional embolic events, debride and remove all the infected tissue and foreign material in case of PVE, and restore the valvular function while maintaining the cardiac integrity.

To achieve adequate exposure of the aortic valve for potential extensive debridement, the gold standard approach is via median sternotomy for both native valve endocarditis (NVE) and PVE. Ministernotomy and right thoracotomy would provide insufficient exposure and compromise on the main objective of the operation, thus are not recommended.

Myocardial protection is critical for both NVE and PVE as the operations can be long and complex. This can be achieved via direct anterograde cardioplegia into the root followed by intermittent coronary ostia cardioplegia delivery. Some surgeons might want to insert an additional retrograde cardioplegia into the coronary sinus. The cardioplegia solution utilised should be at the discretion of the surgeon and their familiarity with it. The key aspect is to ensure a perfect myocardial protection throughout the operation. We advise unnecessary cardiac manipulation before the heart is arrested.

2.3 Native Aortic Valve Endocarditis

In patients with isolated native aortic valve IE, institution of cardiopulmonary bypass should be performed centrally with the standard arterial line towards the arch of the aorta and the venous line into the right atrium towards the inferior vena cava. Bicaval venous cannulation might be warranted in case of endocarditis involving the mitral valve apparatus.

For infections that are limited to the native aortic valve cusps or leaflets, the aortic valve is explored through an oblique aortotomy at the level of the fatpad towards the non-coronary cusp. Complete removal of the native infected valve using "dirty" noncardiotomy suckers should be performed. This is followed by generous irrigation followed by change of contaminated surgical instruments and gloves before handling the new prosthetic valve.

Replacement with a biological or mechanical valve prosthesis is performed according to similar principles as for the non-endocarditis valve surgery. There is no evidence that there is superiority in bioprosthetic to a mechanical valve in patients with active IE (Hammermeister et al. 2000; Byrne et al. 2011). The valve choice follows similar principles as standard valve replacement including taking in consideration patient age, comorbidities, life expectancy and their compliance to anticoagulation. However, in patients who have suffered neurological complications preoperatively or are critically unwell with high risk of anticoagulation-related complications, a biological valve might be better suited. On rare occasions, if there is limited vegetation that resulted in a cusp defect after its removal, repair of the aortic valve with autologous pericardial patch could be enough to restore valvular structure and function (Cohn and Adams 2018). However, if this is not adequate, replacement of the valve must be attempted.

If the infected tissues are more extensive than just the cusps and leaflets, such as involving the annulus, more radical debridement and thus reconstruction might be required. All infected tissues need to be unroofed, opened and cleared out including any necrotic tissues and vegetations without jeopardising the structural integrity around the valve (Pettersson et al. 2014b). Caution is required while debriding and avoiding injuries to coronary arteries, sacrifice healthy left ventricular outflow tract (LVOT) muscle or jeopardising the function of the mitral valve. Reconstruction around the aortic root can be performed by utilising autologous pericardium or bovine pericardium (Pettersson et al. 2014b; Hussain et al. 2014). If more extensive reconstruction is required then aortic root replacement is our preferred choice. In these cases, we ensure all infected tissue is removed, coronary buttons are mobilised and the root is replaced using aortic homografts or mechanical valve conduits or bioprosthetic valve inside a dacron graft. Despite extensive debridement, the LVOT is almost always preserved (Pettersson et al. 2014b) and it is anastomosed to the allograft (proximal anastomosis) at the level of the mitral-aortic intervalvular fibrosa and base of the anterior mitral leaflets and the two trigones.

2.3.1 Prosthetic Aortic Valve Endocarditis

Surgery for PVE follow the generic principles outlined for approaching native valve endocarditis. However, there is additional complexity regarding access to the prosthetic aortic valve as a redo operation and the increased periprosthetic tissue destruction from IE.

In case of emergencies such as in cardiogenic shock, a thorough preoperative planning might not be completed due to the deteriorating condition of the critically unwell patient. In case of redo operation and no CT chest for re-entry planning, it would be advisable to foresee potential resternotomy complications and take the necessary precautions. It would be advisable to perform peripheral femoral cannulation prior to resternotomy to pre-empt any re-entry injury during an emergency and already a critically ill patient.

Dense adhesions are often present around previous suturing sites including aortototomy and right atrium which should be carefully dissected and tissues mobilised while on cardiopulmonary bypass if risks of injury are high. After the redo aortotomy, a meticulous and radical debridement of the infected material is necessary, including also the sutures and pledgetts that were utilised.

In PVE, the infection can extend around the sewing ring and annulus circumference and further develop more posteriorly as a large root abscess. The extension of the abscess can affect the atrioventricular node causing heart block (Pettersson et al. 2014b). Surgically, aortic PVE requires extensive debridement and the surgeon should be prepared for a root replacement similar to the native valve as described above. Similarly, if the root abscess extends deeper and involves the mitral valve, one needs to be prepared for a more extensive operation (Pettersson et al. 2014b).

2.3.2 Double Valve Endocarditis

In case of separate vegetation lesions in the mitral and aortic valve without extensive destruction of the mitral-aortic intervalvular fibrosa tissue (MAIVF), separate replacements of each valve can be performed as usual practice. However, if there is destruction of the MAIVF, more often seen in PVE, a more challenging operation (Commando procedure) is required and the right expertise should be available (De Oliveira et al. 2005; Pettersson et al. 2014a). To gain better exposure of the MAIVF, the left atriotomy incision for the mitral valve can be extended towards the dome of the left atrium. After careful debridement and thorough irrigation of the operative field, the mitral valve prosthesis is implanted first, with posterior valvular sutures inserted from one trigone towards the other covering two thirds of the mitral valve circumference. The MAIVF is then reconstructed using a double-layered autologous or bovine pericardium, with the folded patch sutured to the mitral valve prosthesis ring and anchored to the two trigones (De Oliveira et al. 2005; Pettersson et al. 2014a). The lower pericardium sheet is used to close the dome of the left atrium while the upper layers to reconstruct the aortic root (De Oliveira et al. 2005; Pettersson et al. 2014a). The aortic valve prosthesis is implanted and sutured to the native aortic annulus and the reconstructed MAIVF. It is critical to pay attention to the corners by the central fibrous body and the lateral trigone to ensure that they are sealed and under no tension to prevent tears or leaks (De Oliveira et al. 2005; Pettersson et al. 2014a; Jiang et al. 2020).

2.3.3 TAVR Endocarditis

Treatment options for TAVR IE are complicated by the fact that these patients are older and with significant comorbidities than native valve endocarditis or PVE patients. Similar to PVE, cardiac surgery is the best treatment option for TAVR IE with severe heart failure or prosthetic failure; however it is infrequently performed. Surgery is only performed in around 20% of cases (Regueiro et al. 2016; Mentias et al. 2020) due to some prohibitive surgical risk and potential difficulties with the removal of the TAVR. To date, all studies but one have failed to demonstrate the potential benefits of surgery in IE post TAVR (Regueiro et al. 2016; Mangner et al. 2018; Mentias et al. 2020).

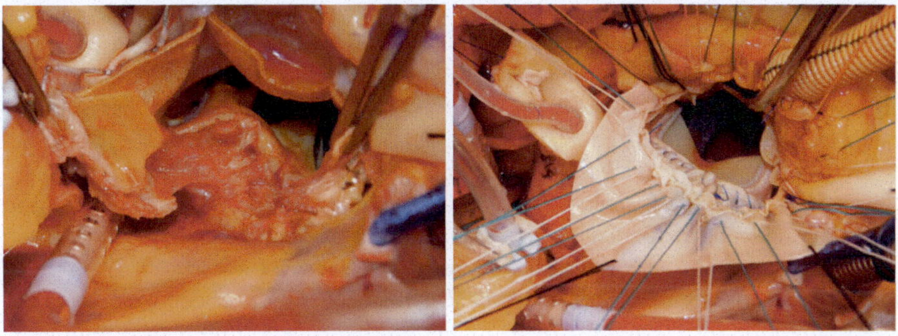

Fig. 1 TAVR endocarditis with extensive destruction of the aortomitral curtain (left). Followed by radical debridement, Commando procedure performed with prosthetic mitral valve in place with patch reconstruction of the aortomitral curtain and ensuring adequate space for new neo-left ventricular outflow tract (right). (Figure caption from Jarral et al. 2024, licensed under CC-BY 4.0)

TAVR explantation is one of the fastest growing procedure in the STS database and it is projected to increase significantly (Bowdish et al. 2024). Removing these devices requires advanced techniques, and surgeons need to be prepared to do more than just an aortic valve replacement. Some cases will require extensive operations such as aortic root replacement, radical debridement of the aortomitral continuity, commando procedures including Cabrol to the coronary buttons and homograft for recurrent infections (Jarral et al. 2024) (Fig. 1).

The only study that showed benefit included surgical intervention focusing on local infection such as abscess or fistula (Panagides et al. 2022). The decision to proceed with surgery in IE post TAVR must be individualised and focus on balancing risks from surgery, patients characteristics, and prognosis with conservative management (Delgado et al. 2023).

2.3.4 Postoperative Outcomes

Postoperative complications after aortic valve endocarditis surgery are common. Patients behave septic with persistent hypotension requiring significant inotropic support. There is severe coagulopathy from prolonged cardiopulmonary bypass causing bleeding, requiring extensive correction and replenishment of coagulation factors intraoperatively and in the immediate postoperative period in intensive care. Occasionally, despite this, these patients return to theatre for exploration for bleeding. The radical debridement required in some cases due to extensive infection in the subvalvular apparatus, predisposes to increased risk of arrhythmias and heart block requiring permanent pacemaker.

Due to the nature of the disease itself, patients can have a protracted course in intensive care associated with multi-organ support including renal filtration or further neurological events. All patients with infective endocarditis will require prolonged intravenous antibiotics with a standard duration of 6 weeks with ongoing

Endocarditis Team consultations to optimise recovery. However, abscess that extends in the para-valvular areas in the native valve endocarditis (such as annular or root abscess) cannot be cured with antibiotics alone and they would require an operative management with higher mortality rate of ≥40% and heart block (Spiliopoulos et al. 2010).

Despite technological advancements, prompt diagnosis, and improvement in surgical outcomes, patients undergoing aortic valve surgery for infective endocarditis still have high in-hospital mortality of 15–20% and approaching 40% at 1-year (Byrne et al. 2011; AATS Surgical Treatment of Infective Endocarditis Consensus Guidelines Writing Committee Chairs et al. 2017). PVE is associated with increased in-hospital mortality (ranging 20–40%) and morbidity with diminished long term survival (Erdem et al. 2019; Luehr et al. 2020) when compared to native valve endocarditis. Factors such as older age, diabetes mellitus, early PVE with infections from staphylococcus and fungi are associated with poorer prognosis for PVE (Chirouze et al. 2004; Luciani et al. 2017).

High volume centres with more extensive surgical experience for IE, have been reporting lower mortality in hospital at around 8% at 30-day mortality (Manne et al. 2012). This might highlight the importance to centralise to a few high volume expert centres to manage the more complex conditions within infective endocarditis.

3 Critical Aortic Stenosis

Critical aortic valve stenosis represents a serious and life-threatening condition that necessitates prompt evaluation and intervention in acutely ill patients.

Aortic stenosis (AS) is one of the most prominent valvular diseases in the developed countries, affecting up to 10% of the population by the eight decade of life (Iung and Vahanian 2011).

When AS progresses to a critical state, it often presents with rapid onset symptoms such as acute pulmonary oedema, which can lead to decompensation, acute heart failure and eventually cardiogenic shock. These patients require emergency intervention including emergency AVR.

Another group of patients requiring emergency intervention includes those with acute thrombosis of a previously implanted prosthetic aortic valve.

Management of severe symptomatic AS is guided by established international guidelines, yet critically aortic stenosis treatment often relies on insights from specialised centres.

This subsection of the chapter will explore the management of patients with decompensated severe aortic stenosis and prosthetic valve thrombosis. It will cover the indications for intervention, diagnostic approaches, and various management strategies for each, drawing on current guidelines and expert practices to provide a comprehensive overview of these challenging clinical scenarios.

3.1 Indications

3.1.1 Decompensated Aortic Stenosis

Critical aortic stenosis complicated by decompensated features, such as reduced left ventricular function or cardiogenic shock, would warrant an emergency intervention. Patients in this category are at very high risk including extremely poor outcomes and hospital mortality of 59.8% (Buchwald et al. 2001; Lang et al. 2021).

Technological advancements have led to significant progress in managing these critically unwell patients. However, there is limited data from current guidelines for management of patients with severe AS presenting acutely with cardiogenic shock (Nair et al. 2024).

Before the widespread availability of transcatheter aortic valve replacement (TAVR), patients with decompensated severe aortic stenosis were often managed with emergency percutenous balloon aortic valvuloplasty (BAV).

While BAV effectively reduced the transvalvular gradients immediately, a substantial proportion of patients experienced recurrence of significant stenosis due to reduction of aortic valve area within 6 months in 15% of patients (Otto et al. 1994) and up to 80% at 15 months (Letac et al. 1991).

BAV is associated with a high all-cause mortality rate of 33% and cardiovascular-related death of 28.6% after 30 days (Bongiovanni et al. 2018). However, it offers the advantage of being a shorter procedure compared to TAVR, requiring less contrast and utilising smaller sheath sizes (8Fr vs 14-16Fr) (Bongiovanni et al. 2018).

Despite the associated procedural morbidities and mortality, BAV has been employed as a temporary measure for managing severe aortic stenosis complicated with refractory pulmonary oedema or cardiogenic shock (Szerlip et al. 2017; Bongiovanni et al. 2018; Nagao et al. 2018). The rapid relief of afterload in these critically ill patients essentially improves haemodynamics, promoting BAV as an attractive option. In these patients, European and US guidelines recommend BAV use as an effective bridging therapy to surgical aortic valve replacement (AVR) or, more recently, TAVR (Otto et al. 2021, p. 202; Vahanian et al. 2022).

Mortality rate at 6 months has been demonstrated to significantly reduce for critically ill patients undergoing BAV alone (55%) compared if having BAV followed by TAVR or surgical AVR (22.3%) (Ben-Dor et al. 2013). However, more recently BAV is less frequently performed due to higher availability and improving outcomes of TAVR in high risks patients (Szerlip et al. 2017; Bongiovanni et al. 2018; Nagao et al. 2018).

Although TAVR is recognised as the accepted standard of care for frail and high-risk patients with severe AS, randomised trials that assess TAVR efficacy have so far excluded patients presenting with cardiogenic shock (Popma et al. 2014).

The advances in TAVR safety and efficacy over the years have contributed to its widespread use in high-risk patients, although its application in decompensated critical aortic stenosis remains less established. It normally would only require a single exposure risk to contrast agent and the associated bleeding or vascular complications, compared to a two-step procedure and risks for having BAV first as bridge to TAVR. One of the limiting factor includes the emergency nature of acute decompensated aortic stenosis which would preclude the time to perform a pre-TAVR CT scan. This is essential to provide comprehensive valvular and aortic assessment without which there would be increased periprocedural risks.

The 30-day mortality rate for patients with decompensated severe aortic stenosis undergoing TAVR remains elevated between 22.6% and 23.8% and it does not significantly differ when compared to those having BAV alone (Bongiovanni et al. 2018; Wernly et al. 2020).

When only focusing on patients with cardiogenic shock, TAVR has been shown to have acceptable device safety and efficacy (94.1%) and 30-day and 1-year mortality were 11.8% and 25.7%, respectively (Frerker et al. 2016).

Although surgical aortic valve replacement has been considered for these critically unwell patients, in the majority of the cases there are contraindications for surgery given their high risk nature. However, excellent outcomes and improved LV functions at follow-ups have been reported in small number of patients with cardiogenic shock, critical aortic valve area of 0.56 ± 0.13 cm^2 and poor left ventricular function of 20 ± 3%, after undergoing emergency surgical AVR (Christ et al. 1997).

More recently, it has been demonstrated that there is survival advantage for patients undergoing surgical AVR for severe aortic stenosis with acute heart failure compared to conservative management (33% vs 75.3%) but the mortality rate remains overall very high.

Analysis from a large registry of patients with severe aortic stenosis and acute heart failure, revealed that overall patients with acute heart failure undergo AVR less frequently than those with chronic symptoms, and continued to have higher 5-year mortality despite undergoing AVR (Nagao et al. 2018).

However, a comparison of surgical AVR and TAVR in a national registry for patients with acute heart failure and aortic stenosis demonstrated no survival difference at 30 days, 1 and 2 years. The surgical patients had longer acute kidney injury, bleeding, and length of stay compared to TAVR (Jalava et al. 2020).

A recent study compared 2754 patients with cardiogenic shock and severe aortic stenosis, undergoing surgical AVR and TAVR and demonstrated favourable short and long term outcomes with mortality of 16% and 18% respectively (Nair et al. 2024). This was similar if patients underwent BAV first followed by either TAVR or surgical AVR. Meanwhile these critically unwell patients who only underwent medical management or BAV alone, mortality was around 50% in each group (Nair et al. 2024).

A possible strategy for managing patients with severe aortic stenosis and cardiogenic shock could involve first performing a BAV to temporise the critical nature of the condition, allowing to investigate the aetiology of the cardiogenic shock. If patients survive this initial period of instability, definitive AVR may be offered and help in improving treatment course (Nair et al. 2024). In terms of timing, a survival advantage has been demonstrated that performing BAV in patients with cardiogenic shock within 48 h of starting inotropes or diagnosis was associated with lower

1-year mortality compared to those patients delayed over 48 h (59% vs 90%) (Debry et al. 2018).

3.1.2 Prosthetic Valve Thrombosis

Prosthetic valve thrombosis (PVT) is a devastating complication, most commonly observed in patients with mechanical heart valves that are poorly anticoagulated. It can present with rapid onset of symptoms including acute pulmonary oedema. While rare in the developed world, PVT has been reported in up to 6.1% of patients within 6 months of a valve replacement (Talwar et al. 2004). The incidence of PVT has been estimated to be between 0.2% and 6% per patient-year in those with left-sided mechanical valve replacements. Operative mortality rates vary widely from 0% to 69% depending on clinical functional status (Lengyel et al. 1997).

The most frequent clinical presentation was severe congestive heart failure in 44% of cases. Studies have reported that at the time of PVT presentation, the international normalised ratio was less than 2.5 in 54%, with inadequate anticoagulation management in 26% and poor compliance in 26% (Dürrleman et al. 2004).

Valve thrombosis has also been reported with biological heart valves in 4% of patients, with 12% having subclinical leaflet thrombosis (Chakravarty et al. 2017). The latter typically manifests as a hypo-attenuated leaflet thickening with normal or reduced leaflet motion (Vahanian et al. 2022).

Bioprosthetic valve thrombosis is most commonly observed in the first 3 months after implantation. Since the increased use in CT imaging there has been a rise in diagnosing subclinical bioprosthetic valve thrombosis. (Chakravarty et al. 2017). Guidelines advise considering anticoagulation in patients with biological heart valves who have leaflet thickening and reduced leaflet motion causing increased gradients (class IIa) (Vahanian et al. 2022).

In case of non-obstructive valve thrombosis, the aim is to first optimise anticoagulation.

While no clear guidance for prosthetic aortic valve thrombosis is described, ESC guidelines specify that in non-obstructive thrombosis of mechanical mitral valves, the management depends on the occurrence of thromboembolic events despite optimal anticoagulation and a thrombus size larger than 10 mm (Laplace et al. 2004).

For obstructive valve thrombosis, the European Society of Cardiology (ESC) and the ACC/AHA recommend emergency aortic valve replacement in critically ill patients without serious comorbidities or contraindications (class Ib) (Karthikeyan et al. 2013; Otto et al. 2021; Vahanian et al. 2022), while fibrinolytic therapy only if surgery is not available or it has prohibitive risks.

Thrombolysis has been demonstrated to have low success rate and high mortality when performed as the sole primary treatment, and it should be reserved for patients who would not tolerate cardiopulmonary bypass. However, reports suggest its use as a medical bridge to surgery, especially in patients with severe haemodynamic compromise to improve cardiac function and to facilitate transfer to a specialist centre for definitive surgical intervention (Dürrleman et al. 2004).

Table 1 Systemic fibrinolysis versus surgery for prosthetic valve thrombosis (Halperin et al. 2016; Levine et al. 2019; Otto et al. 2021)

Favour fibrinolysis	Favour surgery
High surgical risk	Low surgical risk
Surgical expertise not available	Surgical expertise available
No contraindication to fibrinolysis	Contraindication to fibrinolysis
First episode of valve thrombosis	Recurrent valve thrombosis
Small clot ($\leq$0.8 cm^2)	Large clot (>0.8 cm^2)
Absence of left atrium thrombus	Left atrium thrombus
NYHA class I-III	NYHA class IV
No or mild coronary artery disease	Concomitant coronary artery revascularisation
Absence of additional valve disease	Additional valve disease
Thrombus visualised	Possible pannus
Patient choice	Patient choice

NYHA New York Heart Association

Further supporting evidence for urgent surgery preferred over fibrinolytic therapy for left sided PVT is evidenced by a meta-analysis comparing the two interventions and demonstrating that surgery was associated with significant reduced thrombo-embolism (1.6% vs 16%), major bleeding (1.4–5%) and recurrent PVT (7.1% vs 25.4%) (Karthikeyan et al. 2013) The overall 30-day mortality with surgery for PVT has been reported between 10% and 15% and it is significantly reduces to 5% if patients has better functional status with NYHA I or II (Roudaut et al. 2009; Keuleers et al. 2011; Karthikeyan et al. 2013).

The decision for choosing between surgery or systematic fibrinolysis in the case of obstructive PVT should be individualised to each patient and involve Heart Team (Table 1). It needs to take into account shared-decision making and local expertise, such that if there is absence of surgical expertise, thrombolysis should be considered without delay (Otto et al. 2021).

3.2 *Preoperative Planning*

3.2.1 Decompensated Aortic Stenosis

The classic clinical triad of symptoms progression of severe aortic stenosis include angina, syncope and eventually heart failure. Symptoms of heart failure include dyspnoea (NYHA class $\geq$ 3), pulmonary oedema, lower limb oedema, need for intravenous diuretic administration, paroxysmal nocturnal dyspnoea, jugular vein distension and hepatomegaly (Avvedimento et al. 2023).

This progression to heart failure can be rapid and is associated with very poor prognosis (Tandar and Drakos 2019). Acute decompensation develops over a short period, with patient experiencing a sudden deterioration of symptoms or the onset of new symptoms, in contrast to the more gradual decline seen in chronic heart failure. Acute decompensation in severe aortic stenosis coincides with the need for unplanned hospitalisation and/or urgent intervention, and has been reported in up to 20% of patients with severe AS (Wald et al. 2018).

The diagnosis of cardiogenic shock is usually made with the help of pulmonary artery catheterisation; however, echocardiography may also be used to confirm elevation of left ventricular filling pressures (Giannuzzi et al. 1994).

These critically unwell patients would likely be requiring inotropic support, mechanical ventilation, and additional organ support.

Factors that increase the risk for acute decompensation include female sex, advanced age, history of coronary artery disease, prior episodes of congestive heart failure, anaemia, atrial fibrillation, chronic kidney disease, and oxygen-dependent lung diseases (Kolte et al. 2018).

In patients with stable aortic stenosis, left ventricular ejection fraction (LVEF) is typically reduced as decompensation progresses. However, during acute decompensation, LVEF may remain normal despite impaired cardiac function.

Predicting which patients are likely to experience decompensation from severe aortic stenosis is crucial to guide for timely valve intervention. Recent studies indicate that patients with multiple comorbidities, who are frail and exhibit increased cardiac dysfunction, are at greater risk of acute decompensation associated with aortic stenosis (Patel et al. 2023).

By using cardiovascular magnetic resonance (CMR) imaging, it is possible to quantify cardiac fibrosis, which is associated with microcirculatory dysfunction, reduced global longitudinal strain, and elevated brain natriuretic peptide. All these factors have shown to be diagnostic and predictive for onset of heart failure symptoms (Patel et al. 2023). Assessing these parameters through CMR could prove valuable in predicting when the patient might decompensate from aortic stenosis.

Patients with severe aortic stenosis who present with acute heart failure features have extremely high rates of all cause mortality and heart failure related hospitalisation (Nagao et al. 2018). Recognising early acute heart failure and proposing early strategy for management, might improve clinical outcomes in these critically unwell patients (Nagao et al. 2018).

3.2.2 Prosthetic Valve Thrombosis

PVT should be suspected in patients with mechanical aortic valve that present with clinical manifestations from sequela of thromboembolisms resulting in transient ischemic attack, stroke, or pulmonary embolism.

Both ESC and AHA guidelines recommend using TTE or TOE to confirm the diagnosis for suspected PVT and assess valve function, leaflet motion, and extent of thrombosis (Montorsi et al. 2000; Muratori et al. 2006; Lancellotti et al. 2016). Further data on estimated pulmonary pressures, left ventricular size, and systolic function are also informative (Barbetseas et al. 1998).

Diagnosis of PVT includes confirming presence of abnormally elevated velocity or gradients across the prosthetic valve with either limited leaflet motions or presence of thrombus. Obstruction of the prosthetic valve is defined when the mean transvalvular gradient increases by more than 50% from baseline or an increase of more than 10 mmHg across the aortic prosthesis (Otto et al. 2021).

Additionally, it is important to distinguish features between thrombus and pannus when occurring after a prosthetic mechanical valve and their distinct echocardiographic appearances.

Pannus formation typically occurs several years after mechanical valve replacement and symptoms develop gradually over extended periods. In comparison, thrombi may occur at any time and tend to present more acutely. Pannus is more frequently described in the aortic position (70% vs 21%) (Barbetseas et al. 1998). Inadequate anticoagulation with warfarin and acute presentations from PVT should raise suspicion of thrombus instead.

Further distinction between the two can be more accurately assessed by TOE. Thrombosis is suspected in presence of thickened valve leaflets and an increased gradient across the valve. Thrombus also tends to have larger and more mobile characteristics compared to pannus which tends to be more circumferential and growing inward from the valve annulus (Barbetseas et al. 1998). An additional key distinguishing feature is the lower video intensity of the thrombus compared to pannus. In a patient who is febrile and raised infection markers with a background of prosthetic valve, endocarditis must be excluded and TOE would help assessing presence of any mobile vegetations.

The acoustic shadowing from mechanical prosthesis can limit the accurate description of the valve when solely relying on TTE or TOE. Multidetector CT scans can provide additional insights into the causes of prosthetic valve obstruction that constitute indications for surgery, that were missed on echocardiograms or fluoroscopy (Symersky et al. 2009). Cardiac CT scans have been shown to have added diagnostic value (Suh et al. 2016). Fluoroscopy can also be used to visualise leaflet motion in aortic mechanical prosthetic valves and to identify intermittent obstruction, although this might require prolonged periods of observation (Suchá et al. 2015).

3.3 *Operative Considerations*

3.3.1 Decompensated Aortic Stenosis

Treatment of decompensated aortic stenosis can be challenging and it is burdened with higher rates of early mortality. The time from symptoms onset of the acute deterioration to actual treatment is a critical determinant of prognosis (Debry et al. 2018).

Management of cardiogenic shock and decompensated aortic stenosis should be tailored to the individual patient's condition, with initial emphasis placed on haemodynamic stabilisation achieved through pharmacological interventions.

Following stabilisation, percutaneous BAV or TAVR or mechanical circulatory support may be considered as a potential intervention in an emergency setting. If the patient remains stable during this critical state, surgical aortic valve replacement, when feasible, represents the definitive treatment and has been associated with a reduction in mortality (Nair et al. 2024).

Medical Therapy

Initial resuscitative measures are critical for stabilising the critically unwell patient with key objectives including the prevention of tachycardia, optimisation of preload, and maintenance of adequate blood pressure. While ventilatory support may be necessary, intubation should be avoided when possible, as it can exacerbate hypotension.

The use of loop diuretics can effectively reduce fluid retention and alleviate pulmonary congestion in acute scenarios. However, in cases of severe aortic stenosis which is characterised by fixed outflow obstruction, diuretics may lead to excessive intravascular volume depletion, resulting in decreased preload and cardiac output. This, in turn, can precipitate hypotension and peripheral hypoperfusion (Avvedimento et al. 2023).

In cardiogenic shock, the resulting hypotension is managed by administering vasopressors and inotropes which help improving tissue perfusion. However, the resulting vasoconstriction in the context of critical aortic stenosis can increase myocardial oxygen consumption and aggravate myocardial ischaemia. In these settings, there might be a benefit in using levosimendan, which acts a calcium sensitising agent with inotropic and vasodilatory action without affecting oxygen requirement. Despite its use in patients with acute heart failure from severe aortic stenosis and reduced ejection fraction, has been associated with improving haemodynamics and cardiac function, the overall experience is still limited (García-González et al. 2015). IV levosimendan significantly increased cardiac output and decreased filling pressure in decompensated heart failure as demonstrated in large, double-blind, randomised trials and after cardiac surgery in smaller trials (Cohn and Adams 2018). Lastly a perioperative use of pulmonary artery catheter is recommended in patients with cardiogenic shock (class I) and haemodynamic instability (class IIa) as it derives means of calculating cardiac output and left ventricular end diastolic pressure, a marker of LV preload (Lawton et al. 2022).

Balloon Aortic Valvuloplasty (BAV)

Percutaneous balloon aortic valvuloplasty (BAV) was first described by Cribier in 1986 as an alternative to surgical AVR in elderly and/or high-risk patients with symptomatic aortic stenosis (Cribier et al. 1986). This was later employed for patient presented with cardiogenic shock, demonstrating significant improvement in cardiac index and transvalvular gradients. However, its widespread adoption was limited due to unfavourable factors such as a high incidence of early restenosis and elevated in-hospital mortality rates (Otto et al. 1994).

In acute presentations, such as cardiogenic shock, BAV serves as a viable "bail-out" treatment option, especially when clinical information or pre-procedural imaging is insufficient to ensure the safety of TAVR (Otto et al. 2021). Moreover, BAV may be considered a reasonable bridging option to definitive surgical valve replacement (Otto et al. 2021).

BAV is typically conducted by interventional cardiologists in hospitals equipped with cardiothoracic and vascular surgical teams to manage potential complications (Williams and Hildick-Smith 2020).

Preprocedural imaging is essential for assessing the size of the aortic annulus and selecting the appropriate valvuloplasty balloon. Echocardiographic balloon sizing often results in the selection of smaller balloons, as measurements are taken along the anteroposterior axis, representing the minor diameter of the annulus. However, in emergency situations, cardiac CT may not be feasible due to the critical illness.

The procedure is typically performed via the femoral approach under local anaesthesia with conscious sedation. Ultrasound guidance is recommended for identifying the safe puncture site within the common femoral artery. If a CT scan of the peripheral arterial vasculature is performed for preoperative planning, it might help in selecting adequate access sites. A pigtail catheter is inserted and advanced to the aortic root under fluoroscopy. The annulus is then visualised by injecting contrast and performing an aortogram. A catheter with a floating tip is advanced into the aortic root, across the aortic valve orifice, and into the left ventricle (LV). Rapid pacing is briefly initiated, with the goal of reducing blood pressure to $\leq$60 mmHg for a sufficient duration to allow for the inflation and deflation of the valvuloplasty balloon (Williams and Hildick-Smith 2020).

The pressure gradient between the left ventricle and the aorta is typically reassessed after the operator determines that sufficient dilation has been achieved. Aortic regurgitation can be evaluated through aortography, analysis of left ventricular and aortic pressure waveforms, as well as echocardiography.

Transcatheter AVR (TAVR)

In cases of acute clinical decompensation due to aortic stenosis, several key considerations must be taken into account when performing TAVR.

For instance, to expedite the procedure and minimise the use of contrast agents, a pre-procedural CT scan for evaluating vascular access and aortic valve anatomy may be bypassed. Instead, transoesophageal echocardiography can serve as an alternative imaging modality for assessing valve anatomy and guiding prosthesis selection in cases of emergency (Williams and Hildick-Smith 2020).

Procedural volume may significantly influence clinical outcomes. An analysis of more than 25,000 procedures revealed a direct correlation between hospital TAVR volumes and the frequency of urgent or emergent cases outcomes. High-volume hospitals demonstrated markedly lower rates of in-hospital mortality, stroke, and other complications, underscoring the impact of procedural experience on patient outcomes (Bansal et al. 2021).

The procedure should adhere to standardised local protocols, by implementing measures that minimise further haemodynamic instability or complications in these critically unwell patients. Special attention should be given to limiting rapid pacing duration, reducing the risk of residual paravalvular leakage by optimising valve positioning, and ensuring effective haemostasis at the vascular access site (Avvedimento et al. 2023). Continuous monitoring of vital parameters and renal function in the intensive care unit is advised for a minimum of 24–48 h post-procedure (Avvedimento et al. 2023).

Mechanical Circulatory Support

Although evidence supporting their efficacy is limited, escalation to mechanical circulatory support (MCS) devices may be considered in patients having refractory shock. Such devices include the intra-aortic balloon pump (IABP), extracorporeal membrane oxygenation (ECMO) and the Impella system (Abiomed, Inc., Danvers, Massachusetts) which can be brought out through a 10 mm graft from the ascending aorta (Avvedimento et al. 2023). Once considered a contraindication, the Impella device use in severe aortic stenosis has been proven feasible and demonstrates promising results in selected patients who are high risk and in cardiogenic shock (Singh et al. 2018).

These devices aid in reducing left ventricular workload and myocardial oxygen demand while ensuring adequate systemic and coronary perfusion, thereby facilitating prompt haemodynamic stabilisation.

Some technical factors must be considered when selecting an appropriate MCS device. Severe AR and right ventricular failure represents unfavourable conditions for MCS, as it would increase afterload, causing LV dilation, increased filling pressure, and pulmonary congestion. IABP are also contraindicated in aortic disease (Villablanca et al. 2021).

Access site must be also considered and severe calcifications of the peripheral arterial vessels might preclude from inserting ECMO lines or IABP. In case of emergency, having a pre-existing access during TAVR would facilitate insertion of ECMO cannulas over the same wire in the femoral artery.

A systematic evaluation of MCS performance in patients who underwent TAVR revealed significantly rising total hospital costs, extended hospital stay and increased risk of early mortality (Alkhalil et al. 2019). It is crucial to recognise that these concerning findings could be attributed to the critical baseline conditions of these patients, for whom MCS was typically employed as a last-resort intervention.

Surgical Aortic Valve Replacement

Surgical aortic valve replacement in the setting of acute decompensated aortic stenosis or in cardiogenic shock is becoming a limited option given the high procedural risks involved. Important consideration around emergency surgical aortic valve replacements would include optimising periprocedural and anaesthetic risks such as worsening hypotension that could lead to periarrest during induction. The application of defibrillator pads to the patient is advisable. Clear operative strategy is essential to expedite management in such critical scenario.

In addition, a standard median sternotomy with conventional cannulation techniques familiar to the operating surgeon should be employed. It is crucial to utilise optimal cardioplegia strategies to protect the heart effectively. Minimising cross-clamp and cardiopulmonary bypass times will also be advantageous for the patient.

The use of rapid deployment valves such as the Edwards Intuity (Edwards Lifesciences LLC, Irvine, CA) in patients requiring emergency aortic valve replacement has been investigated. These rapidly deployed valves are usually associated with shorter cross clamp time with the advantage of performing annular decalcification before implantation (Kocher et al. 2013). Additionally, the Edwards Intuity valve offers the advantage of very low transvalvular gradients and large effective orifice areas 1-year post-implantation (Kocher et al. 2013).

An additional benefit favouring emergency surgery directly is that no additional diagnostic studies such as CT TAVI would be required, thus reducing any delays for critically ill patients. Intraoperative trans oesophageal echocardiogram would be normally performed for valvular assessment including when coming off cardiopulmonary bypass. If the patient requires emergency surgical aortic valve replacement, the surgeon should be prepared to utilise mechanical assist devices in the event of difficulty weaning from cardiopulmonary bypass.

3.3.2 Prosthetic Valve Thrombosis

Percutaneous Transcatheter Manipulation

Percutaneous transcatheter manipulation of the obstructed mechanical valve has emerged as a potential viable option in patients who fail thrombolytic therapy and are experiencing cardiogenic shock and face prohibitive risks from redo surgery (Soria Jiménez et al. 2023).

This approach might serve as an option for patients presenting in critical conditions, and may offer a temporary therapy as a bridge therapy to subsequent redo surgery. While this technique is not part of guidelines for management of PVT, it has been shown to be safe and effective in small number of cases who fall in the above scenarios. Techniques that have been reported include manipulation of the thrombosed mechanical valve in both aortic and mitral position by using different wires, catheters, and balloons resulting in clinical improvement (Jabbour et al. 1996; Hariram 2014).

Redo Surgery

In emergency cases, redo surgery options are considered in case of prosthetic mechanical valve thrombosis, but it is crucial to balance benefits and associated risks on a case-by-case basis. Careful perioperative planning and Heart Team discussion help to select patients who would benefit from this intervention. In fact, patients presenting with NYHA IV symptoms face a significantly higher perioperative mortality risk of 17.5% compared to 4.7% for those presenting with NYHA II (Deviri et al. 1991). Moreover, undergoing emergency re-operations represents one of the most ominous risk factor and is consistently associated with high early mortality rates ranging from 25% to 44% (Bortolotti et al. 1987). Therefore, it is advisable to perform a detailed consenting of the procedure including benefits and risks and involve patient and next of kin. Emergency redo operations patients carry not only high intraoperative risks but also protracted recovery. During this, patients might require prolonged intensive care stay and need to be consented for potential tracheostomy and feeding tube strategies for optimising nutrition postoperatively.

Redo operations in themselves carry additional operative risks in already critically unwell patients. Optimal preoperative planning is imperative to ensure good outcomes.

Preoperative imaging such as CT scans is the modality of choice to assess relationships of vital structures such as the right ventricle, the aorta, or coronary grafts from previous CABG, to the posterior aspect of the sternum. These structures are at high risk of injury on re-entry. In such cases, exposure of femoral vessels in preparation for emergency femoral-femoral CPB is highly advisable before resternotomy. In particular, it might be a strategy to just insert the percutenous sheaths in the femoral vessels without yet cannulating, but have the CPB lines divided and ready to be connected for rapid cannulation if there is major bleeding on resternotomy. Placement of defibrillator pads before preparing the patient provides additional layer of safety.

The use of oscillating saw should be used to divide the anterior sternal table and reduce risks of injuring structures. Posterior sternal table is normally divided by combination of retraction, scissors, diathermy and opening the pleural spaces. The pericardial dissection plane can be developed by starting at the cardiophrenic angle, advancing slowly cephalad and laterally on the surface of the right heart (Cohn and Adams 2018). Further dissections are then carried around the superior vena cava and the right atrial appendage which often has dense adhesions. Central cannulation sites should be freed of adhesions including around the aorta where re-aortotomy would be performed. If not proceeding for peripheral CPB, aiming to free the dense adhesions around the central cannulation sites first and commencing CPB, would reduce risks of uncontrolled sudden bleeding from additional tissue dissections. Thus, repair of great vessels injury or severe RV injuries are best done when on CPB. These major haemorrhage events often occur at the time of reopening due to severe dense adhesions of the heart or great vessels to the posterior sternum. This incidence of acute bleeding during resternotomy is between 2% and 6% (Wideman et al. 1981; Cohn and Adams 2018).

When major haemorrhage does occur on sternal entry, attempts of resternotomy should be abandoned, the chest should be re-approximated towards the midline, the patient should be heparinised and immediate femoral arterial and venous cannulation should be performed (Cohn and Adams 2018). The blood loss from the resternotomy injury should be aspirated with cardiotomy suction and returned to the CPB pump. Once bypass is established peripherally, the core temperature should be cooled down, flow rates should be reduced for less than a minute and any underlying causative injury should be repaired under direct vision (Dobell and Jain 1984).

Once redo aortotomy is performed, surgical options include valve thrombectomy or redo replacement of the aortic valve. The latter has the advantage to potentially replace older generation valves which are more thrombogenic with newer designs for definitive treatment (Cohn and Adams 2018). When performing redo operations for PVT, the ventricular cavity should be also inspected with a videothoracoscope. Mortality rate of either procedure is reported to be approximately 10–15%, with rate of recurrent thrombosis following de-clotting and thrombectomy occurring in up to 40% of patients (Dürrleman et al. 2004).

Studies have reported that the time interval between the first valve replacement to PVT is around 39 months and patients undergoing emergency surgery have a 30-day operative mortality and total in-hospital mortality of 25% and 41% respectively. The 10-year survival after PVT has been reported as 46 ± 10% (Dürrleman et al. 2004).

Valve thrombectomy is performed in patients with fresh thrombi associated with recent changes in the anticoagulation management, while valve replacement is performed in all other patients.

Existing recommendations advise performing emergency surgery in most patients with PVT with the shortest feasible delay between diagnosis and intervention (Dürrleman et al. 2004).

The risk of re-thrombosis is multifactorial and is closely related to the underlying aetiology of initial thrombotic events. If thrombosis of the prosthetic valve occurred despite strict adherence to INR targets, consultation with a haematologist is recommended to evaluate any hypercoagulable states before deciding on future INR goals or revising anticoagulation strategy (Dürrleman et al. 2004). Additionally, consideration should be given to whether a bioprosthetic valve might be more appropriate in this case. If patient compliance with the medication at long term is an issue, a bioprosthetic valve should be implanted.

Postoperative care often involves close outpatient follow-up with repeat echocardiogram on regular basis and by haemotalogist if necessary. The most common precipitating factors for valve thrombosis are inadequate anticoagulation and poor patient compliance, underscoring the need for both patient- and physician-oriented education. Decisions regarding anticoagulation strategies and choice of second valve prosthesis should be discussed with the patients and require a multidisciplinary team approach in helping patients making informed decisions.

4 Acute Aortic Regurgitation

Acute aortic regurgitation (AR) can manifest with sudden abnormalities of the aortic valve, leading to rapid clinical decline that necessitates emergency surgical intervention.

Acute AR results in sudden aortic valve incompetence, causing immediate volume overload in an unprepared left ventricle that is normal in size. This rapid overload, without adequate time for ventricular remodelling, results in a dramatic increase in left ventricle diastolic pressure which can lead to pulmonary congestion, reduced forward cardiac output and eventually cardiogenic shock. In acute AR the lower aortic diastolic pressure and the higher myocardial oxygen demand results in impaired coronary blood flow in diastole leading to exacerbation of myocardial ischaemia.

4.1 Indications

The most common causes of primary acute AR of the native valve include bacterial endocarditis where destruction of the valve leaflets causes severe regurgitation (discussed within this chapter) and acute aortic dissection (see Chapter "Management of Acute Aortic Dissection"). Less common causes include blunt force chest trauma, spontaneous rupture of congenital fenestrations, and iatrogenic complications from catheter based cardiac interventions, which will be the focus on the following subchapter.

The congenital fenestrations are focal areas of myxomatous degenerations located along the valve commissure line which can rupture and cause severe leaflet dysfunction (Mahara et al. 2017). One of the most relevant catheter-based intervention resulting in acute AR and requiring life-saving emergency cardiac surgery is complications arising during transcatheter aortic valve replacement (TAVR) procedures. Other complications during TAVR, other than acute AR, that require emergency intervention are discussed in Chapter "Emergent Cardiac Surgery Following Transcatheter Aortic Valve Implantation".

Prompt diagnosis, readiness, and swift intervention for acute AR are crucial for improving patient outcomes and can be life-saving.

4.2 Perioperative Considerations

Medical optimisation for acute AR before an emergency intervention can be challenging and must avoid delays before the definitive surgical therapy. Haemodynamic monitoring is recommended for patients in intensive care unit with careful titration of inotropes and vasodilators to optimise cardiac output and end-organ perfusion.

These agents increase the stroke volume, the heart rate and decrease the regurgitation fraction (Voit et al. 2022). Beta blockers are contraindicated in acute severe AR due to the negative inotropic effects causing longer diastole, worsening the severity of AR (Voit et al. 2022). Temporary mechanical support devices such as intra-aortic balloon pumps (IABP) and left ventricular assist devices (LVAD) are not beneficial and contraindicated in acute severe AR. The balloon inflation of the IABP in diastole would worsen the AR, while the efficacy of the LVAD is diminished from the persistent regurgitation of blood into the left ventricle due to an incompetent aortic valve (Voit et al. 2022).

Acute AR with haemodynamic compromise following a TAVR-related complications would most often warrant an emergency cardiac operation and medical therapy is limited. This emergency procedure may be conducted in the hybrid theatre or if time permitted in the standard regular cardiac theatres. Local protocol must be designed and familiarised for such rare and potentially fatal events.

Inducing anaesthesia in a critically unwell patient with severe acute AR is challenging. By reducing the blood pressure further on induction, coronary ischaemia can be exacerbated and worsen the haemodynamic instability (Mokadam et al. 2011). Haemodynamic monitoring, appropriate use of inotropic and anaesthetic agents to prevent tachycardia and hypotension, can help optimise outcomes. Surgeons must be present and scrubbed during induction, ready to operate if the patient has cardiovascular collapse (Mokadam et al. 2011).

Like in all valve operations, perioperative and intraoperative transoeseophageal echocardiogram assessment is helpful to analyse the valve and its characteristics such as number of leaflets, presence of prolapse or fenestrations and to assess size of the aortic root to aid in operative planning.

4.3 Operative Considerations

Prompt surgical intervention in a patient with severe acute AR is lifesaving. Standard median sternotomy is performed followed by initiation of cardiopulmonary bypass through either central or peripheral cannulation, depending on the aetiology of the acute AR.

Placing a left ventricular vent is essential in severe AR to help in ventricular decompression and is most often achieved through the right superior pulmonary vein.

Myocardial protection is crucial and its delivery must be pre-planned. Anterograde delivery of the cardioplegia solution into the root would be ineffective due to an incompetent aortic valve. Placing a cannula into the coronary sinus for retrograde cardioplegia solution delivery is essential to achieve myocardial arrest before opening the aorta and giving direct ostial coronary cardioplegia. If retrograde cannulation is challenging or ineffective, another possible option is to fibrillate the heart, open the aorta and once coronary ostia are identified, deliver the cardioplegia directly to achieve arrest.

4.3.1 Aortic Valve Surgery

Aortic valve can be repaired or replaced depending on the aetiology, the anatomy, and expected long-term outcomes of correcting the acute AR. A careful inspection and assessment of the aortic valve will aid in the decision making.

In case of localised leaflet dysfunction from trauma or ruptured fenestration, a repair of the valve may be attempted by patching with autologous pericardium (Voit et al. 2022). However, there are concerns regarding the durability of using pericardium for leaflet reconstruction as they calcify with time and there is little data on long term durability especially in bicuspid valves (Karliova et al. 2020).

Prolapse of the aortic valve can be addressed with plication where sutures reduce the free margin length of the leaflet and increase the leaflet coaptation (El Khoury and de Kerchove 2013). Valve repairs might necessitate longer cross clamp times which may not be well tolerated in critically ill patients; thus the majority of surgeons in an emergency setting might opt for a valve replacement.

If the aortic valve itself is the reason for the severe regurgitation and is not repairable, then standard aortic valve replacement is preferred. This should be performed as per surgeon's standard practice to avoid unnecessary unaccounted errors from new techniques in an emergency setting.

Patients that have capacity are counselled at the time of consent on the valve choice (mechanical or bioprosthetic) as per standard practice. In patients who are intubated and ventilated in an emergency setting, the valve choice is influenced by demographic factors, psychosocial issues, history of substance abuse, and potential adherence to anticoagulation which are gathered from family members (Voit et al. 2022).

In patients where there is aortic pathology that extends into the aortic sinus including dilated annulus or there is suspicious genetic features for aortopathy, replacement of the aortic root via a modified Bentall procedure is preferred. If there is surgical expertise and the normal aortic valve can be preserved, valve sparing root replacement (David or Yacoub procedures) may be an option. However, in an emergency setting where minimising operative time is crucial, these complex techniques are rarely selected by surgeons.

In patients with acute left ventricular decompensation despite correcting the aortic valve regurgitation, weaning from cardiopulmonary bypass might not be straightforward. Surgeons must be prepared for using mechanical support devices including IABP, extracorporeal membrane oxygenation (ECMO) and the Impella system (Abiomed, Inc., Danvers, Massachusetts). Reversible causes of haemodynamic instability should be ruled out including bleeding, myocardial ischaemia, medication administration, or measurements errors (Nersesian et al. 2023). Despite no uniform guidelines regarding indications for which mechanical support devices to use, recent algorithms based on readily available clinical parameters have been proposed to aid in decision-making in such scenarios (Nersesian et al. 2023). These devices have been associated with survival benefits but it should be also noted that there is significant increase in complications such as bleeding, haemolysis, and limb ischaemia (Schrage and Westermann 2021).

4.3.2 TAVR Explantation

TAVR has been widely used for treating patients with severe aortic stenosis for patients at increased risk from surgery including those who are not candidates for an operation.

At present, TAVR is not recommended for treatment of patients with acute severe native AR. However, recently TAVR therapy has been studied to treat symptomatic patients presenting with severe native AR who are high risk and not surgical candidates. The Trilogy transcatheter heart valve (JenaValve Technology, Irvine, CA, USA) provides a treatment option for these high risk patients and outcomes have been reported in the ALIGN-AR trial (Vahl et al. 2024). The study shows device safety with promising short-term clinical outcomes for patients who would not have an intervention option otherwise, but long-term follow-up is necessary (Vahl et al. 2024).

Most TAVR clinical trials have emphasised on procedural success and specific clinical outcomes, with limited data on the frequency and outcomes of surgical bailout.

Despite its overall safety, TAVR still presents a risk of significant intraoperative complications, which may necessitate an urgent conversion to open heart surgery, known as a "surgical bailout" and emergency aortic valve replacement.

A critical consideration for surgical intervention following TAVR-related complication is the high probability that the device will likely necessitate explantation. Severe paravalvular leaks have been reported to be the leading indication for TAVR explantation in 41.2% via open heart surgery (Fukuhara et al. 2021).

Explantation of a TAVR device in acute settings is technically less challenging than in chronic scenarios, primarily due to the reduced likelihood of adhesion formation. Prostheses implanted for less than 6 months generally exhibit minimal adhesion formation between the stent frame and the aorta. This has been described up to 1 year of TAVR implantation, after which neoendothelisation of the TAVR into the aortic wall would require intense aortic endoarterectomy (Fukuhara et al. 2021).

A method described for explanting a recently inserted TAVR device is by applying a Kocher clamp to the midsection of the stent cage and then distort its round shape, significantly reducing the radial force that holds the valve in place within the annulus. This manoeuvre facilitates the removal of the valve and minimise damage to the annulus, anterior mitral leaflet, or left ventricular outflow tract structures (Fukuhara et al. 2021).

When explanting a prosthesis older than 1 year, the primary challenge lies in addressing the dense endothelial growth that incorporates the aorta and the device, which is more substantial than surgically implanted prosthetic valves. This is most notable for patients having balloon-expandable TAVR in the aortic root or self-expanding prostheses in the sinotubular junction. Both of these cases would require gentle endarterectomy of the aorta while preserving aortic wall integrity (Fukuhara et al. 2021).

In the event of an injury to the aortic root, the surgeon must be prepared for performing a root replacement which is associated with a significantly high mortality rate. In case of an expanding root haematoma, the coronary ostia may become significantly displaced or even avulsed. Therefore, it is important to be prepared to harvest conduits for coronary artery bypass grafting (CABG) if reimplantation of the coronary buttons is not feasible (Pasic et al. 2015).

Despite thorough pre-procedural planning for TAVR including precise measurements of the aortic annulus on preoperative CT scan and improved deployment strategies, complications can still arise. We would like to emphasise the importance of the availability of the cardiac surgical team and cardiopulmonary bypass machine as a bail-out strategy.

5 Conclusions

Emergency aortic valve replacement (AVR) remains a daunting challenge in patients who are critically unwell and face imminent death. It necessitates swift action and a multidisciplinary approach to address life-threatening presentations.

The management of conditions such as infective endocarditis, critical aortic stenosis, and acute severe aortic regurgitation underscores the need for precise and time-sensitive surgical decision-making and tailored interventions for each scenario. Due to the emergency nature of such cases, preoperative optimisation and preparedness is limited compared to less urgent conditions.

While there have been advancements in perioperative care and surgical techniques which have improved outcomes, the inherent complexity of emergency AVR continues to pose significant risks. The absence of robust randomised trials and the reliance on clinical judgement and institutional expertise highlights the importance of global collaboration and innovation to optimise care for these high-risk patients.

Ultimately, the success of emergency AVR relies on the vital role of clinical expertise, evidence-based practices, and multidisciplinary teamwork in overcoming the challenges encountered for acute aortic valve conditions and delivering favourable outcomes for patients.

References

AATS Surgical Treatment of Infective Endocarditis Consensus Guidelines Writing Committee Chairs, Pettersson GB, Coselli JS et al (2017) 2016 The American Association for Thoracic Surgery (AATS) consensus guidelines: surgical treatment of infective endocarditis: executive summary. J Thorac Cardiovasc Surg 153:1241–1258.e29. https://doi.org/10.1016/j.jtcvs.2016.09.093

Alkhalil A, Hajjar R, Ibrahim H, Ruiz CE (2019) Mechanical circulatory support in transcatheter aortic valve implantation in the United States (from the National Inpatient Sample). Am J Cardiol 124:1615–1620. https://doi.org/10.1016/j.amjcard.2019.08.013

Anguera I, Miro JM, Cabell CH et al (2005) Clinical characteristics and outcome of aortic endocarditis with periannular abscess in the International Collaboration on Endocarditis Merged Database. Am J Cardiol 96:976–981. https://doi.org/10.1016/j.amjcard.2005.05.056

Avvedimento M, Angellotti D, Ilardi F et al (2023) Acute advanced aortic stenosis. Heart Fail Rev 28:1101–1111. https://doi.org/10.1007/s10741-023-10312-7

Bansal A, Kumar A, Jain V et al (2021) Impact of hospital procedural volume on use and outcomes of urgent/emergent transcatheter aortic valve replacement. J Am Heart Assoc 10:e019670. https://doi.org/10.1161/JAHA.120.019670

Barbetseas J, Nagueh SF, Pitsavos C et al (1998) Differentiating thrombus from pannus formation in obstructed mechanical prosthetic valves: an evaluation of clinical, transthoracic and transesophageal echocardiographic parameters. J Am Coll Cardiol 32:1410–1417. https://doi.org/10.1016/s0735-1097(98)00385-4

Ben-Dor I, Maluenda G, Dvir D et al (2013) Balloon aortic valvuloplasty for severe aortic stenosis as a bridge to transcatheter/surgical aortic valve replacement. Catheter Cardiovasc Interv 82:632–637. https://doi.org/10.1002/ccd.24682

Bohbot Y, Habib G, Laroche C et al (2022) Characteristics, management, and outcomes of patients with left-sided infective endocarditis complicated by heart failure: a substudy of the ESC-EORP EURO-ENDO (European infective endocarditis) registry. Eur J Heart Fail 24:1253–1265. https://doi.org/10.1002/ejhf.2525

Bongiovanni D, Kühl C, Bleiziffer S et al (2018) Emergency treatment of decompensated aortic stenosis. Heart 104:23–29. https://doi.org/10.1136/heartjnl-2016-311037

Bortolotti U, Guerra F, Magni A et al (1987) Emergency reoperation for primary tissue failure of porcine bioprostheses. Am J Cardiol 60:920–921. https://doi.org/10.1016/0002-9149(87)91052-6

Bowdish ME, Habib RH, Kaneko T et al (2024) Cardiac surgery after transcatheter aortic valve replacement: trends and outcomes. Ann Thorac Surg 118:155–162. https://doi.org/10.1016/j.athoracsur.2024.03.024

Buchwald AB, Meyer T, Scholz K et al (2001) Efficacy of balloon valvuloplasty in patients with critical aortic stenosis and cardiogenic shock—the role of shock duration. Clin Cardiol 24:214–218. https://doi.org/10.1002/clc.4960240308

Byrne JG, Rezai K, Sanchez JA et al (2011) Surgical management of endocarditis: the society of thoracic surgeons clinical practice guideline. Ann Thorac Surg 91:2012–2019. https://doi.org/10.1016/j.athoracsur.2011.01.106

Chakravarty T, Søndergaard L, Friedman J et al (2017) Subclinical leaflet thrombosis in surgical and transcatheter bioprosthetic aortic valves: an observational study. Lancet 389:2383–2392. https://doi.org/10.1016/S0140-6736(17)30757-2

Chirouze C, Cabell CH, Fowler VG et al (2004) Prognostic factors in 61 cases of Staphylococcus aureus prosthetic valve infective endocarditis from the International Collaboration on Endocarditis merged database. Clin Infect Dis 38:1323–1327. https://doi.org/10.1086/383035

Christ G, Zehetgruber M, Mundigler G et al (1997) Emergency aortic valve replacement for critical aortic stenosis. Intensive Care Med 23:297–300. https://doi.org/10.1007/s001340050331

Cohn L, Adams D (2018) Cardiac surgery in the adult, 5th edn. McGraw-Hill Education

Cribier A, Savin T, Saoudi N et al (1986) Percutaneous transluminal valvuloplasty of acquired aortic stenosis in elderly patients: an alternative to valve replacement? Lancet 1:63–67. https://doi.org/10.1016/s0140-6736(86)90716-6

De Oliveira NC, David TE, Armstrong S, Ivanov J (2005) Aortic and mitral valve replacement with reconstruction of the intervalvular fibrous body: an analysis of clinical outcomes. J Thorac Cardiovasc Surg 129:286–290. https://doi.org/10.1016/j.jtcvs.2004.09.032

Debry N, Kone P, Vincent F et al (2018) Urgent balloon aortic valvuloplasty in patients with cardiogenic shock related to severe aortic stenosis: time matters. EuroIntervention 14:e519–e525. https://doi.org/10.4244/EIJ-D-18-00029

Delgado V, Ajmone Marsan N, de Waha S et al (2023) 2023 ESC guidelines for the management of endocarditis: developed by the task force on the management of endocarditis of the European Society of Cardiology (ESC) Endorsed by the European Association for Cardio-Thoracic

Surgery (EACTS) and the European Association of Nuclear Medicine (EANM). Eur Heart J 44:3948–4042. https://doi.org/10.1093/eurheartj/ehad193

Deviri E, Sareli P, Wisenbaugh T, Cronje SL (1991) Obstruction of mechanical heart valve prostheses: clinical aspects and surgical management. J Am Coll Cardiol 17:646–650. https://doi.org/10.1016/s0735-1097(10)80178-0

Dobell AR, Jain AK (1984) Catastrophic hemorrhage during redo sternotomy. Ann Thorac Surg 37:273–278. https://doi.org/10.1016/s0003-4975(10)60728-x

Dürrleman N, Pellerin M, Bouchard D et al (2004) Prosthetic valve thrombosis: twenty-year experience at the Montreal Heart Institute. J Thorac Cardiovasc Surg 127:1388–1392. https://doi.org/10.1016/j.jtcvs.2003.12.013

El Khoury G, de Kerchove L (2013) Principles of aortic valve repair. J Thorac Cardiovasc Surg 145:S26–S29. https://doi.org/10.1016/j.jtcvs.2012.11.071

Erdem H, Puca E, Ruch Y et al (2019) Portraying infective endocarditis: results of multinational ID-IRI study. Eur J Clin Microbiol Infect Dis 38:1753–1763. https://doi.org/10.1007/s10096-019-03607-x

Frerker C, Schewel J, Schlüter M et al (2016) Emergency transcatheter aortic valve replacement in patients with cardiogenic shock due to acutely decompensated aortic stenosis. EuroIntervention 11:1530–1536. https://doi.org/10.4244/EIJY15M03_03

Fukuhara S, Brescia AA, Shiomi S et al (2021) Surgical explantation of transcatheter aortic bioprostheses: results and clinical implications. J Thorac Cardiovasc Surg 162:539–547.e1. https://doi.org/10.1016/j.jtcvs.2019.11.139

García-González MJ, Jorge-Pérez P, Jiménez-Sosa A et al (2015) Levosimendan improves hemodynamic status in critically ill patients with severe aortic stenosis and left ventricular dysfunction: an interventional study. Cardiovasc Ther 33:193–199. https://doi.org/10.1111/1755-5922.12132

Giannuzzi P, Imparato A, Temporelli PL et al (1994) Doppler-derived mitral deceleration time of early filling as a strong predictor of pulmonary capillary wedge pressure in postinfarction patients with left ventricular systolic dysfunction. J Am Coll Cardiol 23:1630–1637. https://doi.org/10.1016/0735-1097(94)90667-x

Habib G, Badano L, Tribouilloy C et al (2010) Recommendations for the practice of echocardiography in infective endocarditis. Eur J Echocardiogr 11:202–219. https://doi.org/10.1093/ejechocard/jeq004

Halperin JL, Levine GN, Al-Khatib SM et al (2016) Further evolution of the ACC/AHA clinical practice guideline recommendation classification system: a report of the American College of Cardiology/American Heart Association Task Force on Clinical Practice Guidelines. J Am Coll Cardiol 67:1572–1574. https://doi.org/10.1016/j.jacc.2015.09.001

Hammermeister K, Sethi GK, Henderson WG et al (2000) Outcomes 15 years after valve replacement with a mechanical versus a bioprosthetic valve: final report of the Veterans Affairs randomized trial. J Am Coll Cardiol 36:1152–1158. https://doi.org/10.1016/s0735-1097(00)00834-2

Hariram V (2014) Percutaneous management of prosthetic valve thrombosis. Indian Heart J 66:427–429. https://doi.org/10.1016/j.ihj.2014.05.008

Hussain ST, Shrestha NK, Gordon SM et al (2014) Residual patient, anatomic, and surgical obstacles in treating active left-sided infective endocarditis. J Thorac Cardiovasc Surg 148:981–988.e4. https://doi.org/10.1016/j.jtcvs.2014.06.019

Iung B, Vahanian A (2011) Epidemiology of valvular heart disease in the adult. Nat Rev Cardiol 8:162–172. https://doi.org/10.1038/nrcardio.2010.202

Jabbour S, Salinger M, Alexander JC (1996) Hemodynamic stabilization of acute prosthetic valve thrombosis using percutaneous catheter manipulation. Catheter Cardiovasc Diagn 39:314–316. https://doi.org/10.1002/(SICI)1097-0304(199611)39:3<314::AID-CCD24>3.0.CO;2-D

Jalava MP, Laakso T, Virtanen M et al (2020) Transcatheter and surgical aortic valve replacement in patients with recent acute heart failure. Ann Thorac Surg 109:110–117. https://doi.org/10.1016/j.athoracsur.2019.05.044

Jarral OA, Pupovac SS, Tseng J-C et al (2024) Transcatheter aortic valve replacement valve endocarditis requiring Commando procedure. JTCVS Techniq. https://doi.org/10.1016/j.xjtc.2024.06.011

Jiang X, Liu J, Khan F et al (2020) Aortic and mitral valve surgery for infective endocarditis with reconstruction of the intervalvular fibrous body: an analysis of clinical outcomes. J Thoracic Dis 12. https://doi.org/10.21037/jtd.2020.03.04

Karliova I, Schneider U, Ehrlich T, Schäfers H-J (2020) Results of pericardial patches in tricuspid and bicuspid aortic cusp repair. Ann Thorac Surg 109:728–735. https://doi.org/10.1016/j.athoracsur.2019.07.025

Karthikeyan G, Senguttuvan NB, Joseph J et al (2013) Urgent surgery compared with fibrinolytic therapy for the treatment of left-sided prosthetic heart valve thrombosis: a systematic review and meta-analysis of observational studies. Eur Heart J 34:1557–1566. https://doi.org/10.1093/eurheartj/ehs486

Keuleers S, Herijgers P, Herregods M-C et al (2011) Comparison of thrombolysis versus surgery as a first line therapy for prosthetic heart valve thrombosis. Am J Cardiol 107:275–279. https://doi.org/10.1016/j.amjcard.2010.09.013

Kiefer T, Park L, Tribouilloy C et al (2011) Association between valvular surgery and mortality among patients with infective endocarditis complicated by heart failure. JAMA 306:2239–2247. https://doi.org/10.1001/jama.2011.1701

Kocher AA, Laufer G, Haverich A et al (2013) One-year outcomes of the Surgical Treatment of Aortic Stenosis With a Next Generation Surgical Aortic Valve (TRITON) trial: a prospective multicenter study of rapid-deployment aortic valve replacement with the EDWARDS INTUITY Valve System. J Thorac Cardiovasc Surg 145:110–115; discussion 115–116. https://doi.org/10.1016/j.jtcvs.2012.07.108

Kolte D, Khera S, Vemulapalli S et al (2018) Outcomes following urgent/emergent transcatheter aortic valve replacement: insights from the STS/ACC TVT registry. JACC Cardiovasc Interv 11:1175–1185. https://doi.org/10.1016/j.jcin.2018.03.002

Lancellotti P, Pibarot P, Chambers J et al (2016) Recommendations for the imaging assessment of prosthetic heart valves: a report from the European Association of Cardiovascular Imaging endorsed by the Chinese Society of Echocardiography, the Inter-American Society of Echocardiography, and the Brazilian Department of Cardiovascular Imaging. Eur Heart J Cardiovasc Imaging 17:589–590. https://doi.org/10.1093/ehjci/jew025

Lang CN, Kaier K, Zotzmann V et al (2021) Cardiogenic shock: incidence, survival and mechanical circulatory support usage 2007-2017-insights from a national registry. Clin Res Cardiol 110:1421–1430. https://doi.org/10.1007/s00392-020-01781-z

Laplace G, Lafitte S, Labèque J-N et al (2004) Clinical significance of early thrombosis after prosthetic mitral valve replacement: a postoperative monocentric study of 680 patients. J Am Coll Cardiol 43:1283–1290. https://doi.org/10.1016/j.jacc.2003.09.064

Lawton JS, Tamis-Holland JE, Bangalore S et al (2022) 2021 ACC/AHA/SCAI guideline for coronary artery revascularization: a report of the American College of Cardiology/American Heart Association Joint Committee on Clinical Practice Guidelines. Circulation 145:e18–e114. https://doi.org/10.1161/CIR.0000000000001038

Lengyel M, Fuster V, Keltai M et al (1997) Guidelines for management of left-sided prosthetic valve thrombosis: a role for thrombolytic therapy. Consensus Conference on Prosthetic Valve Thrombosis. J Am Coll Cardiol 30:1521–1526. https://doi.org/10.1016/s0735-1097(97)00345-8

Letac B, Cribier A, Eltchaninoff H et al (1991) Evaluation of restenosis after balloon dilatation in adult aortic stenosis by repeat catheterization. Am Heart J 122:55–60. https://doi.org/10.1016/0002-8703(91)90758-a

Levine GN, O'Gara PT, Beckman JA et al (2019) Recent innovations, modifications, and evolution of ACC/AHA clinical practice guidelines: an update for our constituencies: a report of the American College of Cardiology/American Heart Association Task Force on

Clinical Practice Guidelines. J Am Coll Cardiol 73:1990–1998. https://doi.org/10.1016/j.jacc.2019.02.012
Luciani N, Mossuto E, Ricci D et al (2017) Prosthetic valve endocarditis: predictors of early outcome of surgical therapy. A multicentric study. Eur J Cardiothorac Surg 52:768–774. https://doi.org/10.1093/ejcts/ezx169
Luehr M, Bauernschmitt N, Peterss S et al (2020) Incidence and surgical outcomes of patients with native and prosthetic aortic valve endocarditis. Ann Thorac Surg 110:93–101. https://doi.org/10.1016/j.athoracsur.2019.10.029
Mahara K, Ota M, Kishiki K, Takanashi S (2017) Acute aortic valve regurgitation due to spontaneous rupture of fenestrated cusp treated with aortic valve repair. Circ J 81:241–242. https://doi.org/10.1253/circj.CJ-16-0959
Mangner N, Leontyev S, Woitek FJ et al (2018) Cardiac surgery compared with antibiotics only in patients developing infective endocarditis after transcatheter aortic valve replacement. J Am Heart Assoc 7:e010027. https://doi.org/10.1161/JAHA.118.010027
Manne MB, Shrestha NK, Lytle BW et al (2012) Outcomes after surgical treatment of native and prosthetic valve infective endocarditis. Ann Thorac Surg 93:489–493. https://doi.org/10.1016/j.athoracsur.2011.10.063
Mentias A, Girotra S, Desai MY et al (2020) Incidence, predictors, and outcomes of endocarditis after transcatheter aortic valve replacement in the United States. JACC Cardiovasc Interv 13:1973–1982. https://doi.org/10.1016/j.jcin.2020.05.012
Mir T, Uddin M, Qureshi WT et al (2022) Predictors of complications secondary to infective endocarditis and their associated outcomes: a large cohort study from the National Emergency Database (2016-2018). Infect Dis Ther 11:305–321. https://doi.org/10.1007/s40121-021-00563-y
Mokadam NA, Stout KK, Verrier ED (2011) Management of acute regurgitation in left-sided cardiac valves. Tex Heart Inst J 38:9–19
Montorsi P, De Bernardi F, Muratori M et al (2000) Role of cine-fluoroscopy, transthoracic, and transesophageal echocardiography in patients with suspected prosthetic heart valve thrombosis. Am J Cardiol 85:58–64. https://doi.org/10.1016/s0002-9149(99)00607-4
Muratori M, Montorsi P, Teruzzi G et al (2006) Feasibility and diagnostic accuracy of quantitative assessment of mechanical prostheses leaflet motion by transthoracic and transesophageal echocardiography in suspected prosthetic valve dysfunction. Am J Cardiol 97:94–100. https://doi.org/10.1016/j.amjcard.2005.07.112
Nadji G, Rusinaru D, Rémadi J-P et al (2009) Heart failure in left-sided native valve infective endocarditis: characteristics, prognosis, and results of surgical treatment. Eur J Heart Fail 11:668–675. https://doi.org/10.1093/eurjhf/hfp077
Nagao K, Taniguchi T, Morimoto T et al (2018) Acute heart failure in patients with severe aortic stenosis—insights from the CURRENT AS registry. Circ J 82:874–885. https://doi.org/10.1253/circj.CJ-17-0610
Nair RM, Chawla S, Abdelghaffar B et al (2024) Comparison of contemporary treatment strategies in patients with cardiogenic shock due to severe aortic stenosis. J Am Heart Assoc 13:e033601. https://doi.org/10.1161/JAHA.123.033601
Nersesian G, Ott S, Fardman A et al (2023) Temporary mechanical circulatory support in cardiogenic shock patients after cardiac procedures: selection algorithm and weaning strategies. Life (Basel) 13:2045. https://doi.org/10.3390/life13102045
Otto CM, Mickel MC, Kennedy JW et al (1994) Three-year outcome after balloon aortic valvuloplasty. Insights into prognosis of valvular aortic stenosis. Circulation 89:642–650. https://doi.org/10.1161/01.cir.89.2.642
Otto CM, Nishimura RA, Bonow RO et al (2021) 2020 ACC/AHA guideline for the management of patients with valvular heart disease: a report of the American College of Cardiology/American Heart Association Joint Committee on Clinical Practice Guidelines. J Thorac Cardiovasc Surg 162:e183–e353. https://doi.org/10.1016/j.jtcvs.2021.04.002

Panagides V, Del Val D, Abdel-Wahab M et al (2022) Perivalvular extension of infective endocarditis after transcatheter aortic valve replacement. Clin Infect Dis 75:638–646. https://doi.org/10.1093/cid/ciab1004

Pasic M, Unbehaun A, Buz S et al (2015) Annular rupture during transcatheter aortic valve replacement: classification, pathophysiology, diagnostics, treatment approaches, and prevention. JACC Cardiovasc Interv 8:1–9. https://doi.org/10.1016/j.jcin.2014.07.020

Patel KP, Chahal A, Mullen MJ et al (2023) Acute decompensated aortic stenosis: state of the art review. Curr Probl Cardiol 48:101422. https://doi.org/10.1016/j.cpcardiol.2022.101422

Pericàs JM, Hernández-Meneses M, Muñoz P et al (2021) Characteristics and outcome of acute heart failure in infective endocarditis: focus on cardiogenic shock. Clin Infect Dis 73:765–774. https://doi.org/10.1093/cid/ciab098

Pettersson GB, Hussain ST, Ramankutty RM et al (2014a) Reconstruction of fibrous skeleton: technique, pitfalls and results. Multimed Man Cardiothorac Surg 2014:mmu004. https://doi.org/10.1093/mmcts/mmu004

Pettersson GB, Hussain ST, Shrestha NK et al (2014b) Infective endocarditis: an atlas of disease progression for describing, staging, coding, and understanding the pathology. J Thorac Cardiovasc Surg 147:1142–1149.e2. https://doi.org/10.1016/j.jtcvs.2013.11.031

Popma JJ, Adams DH, Reardon MJ et al (2014) Transcatheter aortic valve replacement using a self-expanding bioprosthesis in patients with severe aortic stenosis at extreme risk for surgery. J Am Coll Cardiol 63:1972–1981. https://doi.org/10.1016/j.jacc.2014.02.556

Regueiro A, Linke A, Latib A et al (2016) Association between transcatheter aortic valve replacement and subsequent infective endocarditis and in-hospital death. JAMA 316:1083–1092. https://doi.org/10.1001/jama.2016.12347

Roudaut R, Lafitte S, Roudaut M-F et al (2009) Management of prosthetic heart valve obstruction: fibrinolysis versus surgery. Early results and long-term follow-up in a single-centre study of 263 cases. Arch Cardiovasc Dis 102:269–277. https://doi.org/10.1016/j.acvd.2009.01.007

Schrage B, Westermann D (2021) Response by Schrage and Westermann to Letters Regarding Article, "Left ventricular unloading is associated with lower mortality in patients with cardiogenic shock treated with venoarterial extracorporeal membrane oxygenation: results from an International, Multicenter Cohort Study". Circulation 143:e1024. https://doi.org/10.1161/CIRCULATIONAHA.121.053992

Singh V, Mendirichaga R, Inglessis-Azuaje I et al (2018) The role of impella for hemodynamic support in patients with aortic stenosis. Curr Treat Options Cardio Med 20:44. https://doi.org/10.1007/s11936-018-0644-9

Soria Jiménez CE, Papolos AI, Kenigsberg BB et al (2023) Management of mechanical prosthetic heart valve thrombosis: JACC review topic of the week. J Am Coll Cardiol 81:2115–2127. https://doi.org/10.1016/j.jacc.2023.03.412

Spiliopoulos K, Haschemi A, Fink G, Kemkes B-M (2010) Infective endocarditis complicated by paravalvular abscess: a surgical challenge. An 11-year single center experience. Heart Surg Forum 13:E67–E73. https://doi.org/10.1532/HSF98.20081141

Suchá D, Symersky P, Tanis W et al (2015) Multimodality imaging assessment of prosthetic heart valves. Circ Cardiovasc Imaging 8:e003703. https://doi.org/10.1161/CIRCIMAGING.115.003703

Suh YJ, Lee S, Im DJ et al (2016) Added value of cardiac computed tomography for evaluation of mechanical aortic valve: emphasis on evaluation of pannus with surgical findings as standard reference. Int J Cardiol 214:454–460. https://doi.org/10.1016/j.ijcard.2016.04.011

Symersky P, Budde RPJ, de Mol BAJM, Prokop M (2009) Comparison of multidetector-row computed tomography to echocardiography and fluoroscopy for evaluation of patients with mechanical prosthetic valve obstruction. Am J Cardiol 104:1128–1134. https://doi.org/10.1016/j.amjcard.2009.05.061

Szerlip M, Arsalan M, Mack MC et al (2017) Usefulness of balloon aortic valvuloplasty in the management of patients with aortic stenosis. Am J Cardiol 120:1366–1372. https://doi.org/10.1016/j.amjcard.2017.07.024

Talwar S, Kapoor CK, Velayoudam D, Kumar AS (2004) Anticoagulation protocol and early prosthetic valve thrombosis. Indian Heart J 56:225–228

Tandar A, Drakos SG (2019) Cardiogenic shock in aortic stenosis patients: balancing between complexity and simplicity. Hell J Cardiol 60:182–184. https://doi.org/10.1016/j.hjc.2019.06.002

Vahanian A, Beyersdorf F, Praz F et al (2022) 2021 ESC/EACTS Guidelines for the management of valvular heart disease: developed by the Task Force for the management of valvular heart disease of the European Society of Cardiology (ESC) and the European Association for Cardio-Thoracic Surgery (EACTS). Eur Heart J 43:561–632. https://doi.org/10.1093/eurheartj/ehab395

Vahl TP, Thourani VH, Makkar RR et al (2024) Transcatheter aortic valve implantation in patients with high-risk symptomatic native aortic regurgitation (ALIGN-AR): a prospective, multicentre, single-arm study. Lancet 403:1451–1459. https://doi.org/10.1016/S0140-6736(23)02806-4

Villablanca P, Nona P, Lemor A et al (2021) Mechanical circulatory support in cardiogenic shock due to structural heart disease. Interv Cardiol Clin 10:221–234. https://doi.org/10.1016/j.iccl.2020.12.007

Voit J, Otto CM, Burke CR (2022) Acute native aortic regurgitation: clinical presentation, diagnosis and management. Heart 108:1651–1660. https://doi.org/10.1136/heartjnl-2021-320157

Wald DS, Williams S, Bangash F, Bestwick JP (2018) Watchful waiting in aortic stenosis: the problem of acute decompensation. Am J Med 131:173–177. https://doi.org/10.1016/j.amjmed.2017.08.027

Wernly B, Jirak P, Lichtenauer M et al (2020) Systematic review and meta-analysis of interventional emergency treatment of decompensated severe aortic stenosis. J Invasive Cardiol 32:30–36

Wideman FE, Blackstone EH, Kirklin JW et al (1981) Hospital mortality of re-replacement of the aortic valve. Incremental risk factors. J Thorac Cardiovasc Surg 82:692–698

Williams T, Hildick-Smith DJR (2020) Balloon aortic valvuloplasty: indications, patient eligibility, technique and contemporary outcomes. Heart 106:1102–1110. https://doi.org/10.1136/heartjnl-2019-315904

Emergency Mitral Valve Surgery

Arian Arjomandi Rad, Gustavo Antonio Guida, Alexander Weymann, and Peyman Sardari Nia

Abstract Emergency mitral valve surgery is a critical, high-stakes procedure performed to manage acute mitral valve dysfunction threatening patient survival. This chapter explores the surgical challenges and decision-making strategies unique to urgent interventions, encompassing conditions such as infective endocarditis, acute mitral regurgitation, and critical mitral stenosis. Rapid diagnosis, advanced imaging, and timely haemodynamic stabilisation are crucial for preoperative planning. Surgical techniques should be tailored to the specific pathology and patient condition, prioritising repair over replacement when feasible. Postoperative care focuses on managing complications and optimising recovery, underscoring the role of a multidisciplinary approach in improving outcomes in these complex cases.

Keywords Emergency mitral valve surgery · Infective endocarditis · Acute mitral regurgitation · Papillary muscle rupture · Chordal rupture · Mitral leaflet prolapse · Critical mitral stenosis · Prosthetic mitral valve complications · Paravalvular leak · Transcatheter mitral interventions

---

A. Arjomandi Rad
Department of Cardiothoracic Surgery, Oxford Heart Centre, Oxford University Hospitals NHS Foundation Trust, Oxford, UK

Department of Cardio-thoracic Surgery, Maastricht University Medical Center, Maastricht, the Netherlands

G. A. Guida
Department of CardioThoracic Surgery, Bristol Heart Institute, University Hospitals Bristol and Weston NHS Foundation Trust, Bristol, UK

A. Weymann
Department of Cardiothoracic, Transplantation and Vascular Surgery, Hannover Medical School, Hannover, Germany

P. Sardari Nia (✉)
Department of Cardio-thoracic Surgery, Maastricht University Medical Center, Maastricht, the Netherlands
e-mail: peyman.sardarinia@mumc.nl

A. Kourliouros (ed.), *Emergency Cardiac Surgery*,
https://doi.org/10.1007/978-3-032-15787-4_10

1 Introduction

Emergency mitral valve surgery represents one of the most demanding scenarios in cardiac surgery, requiring immediate intervention to address acute mitral valve dysfunction that threatens patient survival (Arjomandi Rad et al. 2024; Lorusso et al. 2008). The mitral valve, integral to left ventricular function and systemic circulation, can be compromised suddenly due to various etiologies such as infective endocarditis with rapid tissue destruction, acute ischemic events leading to papillary muscle rupture, or prosthetic valve complications like thrombosis or dehiscence.

The urgency in these cases stems from the haemodynamic instability caused by abrupt changes in mitral valve function. Acute severe mitral regurgitation, for instance, precipitates a sudden volume load on the left atrium and ventricle, leading to pulmonary oedema and cardiogenic shock. Similarly, obstructive lesions like prosthetic valve thrombosis can cause rapid increases in left atrial pressure and subsequent pulmonary hypertension.

Managing these emergencies requires not only surgical expertise but also swift diagnostic acumen and multidisciplinary coordination. Advanced imaging modalities such as transoesophageal echocardiography (TEE) are indispensable for rapid assessment of valvular pathology and guiding surgical planning. Haemodynamic support, including intra-aortic balloon pump (IABP) or extracorporeal membrane oxygenation (ECMO), may be necessary to stabilise patients preoperatively.

The surgical approach in emergency settings often differs from elective procedures due to the acute nature of tissue pathology and haemodynamic compromise. Decisions between repair and replacement must consider the extent of structural damage, the presence of infection, and the patient's haemodynamic status. Techniques such as aggressive debridement in endocarditis or the use of artificial chordae in cases of chordal rupture demand a high level of surgical proficiency.

Postoperative management is equally critical, with attention to haemodynamic monitoring, management of ventricular function, and in cases of infective endocarditis, prolonged antimicrobial therapy. The risk of postoperative complications, including low cardiac output syndrome, arrhythmias, and recurrent infection, necessitates vigilant ICU care.

This chapter aims to provide an in-depth analysis of emergency mitral valve surgery tailored for the expert cardiac surgeon. It will delve into:

- **Infective Endocarditis**: Discussing the indications for surgery, the impact of various pathogens on surgical timing and technique, and advanced operative strategies for both native and prosthetic valve involvement.
- **Acute Mitral Regurgitation**: Exploring surgical management of papillary muscle rupture and chordal rupture or prolapse, including contemporary repair techniques and the role of mechanical circulatory support.
- **Critical Mitral Stenosis**: Examining urgent interventions for decompensated stenosis and prosthetic valve obstruction, with emphasis on surgical versus percutaneous approaches and management of associated comorbidities.

- **Acute Prosthetic Valve Complications**: Addressing the surgical management of prosthetic valve thrombosis, pannus formation, and dehiscence, including considerations for re-replacement and techniques to ensure annular integrity.
- **Transcatheter Interventions for Emergency Mitral Valve Scenarios**: a brief overview of transcatheter interventions for emergency mitral valve scenarios where these technologies could be also useful to the mitral valve surgeon.

2 Infective Endocarditis

(a) ***Indications for Emergency Surgery***

Infective endocarditis of the mitral valve is a life-threatening condition that can rapidly progress to severe cardiac and systemic complications (Arjomandi Rad et al. 2024). Emergency surgical intervention is indicated in specific scenarios where immediate action is necessary to prevent mortality (Delgado et al. 2023). Details about guidelines related IE indications are covered in details in the IE chapter. Herein we focus on mitral valve related specific scenarios.

According to the 2023 ESC guidelines for the management of IE (Delgado et al. 2023), urgent surgical intervention in mitral valve IE is generally warranted in three overlapping categories: patients with acute heart failure due to valvular dysfunction, those with ongoing infection not responding to antibiotics, and individuals at high risk of, or already experiencing, embolic complications:

1. **Heart Failure due to Acute Valvular Dysfunction**

Severe Mitral Regurgitation or Obstruction Caused by Vegetations

- **Haemodynamic Instability**: Large vegetations can cause acute mitral regurgitation by interfering with leaflet coaptation or by physically destroying leaflet tissue. This leads to sudden volume overload of the left atrium and ventricle, pulmonary oedema, and cardiogenic shock (Arjomandi Rad et al. 2024).
- **Obstructive Vegetations**: Rarely, large vegetations may obstruct the mitral orifice, mimicking mitral stenosis and causing elevated left atrial pressures and decreased cardiac output.
- **Surgical Implications**: Emergency surgery aims to remove infective material, restore valvular function, and prevent haemodynamic collapse. Preservation of viable valvular tissue is critical, but extensive destruction may necessitate valve replacement.

2. ***High Risk of Embolisation or Established embolisation***

Recurrent Embolic Events Despite Optimal Antibiotic Therapy

- **Embolic Risk Factors**: Vegetations >10 mm, mobile vegetations, and those located on the anterior mitral leaflet are associated with higher embolic potential.
- **Neurological Complications**: Cerebral emboli can lead to ischemic stroke, intracerebral haemorrhage, or mycotic aneurysms. Timing of surgery post-stroke

requires careful consideration to balance the risks of haemorrhagic transformation versus ongoing embolisation (Arjomandi Rad et al. 2024).

- **Other Systemic Emboli**: Renal, splenic, and peripheral emboli can cause organ infarction and sepsis.
- **Surgical Decision-Making**: Emergency surgery is indicated when there are recurrent embolic events or a single embolic event with large, mobile vegetations. Rapid removal of the source of emboli is essential.

3. **Uncontrolled Infection**

Periannular Extension Leading to Abscesses Threatening Structural Integrity

- **Anatomical Considerations**: Abscesses can develop in the mitral annulus, intervalvular fibrosa, or extend into adjacent cardiac structures, leading to fistula formation or conduction abnormalities.
- **Diagnostic Indicators**: Transoesophageal echocardiography (TEE) is crucial for identifying abscess cavities, pseudoaneurysms, and perivalvular complications.
- **Clinical Consequences**: Abscess formation can result in severe valvular dysfunction, heart block due to involvement of conduction tissue, and persistent infection despite antibiotic therapy.
- **Surgical Challenges**: Management includes radical debridement of infected and necrotic tissue, reconstruction of the annulus or surrounding structures, and often valve replacement. Homografts or prosthetic materials may be utilised for reconstruction.

(b) ***Preoperative Planning***

Effective preoperative planning is crucial in emergency mitral valve surgery for infective endocarditis to optimise surgical outcomes and minimise perioperative risks. This involves a multidisciplinary approach focusing on the identification of the causative organism, detailed imaging to assess the extent of infection, and meticulous coordination among various specialties.

1. **Microbiological Assessment**

Impact of Pathogen Type on Surgical Timing and Antibiotic Therapy

- **Staphylococcus aureus** (Arjomandi Rad et al. 2024):
  - *Characteristics*: Highly virulent, leading to rapid valvular destruction and abscess formation.
  - *Surgical Timing*: Requires urgent surgical intervention due to aggressive tissue invasion and high embolic risk.
  - *Antibiotic Therapy*: Empiric therapy often includes vancomycin; adjust based on sensitivity to methicillin (MRSA vs. MSSA).
- **Streptococcus species** (Arjomandi Rad et al. 2024):
  - *Characteristics*: Generally less aggressive than S. aureus but can cause significant damage in native valves.
  - *Surgical Timing*: Surgery is indicated in cases of heart failure or large vegetations (>10 mm) with embolic potential (Delgado et al. 2023).

- *Antibiotic Therapy*: Penicillin or ceftriaxone-based regimens; consider synergistic aminoglycosides in some cases.

- **Enterococcus species** (Arjomandi Rad et al. 2024):
  - *Characteristics*: Often affects elderly patients with comorbidities; may exhibit antibiotic resistance.
  - *Surgical Timing*: Early surgery considered if there is evidence of heart failure or uncontrolled infection.
  - *Antibiotic Therapy*: Ampicillin or vancomycin with gentamicin; linezolid or daptomycin for resistant strains.

- **Fungal Endocarditis** (Arjomandi Rad et al. 2024):
  - *Characteristics*: Rare but associated with large vegetations and high mortality; often in immunocompromised patients.
  - *Surgical Timing*: Immediate surgery is typically required due to poor response to antifungal therapy alone.
  - *Antibiotic Therapy*: Amphotericin B or echinocandins; long-term suppressive therapy may be necessary postoperatively.

- **Culture-Negative Endocarditis** (Arjomandi Rad et al. 2024):
  - *Characteristics*: May result from prior antibiotic use or fastidious organisms (e.g. HACEK, Bartonella).
  - *Surgical Timing*: Based on clinical criteria; surgery is not delayed for microbiological identification.
  - *Antibiotic Therapy*: Broad-spectrum coverage including agents effective against common fastidious organisms.

Considerations

- Obtain multiple sets of blood cultures before initiating antibiotics.
- Use molecular diagnostic tools (e.g. PCR, 16S rRNA sequencing) for pathogen identification when cultures are negative.
- Collaboration with infectious disease specialists to tailor antimicrobial therapy.

(c) ***Native Mitral Valve Endocarditis:*** **Valve Preservation versus Replacement**

In the surgical management of native mitral valve infective endocarditis, valve preservation through repair is generally preferred over replacement when feasible. MV repair offers significant advantages, including better preservation of left ventricular function, avoidance of prosthesis-related complications, and improved long-term survival rates (Shimokawa et al. 2009; Zegdi et al. 2005; Muehrcke et al. 1997). The feasibility and benefits of MV repair in degenerative mitral regurgitation due to chordal rupture or leaflet prolapse have been well documented in multiple large-scale studies, leading to current guidelines that recommend repair whenever possible (Delgado et al. 2023).

The debate over repair versus replacement in the context of IE centres on concerns about the durability of repair and long-term outcomes. MV repair in IE involves a spectrum of techniques tailored to the lesion's location, the extent of leaflet destruction, and associated complications such as paravalvular abscesses (Arjomandi Rad et al. 2024). The resection technique necessitates the removal of sufficient leaflet tissue to ensure complete eradication of the infectious process. However, the specific surgical approach varies significantly. Lesions on the anterior leaflet, commissural lesions, and scenarios involving extensive leaflet destruction or paravalvular abscess may require distinct and often more complex repair techniques (Arjomandi Rad et al. 2024).

For instance, in cases of anterior leaflet involvement, complex reconstruction using pericardial patches may be necessary due to the leaflet's critical role in valve competence. Commissural lesions might necessitate commissuroplasty or patch augmentation to restore valve function. Extensive destruction may challenge the feasibility of repair and may necessitate valve replacement.

Annuloplasty plays a pivotal role in achieving stable long-term surgical outcomes. It involves the use of a prosthetic ring to provide leaflet coaptation, limit suture tension, and prevent further annular dilation. The choice of annuloplasty ring is crucial; complications such as ring dehiscence have been reported to be higher with rigid rings compared to flexible rings (Arjomandi Rad et al. 2021). Therefore, flexible or semi-rigid rings are often preferred due to their ability to accommodate the dynamic nature of the mitral annulus. Additionally, in patients with active IE, the utilisation of autologous pericardium as an alternative material for annuloplasty represents an adaptation to the unique challenges posed by the infectious environment, potentially reducing the risk of prosthetic-related reinfection (Kazaz et al. 2005).

Early clinical evidence for mitral valve repair in infective endocarditis was described by Dreyfus and colleagues in 1990, who reported 17 cases with low operative mortality and encouraging follow-up outcomes (Dreyfus et al. 1990). Broader support for repair came from Ferringa et al., whose systematic review of 24 studies demonstrated that repair was linked with improved survival and reduced complication rates compared with replacement (Feringa et al. 2007). These conclusions were reinforced by a Taiwanese nationwide cohort study in 2018, which analysed nearly 2000 patients and showed that repair was associated with superior perioperative and long-term outcomes, with the most significant benefit observed in high-volume surgical centres (Lee et al. 2018).

The impact of centre experience on MV repair outcomes has been well documented in the cardiac surgical literature, illustrating the importance of the learning curve and the variability of results among centres with different levels of expertise (Badhwar et al. 2020). The beneficial effects of MV repair have been attributed to the maintenance of the mitral valve apparatus and left ventricular function. Moreover, MV repair avoids or minimises the introduction of prosthetic material, which is advantageous in an infectious setting. MV replacement with a mechanical valve increases the risk of thromboembolic events and necessitates lifelong anticoagulation, while bioprosthetic valves are prone to inevitable structural deterioration.

It must be noted that the feasibility of repair must be assessed in the context of the extent of valvular and extravalvular destruction, with careful intraoperative evaluation of the valve following thorough debridement (El Gabry et al. 2019). Extensive involvement and damage of the anterior mitral leaflet, perivalvular structures, and annular abscess formation may complicate the feasibility of repair, especially in less experienced centres (Arjomandi Rad et al. 2024). In such cases, valve replacement may become necessary.

The lack of standardisation in MV repair techniques for IE is noteworthy and can largely be attributed to the variability in clinical presentations and the extent of complications associated with valvular infection. This diversity necessitates a high degree of customisation in surgical strategies, underscoring the importance of surgical expertise and experience in determining the most appropriate course of action. Furthermore, there is a scarcity of comprehensive long-term data on patients who have undergone MV repair for IE. Information regarding long-term valve function, recurrence of endocarditis, and overall patient outcomes remains limited, highlighting a significant gap in our current understanding. This lack of data underscores the urgent need for systematic follow-up studies and registries to better inform clinical practice and improve patient care strategies in this challenging domain.

(d) ***Mitral Valve Repair Options: Techniques for repair***

1. **Pericardial Patch Reconstruction**

Pericardial patching is a versatile technique used when leaflet perforations or significant tissue loss has occurred due to IE. This approach is particularly useful for repairing large defects on the anterior or posterior leaflets, where direct suturing would compromise the valve's function.

Materials Used

- **Autologous Pericardium**: Fresh autologous pericardium is commonly harvested from the patient and is generally preferred due to its low antigenicity, flexibility, and durability. Autologous patches offer a more compatible biological structure, reducing the risk of calcification or degradation over time.
- **Bovine Pericardium**: Bovine pericardium is another widely used material, favoured for its ready availability and structural integrity. However, its biocompatibility is slightly lower than autologous tissue, which may make it more prone to calcification in younger patients.

Technique

1. **Patch Sizing and Shaping**: The patch is carefully tailored to fit the size and shape of the leaflet defect. A slightly oversized patch is often used to ensure adequate coverage of the damaged area and avoid tension at the suture lines.
2. **Attachment**: The patch is secured to the healthy leaflet edges using fine 5-0 or 6-0 monofilament sutures in a continuous or interrupted fashion, depending on the surgeon's preference and the defect's location. Continuous sutures offer a smoother surface and reduce the risk of thrombogenicity, while interrupted sutures may provide enhanced tensile strength.

3. **Edge Alignment and Coaptation**: Precise placement is critical to ensure that the patch integrates seamlessly with the leaflet and does not interfere with the opposing leaflet during closure. Careful alignment and tensioning help maintain a smooth leaflet surface, facilitating effective coaptation with the opposite leaflet.

Benefits and Considerations Pericardial patches are highly effective in restoring structural integrity to leaflet segments compromised by infection. They provide strength while preserving leaflet mobility, critical for maintaining normal valve dynamics. However, ensuring that the patch material aligns well with the leaflet and avoids excess bulk is essential to minimise the risk of postoperative complications, such as mitral regurgitation or thrombogenesis.

2. **Segmental Leaflet Resection and Reconstruction**

For cases where leaflet damage is localised, particularly on the posterior leaflet, segmental resection allows for the removal of infected or necrotic tissue while retaining functional portions of the leaflet (Arjomandi Rad et al. 2024). This technique is effective in cases where lesions are confined to one segment, enabling the preservation of most of the leaflet structure.

Types of Resection

- **Triangular Resection**: This approach is commonly used for smaller, localised lesions. The triangular section of damaged leaflet tissue is excised, creating two opposing edges that can then be sutured together to restore continuity. Triangular resections are advantageous due to their simplicity and minimal impact on leaflet surface area.
- **Quadrangular Resection**: Used for larger lesions, quadrangular resection involves removing a rectangular section of the leaflet. The free edges are then approximated, sometimes with additional sliding techniques to prevent tension. This technique is often applied to the posterior leaflet, where increased leaflet mobility allows for easier reconstruction.

Reattachment Techniques

- **Direct Suturing of Free Edges**: After resection, the remaining leaflet edges are sutured together using interrupted or continuous 5-0 or 6-0 sutures. Care is taken to align the edges precisely, avoiding excessive tightening that might lead to restricted leaflet motion.
- **Sliding Leaflet Technique**: When a large segment of the posterior leaflet is resected, a sliding technique may be employed to avoid tension at the suture line. This approach involves advancing adjacent leaflet tissue to cover the defect, effectively redistributing the tension and ensuring a more robust repair.

Benefits and Considerations

Segmental resection preserves the overall function of the mitral valve by retaining native tissue and avoiding the use of foreign materials. This method also maintains natural leaflet flexibility, essential for the valve's dynamic movements. However, achieving proper alignment and ensuring adequate coaptation post-repair are critical, as any misalignment can lead to residual mitral regurgitation.

3. **Commissural Repair**

Commissural lesions in IE require particular attention due to their proximity to the mitral annulus and their potential impact on valve function. Commissural repair is more challenging due to the complex geometry and the risk of compromising coaptation.

Techniques for Commissural Repair

- **Commissuroplasty**: This technique involves suturing the damaged leaflet edges at the commissure to restore coaptation without the need for extensive reconstruction. Commissuroplasty is ideal for small, localised defects at the commissure where preservation of leaflet mobility is possible (Arjomandi Rad et al. 2024).
- **Pericardial Patch in Commissure**: When more extensive damage exists, a small pericardial patch may be inserted into the commissural area to reinforce the structure. This patch is carefully trimmed to avoid interference with the neighbouring leaflet and sutured along the leaflet edge, ensuring it provides strength without adding bulk.

Challenges and Solutions

- **Maintaining Annular Flexibility**: The commissure is closely associated with the mitral annulus, and any repair must respect the natural annular flexibility. Rigid or excessive suturing in this area can restrict annular motion, adversely affecting valve dynamics.
- **Avoiding Excessive Tension**: Repairing the commissure with minimal tension is essential to prevent dehiscence or restricted movement, which can compromise valve competency. Fine sutures and careful positioning help minimise tension in this delicate area.

4. **Annuloplasty**

- **Annular Stabilisation**: Application of annuloplasty rings or bands restores annular geometry and ensures proper leaflet coaptation.
- **Choice of Device**:
  - **Flexible or Semi-Rigid Rings**: Preferred due to their accommodation of the mitral annulus's dynamic nature.
  - **Biologic Annuloplasty**: Using autologous pericardium may reduce the risk of prosthetic infection in active IE.

Considerations on the choice of annuloplasty ring are important. Complications such as ring dehiscence have been reported to be higher with rigid rings compared to flexible ones (Arjomandi Rad et al. 2021). Additionally, the use of autologous pericardium for annuloplasty represents an adaptation to the challenges posed by the infectious environment.

(e) ***Prosthetic Mitral Valve Endocarditis: Challenges with Infected Prosthesis and Re-replacement***

Prosthetic Mitral Valve Endocarditis (PMVE)
Introduction

Prosthetic mitral valve endocarditis (PMVE) represents one of the most formidable challenges in cardiac surgery due to its complex pathology and the high-risk nature of reoperative procedures (Arjomandi Rad et al. 2024). PMVE is associated with higher morbidity and mortality rates compared to native valve endocarditis, largely due to the aggressive nature of the infection, the involvement of prosthetic material, and the technical difficulties associated with re-replacement surgery (Arjomandi Rad et al. 2024). Successful management requires a multidisciplinary approach, meticulous surgical technique, and adherence to evidence-based practices.

Pathogenesis and Risk Factors
PMVE can be classified based on the timing of onset after valve implantation:

- **Early PMVE**: Occurs within 12 months of surgery, often within the first 60 days. It is typically nosocomial and associated with perioperative contamination. Common causative organisms include *Staphylococcus aureus* and coagulase-negative staphylococci (Delgado et al. 2023).
- **Late PMVE**: Occurs after 12 months post-implantation. It is more likely due to community-acquired infections with organisms such as *Streptococcus viridans*, *Enterococcus* species, and occasionally fungi (Delgado et al. 2023).

Risk factors for PMVE include previous endocarditis, immunosuppression, diabetes mellitus, prolonged hospitalisation, and the presence of other prosthetic devices or intravascular lines. The prosthetic material provides a surface conducive to bacterial adherence and biofilm formation, making eradication of infection challenging (Arjomandi Rad et al. 2024).

Surgical Challenges
Removal of Infected Prosthesis

Complete excision of the infected prosthesis and all associated foreign material is essential to eradicate the infection. This involves meticulous debridement of the prosthetic sewing ring, sutures, and any infected surrounding tissue. The presence of friable tissue and adhesions from prior surgery increases the risk of intraoperative complications such as bleeding and damage to adjacent cardiac structures. According to Musci et al. (2010), aggressive surgical debridement is crucial for successful outcomes in PMVE (Musci et al. 2010).

Reconstruction of Annular and Periannular Structures
Extensive infection may result in annular destruction, periannular abscesses, or fistula formation, necessitating complex reconstructive procedures:

- **Pericardial Patch Reconstruction**: Autologous or bovine pericardium is used to rebuild the annulus and adjacent structures. This provides a scaffold for prosthesis implantation but may be technically demanding due to the need for precise sizing and shaping to fit the defect.
- **Use of Allografts or Homografts**: Cryopreserved mitral homografts can be considered, especially in cases with extensive destruction. Homografts offer several advantages, including reduced immunogenicity and better resistance to reinfection. However, their availability is limited, and implantation requires specialised expertise. Ali et al. (2004) reported favourable outcomes using homografts in mitral positions (Ali et al. 2004).

Re-replacement Considerations

The choice of prosthesis for re-replacement must consider the risk of reinfection, patient factors, and the potential need for future interventions:

- **Mechanical Valves**: Offer durability but require lifelong anticoagulation. They may be associated with a higher risk of recurrent infection due to the presence of synthetic materials. However, some studies have not demonstrated a significant difference in reinfection rates between mechanical and biological prostheses (Hogan et al. 2024).
- **Bioprosthetic Valves**: Reduce the need for anticoagulation and may have a lower risk of reinfection. Bioprostheses are often preferred in older patients or those with contraindications to anticoagulation. However, they are less durable, particularly in younger patients.
- **Stentless Bioprostheses and Homografts**: May reduce the foreign material burden and potentially lower infection risk. Long-term data are limited, but they may be beneficial in selected patients with extensive infection.

Technical Considerations

Reoperative surgery poses increased risks due to:

- **Adhesions**: Previous sternotomy leads to scar tissue formation, increasing the risk of injury during re-entry. Strategies to mitigate this risk include careful dissection techniques and the use of femoral cannulation for cardiopulmonary bypass initiation before sternotomy.
- **Calcification**: Calcified prosthetic material and annular calcification complicate debridement and prosthesis removal. Ultrasonic decalcification devices may be employed to aid in the safe removal of calcific deposits.
- **Haemodynamic Instability**: Patients may be haemodynamically compromised preoperatively, necessitating rapid surgical intervention and careful intraoperative management, including the use of inotropes and mechanical circulatory support if needed.

Outcomes and Prognosis

PMVE is associated with high mortality rates, with in hospital mortality ranging from 20% to 40%, which is higher than that observed in native valve endocarditis (Arjomandi Rad et al. 2024). Factors influencing outcomes include:

- **Timing of Surgery**: Early surgical intervention after diagnosis is associated with improved survival rates. Lalani et al. (2013) demonstrated that early surgery in infective endocarditis patients reduced mortality (Lalani et al. 2013).
- **Microbiological Etiology**: Infections caused by *Staphylococcus aureus* and fungal organisms carry worse prognoses due to their aggressive nature and resistance to antimicrobial therapy.
- **Complete Eradication of Infection**: Successful removal of all infected material reduces the risk of persistent or recurrent infection. Kim et al. (2016) emphasised the importance of radical debridement in reducing recurrence rates (Kim et al. 2016).

Long-term outcomes depend on patient comorbidities, the extent of infection, and the success of surgical reconstruction. Recurrent endocarditis remains a concern, emphasising the need for diligent postoperative management, including prolonged antibiotic therapy and regular follow-up.

Postoperative Management

- **Antimicrobial Therapy**: Tailored antibiotic regimens based on culture and sensitivity results are critical. A minimum of 6 weeks of intravenous antibiotics is generally recommended, following guidelines from the American Heart Association (AHA) (Nishimura et al. 2014). New guidelines from ESC suggest a combination of intravenous and oral antibiotics can be a viable alternative in selected cases, offering the patient the possibility of an earlier discharge and therefore a quicker recovery (Delgado et al. 2023).
- **Monitoring for Complications**: Regular follow-up with echocardiography is essential to assess prosthesis function and detect early signs of reinfection or prosthesis dysfunction.
- **Anticoagulation Management**: In patients with mechanical prostheses, careful balancing of anticoagulation is necessary to prevent thromboembolic events while minimising bleeding risks.
- **Antibiotic prophylaxis**: Patients with prosthetic valves are already at a higher risk of IE than the general population; however patients with previous endocarditis are at the highest risk of endocarditis; both AHA and ESC recommend antibiotic prophylaxis for dental treatments involving manipulation of the gum in these patients.

3 Acute Mitral Regurgitation

(a) ***Aetiology***

Papillary Muscle Rupture

Acute mitral regurgitation due to papillary muscle rupture is a life-threatening condition that typically occurs following an acute myocardial infarction (AMI) (Güvenç and Güvenç 2016). The posteromedial papillary muscle is more commonly affected because it receives blood supply solely from the posterior descending artery, making it particularly vulnerable to ischaemia during inferior or posterior infarctions involving the right coronary artery (Burton and Beier 2023). Rupture of the papillary muscle leads to abrupt loss of mitral valve competency, resulting in sudden and severe regurgitation.

This catastrophic event causes an immediate increase in left atrial pressure and volume overload, leading to pulmonary oedema and cardiogenic shock. Patients often present with acute dyspnea, hypotension, and signs of low cardiac output. Given the rapid haemodynamic deterioration, prompt recognition and emergency surgical intervention are critical. Without surgery, mortality rates are exceedingly high due to the inability of the compromised heart to compensate for the sudden regurgitant volume.

Chordae Tendineae Rupture or Leaflet Prolapse

Chordal rupture or leaflet prolapse is another cause of acute severe mitral regurgitation leading to haemodynamic instability. Chordae tendineae may rupture due to various etiologies, including:

- **Myxomatous Degeneration**: In patients with mitral valve prolapse syndrome, elongated and weakened chordae are prone to rupture.
- **Infective Endocarditis**: Destruction of chordae by infective processes can lead to sudden leaflet flail.
- **Trauma**: Blunt chest trauma can directly damage the chordal structures.
- **Iatrogenic Causes**: Injury during interventional procedures such as percutaneous mitral balloon valvotomy.

The sudden loss of chordal support results in leaflet flail and significant mitral regurgitation. Clinically, patients may exhibit acute onset of dyspnea, tachycardia, and signs of pulmonary congestion. Haemodynamic instability arises due to decreased forward stroke volume and increased regurgitant flow into the left atrium, overwhelming pulmonary circulation. Emergency surgical repair or replacement of the mitral valve is indicated to restore valve function and stabilise the patient.

(b) ***Preoperative Planning***

Haemodynamic Support

Patients presenting with acute severe mitral regurgitation require immediate haemodynamic stabilisation to optimise conditions before surgical intervention. Strategies include:

- **Intra-Aortic Balloon Pump (IABP) Counterpulsation**:
  - *Mechanism*: IABP reduces afterload by inflating during diastole and deflating just before systole, decreasing left ventricular workload and regurgitant volume.
  - *Benefits*: Improves coronary artery perfusion, augments systemic perfusion, and alleviates pulmonary congestion.
  - *Considerations*: Placement should not delay surgical intervention; contraindicated in patients with significant aortic regurgitation or aortic dissection.

- **Extracorporeal Membrane Oxygenation (ECMO)**:
    - *Indications*: Reserved for patients with refractory cardiogenic shock unresponsive to conventional therapies.
    - *Types*: Veno-arterial ECMO provides both cardiac and respiratory support. Veno-venous ECMO is of limited use in these cases.
    - *Benefits*: Stabilises haemodynamics, allows time for end-organ recovery, and serves as a bridge to surgery.
    - *Considerations*: Requires specialised equipment and expertise; associated with risks such as bleeding, thrombosis, and infection.
- **Pharmacological Management**:
    - *Vasodilators*: Agents like nitroprusside reduce systemic vascular resistance, decreasing afterload and regurgitant fraction.
    - *Inotropes*: Medications such as dobutamine enhance myocardial contractility but must be used cautiously to avoid increasing regurgitant flow.
    - *Diuretics*: Alleviate pulmonary congestion but may lead to hypotension if not carefully managed.

(c) ***Papillary Muscle Rupture***

Papillary muscle rupture is a catastrophic mechanical complication of acute myocardial infarction that necessitates emergent surgical intervention due to the severe haemodynamic instability it precipitates. The rupture leads to acute severe mitral regurgitation, resulting in rapid volume overload of the left atrium and pulmonary congestion, often culminating in cardiogenic shock. The surgical management involves a critical decision between reattachment of the ruptured papillary muscle and mitral valve replacement, contingent upon factors such as the extent of rupture (partial or complete), viability of the remaining papillary muscle tissue, condition of the mitral valve leaflets and chordae tendineae, and the patient's overall clinical status. The overarching surgical objectives are to restore mitral valve competence, preserve LV function, and ensure long-term durability of the repair or replacement.

Techniques for Papillary Muscle Reattachment

Reattachment of the ruptured papillary muscle is feasible and preferred when the muscle head remains viable and the rupture is partial. This approach preserves the native mitral valve and maintains the subvalvular apparatus, which is crucial for optimal LV function. Several techniques are employed (Hamid et al. 2022; Athanasopoulos et al. 2017; Dreyfus et al. 2006):

1. **Direct Reimplantation**

This technique involves reattaching the ruptured papillary muscle directly to its original position on the LV wall or adjacent viable myocardium using pledgeted, non-absorbable sutures such as 4-0 or 5-0 polypropylene (Prolene) or polyester (Ethibond) sutures. Deep bites are taken into healthy myocardial tissue to ensure secure fixation, and pledgets (e.g. Teflon felt) are used to distribute the stress and prevent suture pull-through. Careful attention is required to avoid ventricular perforation and ensure haemostasis at suture sites.

2. **Papillary Muscle Shortening or Relocation**

In cases where papillary muscle elongation or displacement contributes to leaflet malcoaptation, the muscle can be shortened or repositioned. This may involve plicating the papillary muscle or securing it to the ventricular wall at an appropriate position using sutures. This adjustment restores the correct tension on the chordae tendineae, facilitating proper leaflet coaptation. Oi et al. (2022) demonstrated that papillary muscle relocation can effectively address functional MR by restoring the geometric relationship between the papillary muscles and mitral valve leaflets.

3. **Use of Artificial Chordae**

When native chordae are damaged or insufficient, artificial chordae constructed from expanded polytetrafluoroethylene (ePTFE) sutures (e.g. Gore-Tex) are utilised. The ePTFE sutures are anchored to the papillary muscle remnant or the LV wall and attached to the free edge of the mitral leaflet. The length of the artificial chordae is carefully adjusted intraoperatively to ensure optimal leaflet coaptation without tension. David et al. (2020) reported favourable long-term results using ePTFE sutures for chordal replacement in mitral valve repair.

4. **Papillary Muscle Approximation**

If the papillary muscle is split or bifurcated, approximation of the muscle heads can restore functional anatomy. Sutures are used to approximate and secure the separated segments, re-establishing the normal configuration and tension of the subvalvular apparatus. This technique helps in achieving effective leaflet coaptation and mitral competence.

Additional Aspects of Mitral Valve Repair

Following successful reattachment of the papillary muscle, additional mitral valve repair techniques may be necessary to address any residual regurgitation. Annuloplasty is an integral component, involving the implantation of an annuloplasty ring or band to restore the normal size and shape of the mitral annulus, thereby enhancing leaflet coaptation. Flexible or semi-rigid rings, such as the Carpentier-Edwards Physio ring, are preferred as they accommodate the dynamic motion of the annulus and reduce stress on the repair. Leaflet repair techniques, such as triangular resection of prolapsing segments, sliding plasty, or edge-to-edge repair (Alfieri stitch), may also be employed based on the specific pathology.

Mitral Valve Replacement

When reattachment of the papillary muscle is not feasible—due to complete rupture with extensive damage, non-viable myocardial tissue, or when repair is unlikely to yield a durable result—mitral valve replacement becomes necessary. Preservation of the subvalvular apparatus during replacement is crucial for maintaining LV function. Techniques involve retaining as much of the native chordae and papillary muscles as possible, reattaching them to the prosthetic valve sewing ring. Generally evidence shows that preservation of chordal structures during mitral valve replacement significantly improves postoperative LV function and survival (Popovic et al. 1996; Solomon et al. 2006).

Outcomes and Prognosis
Early surgical intervention in papillary muscle rupture is associated with improved survival rates. In a series reported by Russo et al. (2008), operative mortality ranged from 20% to 30%, but survivors had good long-term outcomes with appropriate surgical management (Russo et al. 2008). The choice of repair versus replacement should be individualised, considering patient-specific factors and the surgeon's expertise.

(d) ***Chordal Rupture or Prolapse***

Acute mitral regurgitation resulting from chordal rupture or prolapse represents a surgical emergency characterised by sudden haemodynamic instability due to severe mitral valve dysfunction. The loss of chordal support leads to flail leaflet segments, causing significant regurgitant flow into the left atrium, which precipitates pulmonary oedema and cardiogenic shock.

Etiology and Pathophysiology
Chordal rupture or prolapse can result from several etiologies:

1. **Myxomatous Degeneration (Degenerative Mitral Valve Disease)**

   - *Mitral Valve Prolapse (MVP)*: This is the most common cause in developed countries. Myxoid degeneration leads to elongation or rupture of chordae tendineae, resulting in leaflet prolapse. Freed et al. (1999) reported that MVP affects approximately 2–3% of the population (Freed et al. 1999).
   - *Barlow's Disease*: Characterised by diffuse myxomatous changes, excessive leaflet tissue, and redundant chordae, leading to multisegmental prolapse.

2. **Infective Endocarditis**

Destructive vegetations can erode chordal structures, causing rupture and acute MR.

3. **Trauma**

Blunt chest trauma can directly injure the chordae tendineae, leading to acute MR. This is relatively rare but must be considered in the context of chest injuries.

4. **Rheumatic Heart Disease**

Chronic inflammatory processes result in fibrosis and weakening of chordae over time, making them susceptible to rupture.

5. **Iatrogenic Causes**

Complications from percutaneous interventions, such as mitral valvuloplasty, or surgical procedures involving the mitral valve can lead to chordal injury.

Surgical Techniques

1. **Artificial Chordae Replacement with ePTFE Sutures**

This technique involves the creation of artificial chordae using ePTFE sutures to replace ruptured or elongated native chordae, effectively restoring normal leaflet position and function.

- **Technique**

ePTFE sutures (4-0 or 5-0) are anchored to the papillary muscle head using pledgeted mattress sutures. The free ends are passed through the fibrous portion of the prolapsed leaflet edge multiple times to prevent cutting through the tissue. Accurate adjustment of chordal length is achieved by filling the left ventricle with saline to mimic physiological conditions (saline test) and adjusting the sutures until optimal leaflet coaptation is observed.

2. **Leaflet Resection Techniques**

- **Quadrangular Resection**

Indicated for isolated prolapse of the middle scallop (P2) of the posterior leaflet. The prolapsed segment is excised, and the adjacent leaflet edges are approximated. This may be combined with a sliding plasty to prevent annular distortion.

- **Triangular Resection**

Suitable for smaller prolapsing areas or when leaflet preservation is critical. A triangular segment is excised, and the leaflet edges are sutured together, maintaining appropriate leaflet height.

3. **Folding Plasty (Posterior Leaflet Folding)**

This technique addresses excessive posterior leaflet height contributing to prolapse by folding and suturing the redundant leaflet tissue onto itself, reducing height while preserving leaflet tissue. This method avoids resection and maintains leaflet mobility.

4. **Edge-to-Edge Repair (Alfieri Stitch)**

Used in complex or multifocal prolapse cases, bileaflet prolapse, or as a secondary technique when other repairs are inadequate. The free edges of the anterior and posterior leaflets are sutured together at the site of regurgitation, creating a double-orifice valve. This technique, introduced by Alfieri et al., provides a simple and quick solution but may result in mitral stenosis if not carefully performed (Alfieri et al. 2001).

5. **Commissuroplasty**

Indicated for prolapse involving the commissural scallops (e.g. P3 or A3 segments). Suturing the affected commissure eliminates the regurgitant orifice but requires caution to maintain adequate mitral orifice area.

6. **Annuloplasty**

An annuloplasty is essential in all repair procedures to restore annular size and shape, ensuring proper leaflet coaptation. The annuloplasty ring is selected based on the anterior leaflet height and secured to the annulus with interrupted sutures for even distribution. Flexible or semi-rigid rings are preferred to accommodate dynamic annular motion and reduce stress on the repair. Inappropriate ring sizing can lead to systolic anterior motion or residual MR.

Outcomes and Prognosis

Mitral valve repair for chordal rupture or prolapse has been associated with excellent long-term outcomes. According to David et al. (2020), the 20-year freedom from reoperation was approximately 90% in patients who underwent mitral valve repair with chordal replacement (David et al. 2020). Preservation of the native mitral valve and subvalvular apparatus contributes to better postoperative LV function and survival compared to valve replacement.

(e) ***Concomitant Coronary Artery Bypass Grafting (CABG) with Mitral Valve Replacement in Ischemic Mitral Regurgitation***

Ischemic MR is a complex condition resulting from LV remodelling due to coronary artery disease (CAD), leading to dysfunction of the mitral valve apparatus. When severe MR coexists with significant multivessel CAD, surgical intervention often necessitates both mitral valve replacement and coronary revascularisation. Concomitant CABG addresses the underlying myocardial ischaemia while MVR corrects the valvular insufficiency, aiming to improve haemodynamics, alleviate symptoms, and enhance long-term survival (Naruka et al. 2024).

Guidelines and Recommendations

Current clinical guidelines support the combined approach of CABG and MVR in patients with severe ischemic MR. The American College of Cardiology (ACC) and the American Heart Association (AHA) recommend that in patients with chronic severe secondary (ischemic) MR undergoing CABG, mitral valve surgery is indicated (Class I recommendation) (Otto et al. 2020). The guidelines emphasise that addressing both the valvular lesion and the myocardial ischaemia in a single operative session optimises patient outcomes by reducing the risk of heart failure progression and improving survival rates. There is still no clear evidence to indicate that the same applies to moderate ischemic MR in patients undergoing CABG, there is a high degree of controversy in this topic.

Evidence Supporting Concomitant CABG and MVR

Clinical studies and meta-analyses have demonstrated the benefits of concomitant CABG and MVR in patients with severe ischemic MR (Sá et al. 2013; Virk et al. 2017; Pienta et al. 2023; Chan et al. 2012):

- **Improved Survival**: The addition of MVR to CABG has been associated with enhanced long-term survival compared to CABG alone.
- **Enhanced Left Ventricular Function**: Correcting severe MR reduces volume overload on the left ventricle, promoting reverse remodelling and improving ejection fraction over time.

- **Symptomatic Relief**: Patients experience significant reductions in heart failure symptoms, such as dyspnea and fatigue, leading to improved quality of life.
- **Reduction in Hospitalisations**: Combined surgery decreases the frequency of hospital readmissions for heart failure exacerbations.

Surgical Considerations

Performing concomitant CABG and MVR involves several technical considerations:

- **Operative Strategy**: The surgical team must decide on the sequence of procedures. Most surgeons prefer completing the distal coronary anastomoses before addressing the mitral valve to restore myocardial perfusion early in the operation and avoid mobilisation of the heart after a prosthesis has been implanted.
- **Preservation of Subvalvular Apparatus**: During MVR, it is crucial to preserve as much of the subvalvular apparatus (chordae tendineae and papillary muscles) as possible. Chordal-sparing techniques maintain LV geometry and function, reducing the risk of postoperative ventricular dysfunction.
- **Myocardial Protection**: Given the extended cross-clamp time required for combined procedures, meticulous myocardial protection using cold blood cardioplegia and systemic hypothermia is essential. New studies will show if the use of more modern cardioplegia solutions like Del Nido or Custodiol will improve outcomes for these patients.
- **Graft Selection and Placement**: Emphasis on complete revascularisation, especially of vessels supplying viable myocardium and areas related to the mitral apparatus.

4 Critical Mitral Stenosis

(a) ***Indications***

Severe Decompensated Stenosis: Symptomatic Patients with Haemodynamic Instability

Critical mitral stenosis is characterised by a markedly reduced mitral valve orifice area, leading to significant obstruction of blood flow from the left atrium to the left ventricle during diastole. The normal mitral valve area ranges from 4 to 6 cm^2. Symptoms typically manifest when the valve area decreases below 1.5 cm^2, with severe stenosis defined as an area less than 1.0 cm^2.

Clinical Presentation

Indications for Emergency Surgical Intervention

Emergency surgery is indicated in patients with critical mitral stenosis who exhibit (Beyersdorf et al. 2021):

- **Severe Symptomatic Decompensation**: NYHA Class III-IV symptoms refractory to medical therapy.
- **Haemodynamic Instability**: Evidence of cardiogenic shock or pulmonary oedema requiring ventilatory support.

- **Refractory Symptoms**: Persistent symptoms despite aggressive diuretic therapy and afterload reduction.
- **Thromboembolic Events**: Recent cerebrovascular accidents or systemic emboli associated with left atrial thrombus.
- **Contraindications to Percutaneous Intervention**: Patients unsuitable for percutaneous mitral balloon valvotomy (PMBV) due to unfavourable valve morphology or presence of left atrial thrombus.

Assessment of Valve Anatomy and Suitability for Surgery
Comprehensive preoperative evaluation is crucial to determine the optimal surgical approach:

- **Echocardiography**: Transthoracic and transoesophageal echocardiography provide detailed assessment of:
    - **Valve Morphology**: Leaflet mobility, thickness, calcification, and commissural fusion.
    - **Subvalvular Apparatus**: Degree of chordal thickening and fusion.
    - **Left Atrial Size and Thrombus**: Identification of thrombus contraindicates PMBV.
    - **Pulmonary Artery Pressures**: Estimation of pulmonary hypertension severity.
- **Wilkins Score**: A scoring system evaluating valve anatomy to predict suitability for PMBV versus surgical intervention.
- **Cardiac Catheterisation**: Haemodynamic measurements and coronary angiography in patients with risk factors for coronary artery disease.

(b) ***Operative Considerations***

Stenotic Native Valve Repair vs. Replacement
The decision between mitral valve repair and replacement hinges on the anatomical features of the valve, the extent of pathological changes, and the likelihood of achieving a durable, satisfactory result. The primary objective is to relieve the obstruction, alleviate symptoms, and improve haemodynamics while minimising surgical risks and preserving left ventricular function.

Mitral Valve Repair
Mitral valve repair aims to restore normal valve function by correcting structural abnormalities without replacing the native valve. Surgical commissurotomy is the most common repair technique for mitral stenosis.

Indications for Repair
- **Favourable Valve Anatomy**:
    - **Mobile Leaflets**: Minimal leaflet thickening and calcification.
    - **Commissural Fusion**: Predominant commissural involvement without extensive calcification.
    - **Mild Subvalvular Disease**: Limited chordal fusion or thickening.

- **Younger Patients**: Valve preservation is preferred to avoid prosthesis-related complications and the need for anticoagulation.

Surgical Techniques

1. **Open Surgical Commissurotomy**
   - **Procedure Overview**: Direct visualisation and separation of fused commissures and mobilisation of the leaflets and subvalvular apparatus.
   - **Technique Details**:
     - **Access**: Median sternotomy followed by cardiopulmonary bypass and cardioplegic arrest. Left atriotomy is performed through the interatrial groove.
     - **Commissural Incision**: Fused commissures are incised using a scalpel or fine scissors, extending from the annulus to the leaflet tips.
     - **Leaflet Mobilisation**: Calcific deposits are carefully debrided, and leaflet mobility is restored. Care is taken to avoid creating leaflet perforations.
     - **Subvalvular Release**: Chordae tendineae are separated if fused, and papillary muscle mobility is assessed.
   - **Advantages**:
     - **Valve Preservation**: Maintains native valve structures and function.
     - **Avoidance of Prosthesis**: Eliminates risks associated with prosthetic valves, such as thrombosis and endocarditis.
   - **Limitations**:
     - **Durability**: Potential for restenosis due to progressive rheumatic disease or re-fusion of commissures.
     - **Technical Complexity**: Requires meticulous surgical technique to prevent regurgitation or residual stenosis.
2. **Valvuloplasty with Patch Augmentation**
   - **Indications**: Cases with limited leaflet area or when significant calcification prevents adequate commissurotomy.
   - **Technique**:
     - **Leaflet Augmentation**: Diseased leaflet segments are excised, and patches of autologous pericardium or bovine pericardium are used to enlarge the leaflet area.
     - **Annular Enlargement**: The mitral annulus may be enlarged using patch material to increase the valve orifice.
   - **Considerations**:
     - **Complexity**: Technically demanding and may not be suitable in emergency settings.
     - **Risk of Regurgitation**: Increased if leaflet coaptation is not adequately achieved.

Mitral Valve Replacement

Mitral valve replacement the most common performed procedure for this patients as in most of them repair is not feasible or unlikely to provide a durable result due to extensive pathological changes.

Indications for Replacement

- **Extensive Leaflet Thickening and Calcification**: Rigid, immobile leaflets with heavy calcification.
- **Severe Subvalvular Disease**: Marked chordal fusion, shortening, or calcification.
- **Failed Previous Repairs**: Recurrent stenosis after prior commissurotomy or valvuloplasty.
- **Mixed Valve Disease**: Presence of both significant stenosis and regurgitation.

Excision of Native Valve

- **Leaflet Removal**: Diseased anterior and posterior leaflets are excised. Preservation of posterior leaflet and chordae may be considered to maintain left ventricular function.
- **Subvalvular Apparatus Management**:
    - **Chordal Preservation**: Retaining chordae tendineae when possible to preserve ventricular geometry.
    - **Calcification Debridement**: Meticulous removal of calcific deposits from the annulus and subvalvular structures.

5 Acute Complications of Mitral Valve Prosthesis and Post-repair

Management of Prosthetic Valve Thrombosis and Obstruction

Prosthetic valve thrombosis is a severe complication that can occur after mitral valve replacement with mechanical prostheses. It leads to obstruction of the valve orifice due to thrombus formation on or around the prosthetic valve, resulting in impaired leaflet or occluder motion. Prompt surgical intervention is often required because delayed treatment increases the risk of mortality and morbidity.

The primary surgical options are thrombectomy and prosthetic valve replacement. Thrombectomy involves the surgical removal of thrombotic material obstructing the prosthesis while preserving the existing valve. This approach is considered when the thrombus is small, localised, and the prosthesis is structurally intact. Surgical thrombectomy allows for the restoration of valve function without the risks associated with re-replacement, such as prosthesis-patient mismatch or additional complications from reoperative surgery.

However, in cases where the thrombus is extensive, the prosthesis is damaged, or there is significant pannus formation—a fibrovascular overgrowth that obstructs the valve—prosthetic valve replacement becomes necessary. The existing prosthesis is carefully explanted, and a new valve is implanted. According to a study by Durrleman et al. (2004), surgical replacement for prosthetic valve thrombosis had a mortality rate of approximately 20%, underscoring the seriousness of this complication and the need for timely intervention (Dürrleman et al. 2004).

Postoperative management focuses on optimising anticoagulation therapy to prevent recurrent thrombosis. Warfarin is typically used to maintain an appropriate international normalised ratio (INR), with target levels adjusted based on the type of prosthesis and patient-specific factors. Close monitoring of anticoagulation status is essential, as subtherapeutic levels increase the risk of thrombus formation, while supratherapeutic levels raise the risk of bleeding.

Management of Prosthetic Valve Endocarditis with Dehiscence

Prosthetic valve endocarditis is a life-threatening infection involving the prosthetic material and surrounding cardiac tissue. It can lead to prosthetic dehiscence, where the valve becomes partially or completely detached from the annulus, causing severe regurgitation and haemodynamic instability. Surgical intervention is critical to eradicate the infection and restore valve function.

The management of PVE with dehiscence involves complete removal of the infected prosthesis and extensive debridement of all infected and necrotic tissue. This step is crucial to eliminate the source of infection and prevent recurrence. Annular reconstruction may be required if there is significant destruction of the mitral annulus. Techniques such as the use of autologous pericardial patches or bovine pericardium can help rebuild the annular structure, providing a secure foundation for the new prosthesis.

Implantation of a new prosthetic valve follows, with careful consideration given to the type of prosthesis. Bioprosthetic valves are often favoured in this context due to their lower thrombogenicity and reduced need for long-term anticoagulation, which is beneficial in patients recovering from infection.

Management of Left Ventricular Outflow Tract (LVOT) Obstruction Post-repair

LVOT obstruction is a recognised complication following mitral valve repair, particularly when surgical techniques inadvertently alter the geometry of the mitral apparatus. SAM of the anterior mitral leaflet can occur, leading to dynamic obstruction of the LVOT and significant haemodynamic compromise.

Preventive strategies during surgery are paramount. Preserving the posterior leaflet and chordae tendineae helps maintain normal subvalvular geometry and prevents anterior displacement of the mitral apparatus. Avoiding excessive resection of leaflet tissue and careful sizing of annuloplasty rings are critical to minimise the risk of SAM. Techniques such as the "respect rather than resect" approach advocated by Perier et al. (2015) emphasise the importance of leaflet preservation (Perier et al. 2015).

Intraoperative TEE allows for immediate detection of LVOT obstruction. If identified, surgical adjustments can be made, such as resizing the annuloplasty ring or modifying leaflet repair techniques. Postoperatively, medical management with beta-blockers can reduce heart rate and contractility, decreasing the degree of obstruction. In refractory cases, reoperation may be necessary to revise the repair.

Management of Paravalvular Leaks

Paravalvular leaks occur when there is a gap between the prosthetic valve sewing ring and the native annulus, leading to regurgitation around the valve. Significant PVLs can cause haemolysis, heart failure symptoms, and increase the risk of endocarditis. Surgical repair is indicated for symptomatic PVLs or those causing significant haemolysis.

Surgical management involves reoperation with removal of the existing prosthesis, thorough debridement of the annulus to remove fibrous tissue or calcifications, and implantation of a new prosthesis. Reinforcement of the annulus using patches of pericardium or synthetic materials may be necessary to provide a solid anchoring surface. Pledgeted sutures are employed to secure the prosthesis and distribute tension evenly, reducing the risk of recurrent leaks.

Transcatheter closure has emerged as an alternative for high-risk surgical patients. Devices such as occluder systems can be deployed via catheterisation to seal the leak. Studies reported a procedural success rate of around 80% with transcatheter PVL closure, along with significant symptom relief and improvement in quality of life (Taramasso et al. 2016). However, this approach is not suitable for all patients, particularly those with large or irregular defects.

6 Transcatheter Interventions for Emergency Mitral Valve Scenarios

Transcatheter therapies, particularly the MitraClip system, have emerged as a critical tool in the management of acute mitral regurgitation (MR) in emergency settings. These techniques are especially valuable for high-risk patients who cannot tolerate conventional surgical intervention, providing both immediate haemodynamic stabilisation and a bridge to definitive treatment or recovery.

Clinical Applications and Evidence

1. **MitraClip as a Bridge to Surgery or Recovery**:
    - The **MitraBridge Registry** provides compelling evidence for MitraClip's use in bridging high-risk patients with severe MR to heart transplantation (HTx) or recovery. Among 119 patients treated with MitraClip, procedural success was 87.5%, and survival at 30 days reached 100%. At follow-up, 15% underwent elective HTx, while 23.5% showed such clinical improvement that HTx was no longer required. This demonstrates MitraClip's potential to stabilise patients with advanced heart failure and significant MR while mitigating perioperative risks (Godino et al. 2020)
2. **MitraClip in Cardiogenic Shock**:
    - In patients with cardiogenic shock secondary to acute MR, MitraClip has been successfully used in combination with mechanical circulatory support devices such as Impella. This strategy reduced MR severity and facilitated stabilisation, enabling successful weaning from mechanical ventilation. Survival to discharge

reached 86% in critically ill patients unsuitable for immediate surgery, with 80% survival at 6 months (Vandenbriele et al. 2020, 2021)

3. **Preoperative Stabilisation**:

    - A case report highlights MitraClip's use in a patient listed for HTx who had severe MR and refractory heart failure. The device significantly improved functional status and reduced pulmonary hypertension, enabling a successful transplant 8 months later. This underscores MitraClip's utility in stabilising patients as a bridge-to-transplant therapy (Garatti et al. 2015).

Technical Advantages

- **Minimally Invasive Approach**: MitraClip eliminates the need for cardiopulmonary bypass, reducing perioperative morbidity in high-risk patients.
- **Rapid Deployment**: These procedures can be performed emergently under echocardiographic guidance, ensuring timely intervention in acute settings.
- **Preservation of Surgical Options**: MitraClip often serves as a temporary solution, preserving the anatomy for future surgical repair or replacement.

Limitations and Challenges

1. **Anatomical Feasibility**:

    - MitraClip is most effective in cases where leaflet coaptation can be restored without excessive tethering or annular dilation. Cases involving extensive tissue destruction or severe calcification may require open surgery.

2. **Durability of Repair**:

    - While MitraClip provides immediate relief, recurrent MR may occur over time, particularly in cases with suboptimal clip positioning or progressive valvular pathology.

3. **Learning Curve**:

    - Successful outcomes require expertise in transoesophageal echocardiography (TEE) and procedural techniques, emphasising the importance of a multidisciplinary heart team.

7 Conclusion

Emergency mitral valve surgery represents a challenging yet essential intervention in cases of acute mitral dysfunction where rapid deterioration threatens patient survival. Through rigorous preoperative assessment, innovative surgical techniques, and comprehensive postoperative care, cardiac surgeons can significantly improve patient outcomes. This chapter highlights the need for surgical expertise and a coordinated multidisciplinary approach to manage these high-risk situations effectively. As knowledge advances, integrating evidence-based practices with clinical experience will be key to further refining the strategies and protocols that support successful outcomes in emergency mitral valve surgery.

References

Alfieri O, Maisano F, De Bonis M, Stefano PL, Torracca L, Oppizzi M et al (2001) The double-orifice technique in mitral valve repair: a simple solution for complex problems. J Thorac Cardiovasc Surg 122:674–681. https://doi.org/10.1067/MTC.2001.117277

Ali M, Iung B, Lansac E, Bruneval P, Acar C (2004) Homograft replacement of the mitral valve: eight-year results. J Thorac Cardiovasc Surg 128:529–534. https://doi.org/10.1016/j.jtcvs.2003.11.076

Arjomandi Rad A, Naruka V, Vardanyan R, Viviano A, Salmasi MY, Magouliotis D et al (2021) Mitral and tricuspid annuloplasty ring dehiscence: a systematic review with pooled analysis. Eur J Cardiothorac Surg 60:801. https://doi.org/10.1093/EJCTS/EZAB178

Arjomandi Rad A, Zubarevich A, Osswald A, Vardanyan R, Magouliotis DE, Ansaripour A et al (2024) The surgical treatment of infective endocarditis: a comprehensive review. Diagnostics 14:464. https://doi.org/10.3390/DIAGNOSTICS14050464

Athanasopoulos LV, Casula RP, Punjabi PP, Abdullahi YS, Athanasiou T (2017) A technical review of subvalvular techniques for repair of ischaemic mitral regurgitation and their associated echocardiographic and survival outcomes. Interact Cardiovasc Thorac Surg 25:975–982. https://doi.org/10.1093/ICVTS/IVX187

Badhwar V, Vemulapalli S, Mack MA, Gillinov AM, Chikwe J, Dearani JA et al (2020) Volume-outcome association of mitral valve surgery in the United States. JAMA Cardiol 5:1092–1101. https://doi.org/10.1001/JAMACARDIO.2020.2221

Beyersdorf F, Vahanian A, Milojevic M, Praz F, Baldus S, Bauersachs J et al (2021) 2021 ESC/EACTS Guidelines for the management of valvular heart disease: developed by the Task Force for the management of valvular heart disease of the European Society of Cardiology (ESC) and the European Association for Cardio-Thoracic Surgery (EACTS). Eur J Cardiothorac Surg 60:727–800. https://doi.org/10.1093/EJCTS/EZAB389

Burton LV, Beier K (2023) Papillary muscle rupture. StatPearls

Chan KMJ, Punjabi PP, Flather M, Wage R, Symmonds K, Roussin I et al (2012) Coronary artery bypass surgery with or without mitral valve annuloplasty in moderate functional ischemic mitral regurgitation: final results of the Randomized Ischemic Mitral Evaluation (RIME) trial. Circulation 126:2502–2510. https://doi.org/10.1161/CIRCULATIONAHA.112.143818/-/DC1

David TE, David CM, Lafreniere-Roula M, Manlhiot C (2020) Long-term outcomes of chordal replacement with expanded polytetrafluoroethylene sutures to repair mitral leaflet prolapse. J Thorac Cardiovasc Surg 160:385–394.e1. https://doi.org/10.1016/J.JTCVS.2019.08.006

Delgado V, Ajmone Marsan N, de Waha S, Bonaros N, Brida M, Burri H et al (2023) 2023 ESC Guidelines for the management of endocarditis: developed by the task force on the management of endocarditis of the European Society of Cardiology (ESC) Endorsed by the European Association for Cardio-Thoracic Surgery (EACTS) and the European Association of Nuclear Medicine (EANM). Eur Heart J 44:3948–4042. https://doi.org/10.1093/EURHEARTJ/EHAD193

Dreyfus G, Serraf A, Jebara VA, Deloche A, Chauvaud S, Couetil JP et al (1990) Valve repair in acute endocarditis. Ann Thorac Surg 49:706–713. https://doi.org/10.1016/0003-4975(90)90007-S

Dreyfus GD, Neto OS, Aubert S (2006) Papillary muscle repositioning for repair of anterior leaflet prolapse caused by chordal elongation. J Thorac Cardiovasc Surg 132:578–584. https://doi.org/10.1016/J.JTCVS.2006.06.003

Dürrleman N, Pellerin M, Bouchard D, Hébert Y, Cartier R, Perrault LP et al (2004) Prosthetic valve thrombosis: twenty-year experience at the Montreal Heart Institute. J Thorac Cardiovasc Surg 127:1388–1392. https://doi.org/10.1016/j.jtcvs.2003.12.013

El Gabry M, Haidari Z, Mourad F, Nowak J, Tsagakis K, Thielmann M et al (2019) Outcomes of mitral valve repair in acute native mitral valve infective endocarditis. Interact Cardiovasc Thorac Surg 29:823–829. https://doi.org/10.1093/ICVTS/IVZ187

Feringa HHH, Shaw LJ, Poldermans D, Hoeks S, van der Wall EE, Dion RAE et al (2007) Mitral valve repair and replacement in endocarditis: a systematic review of literature. Ann Thorac Surg 83:564–570. https://doi.org/10.1016/J.ATHORACSUR.2006.09.023

Freed LA, Levy D, Levine RA, Larson MG, Evans JC, Fuller DL et al (1999) Prevalence and clinical outcome of mitral-valve prolapse. N Engl J Med 341:1–7. https://doi.org/10.1056/NEJM199907013410101

Garatti A, Castelvecchio S, Bandera F, Medda M, Menicanti L (2015) Mitraclip procedure as a bridge therapy in a patient with heart failure listed for heart transplantation. Ann Thorac Surg 99(5):1796–1799. https://doi.org/10.1016/J.ATHORACSUR.2014.07.079

Godino C, Munafò A, Scotti A, Estévez-Loureiro R, Portolés Hernández A, Arzamendi D et al (2020) MitraClip in secondary mitral regurgitation as a bridge to heart transplantation: 1-year outcomes from the International MitraBridge Registry. J Heart Lung Transplant 39:1353–1362. https://doi.org/10.1016/j.healun.2020.09.005

Güvenç RÇ, Güvenç TS (2016) Clinical presentation, diagnosis and management of acute mitral regurgitation following acute myocardial infarction. J Acute Dis 5:96–101. https://doi.org/10.1016/J.JOAD.2015.11.001

Hamid UI, Aksoy R, Nia PS (2022) Mitral valve repair in papillary muscle rupture. Ann Cardiothorac Surg 11:28189–28289. https://doi.org/10.21037/ACS-2021-AMI-23

Hogan KJ, Sylvester CB, Wall MJ, Rosengart TK, Coselli JS, Moon MR et al (2024) Outcomes after bioprosthetic versus mechanical mitral valve replacement for infective endocarditis in the United States. JTCVS Open 17:74–83. https://doi.org/10.1016/J.XJON.2023.11.019

Kazaz H, Celkan MA, Ustunsoy H, Baspinar O, Mestres CA (2005) Mitral annuloplasty with biodegradable ring for infective endocarditis: a new tool for the surgeon for valve repair in childhood. Interact Cardiovasc Thorac Surg 4:378–380. https://doi.org/10.1510/ICVTS.2005.105833

Kim JB, Ejiofor JI, Yammine M, Ando M, Camuso JM, Youngster I et al (2016) Surgical outcomes of infective endocarditis among intravenous drug users. J Thorac Cardiovasc Surg 152:832–841.e1. https://doi.org/10.1016/J.JTCVS.2016.02.072

Lalani T, Chu VH, Park LP, Cecchi E, Corey GR, Durante-Mangoni E et al (2013) In-hospital and 1-year mortality in patients undergoing early surgery for prosthetic valve endocarditis. JAMA Intern Med 173:1495–1504. https://doi.org/10.1001/JAMAINTERNMED.2013.8203

Lee HA, Cheng YT, Wu VCC, Chou AH, Chu PH, Tsai FC et al (2018) Nationwide cohort study of mitral valve repair versus replacement for infective endocarditis. J Thorac Cardiovasc Surg 156:1473–1483.e2. https://doi.org/10.1016/J.JTCVS.2018.04.064

Lorusso R, Gelsomino S, De Cicco G, Beghi C, Russo C, De Bonis M et al (2008) Mitral valve surgery in emergency for severe acute regurgitation: analysis of postoperative results from a multicentre study. Eur J Cardiothorac Surg 33:573–582. https://doi.org/10.1016/J.EJCTS.2007.12.050

Muehrcke DD, Cosgrove DM, Lytle BW, Taylor PC, Burgar AM, Durnwald CP et al (1997) Is there an advantage to repairing infected mitral valves? Ann Thorac Surg 63:1718–1724. https://doi.org/10.1016/S0003-4975(97)00271-3

Musci M, Hübler M, Amiri A, Stein J, Kosky S, Meyer R et al (2010) Surgical treatment for active infective prosthetic valve endocarditis: 22-year single-centre experience. Eur J Cardiothorac Surg 38:528–538. https://doi.org/10.1016/J.EJCTS.2010.03.019

Naruka V, Arjomandi Rad A, Chacko J, Liu G, Afoke J, Punjabi PP (2024) Concomitant interventions in mitral valve surgery—a European perspective. Perfusion. https://doi.org/10.1177/02676591241237130

Nishimura RA, Otto CM, Bonow RO, Carabello BA, Erwin JP, Guyton RA et al (2014) AHA/ACC guideline for the management of patients with valvular heart disease: a report of the american college of cardiology/american heart association task force on practice guidelines. Circulation 2014:129. https://doi.org/10.1161/CIR.0000000000000031

Oi K, Arai H, Nagaoka E, Fujiwara T, Oishi K, Takeshita M et al (2022) Long-term outcomes of papillary muscle relocation anteriorly for functional mitral regurgitation. Interact Cardiovasc Thorac Surg:35. https://doi.org/10.1093/ICVTS/IVAC245

Otto CM, Nishimura RA, Bonow RO, Carabello BA, Irwin JP, Gentile F et al (2020) ACC/AHA guideline for the management of patients with valvular heart disease: a report of the American College of Cardiology/American Heart Association Joint Committee on Clinical Practice Guidelines. Circulation 2021(143):E72–E227. https://doi.org/10.1161/CIR.0000000000000923/SUPPL_FILE/DATA

Perier P, Hohenberger W, Lakew F, Diegeler A (2015) Prolapse of the posterior leaflet: resect or respect. Ann Cardiothorac Surg 4:27377–27277. https://doi.org/10.3978/J.ISSN.2225-319X.2014.11.16

Pienta MJ, Theurer P, He C, Clark M, Haft J, Bolling SF et al (2023) Contemporary management of ischemic mitral regurgitation at coronary artery bypass grafting. Ann Thorac Surg 115:88–95. https://doi.org/10.1016/j.athoracsur.2022.08.046

Popovic Z, Barac I, Jovic M, Ristic M, Panic G, Miric M et al (1996) Chordal preservation improves postoperative ventricular performance following valve replacement for chronic mitral regurgitation. Cardiovasc Surg 4:628–634. https://doi.org/10.1016/0967-2109(96)00039-7

Russo A, Suri RM, Grigioni F, Roger VL, Oh JK, Mahoney DW et al (2008) Clinical outcome after surgical correction of mitral regurgitation due to papillary muscle rupture. Circulation 118:1528–1534. https://doi.org/10.1161/CIRCULATIONAHA.107.747949

Sá MPBO, Soares EF, Santos CA, Figueiredo OJ, Lima ROA, Escobar RR et al (2013) Mitral valve replacement combined with coronary artery bypass graft surgery in patients with moderate-to-severe ischemic mitral regurgitation. Rev Port Cardiol 32:131–137. https://doi.org/10.1016/J.REPC.2012.12.002

Shimokawa T, Kasegawa H, Matsuyama S, Seki H, Manabe S, Fukui T et al (2009) Long-term outcome of mitral valve repair for infective endocarditis. Ann Thorac Surg 88:733–739. https://doi.org/10.1016/j.athoracsur.2009.05.033

Solomon NAG, Pranav SK, Naik D, Sukumaran S (2006) Importance of preservation of chordal apparatus in mitral valve replacement. Expert Rev Cardiovasc Ther 4:253–261. https://doi.org/10.1586/14779072.4.2.253

Taramasso M, Maisano F, Pozzoli A, Alfieri O, Meier B, Nietlispach F (2016) Catheter-based treatment of paravalvular leaks. EuroIntervention 12:X55–X60. https://doi.org/10.4244/EIJV12SXA11

Vandenbriele C, Balthazar T, Wilson J, Ledot S, Smith R, Caetano AF et al (2020) Left heart Impella-device to bridge acute mitral regurgitation to MitraClip-procedure: a novel implementation of percutaneous mechanical circulatory support. Eur Heart J 41. https://doi.org/10.1093/EHJCI/EHAA946.1849

Vandenbriele C, Balthazar T, Wilson J, Adriaenssens T, Davies S, Droogne W et al (2021) Left Impella®-device as bridge from cardiogenic shock with acute, severe mitral regurgitation to MitraClip®-procedure: a new option for critically ill patients. Eur Heart J Acute Cardiovasc Care 10:415–421. https://doi.org/10.1093/EHJACC/ZUAA031

Virk SA, Tian DH, Sriravindrarajah A, Dunn D, Wolfenden HD, Suri RM et al (2017) Mitral valve surgery and coronary artery bypass grafting for moderate-to-severe ischemic mitral regurgitation: meta-analysis of clinical and echocardiographic outcomes. J Thorac Cardiovasc Surg 154:127–136. https://doi.org/10.1016/j.jtcvs.2017.03.039

Zegdi R, Debièche M, Latrémouille C, Lebied D, Chardigny C, Grinda JM et al (2005) Long-term results of mitral valve repair in active endocarditis. Circulation 111:2532–2536. https://doi.org/10.1161/01.CIR.0000165122.08660.1A

Emergency Surgery for Mechanical Complications of Myocardial Infarction

Olatoye Olutola and Yasir Abu-Omar

Abstract Acute myocardial infarction (AMI) may necessitate surgical intervention for a range of complications. The most common indication is significant coronary artery stenosis, which may be addressed through coronary artery bypass grafting (CABG) to mitigate infarct progression and prevent subsequent angina, reinfarction, or mortality. In cases of refractory congestive heart failure or circulatory shock resulting from left and/or right ventricular dysfunction, advanced therapies such as cardiac transplantation, extracorporeal membrane oxygenation (ECMO), or implantation of left and/or right ventricular assist devices (VADs) may be required. Furthermore, AMI can lead to mechanical complications including ischemic mitral regurgitation, papillary muscle rupture, and functional tricuspid regurgitation. Severe, life-threatening complications, such as postinfarction ventricular septal defect, cardiac rupture, and left ventricular aneurysm, may also require urgent surgical management.

Keywords Mechanical complications of AMI · Papillary muscle rupture · Acute mitral regurgitation · Postinfarction ventricular septal defect (VSD) · Left ventricular free wall rupture · Left ventricular aneurysm and pseudoaneurysm · Mechanical circulatory support · Heart transplantation after AMI

1 Epidemiology

In the United States, the AHA estimates that the overall prevalence of acute myocardial infarction (AMI) is 3% (Benjamin et al. 2018). While primary prevention has significantly reduced the age- and sex-adjusted incidence of AMI, factors such as large infarcts, delayed presentation, and inadequate reperfusion following PCI still

O. Olutola · Y. Abu-Omar (✉)
Division of Cardiac Surgery, University Hospitals Cleveland Medical Center, Cleveland, OH, USA
e-mail: Olatoye.Olutola@uhhospitals.org

A. Kourliouros (ed.), *Emergency Cardiac Surgery*,
https://doi.org/10.1007/978-3-032-15787-4_11

contribute to mechanical complications, haemodynamic instability, and pump failure (Peterson et al. 2008).

Over the past 30 years, improved reperfusion and medical therapies have reduced AMI mortality. However, an aging population and increased comorbidities pose challenges, as they are key risk factors for post-AMI mechanical complications (Rogers et al. 2008). Despite the decreasing incidence of ST Elevation Myocardial Infarction (STEMI) presentations, contemporary patients who experience mechanical complications are typically older, female, have pre-existing heart failure or chronic kidney disease, and frequently present with their first acute myocardial infarction (French et al. 2010). Socioeconomic factors also significantly impact AMI outcomes (Rao et al. 2004). There is evidence that higher-income Medicare beneficiaries tend to present earlier, receive care from specialised staff, and are more likely to receive guideline-directed medical therapy compared to those from lower socioeconomic backgrounds.

The introduction of early fibrinolytic therapy for treating STEMI over the past two decades resulted in a 40% overall reduction in mortality rate, and a reduction in the global incidence of mechanical complications of Acute Myocardial Infarction (AMI) (Keeley et al. 2003).

Contemporary studies demonstrate that nearly three-fourths of patients with AMI and mechanical complications present with cardiogenic shock, requiring interventions such as vasopressors, balloon pumps, or percutaneous left ventricular support devices (Lanz et al. 2019). Cardiogenic shock leads to systemic hypoperfusion and a cycle of ischaemia, inflammation, vasoconstriction, and volume overload, ultimately resulting in multisystem failure and death. Clinical trials indicate no significant mortality difference between primary PCI and fibrinolysis with adjunctive therapy (Armstrong et al. 2013). The stable incidence of mechanical complications despite improved AMI management may be attributed to factors such as the aging population, advances in cardiac imaging for detecting complications, and the expansion of specialised cardiac centres with advanced haemodynamic support.

1.1 Acute Mitral Regurgitation Secondary to Papillary Muscle Rupture

In the reperfusion era, the incidence of acute severe mitral regurgitation (MR) secondary to papillary muscle rupture (PMR) has declined to 0.05–0.26%, yet in-hospital mortality remains substantial at 10–40% (Bhardwaj et al. 2020; Valle et al. 2017). The mitral valve is anchored by two papillary muscles: the anterolateral, which receives dual blood supply from the left anterior descending and circumflex arteries, and the posteromedial, which is supplied solely by either the circumflex or right coronary artery. Consequently, anterolateral papillary muscle rupture (PMR) is uncommon, whereas posteromedial PMR typically follows inferior or lateral STEMIs. PMR may be complete or partial, with clinical severity determined by the extent of rupture.

Risk factors for papillary muscle rupture (PMR) include advanced age, female sex, pre-existing heart failure, chronic kidney disease, and delayed presentation with an initial acute myocardial infarction (Gueret et al. 2008). PMR typically develops within several days of acute myocardial infarction, with approximately half of patients presenting with pulmonary oedema that may progress to cardiogenic shock. A murmur may be absent owing to the rapid equalisation of intracardiac pressures. Bedside echocardiography or point-of-care ultrasound can help diagnose acute MR from PMR, though transoesophageal echocardiography has higher sensitivity. Left ventricular ejection fraction is generally preserved or mildly reduced, and coronary angiography often demonstrates single- or two-vessel disease with occlusion of the infarct-related artery (Table 1) (Elbadawi et al. 2019).

Table 1 Clinical characteristics, diagnostic features and management of complications associated with Acute Myocardial Infarction

Complication	Presentation	Diagnosis	Management	Mortality rate (%)
Papillary muscle rupture and acute mitral regurgitation	3–5 days after transmural infarct (inferior or lateral). Acute pulmonary oedema and shock	Echocardiogram shows severe and often eccentric jet of mitral regurgitation and mobile mass in left ventricle sometimes prolapsing into left atrium	Surgical replacement (or repair in select cases; preferably emergency operation within 24 h)	10–40
Ventricular septal defect	Commonly 3–5 days after transmural infarct. Symptoms range from isolated murmur to circulatory collapse	Echocardiogram shows left-to-right shunt across septum. Mixed venous O_2 saturations > right atrial, i.e. step up in O_2 saturation	Initial afterload reduction with intra-aortic balloon pump or LV assist device. Urgent surgical or percutaneous repair, [a]timing depends on cardiogenic shock and end-organ function	30–40
Rupture of the ventricular free wall	Commonly 3–5 days after transmural infarct. Tamponade and shock	Echocardiogram shows tamponade and may visualise flow across defect in free wall	Immediate surgical repair unless prohibitive surgical risk	>50
Pseudoaneurysm	Weeks to years after infarct. May be asymptomatic or present with chronic heart failure	Computerised tomography scan or echocardiogram shows large aneurysm cavity with flow from left ventricle across small neck	Urgent surgical or percutaneous repair, [a]depending on symptoms	<10

[a]Percutaneous repair needs discussion by the multidisciplinary heart team because only few cases are reported in the literature

Initial care for PMR and severe MR in the CICU may involve vasoactive drugs, respiratory support, and invasive mechanical ventilation to improve gas exchange and reduce LV afterload (van Diepen et al. 2017). In stable patients, nitroglycerin or nitroprusside can reduce afterload, while norepinephrine or dopamine are used for haemodynamic support. Inotropic agents may be initiated once the patient is haemodynamically stable. The use of vasopressors and inotropes in AMI-related mechanical complications is not well-studied. For all patients with advanced cardiogenic shock, a Heart Team approach is strongly recommended to plan medical optimisation and temporary mechanical support.

Mechanical circulatory support, such as IABP, is recommended as a bridge to therapy, despite limited evidence for its benefit in large trials like IABP-Shock II (Thiele et al. 2012). IABP therapy reduces afterload and augments coronary perfusion, thereby improving outcomes in severe MR secondary to PMR. Balloon counterpulsation provides approximately 0.5 L/min of mechanical circulatory support, increasing aortic pressure during diastole while lowering mean arterial pressure during systole (Tehrani et al. 2020).

Surgical intervention for PMR significantly improves survival compared with medical therapy alone (69% vs. 33%), as demonstrated in the APEX-AMI trial (Assessment of Pexelizumab in Acute Myocardial Infarction) (APEX AMI Investigators et al. 2007). Mechanical support, including ECMO and percutaneous devices, may also be used as a bridge to surgery or definitive therapy (DiVita et al. 2020).

Acute PMR constitutes a surgical emergency requiring prompt surgical evaluation. Respiratory failure due to mechanical complications necessitates prompt consultation with both surgical and shock teams. As already mentioned, preoperative use of temporary mechanical circulatory support may help mitigate haemodynamic and respiratory deterioration. Mitral valve replacement is typically performed as it is a predictable procedure with established durability. The technical details are discussed in a separate chapter. However, surgical outcomes for PMR patients are highly selective, and many with PMR are not candidates for surgery. For instance, in the SHOCK (Should We Emergently Revascularize Occluded Coronaries for Cardiogenic Shock) Trial Registry, only 38% of patients with AMI and cardiogenic shock secondary to acute MR underwent surgical intervention (Thompson et al. 2000). Similarly, only 58% of PMR patients in a National Inpatient Sample analysis underwent mitral valve surgery. Factors influencing the decision to proceed with surgery include advanced age, comorbidities, and the patient's haemodynamic stability. The optimal surgical approach for severe MR due to PMR remains controversial. Generally, chordal-sparing mitral valve replacement is preferred due to its predictability and established durability. In younger patients, a mechanical valve may offer better long-term survival compared to a bioprosthetic valve (Kaneko et al. 2014, Chikwe et al. 2015). Repair techniques are typically considered for partial PMR with less severe haemodynamic impairment, though operative mortality can approach 20% (Lee et al. 2015). The choice between bioprosthetic and mechanical valves also depends on the need for mechanical circulatory support or advanced heart failure therapies, as the risk of valve thrombosis is higher with mechanical valves when used with devices like LV assist devices or ECMO.

Concomitant coronary artery bypass grafting (CABG) should be considered in patients with PMR and obstructive coronary disease; however, the surgeon must carefully balance the risks associated with prolonged operative time against the potential benefits of revascularisation. While some studies suggest improved outcomes with CABG, a large analysis from the Society of Thoracic Surgeons (STS) Database demonstrated comparable operative mortality in patients undergoing mitral valve surgery with or without CABG (20.1% vs. 19.8%, $P = 0.91$) (Schroeter et al. 2013). Many patients with PMR have multivessel coronary disease requiring revascularisation. Although high-quality evidence is limited, failure to address severe multivessel coronary disease during surgery may hinder weaning from cardiopulmonary bypass. Moreover, low cardiac output syndrome and the requirement for postoperative venoarterial extracorporeal membrane oxygenation (VA-ECMO) are associated with increased mortality following PMR surgery.

Surgical treatment remains the standard for severe MR due to PMR, but surgical risk may be prohibitive in certain patients. In cases of chronic mitral regurgitation, percutaneous edge-to-edge repair using the MitraClip may be considered for patients deemed high risk for surgical intervention (Stone et al. 2018). Although MitraClip has been used for severe MR due to PMR, these results should be interpreted cautiously due to publication bias. In select patients with PMR complicated by cardiogenic shock and pump failure, percutaneous mitral valve repair may be considered; however, multidisciplinary discussions that incorporate patient and family preferences are essential in guiding the optimal treatment strategy. Alternatives for patients ineligible for surgery include medical management as a bridge to surgery or temporary mechanical support, with eventual transition to a ventricular assist device or heart transplantation.

1.2 Summary

According to AHA guidelines, emergency mitral valve replacement is the preferred treatment for severe MR due to PMR, though repair may be considered for partial PMR with stable haemodynamics. Medical management can bridge patients with severe MR and cardiogenic shock to more advanced therapies. The choice between bioprosthetic and mechanical mitral valve replacement should consider age, anticoagulation needs, and patient preferences. In patients with prohibitive surgical risk, transcatheter edge-to-edge mitral valve repair may be considered within a Heart Team framework. For those with concomitant coronary artery disease, CABG can be performed alongside mitral valve surgery with operative mortality comparable to valve surgery alone. Patient preferences are critical in treatment decisions for high-risk cases. In cases where there are major contraindications for surgery, medical management, transcatheter repair, or temporary mechanical support (e.g. LVAD or heart transplant) can be considered.

1.3 Ventricular Septal Defect (VSD)

The incidence of postinfarct VSD is ~0.31%, with risk factors that include advanced age, female sex, and delayed reperfusion. (Jones et al. 2014) VSD typically develops 3–5 days after myocardial infarction, with clinical presentations ranging from an incidental murmur to full circulatory collapse. Patients may exhibit dyspnea, orthopnea, hypotension, cool extremities, oliguria, and a new pansystolic murmur—often best heard at the lower left sternal border—accompanied by signs of pulmonary venous congestion. A 12-lead ECG may reveal ongoing ischaemia, evolving infarction, Q waves in the affected territory (anterior or inferior), and associated ventricular arrhythmias.

Echocardiography is crucial for diagnosing VSDs, evaluating the shunt size, biventricular function, and MR. Right heart catheterisation shows a diagnostic oxygen step-up and elevated pulmonary-to-systemic flow ratio. Left heart catheterisation reveals coronary obstruction and guides revascularisation. Anterior and apical ischemic VSDs are linked to LAD infarcts, while posterior VSDs result from inferior infarcts. Right ventricular infarction is common with acute right coronary occlusion. VSDs are more frequent in the anterior wall (70%) than in the inferior wall (29%), with inferior infarcts often leading to complex VSDs (Crenshaw et al. 2000). Due to the high mortality rate (up to 80% at 30 days) associated with uncorrected VSDs, conservative medical therapy is typically reserved for patients with haemodynamically minor defects or for those deemed high risk for surgical intervention (Calvert et al. 2014).

Effective afterload reduction is essential to diminish the left-to-right shunt in VSDs, with IABPs and pharmacotherapy used in more than 80% of emergent cases and 60% of urgent repairs (Ibanez et al. 2018). The SHOCK Trial Registry reported IABP use in up to 75% of postinfarct VSDs, with median systolic blood pressure increasing from 81 to 102 mm Hg within 30 min (Menon et al. 2000). In patients with multiorgan failure, ECMO may be employed to support end-organ function as a bridge to surgery. For those without evidence of end-organ compromise, delayed intervention can allow for connective tissue or scar formation, enhancing suture anchorage and reducing the risk of patch dehiscence. Patients presenting with early shock but without multiorgan failure are often optimal candidates for emergency surgery, as they have a greater likelihood of favourable outcomes and uncomplicated recovery (Vondran et al. 2021). ECMO, Impella, and TandemHeart have all been reported to provide similar haemodynamic stability as a bridge to definitive therapy (Rob et al. 2017) (Arnaoutakis et al. 2012).

Patients with multiorgan failure may benefit from biventricular support or ECMO with LV venting to improve end-organ recovery before surgery. LV venting reduces afterload, pulmonary oedema, harlequin syndrome, and thrombosis risk but may cause complications like aspiration of deoxygenated blood or embolisation of LV debris in VSD patients. Careful assessment by a multidisciplinary team is essential. Surgery is indicated for refractory cardiogenic shock, but delaying surgery for a week can lower mortality by minimising bleeding risks and allowing stabilisation

(Jaswaney et al. 2022). Surgical techniques include primary repair or, more commonly in recent years, infarct exclusion (Fig. 1).

In the primary repair of anterior VSDs, the infarcted anterolateral LV surface is incised parallel to the LAD, with the defect typically located beneath the incision. A patch repair using pericardium or synthetic material is carried out with mattress sutures that traverse the healthy portion of the septum circumferentially. The repair starts with pledgeted sutures placed at the posterior aspect of the septum, offering transseptal fixation of the patch at its inferior border as a first step, followed by sutures through the patch and around the rest of the healthy septal circumference, which are exteriorised through the right ventricle i.e. placed transmurally and then also fixed with pledgets on the surface of the heart. The left ventriculotomy is closed with large mattress sutures reinforced with pericardium or felt, followed by a second layer of continuous sutures and BioGlue to ensure haemostasis.

In the VSD exclusion technique, as shown in Fig. 1, a left ventriculotomy is made lateral to the LAD. This is followed by suturing a bovine patch to the endocardium of the healthy inferior portion of the septum, with the patch's generous extension and suture fixation onto healthy septum and adjacent ventricular muscle, including part of the anterior wall of the left ventricle. The remaining free edge of the patch is often fixed to the medial side of the left ventriculotomy incision. The ventriculotomy is subsequently closed similarly, as previously described. With the exclusion technique, a new internal surface of the left ventricle is constructed using pericardial tissue, thereby avoiding any tension on potentially necrotic myocardium, a limitation often encountered with primary patch repair.

Apical VSDs may be repaired by apex amputation. Posterior VSDs are typically approached via a ventriculotomy through the infarcted posterior left ventricular wall, with patch or primary closure depending on the extent of infarction. Temporary left ventricular assist devices may be employed to decompress the ventricle and reduce the risk of rupture. Modified surgical techniques, such as the double-patch repair, have also been described for postinfarction VSDs. For anterior VSDs, a left ventriculotomy is generally performed approximately 2 cm from the LAD artery,

Fig. 1 Surgical repair of postinfarct ventricular septal defect with the exclusion technique

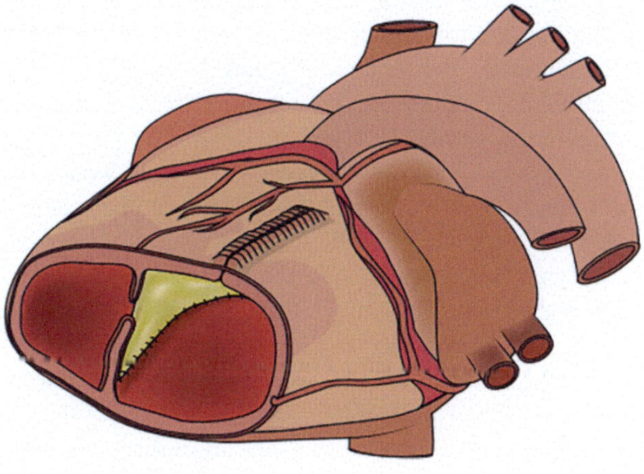

through the infarcted region. The first bovine pericardial patch is sutured to healthy endocardium to exclude the infarcted muscle, while a second smaller patch is used to directly close the VSD with running sutures, preventing right-to-left shunting (Tabuchi et al. 2004). BioGlue or fibrin is inserted between the patches to secure the closure. Finally, the left ventriculotomy site is closed. This double-patch technique can also be applied to posterior VSDs (Balkanay et al. 2005). Despite advancements, operative mortality remains around 40% (Abu-Omar et al. 2012).

In patients undergoing surgical repair of postinfarct VSD, preoperative prognostic factors associated with in-hospital mortality include impaired ventricular function, progressive cardiovascular deterioration, cardiogenic shock, inferior myocardial infarction, dependence on inotropic support, and complete occlusion of the infarct-related artery (Barker et al. 2003). Long-term survival after surgical closure of postinfarct VSD is influenced by factors such as right ventricular dysfunction, residual LV function, and the patient's New York Heart Association functional class at presentation (Pang et al. 2013).

For patients at prohibitive risk for surgical ventricular septal defect (VSD) repair, percutaneous closure may serve as an alternative. The procedure is generally performed under general anaesthesia with transoesophageal echocardiographic guidance to aid in device sizing. The defect is typically crossed with a hydrophilic wire from the left ventricle to the right ventricle and into the pulmonary trunk, where it is snared and exteriorised through venous access (femoral or jugular). A shuttle sheath is then advanced across the interventricular septum, allowing deployment of an occluder device. If crossing from left to right proves challenging, a right-to-left approach with subsequent exteriorisation may be utilised. Although procedural success rates are high in specialised centres (89%, range 80–100%), hospital mortality remains substantial, and complications—including device embolisation, arrhythmia, haemolysis, and incomplete occlusion necessitating surgical intervention—are relatively common (Holzer et al. 2004). Adverse outcomes are predicted by delayed diagnosis, Model for End-Stage Liver Disease (MELD) score, increased pulmonary-to-systemic flow ratio at the time of closure, and residual defects. In cases of severe refractory shock and biventricular failure where surgical or transcatheter repair is not feasible, consideration of durable mechanical circulatory support, heart transplantation, or a total artificial heart may be warranted (Gregoric 2020).

In summary, the American Heart Association provides the following guidance for clinical practice: postinfarction VSD, a consequence of rupture of infarcted myocardium, occurs in fewer than 0.3% of patients in the current era of routine primary revascularisation, typically within 3–5 days of a transmural acute myocardial infarction. Initial management should emphasise prompt afterload reduction, with temporary mechanical circulatory support used perioperatively to decompress the left ventricle and stabilise cardiac output. The optimal timing for surgical intervention should be determined through consultation among a cardiac surgeon, cardiologist, and intensivist, considering factors such as the severity of cardiogenic shock, organ failure, and the risk of coagulopathy due to antiplatelet therapy. Urgent surgical repair of postinfarct VSD in patients with cardiogenic shock and respiratory failure is associated with a 40% mortality rate, while percutaneous closure is an emerging option for patients at high surgical risk. We recommend delaying surgery, when feasible, in haemodynamically stable patients without respiratory failure, to optimise patient selection and minimise complications related to oral antiplatelet therapy. For patients ineligible for VSD repair, treatment options include percutaneous closure, mechanical circulatory support, heart transplantation, or palliative medical therapy.

1.4 Free Wall Rupture

Free wall rupture is the most reported mechanical complication of acute myocardial infarction (AMI), yet its true incidence remains uncertain, as it frequently presents as out-of-hospital sudden cardiac death and is seldom detected at routine autopsy. Although the overall incidence has decreased with the advent of timely reperfusion therapy for STEMI, early trials comparing fibrinolysis with placebo demonstrated a higher risk of rupture when fibrinolytic therapy was administered beyond 24 h, suggesting that delayed reperfusion promotes rupture through mechanisms such as intramyocardial haemorrhage, myocardial dissection, and subsequent structural failure.

Free wall rupture should be suspected in patients with haemodynamic instability after AMI, especially with delayed reperfusion. Clinical signs include jugular venous distension, pulsus paradoxus, muffled heart sounds, and possible ST-segment elevation. While rapidly fatal, it can be diagnosed with a bedside echocardiogram, prompting emergency surgery. However, hospital mortality after surgical repair remains over 35% (Matteucci et al. 2019). A variant of frank rupture, characterised by a friable infarct zone with oozing haemorrhagic pericardial effusion, should be recognised. In patients presenting with circulatory collapse, the immediate initiation of ECMO can stabilise haemodynamics and facilitate definitive repair, resulting in acceptable outcomes. However, in the setting of tamponade, impaired venous return may limit ECMO flow (Formica et al. 2018).

Left ventricular free wall rupture (FWR) is classified into two forms: the "blowout" type, presenting with profound cardiogenic shock and cardiac arrest, and the "oozing" type, associated with less dramatic yet significant haemodynamic compromise and pericardial effusion. Depending on clinical status, patients may require temporary stabilisation with intra-aortic balloon pump (IABP) or extracorporeal membrane oxygenation (ECMO); however, definitive management invariably necessitates surgical repair.

The surgical objectives in left ventricular free wall rupture (FWR) are to relieve tamponade, close the defect, secure the repair to viable myocardium, preserve ventricular geometry, and prevent pseudoaneurysm formation or re-rupture. Two principal surgical strategies are employed: sutured and sutureless repair. Sutured techniques include linear closure, infarctectomy with closure, and patch repair. If LV depressurisation is achieved with cardiopulmonary bypass and cardioplegic arrest or LV venting, sutureless repair can be an effective adjunctive therapeutic approach. Sutureless repair involves applying a patch, often with surgical glue or a collagen sponge patch like TachoSil, and is more commonly used for oozing-type FWR. However, it has limitations in controlling bleeding and preventing re-rupture in the blow-out type (Yousef et al. 2022). Ventricular assist devices may be considered for mechanical circulatory support to facilitate weaning from cardiopulmonary bypass following surgical closure of LV free wall rupture and to provide LV decompression.

Sutureless repair offers advantages, including the avoidance of cardiopulmonary bypass (CPB), systemic heparinisation, and suturing fragile, infarcted myocardium. A recent review by Nasir et al. highlighted improved short- and mid-term survival with sutureless repair without CPB, although long-term outcomes remain unclear (Nasir et al. 2014). The goals of surgical intervention are to repair the defect, resolve tamponade, and preserve sufficient healthy tissue to minimise late complications.

In summary, free wall rupture is a life-threatening complication of AMI with delayed reperfusion, often causing sudden cardiac death. Early diagnosis, echocardiography, and urgent surgery are essential, with ECMO for preoperative stabilisation if needed. Primary patch repair is standard, with sutureless options in select cases.

1.5 LV Pseudoaneurysm and LV Aneurysms

Left ventricular pseudoaneurysms can develop after transmural infarction, leading to cardiac rupture contained by pericardial adhesions (Atik et al. 2007). Pseudoaneurysms are most associated with prior AMI, though they can also result from cardiovascular surgery, chest trauma, or infective endocarditis (Mackenzie and Lemole 1994). Unlike a true aneurysm, a ventricular pseudoaneurysm is enclosed by the pericardium, pericardial adhesions, or a thrombus. In contrast, a true ventricular aneurysm retains endocardium and myocardium within an intact heart wall (Inayat et al. 2018). Pseudoaneurysms more commonly affect the inferior or lateral wall, likely due to dependent pericardial adhesions forming in the recumbent, recovering patient after infarction (Frances et al. 1998). Although acute rupture of the anterior wall is usually fatal, pseudoaneurysms of the inferior or lateral wall can remain clinically silent and undetected for months.

Patients with left ventricular pseudoaneurysms may remain asymptomatic or present with clinical features such as heart failure, chest pain, dyspnea, arrhythmias, systemic embolisation, or signs of tamponade (Mahesh et al. 2015) or sudden cardiac death. Most are male and show electrocardiographic and radiographic abnormalities. Diagnosis requires high suspicion and often involves multiple imaging techniques, including echocardiography, coronary angiography, CT, and MRI. Pseudoaneurysms typically have a narrow neck and lack the normal structural elements of an intact cardiac wall.

Due to the high risk of rupture, pseudoaneurysms following AMI typically require urgent surgical repair. This can be done using pledgeted sutures or with patches such as GoreTex, Dacron, autologous, or bovine pericardium. A Mayo Clinic series found most medically treated LV pseudoaneurysm patients died from ischaemia or heart failure, not haemorrhage (Yeo et al. 1998). Immediate surgery is preferred, with repair options including PTFE felt for small-neck aneurysms and heavy fibrotic edges. Gore-Tex, Dacron, or autologous pericardial patches should be used for basal LV pseudoaneurysms (Prifti et al. 2017). For remote myocardial infarctions, incidental LV pseudoaneurysms can be addressed urgently, but not as emergencies.

The 2004 ACC/AHA guidelines recommended aneurysmectomy during CABG for refractory arrhythmias or heart failure (Class IIa, Level B) (Antman et al. 2004). The 2013 guidelines suggested surgery for LV aneurysms with refractory heart failure, unresponsive arrhythmias, or recurrent thromboembolisms despite anticoagulation. Surgical options include plication, excision, and endoventricular patch reconstruction.

Percutaneous repair of LV pseudoaneurysms involves a retrograde approach across the aortic valve under general anaesthesia, guided by imaging techniques like transoesophageal echocardiography and fluoroscopy (Dundon et al. 2008). A guidewire is used to access the pseudoaneurysm neck, and an Amplatzer Septal Occluder is deployed across it under real time TEE guidance. Spontaneous echocardiographic contrast indicates decreased flow in the pseudoaneurysm. Successful technical outcomes depend on defect size and tissue thickness, while clinical outcomes are influenced by pseudoaneurysm chronicity and LV function. The PARACHUTE III study showed high procedural success with the Parachute device for LV aneurysms, but 7% of patients had major adverse events. As a result, the PARACHUTE IV study was terminated early in 2017 after enrolling 331 subjects, and it is uncertain if further evaluation will continue (Costa et al. 2013).

In summary, LV pseudoaneurysms are a rare complication of myocardial infarction, often in the posterior or lateral walls, and require a high index of suspicion for diagnosis. Urgent surgical intervention is recommended, though the outcomes of medical management are unclear. Small-neck pseudoaneurysms can be repaired with pledgeted sutures and PTFE felt, or with Gore-Tex, pericardium, or double-patch Dacron. A Heart Team approach may allow for percutaneous repair in specialised centres.

2 Cardiac Replacement Therapy

In patients who are not candidates for surgical or transcatheter therapies—such as those with severe biventricular failure and end-organ dysfunction—consideration may be given to orthotopic heart transplantation (see Chapter "Donor Heart Allocation Systems for Adult Recipients Incorporating Clinical Urgency—An International Comparison") or mechanical circulatory support. Under the updated United Network for Organ Sharing (UNOS) allocation system, the highest priority is assigned to patients receiving full circulatory support with venoarterial

ECMO. Increasingly, heart transplantation is being performed in patients supported with advanced circulatory devices, including those classified as INTERMACS 1 or SCAI stage E (Cogswell et al. 2020).

3 Future Studies

Mechanical complications of AMI are rare (<1%) and require specialised care, often only available at advanced centres, making clinical trials challenging. Factors such as diagnostic delays, limited LV assist devices, and risk-averse behaviours contribute to care variability. Randomised trials are difficult, and observational data are insufficient. Studying these complications as rare diseases with smaller, more focused trials could be useful. A registry modelled after the International Registry of Acute Aortic Dissection could enhance care pathways. Key gaps include the use of point-of-care echocardiography, advanced imaging, timing of LV support or ECMO, and corrective interventions. Advances in structural heart disease procedures, including 3D printing, may offer tailored solutions (Vukicevic et al. 2017).

4 Conclusion

Most mechanical complications of AMI are surgical emergencies, requiring early cardiac surgeon involvement. Multidisciplinary teams, including cardiac intensivists, improve adherence to best practices, reduce adverse events, and enhance survival. Given the high prevalence of multisystem organ injury, cross-specialty collaboration is essential. Active engagement of patients, families, and palliative care specialists in decision-making is crucial in the CICU.

References

Abu-Omar Y, Bhinda P, Choong CK, Nashef SA, Nair S (2012) Survival after surgical repair of ischemic ventricular septal rupture. Asian Cardiovasc Thorac Ann 20(4):404–408. https://doi.org/10.1177/0218492312438739. PMID: 22879546

Antman EM, Anbe DT, Armstrong PW et al (2004) ACC/AHA guidelines for the management of patients with ST-elevation myocardial infarction: a report of the American College of Cardiology/American Heart Association Task Force on Practice Guidelines (Committee to Revise the 1999 Guidelines for the Management of Patients with Acute Myocardial Infarction) [published correction appears in Circulation. 2005 Apr 19;111(15):2013-4] [published correction appears in Circulation. 2007 Apr 17;115(15):e411] [published correction appears in Circulation. 2010 Jun 15;121(23):e441]. Circulation 110(9):e82–e292

APEX AMI Investigators, Armstrong PW, Granger CB et al (2007) Pexelizumab for acute ST-elevation myocardial infarction in patients undergoing primary percutaneous coronary intervention: a randomized controlled trial. JAMA 297(1):43–51. https://doi.org/10.1001/jama.297.1.43

Armstrong PW, Gershlick AH, Goldstein P et al (2013) Fibrinolysis or primary PCI in ST-segment elevation myocardial infarction. N Engl J Med 368(15):1379–1387. https://doi.org/10.1056/NEJMoa1301092

Arnaoutakis GJ, Zhao Y, George TJ, Sciortino CM, McCarthy PM, Conte JV (2012) Surgical repair of ventricular septal defect after myocardial infarction: outcomes from the Society of Thoracic Surgeons National Database. Ann Thorac Surg 94(2):436–444. https://doi.org/10.1016/j.athoracsur.2012.04.020

Atik FA, Navia JL, Vega PR et al (2007) Surgical treatment of postinfarction left ventricular pseudoaneurysm. Ann Thorac Surg 83(2):526–531. https://doi.org/10.1016/j.athoracsur.2006.06.080

Balkanay M, Eren E, Keles C, Toker ME, Guler M (2005) Double-patch repair of postinfarction ventricular septal defect. Tex Heart Inst J 32(1):43–46

Barker TA, Ramnarine IR, Woo EB et al (2003) Repair of post-infarct ventricular septal defect with or without coronary artery bypass grafting in the northwest of England: a 5-year multi-institutional experience. Eur J Cardiothorac Surg 24(6):940–946. https://doi.org/10.1016/s1010-7940(03)00465-2

Benjamin EJ, Virani SS, Callaway CW et al (2018) Heart Disease and Stroke Statistics-2018 update: a report from the American Heart Association [published correction appears in Circulation. 2018 Mar 20;137(12):e493. doi: 10.1161/CIR.0000000000000573]. Circulation 137(12):e67–e492. https://doi.org/10.1161/CIR.0000000000000558

Bhardwaj B, Sidhu G, Balla S et al (2020) Outcomes and hospital utilization in patients with papillary muscle rupture associated with acute myocardial infarction. Am J Cardiol 125(7):1020–1025. https://doi.org/10.1016/j.amjcard.2019.12.051

Calvert PA, Cockburn J, Wynne D et al (2014) Percutaneous closure of postinfarction ventricular septal defect: in-hospital outcomes and long-term follow-up of UK experience. Circulation 129(23):2395–2402. https://doi.org/10.1161/CIRCULATIONAHA.113.005839

Chikwe J, Chiang YP, Egorova NN, Itagaki S, Adams DH (2015) Survival and outcomes following bioprosthetic vs mechanical mitral valve replacement in patients aged 50 to 69 years. JAMA 313(14):1435–1442. https://doi.org/10.1001/jama.2015.3164

Cogswell R, John R, Estep JD et al (2020) An early investigation of outcomes with the new 2018 donor heart allocation system in the United States. J Heart Lung Transplant 39(1):1–4. https://doi.org/10.1016/j.healun.2019.11.002

Costa MA, Pencina M, Nikolic S, Engels T, Templin B, Abraham WT (2013) The PARACHUTE IV trial design and rationale: percutaneous ventricular restoration using the parachute device in patients with ischemic heart failure and dilated left ventricles. Am Heart J 165(4):531–536. https://doi.org/10.1016/j.ahj.2012.12.022

Crenshaw BS, Granger CB, Birnbaum Y et al (2000) Risk factors, angiographic patterns, and outcomes in patients with ventricular septal defect complicating acute myocardial infarction. GUSTO-I (Global Utilization of Streptokinase and TPA for Occluded Coronary Arteries) Trial Investigators. Circulation 101(1):27–32. https://doi.org/10.1161/01.cir.101.1.27

DiVita M, Visveswaran GK, Makam K, Naji P, Cohen M, Kapoor S, Saunders CR, Zucker MJ (2020) Emergent TandemHeart-ECMO for acute severe mitral regurgitation with cardiogenic shock and hypoxaemia: a case series. Eur Heart J Case Rep 4:1–6. https://doi.org/10.1093/ehjcr/ytz234

Dundon BK, Yeend RA, Worthley SG (2008) Percutaneous closure of a large peri-prosthetic left ventricular pseudoaneurysm in a high-risk surgical candidate. Heart 94(8):1043. https://doi.org/10.1136/hrt.2007.128405

Elbadawi A, Elgendy IY, Mahmoud K et al (2019) Temporal trends and outcomes of mechanical complications in patients with acute myocardial infarction. JACC Cardiovasc Interv 12(18):1825–1836. https://doi.org/10.1016/j.jcin.2019.04.039

Formica F, Mariani S, Singh G et al (2018) Postinfarction left ventricular free wall rupture: a 17-year single-centre experience. Eur J Cardiothorac Surg 53(1):150–156. https://doi.org/10.1093/ejcts/ezx271

Frances C, Romero A, Grady D (1998) Left ventricular pseudoaneurysm. J Am Coll Cardiol 32(3):557–561. https://doi.org/10.1016/s0735-1097(98)00290-3
French JK, Hellkamp AS, Armstrong PW et al (2010) Mechanical complications after percutaneous coronary intervention in ST-elevation myocardial infarction (from APEX-AMI). Am J Cardiol 105(1):59–63. https://doi.org/10.1016/j.amjcard.2009.08.653
Gregoric ID (2020) Total artificial heart in patients with post-infarction ventricular septal defect. Ann Cardiothorac Surg 9(2):116–117. https://doi.org/10.21037/acs.2020.01.04
Gueret P, Khalife K, Jobic Y et al (2008) Echocardiographic assessment of the incidence of mechanical complications during the early phase of myocardial infarction in the reperfusion era: a French multicentre prospective registry. Arch Cardiovasc Dis 101(1):41–47. https://doi.org/10.1016/s1875-2136(08)70254-7
Holzer R, Balzer D, Amin Z et al (2004) Transcatheter closure of postinfarction ventricular septal defects using the new Amplatzer muscular VSD occluder: Results of a U.S. Registry. Catheter Cardiovasc Interv 61(2):196–201. https://doi.org/10.1002/ccd.10784
Ibanez B, James S, Agewall S et al (2018) 2017 ESC Guidelines for the management of acute myocardial infarction in patients presenting with ST-segment elevation: The Task Force for the management of acute myocardial infarction in patients presenting with ST-segment elevation of the European Society of Cardiology (ESC). Eur Heart J 39(2):119–177. https://doi.org/10.1093/eurheartj/ehx393
Inayat F, Ghani AR, Riaz I et al (2018) Left ventricular pseudoaneurysm: an overview of diagnosis and management. J Investig Med High Impact Case Rep 6:2324709618792025. https://doi.org/10.1177/2324709618792025. Published 2018 Aug 2
Jaswaney R, Arora S, Khwaja T, Shah N, Osman MN, Abu-Omar Y, Shishehbor MH (2022 Jul) Timing of repair in postinfarction ventricular septal defect. Am J Cardiol 15(175):44–51. https://doi.org/10.1016/j.amjcard.2022.04.017. Epub 2022 May 18. PMID: 35597625
Jones BM, Kapadia SR, Smedira NG et al (2014) Ventricular septal rupture complicating acute myocardial infarction: a contemporary review. Eur Heart J 35(31):2060–2068. https://doi.org/10.1093/eurheartj/ehu248
Kaneko T, Aranki S, Javed Q et al (2014) Mechanical versus bioprosthetic mitral valve replacement in patients <65 years old. J Thorac Cardiovasc Surg 147(1):117–126. https://doi.org/10.1016/j.jtcvs.2013.08.028
Keeley EC, Boura JA, Grines CL (2003) Primary angioplasty versus intravenous thrombolytic therapy for acute myocardial infarction: a quantitative review of 23 randomised trials. Lancet 361(9351):13–20. https://doi.org/10.1016/S0140-6736(03)12113-7
Lanz J, Wyss D, Räber L et al (2019) Mechanical complications in patients with ST-segment elevation myocardial infarction: a single centre experience. PLoS One 14(2):e0209502. https://doi.org/10.1371/journal.pone.0209502. Published 2019 Feb 22
Lee SK, Heo W, Min HK, Kang DK, Jun HJ, Hwang YH (2015) A new surgical repair technique for ischemic total papillary muscle rupture. Ann Thorac Surg 100(5):1891–1893. https://doi.org/10.1016/j.athoracsur.2014.12.091
Mackenzie JW, Lemole GM (1994) Pseudoaneurysm of the left ventricle. Tex Heart Inst J 21(4):296–301
Mahesh B, Ong P, Kutty R, Abu-Omar Y (2015) Tamponade by an expanding left ventricular pseudoaneurysm: a unique presentation. Asian Cardiovasc Thorac Ann 23(8):976–978. https://doi.org/10.1177/0218492314530135. Epub 2014 Apr 1. PMID: 24692597
Matteucci M, Fina D, Jiritano F et al (2019) Treatment strategies for post-infarction left ventricular free-wall rupture. Eur Heart J Acute Cardiovasc Care 8(4):379–387. https://doi.org/10.1177/2048872619840876
Menon V, Webb JG, Hillis LD et al (2000) Outcome and profile of ventricular septal rupture with cardiogenic shock after myocardial infarction: a report from the SHOCK Trial Registry. SHould we emergently revascularize Occluded Coronaries in cardiogenic shocK? J Am Coll Cardiol 36(3 Suppl A):1110–1116. https://doi.org/10.1016/s0735-1097(00)00878-0

Nasir A, Gouda M, Khan A, Bose A (2014) Is it ever possible to treat left ventricular free wall rupture conservatively? Interact Cardiovasc Thorac Surg 19(3):488–493. https://doi.org/10.1093/icvts/ivu140

Pang PY, Sin YK, Lim CH et al (2013) Outcome and survival analysis of surgical repair of post-infarction ventricular septal rupture. J Cardiothorac Surg 8:44. https://doi.org/10.1186/1749-8090-8-44. Published 2013 Mar 9

Peterson ED, Shah BR, Parsons L et al (2008) Trends in quality of care for patients with acute myocardial infarction in the National Registry of Myocardial Infarction from 1990 to 2006. Am Heart J 156(6):1045–1055. https://doi.org/10.1016/j.ahj.2008.07.028

Prifti E, Bonacchi M, Baboci A et al (2017) Surgical treatment of post-infarction left ventricular pseudoaneurysm: case series highlighting various surgical strategies. Ann Med Surg (Lond) 16:44–51. https://doi.org/10.1016/j.amsu.2017.03.013. Published 2017 Mar 9

Rao SV, Schulman KA, Curtis LH, Gersh BJ, Jollis JG (2004) Socioeconomic status and outcome following acute myocardial infarction in elderly patients. Arch Intern Med 164(10):1128–1133. https://doi.org/10.1001/archinte.164.10.1128

Rob D, Špunda R, Lindner J et al (2017) A rationale for early extracorporeal membrane oxygenation in patients with postinfarction ventricular septal rupture complicated by cardiogenic shock. Eur J Heart Fail 19(Suppl 2):97–103. https://doi.org/10.1002/ejhf.852

Rogers WJ, Frederick PD, Stoehr E et al (2008) Trends in presenting characteristics and hospital mortality among patients with ST elevation and non-ST elevation myocardial infarction in the National Registry of Myocardial Infarction from 1990 to 2006. Am Heart J 156(6):1026–1034. https://doi.org/10.1016/j.ahj.2008.07.030

Schroeter T, Lehmann S, Misfeld M et al (2013) Clinical outcome after mitral valve surgery due to ischemic papillary muscle rupture. Ann Thorac Surg 95(3):820–824. https://doi.org/10.1016/j.athoracsur.2012.10.050

Stone GW, Lindenfeld J, Abraham WT et al (2018) Transcatheter Mitral-valve repair in patients with heart failure. N Engl J Med 379(24):2307–2318. https://doi.org/10.1056/NEJMoa1806640

Tabuchi N, Tanaka H, Arai H et al (2004) Double-patch technique for postinfarction ventricular septal perforation. Ann Thorac Surg 77(1):342–343. https://doi.org/10.1016/s0003-4975(03)01008-7

Tehrani BN, Truesdell AG, Psotka MA et al (2020) A standardized and comprehensive approach to the management of cardiogenic shock. JACC Heart Fail 8(11):879–891. https://doi.org/10.1016/j.jchf.2020.09.005

Thiele H, Zeymer U, Neumann FJ et al (2012) Intraaortic balloon support for myocardial infarction with cardiogenic shock. N Engl J Med 367(14):1287–1296. https://doi.org/10.1056/NEJMoa1208410

Thompson CR, Buller CE, Sleeper LA et al (2000) Cardiogenic shock due to acute severe mitral regurgitation complicating acute myocardial infarction: a report from the SHOCK Trial Registry. SHould we use emergently revascularize Occluded Coronaries in cardiogenic shocK? J Am Coll Cardiol 36(3 Suppl A):1104–1109. https://doi.org/10.1016/s0735-1097(00)00846-9

Valle JA, Miyasaka RL, Carroll JD (2017) Acute Mitral regurgitation secondary to papillary muscle tear: is transcatheter edge-to-edge mitral valve repair a new paradigm? Circ Cardiovasc Interv 10(6):e005050. https://doi.org/10.1161/CIRCINTERVENTIONS.117.005050

van Diepen S, Katz JN, Albert NM et al (2017) Contemporary management of cardiogenic shock: a scientific statement from the American Heart Association. Circulation 136(16):e232–e268. https://doi.org/10.1161/CIR.0000000000000525

Vondran M, Wehbe MS, Etz C et al (2021) Mechanical circulatory support for early surgical repair of postinfarction ventricular septal defect with cardiogenic shock. Artif Organs 45(3):244–253. https://doi.org/10.1111/aor.13808

Vukicevic M, Mosadegh B, Min JK, Little SH (2017) Cardiac 3D printing and its future directions. JACC Cardiovasc Imaging 10(2):171–184. https://doi.org/10.1016/j.jcmg.2016.12.001

Yeo TC, Malouf JF, Oh JK, Seward JB (1998) Clinical profile and outcome in 52 patients with cardiac pseudoaneurysm. Ann Intern Med 128(4):299–305. https://doi.org/10.7326/0003-4819-128-4-199802150-00010

Yousef S, Sultan I, VonVille HM, Kahru K, Arnaoutakis GJ (2022) Surgical management for mechanical complications of acute myocardial infarction: a systematic review of long-term outcomes. Ann Cardiothorac Surg 11(3):239–251. https://doi.org/10.21037/acs-2021-ami-20

Emergency Surgery for Infective Endocarditis

Arian Arjomandi Rad, Marinos Koulouroudias, Mohammad Yousuf Salmasi, and Thanos Athanasiou

Abstract This chapter provides a comprehensive overview of the surgical management of infective endocarditis (IE), emphasising its prevalence, urgency, and the critical role of timely intervention in optimising patient outcomes. Despite its relatively low incidence, IE can rapidly lead to severe complications, including valvular destruction, systemic embolisation, and haemodynamic collapse, necessitating urgent or emergency surgery in many cases. The chapter highlights the importance of early surgical intervention—often within 48–72 h for high-risk patients—as data demonstrate significant reductions in mortality, recurrent embolic events, and chronic heart failure. Surgical timing is discussed in the context of heart failure, uncontrolled infection, and prevention of embolic events, guided by the latest ESC guidelines. Special attention is given to surgical timing post-stroke, considering the risks of haemorrhagic transformation. Multidisciplinary collaboration between cardiologists, surgeons, and infectious disease specialists is crucial in decision-making, particularly when balancing the risks of early surgery with the potential for improved long-term outcomes. This chapter also addresses the practical challenges of managing IE, offering guidance on handling complex cases involving haemodynamic instability, recurrent infection, and multi-organ dysfunction, thus providing a valuable resource for cardiac surgeons navigating the intricacies of IE surgery.

Keywords Emergency surgery for infective endocarditis (IE) · Timing of surgery after stroke in IE · Stroke and haemorrhagic transformation risk in IE · Perivalvular abscess · Prosthetic valve endocarditis (PVE) · Risk prediction in IE · Surgery for IE in intravenous drug users · Elderly and endocarditis surgery · Multiorgan dysfunction in IE · ESC endocarditis guidelines · Imaging for surgical planning in IE · Outcomes for IE surgery

---

A. Arjomandi Rad · M. Koulouroudias
Department of Cardiothoracic Surgery, John Radcliffe Hospital, Oxford University Hospitals NHS Foundation Trust, Oxford, UK

M. Y. Salmasi · T. Athanasiou (✉)
Department of Surgery and Cancer, Imperial College London, London, UK
e-mail: t.athanasiou@imperial.ac.uk

A. Kourliouros (ed.), *Emergency Cardiac Surgery*,
https://doi.org/10.1007/978-3-032-15787-4_12

1 Overview of Infective Endocarditis in Surgical Practice

1.1 Prevalence and Urgency

While the incidence of infective endocarditis (IE) remains relatively low compared to other cardiovascular conditions, its propensity to cause severe valvular destruction, systemic embolisation, and rapid haemodynamic deterioration demands prompt and decisive surgical intervention (Delgado et al. 2023). The increasing incidence of IE in older populations, those with prosthetic valves, and patients with intracardiac devices has heightened the frequency with which cardiac surgeons must address this condition surgically (Pant et al. 2015) (Fig. 1). IE can rapidly progress from a controlled infection to a life-threatening emergency, particularly in the presence of cardiogenic shock, recalcitrant pulmonary oedema, large vegetations, abscess formation, or extensive annular involvement. Given these risks, the surgical management of IE often cannot be delayed (Arjomandi Rad et al. 2024).

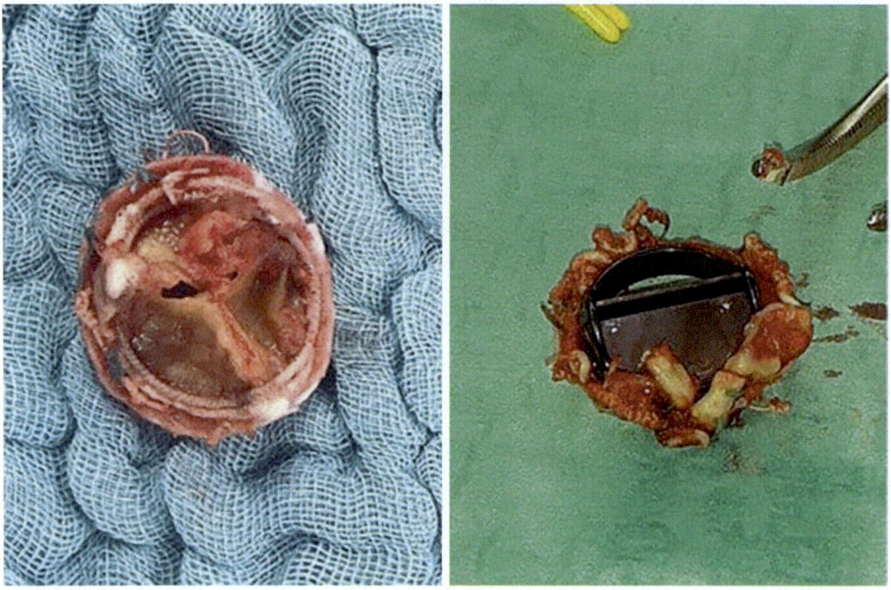

Fig. 1 Bioprosthetic (*left*) and mechanical (*right*) PVE. (Reproduced from Arjomandi Rad et al. with permission from the authors (Arjomandi Rad et al. 2024))

1.2 Impact on Outcomes

Data consistently show that early surgery—typically within 48–72 h of diagnosis in high-risk patients—significantly reduces mortality, particularly in those with heart failure or large vegetations (Habib et al. 2019). In the long term, early surgical intervention has been associated with reduced rates of recurrent endocarditis and improved functional status, particularly when performed before significant structural damage occurs (Revilla et al. 2007). Patients who undergo early surgery are less likely to develop chronic heart failure and other sequelae of prolonged infection, thereby improving their quality of life and reducing the burden on healthcare resources (Thuny et al. 2012).

For cardiac surgeons, the management of IE requires a judicious approach that balances the risks of early surgery with the potential benefits of preventing further deterioration. This underscores the importance of multidisciplinary collaboration, with close communication between surgeons, cardiologists, and infectious disease specialists to ensure that surgical interventions are performed at the optimal time for each individual patient (Gammie et al. 2023).

1.3 Focus

This chapter is designed to serve as a detailed guide for cardiac surgeons managing the complexities of IE, particularly in emergency settings where rapid decision-making and precise surgical execution are crucial. The focus is on providing an in-depth exploration of the various conundrums and requirements for complex decision making in the timely and efficient management of IE.

1.4 Practical Guidance

Recognising the urgent and often unpredictable nature of IE, this chapter also aims to offer practical guidance for real-world surgical scenarios. This includes addressing common pitfalls and providing strategic advice on how to navigate the complexities of IE surgery under various clinical conditions.

The chapter will include discussion on the management of patients who present with haemodynamic instability, multi-organ dysfunction, or recurrent infection after initial surgery. The guidance provided will help surgeons anticipate challenges, make informed intraoperative decisions, and optimise postoperative care to improve patient outcomes.

2 Pathophysiology and Clinical Presentation of Acute Infective Endocarditis

2.1 Clinical Presentation

A patient with endocarditis can present with non-specific symptoms of systemic infection, heart failure, haemodynamic collapse, or because of the sequelae of embolisation (Delgado et al. 2023; Arjomandi Rad et al. 2024). The exact clinical presentation can vary widely depending on the affected valve/chamber, the causative organism, the patient's cardiovascular reserve, and their underlying comorbidities (Arjomandi Rad et al. 2024) (Table 1).

In the European Infective Endocarditis Registry, fever is the predominant presenting complaint, followed by the finding of a new murmur, features of heart failure, and embolic phenomena (Habib et al. 2019).

Heart failure features: Endocarditis will commonly lead to varying degrees of valvular insufficiency. In cases of serious valve dysfunction, the regurgitant volume load can lead to symptoms of both congestion and poor perfusion. The exact constellation of symptoms will vary depending on the valve involved, the acuity of valve destruction, and the compliance of the receiving chamber of the regurgitant volume load (Revilla et al. 2007; Thuny et al. 2012). Occasionally, a valve will be rendered stenotic by a large vegetation, presenting in a similar manner to native valve stenosis. Finally, a haemodynamically significant shunt from a fistula can contribute to heart failure symptoms (Habib et al. 2019; Revilla et al. 2007).

Presentation due to embolisation: Left-sided valve endocarditis has the propensity to present with embolic phenomena that can affect the cerebral, coronary, visceral, and peripheral extremity vasculature (Delgado et al. 2023; Habib et al. 2019). Right-sided endocarditis can present with septic pulmonary emboli (Pant et al. 2015).

Systemic infection and immunologic sequelae: Fever is the most common presenting complaint. Varying degrees of the systemic inflammatory response syndrome might be present, including fulminant septic shock with multi-organ dysfunction. Immune phenomena, including glomerulonephritis, can occasionally be a feature on presentation (Baddour et al. 2015; Moreillon and Que 2004).

2.2 Diagnostic Criteria

Table 1 Comparison of diagnostic criteria for infective endocarditis: 2015 vs. 2023 guidelines

Diagnostic criteria	2015 guidelines	2023 guidelines
Major criteria		
Positive blood cultures	Persistent bacteremia with typical IE organisms. Use of serology or PCR for culture-negative cases	Expanded to include molecular diagnostic methods (e.g. PCR, 16S rRNA sequencing) for pathogen identification
Evidence of endocardial involvement		
Echocardiographic evidence	Oscillating intracardiac mass, abscess, or new prosthetic valve dehiscence	Use of advanced imaging modalities for detecting new lesions, particularly in high-risk patients
	Focus on vegetation size, valve destruction, and mobility	Incorporation of 3D echocardiography and strain imaging for detailed assessment
New valvular regurgitation	New murmur consistent with valve dysfunction	
Minor criteria		
Predisposing heart condition	Valvular heart disease, IV drug use	Includes post-transcatheter valve interventions and cardiac device implantation
Fever ≥38.0 °C	Unexplained fever in patients with risk factors	
Vascular phenomena	Major arterial emboli, septic pulmonary infarcts, mycotic aneurysm, etc.	Addition of asymptomatic peripheral embolic events detected by PET/CT or MRI
Immunologic phenomena	Glomerulonephritis, Osler's nodes, Roth spots, rheumatoid factor	Expanded consideration of immune-mediated conditions with molecular confirmation
Microbiological evidence	Positive cultures not meeting major criteria or serological evidence	Enhanced role of serological and molecular testing for fastidious organisms
New diagnostic algorithms	Basic algorithms for native and prosthetic valve endocarditis	Comprehensive algorithms for native valve, prosthetic valve, and device-related endocarditis

3 Indications and Timing of Surgery in Acute Infective Endocarditis

3.1 Indications and Timing of Surgery in Acute Infective Endocarditis

Based on the latest IE guidelines (ESC 2023), these are the indications for surgical management of left-sided Infective Endocarditis (Delgado et al. 2023):

1. Heart failure
2. Uncontrolled infection
3. Prevention of recurrent (especially cerebral) embolic events

With reference to timings, urgent implies 3–5 days, but without unnecessary delays if the indication is clear. Emergency is defined in the guidelines as within 24 h of establishing the indication (Delgado et al. 2023; Habib et al. 2019).

Some patients can have non-urgent inpatient surgery or elective outpatient surgery after antibiotic treatment has completely healed the vegetation—any residual valve pathology is treated as per the native valve guidelines (Delgado et al. 2023; Thuny et al. 2012).

1. **Heart failure**:
   (a) Emergency surgery should be undertaken with severe/rest symptoms (NYHA IV), pulmonary oedema, or cardiogenic shock secondary to valve insufficiency/stenosis, prosthetic valve dehiscence, or significant fistula. This is irrespective of antibiotic treatment duration (Delgado et al. 2023; Habib et al. 2019).
   (b) Urgent surgery should be undertaken if there is severe regurgitation/stenosis and milder symptoms (NYHA II-III) after a period of optimisation. Some delay to continue intravenous antibiotic therapy might be tolerated, but very close clinical and echocardiographic follow-up is necessary (Delgado et al. 2023; Revilla et al. 2007).
2. **Uncontrolled infection**:
   (a) Persistent infection: Fever and blood culture positivity after 7 days of appropriate antibiotics, as infection is unlikely to dissipate without surgery. Surgery should happen on an urgent basis if there are no other indications for emergency surgery (Delgado et al. 2023; Moreillon and Que 2004). Some time can be afforded to rule out alternative causes for persistent fever/bacteremia but with very close observation (Moreillon and Que 2004).

       If basing a decision on persistent infection, one should be certain that the patient is indeed receiving an appropriate dose of the correct antibiotics via the appropriate route and that there are no extracardiac infective foci (distant abscesses, concurrent hospital-acquired infections, etc.) (Baddour et al. 2015).

(b) Locally uncontrolled infection: Peri-valvular extension with abscess formation (and/or fistulation). This is more common in prosthetic valve endocarditis and in aortic more than mitral. It can be challenging to identify on transthoracic echocardiography, and where a patient fails to improve or develops new features (conduction block, chest pain, persistent fever), there should be a low threshold to acquire further imaging to rule out these complications (Gated cardiac CT, PET-CT, TOE) (Moreillon and Que 2004).

    In the vast majority of cases, the patient should undergo urgent surgery (unless these lesions are causing severe heart failure and dictate emergency surgery) (Moreillon and Que 2004).

(c) Difficult to treat organisms: Fungal endocarditis, MRSA, VRE, and *Staphylococcus aureus* that fails to demonstrate an early response to antibiotics should all be considered by the endocarditis team for urgent surgery, to prevent complications from uncontrolled infection (Delahaye et al. 2023).

(d) Septic shock: Fulminant vasodilatory/septic shock is an uncommon presentation but highly lethal. It's more likely with *Staphylococcus aureus* and in debilitated/multi-morbid patients. Careful echocardiographic and haemodynamic assessment is necessary to delineate whether this is cardiogenic (i.e. from valve failure) or septic shock (Baddour et al. 2015). Where surgery is not deemed futile due to co-morbidities or severity of multi-organ dysfunction, urgent surgery should be performed (Delgado et al. 2023). The ESC guidelines do not recommend emergency surgery for purely septic shock, allowing more time for resuscitation and antibiotic coverage where possible (Delgado et al. 2023).

3. **Prevention of recurrent embolism**: Vegetation embolisation is very common and tends to occur within the first 2 weeks of initiation of antimicrobial therapy. It's difficult to prognosticate which vegetations will embolise, but bulkier, more mobile, longer mitral vegetations associated with *Staphylococcus aureus* probably have a higher risk than a sessile, immobile tricuspid vegetation (Delgado et al. 2023; Moreillon and Que 2004). Left-sided vegetations ≥10mm associated with one or more embolic events should undergo urgent surgery (Delgado et al. 2023). Urgent surgery should also be performed without previous embolic events if there are other indications for surgery and the vegetation is ≥10 mm (Delgado et al. 2023). Finally, urgent surgery can be considered for an isolated vegetation ≥10 mm even without any other indications if this can be offered at very low risk (Moreillon and Que 2004).

The effects of neurological and septic sequelae of embolic events on the timing of surgery are further discussed later (Moreillon and Que 2004).

3.2 Indications in Right-Sided Endocarditis

The indications for surgical intervention in right-sided endocarditis are more limited and include:

1. RV failure secondary to TR not responding to diuresis (Moreillon and Que 2004).
2. Recurrent septic emboli leading to ventilatory dependence (Moreillon and Que 2004).
3. Vegetations >20 mm and recurrent septic emboli (Moreillon and Que 2004).

3.3 Key Considerations for Timing Surgery After Ischemic and Haemorrhagic Stroke in IE Patients

The class recommendations for the timing of surgery after stroke in infective endocarditis as of the 2023 ESC guidelines are (Delgado et al. 2023):

1. **Class I, Level B**: After a transient ischemic attack (TIA), cardiac surgery is recommended without delay if indicated.
2. **Class I, Level B**: After a stroke, surgery should proceed without delay in the presence of heart failure, uncontrolled infection, abscess, or persistent high embolic risk, as long as coma is absent and cerebral haemorrhage has been excluded.
3. **Class IIa, Level C**: For intracranial haemorrhage, delaying surgery for more than 1 month should be considered, with regular reassessment through imaging.
4. **Class IIa, Level C**: In patients with intracranial haemorrhage and unstable clinical status due to HF, uncontrolled infection, or persistent high embolic risk, urgent or emergency surgery should be considered.

Large-scale studies have investigated the optimal timing for cardiac surgery in patients with infective endocarditis complicated by stroke, providing mixed results on the safety and outcomes of early surgical intervention (Eishi et al. 2020; Durante-Mangoni et al. 2022).

One significant study from the International Collaboration on Endocarditis demonstrated that early surgery within the first week of an ischemic stroke does not increase the risk of 1-year mortality, even in cases with severe complications such as meningitis or brain abscesses. This suggests that early surgery might be safely performed in selected cases without a heightened risk of haemorrhagic transformation (Eishi et al. 2020; Kowalski et al. 2022).

A meta-analysis reviewed the literature on this topic, highlighting that early surgery (within 1–2 weeks) is generally safe in patients with ischemic stroke without severe neurological damage, provided the patient is haemodynamically unstable or has high embolic risk due to large vegetations (Durante-Mangoni et al. 2022).

However, in cases of haemorrhagic stroke, a delay of at least 4 weeks is recommended to reduce the risk of re-bleeding during surgery (Thuny et al. 2011a).

Another study supports the timing guidelines for early surgery in ischemic stroke patients, showing that early intervention reduces the risk of recurrent embolism and severe cardiac complications. In contrast, the risk of neurological worsening was not significantly elevated when surgery was performed early, especially if the neurological event was minor (Durante-Mangoni et al. 2022).

These findings emphasise the importance of individualised decision-making, taking into account the severity of the stroke, the risk of embolism, and the patient's overall clinical status. A multidisciplinary team approach involving cardiologists, cardiac surgeons, neurologists, and infectious disease specialists is crucial to optimise the timing and outcomes of surgery in these complex cases (Kowalski et al. 2022).

(a) **Assessing Stroke Severity**:

The severity of the ischemic or haemorrhagic stroke is a crucial determinant in timing surgical intervention. The classification of stroke severity can be guided by clinical scales such as the National Institutes of Health Stroke Scale (NIHSS) for ischemic stroke and modified Rankin Scale for haemorrhagic stroke. Severity can be broadly categorised into:

- **Minor Ischemic Stroke (NIHSS $\leq$ 5)**: Patients with minor strokes usually exhibit mild neurological deficits and often have better chances of recovery without significant disability. In these cases, the risk of haemorrhagic transformation is relatively low.
- **Moderate Ischemic Stroke (NIHSS 6–15)**: Patients with moderate strokes have more pronounced neurological deficits. The risk of haemorrhagic transformation is higher (Durante-Mangoni et al. 2022).
- **Severe Ischemic Stroke (NIHSS > 15)**: Severe strokes are associated with significant neurological impairment and a high risk of haemorrhagic transformation. Surgery should proceed urgently in cases of heart failure, uncontrolled infection, abscess or embolic risk. However, for stable cases, while the guidelines do not specify a timeline for delay, a 4–6-week delay with regular reassessments could be considered due to risk of haemorrhagic transformation. (Thuny et al. 2011a).
- **Haemorrhagic Stroke**: Haemorrhagic strokes require a more cautious approach due to the inherent risk of re-bleeding during surgery. Patients should be stabilised for at least 4–6 weeks if possible, with regular re-imaging to assess the resolution of the haemorrhage and any associated mass effect or oedema. Surgery should only be considered earlier if there is a compelling cardiac indication such as uncontrolled infection or severe heart failure (Kowalski et al. 2022).

(b) **Risk of Haemorrhagic Transformation in Ischemic Stroke**:

Haemorrhagic transformation of an ischemic stroke is a critical concern when considering surgery. The following factors increase the risk:

- **Large Cerebral Infarcts**: Infarcts affecting more than 50% of the middle cerebral artery territory are at a higher risk of haemorrhagic transformation (Thuny et al. 2011a).
- **Use of Anticoagulation or Antiplatelet Therapy**: Patients on anticoagulation for other comorbidities, such as atrial fibrillation, may be at an increased risk. If anticoagulation is necessary, careful management and monitoring are required (Durante-Mangoni et al. 2022).
- **Uncontrolled Hypertension**: Elevated blood pressure in the perioperative period increases the likelihood of haemorrhagic transformation. Blood pressure control is essential before considering surgery (Eishi et al. 2020).
- **Presence of Severe Septicemia**: Sepsis-related coagulopathy can exacerbate the risk of haemorrhagic transformation. Stabilising the septic state before surgery is crucial (Eishi et al. 2020; Thuny et al. 2011a).

(c) **Haemorrhagic Stroke-Specific Considerations**:

- **Timing of Surgery After Haemorrhagic Stroke**: In patients with a recent haemorrhagic stroke, surgery should be postponed for a minimum of 4 weeks, ideally up to 6 weeks, to allow the haemorrhage to stabilise and the risk of re-bleeding to decrease. This period also permits the resolution of any mass effect or hydrocephalus, which could complicate surgery (Durante-Mangoni et al. 2022; Thuny et al. 2011a).
- **Re-imaging Protocol**: Regular imaging (CT or MRI) every 1–2 weeks is recommended to monitor the resolution of the haemorrhage and to assess the stability of the patient's neurological status (Kowalski et al. 2022). Significant residual haematoma or persistent oedema should prompt

(d) **The evidence base for timing of Surgical Intervention**

This section provides a detailed analysis of the benefits and risks of early versus delayed surgery, supported by data from randomised controlled trials (RCTs) and key studies that guide current clinical practice.

3.4 Review of Studies

Several key studies have shaped current understanding and practice regarding the timing of surgery in infective endocarditis:

1. **EASE Trial** (Kang et al. 2012):
    - **Study Design**: A randomised controlled trial comparing early surgery (within 48 h of randomisation) to conventional treatment in patients with left-sided IE and large vegetations at high risk of embolism.
    - **Findings**: The trial showed that early surgery significantly reduced the composite endpoint of death, embolic events, and recurrence of IE (3% in the early surgery group vs. 28% in the conventional group; $P = 0.02$). However,

patients with major strokes were excluded, limiting its application to patients with recent cerebrovascular events (Kang et al. 2012).
- **Impact on Practice**: The EASE trial provides strong evidence supporting early surgery in patients with large vegetations and high embolic risk, particularly in the absence of recent major stroke (Kang et al. 2012).

2. Revilla et al. (2007):
   - **Study Design**: A cohort study of 546 patients with left-sided IE, focusing on the outcomes of early surgical intervention in those presenting with heart failure.
   - **Findings**: Surgery was performed in 72% of patients with heart failure. Early surgery was associated with a significant reduction in mortality compared to those managed conservatively (Revilla et al. 2007).
   - **Impact on Practice**: The study underscores the critical importance of early surgery in patients with heart failure due to IE, highlighting the need for timely intervention to improve survival (Revilla et al. 2007).

3. Nadji et al. (2009):
   - **Study Design**: This study included 259 patients with IE and evaluated the impact of early surgery on patient outcomes.
   - **Findings**: 46% of patients underwent early surgery, and the perioperative mortality rate was 10%. Early surgery was an independent predictor of reduced mortality at 1-year follow-up (HR 0.45; $P = 0.03$) (Nadji et al. 2009).
   - **Impact on Practice**: Nadji et al.'s study supports early surgical intervention in reducing long-term mortality, particularly in patients with severe complications like heart failure (Nadji et al. 2009).

4. **EuroEndo Registry (2022)**:
   - **Study Design**: The EuroEndo registry is one of the largest contemporary datasets on IE in Europe, involving more than 3,000 patients across multiple countries.
   - **Findings**: The registry showed that early surgery (within the first week) was associated with improved outcomes, particularly in terms of reduced in-hospital mortality and embolic events. However, the study also noted lower rates of surgical intervention in older patients and those with comorbidities (Habib et al. 2019).
   - **Impact on Practice**: The EuroEndo registry highlights the importance of early surgical intervention in reducing mortality and morbidity, while also calling attention to the underutilisation of surgery in elderly and high-risk patients (Habib et al. 2019).

5. **Timing of Surgery in Stroke Patients with IE** (Durante-Mangoni et al. 2022):
   - **Study Design**: This study reviewed the impact of surgical timing in patients with IE who had suffered a stroke.

- **Findings**: Early surgery (within 2 weeks) was associated with a lower risk of recurrent embolism, especially in patients with ischemic stroke, while delayed surgery was recommended for those with severe neurological events to reduce the risk of haemorrhagic transformation (Durante-Mangoni et al. 2022).
- **Impact on Practice**: This study supports early surgery in IE patients with minor ischemic strokes, while advocating for a more conservative approach in patients with severe strokes (Durante-Mangoni et al. 2022).

6. Kowalski et al. (2022)—**Neurological Considerations in Surgical Timing**:
   - **Study Design**: Published in *Clinical Neurology and Neurosurgery*, this study examined surgical outcomes in IE patients with cerebrovascular complications.
   - **Findings**: Patients with minor strokes benefitted from early surgery, while those with haemorrhagic strokes required delayed intervention (at least 4 weeks) to mitigate the risk of haemorrhagic transformation (Kowalski et al. 2022).
   - **Impact on Practice**: This study suggests that early surgery is feasible and beneficial in patients with minor ischemic strokes, while delayed surgery should be reserved for those with haemorrhagic strokes (Kowalski et al. 2022).
7. **Stroke and Surgery in IE (2023, EJCTS)**:
   - **Study Design**: This study, published in the *European Journal of Cardio-Thoracic Surgery*, examined the timing of surgery in patients with stroke and IE.
   - **Findings**: Early surgery in patients with minor or moderate strokes did not increase the risk of neurological worsening, while delaying surgery in these patients was linked to higher embolic events and worse outcomes. However, for severe strokes, a delayed approach was recommended to minimise the risk of haemorrhagic transformation (Thuny et al. 2011a).
   - **Impact on Practice**: This paper provides key insights, supporting early surgery in patients with minor strokes but recommending a more cautious approach in severe stroke cases (Thuny et al. 2011a).

4 Risk Stratification Tools

Risk stratification (Table 2) is essential for guiding the timing of surgery in IE and predicting perioperative outcomes. Two widely used tools are the EuroSCORE II and the Society of Thoracic Surgeons (STS) score.

EuroSCORE II EuroSCORE II is a widely used risk model that estimates the risk of mortality from cardiac surgery based on patient demographics, comorbid conditions, and the complexity of the surgery. Although not specific to IE, EuroSCORE II provides a framework for understanding the overall surgical risk in these patients.

Table 2 Summary of major risk prediction tools in infective endocarditis

Tool name	Purpose	Main parameters	Application	Reference/validation	Limitations
International collaboration on endocarditis (ICE) risk score	Prediction of in-hospital mortality	Age > 40 years, Health-care associated infection, Cerebrovascular accident, Diabetes, *Staphylococcus aureus* infection, Prosthetic valve endocarditis	Predicts in-hospital mortality in patients with IE based on clinical and microbiological data	ICE Prospective Cohort Study, Thuny et al. (2011b)	Limited to in-hospital mortality only, Not validated for post-discharge mortality
PALSUSE score	Risk of mortality in prosthetic valve IE	Prosthetic valve endocarditis, Age > 70 years, Large vegetations (>10 mm), *Staphylococcus aureus* infection, Urgent surgery, Septic shock, Embolism	Specifically stratifies risk for surgical mortality in patients with prosthetic valve endocarditis	Chirillo et al., Circulation (2010)	Only applicable to prosthetic valve endocarditis, Does not account for non-surgical management
VIRSTA score	Predicts in-hospital mortality in *Staphylococcus aureus* IE	Age > 65 years, Male sex, Charlson comorbidity index > 3, Community-acquired infection, Presence of prosthetic valve, Stroke or septic shock at diagnosis	Evaluates severity and predicts outcome specifically in patients with *Staphylococcus aureus* endocarditis	VIRSTA Study Group, JAMA Cardiology (2016)	Limited to *Staphylococcus aureus* infection, Focuses on in-hospital mortality, not long-term outcomes
EuroSCORE II	Surgical risk stratification in IE	Age, Sex, Renal function (creatinine clearance), NYHA functional class, Extracardiac arteriopathy, Pulmonary hypertension, Urgency of surgery, Critical preoperative state	Predicts surgical risk for patients undergoing IE surgery, applicable for various cardiac surgeries	Updated EuroSCORE II, Nashef et al., EJCTS (2012)	General surgical risk tool, may not capture IE-specific factors, Developed for broader cardiac surgery, less specific to IE

(continued)

Table 2 (continued)

Tool name	Purpose	Main parameters	Application	Reference/validation	Limitations
Liestøl risk model	Predicts surgical mortality in IE patients	Age > 65 years, Preoperative critical condition, Reoperation, Type of infecting organism, Prosthetic valve, Duration of cardiopulmonary bypass, Left ventricular function	Risk stratification tool for mortality prediction in patients undergoing IE surgery, with emphasis on preoperative and intraoperative factors	Liestøl et al., The Annals of Thoracic Surgery (1997)	Developed on a relatively small cohort, May not account for newer surgical techniques and medical management advances
STS-IE score	Risk of mortality and morbidity for IE surgery	Age, Gender, Urgency of surgery, Renal failure, Hepatic failure, NYHA class, Pulmonary hypertension, Preoperative shock, Endocarditis type (native vs prosthetic valve)	Estimates 30-day mortality and major morbidity after IE surgery, aiding in preoperative risk assessment and decision-making	Society of Thoracic Surgeons Database, Gammie et al., The Annals of Thoracic Surgery (2011)	Data largely from North American population, Focuses on short-term (30-day) outcomes, limited information on long-term prognosis

- **Data:** EuroSCORE II tends to overestimate risk in IE patients, with studies suggesting that while it is useful for assessing relative risk, it should not be the sole determinant of surgical timing.
  - **Example:** A 72-year-old female with severe aortic regurgitation due to IE and a large annular abscess has a EuroSCORE II of 18%, reflecting high surgical risk. Despite this, the presence of uncontrolled infection and heart failure necessitates urgent surgery, highlighting the importance of clinical judgement alongside risk scores.

STS Score The STS score is another risk prediction model that is more specific to valve surgery, incorporating variables such as pulmonary hypertension, reoperation status, and active endocarditis.

Multidisciplinary Approach The decision to proceed with surgery, particularly in high-risk IE patients, should involve a multidisciplinary team, including cardiologists, infectious disease specialists, anaesthesiologists, and surgeons. This approach ensures that all aspects of the patient's condition are considered, optimising the decision-making process and improving patient outcomes (Baddour et al. 2015).

5 Preoperative Imaging

5.1 Imaging and Diagnostic Workup Echocardiography: Primary Diagnostic Tool with Nuanced Use

Echocardiography remains central to diagnosing IE due to its immediate availability, non-invasive nature, and the ability to provide detailed anatomical and functional information. However, the 2023 ESC guidelines emphasise a more nuanced use of TTE and TOE, tailoring the choice based on the type of valve, location of infection, and suspected complications (Delgado et al. 2023).

- **Transthoracic Echocardiography (TTE)**: TTE is the first-line imaging modality in most cases of suspected IE, particularly in native valve endocarditis (NVE). Its sensitivity is around 50–60% in detecting vegetations and valvular destruction but increases significantly when used for large vegetations (>10 mm). The guidelines recommend TTE as a screening tool but highlight that its sensitivity is reduced in patients with prosthetic valves and poor acoustic windows, such as in patients with obesity or chronic lung disease (Delgado et al. 2023; Evangelista and González-Alujas 2004).
- **Transoesophageal Echocardiography (TOE)**: For prosthetic valve endocarditis (PVE) and cases where TTE is inconclusive, TOE becomes the definitive test, with a sensitivity of up to 90% for detecting valvular vegetations, abscesses, and perivalvular involvement (Sonne and Bonow 2009). TOE's higher sensitivity for

detecting smaller vegetations (less than 10 mm), valve perforation, and periannular complications makes it indispensable in diagnostic protocols. The guidelines recommend TOE in all patients with suspected PVE and for those with negative TTE but ongoing suspicion of IE based on persistent bacteremia and clinical deterioration. Repeated TOE is also emphasised if initial findings are negative but clinical suspicion remains high (Delgado et al. 2023; Sonne and Bonow 2009).

- **Intraoperative TOE**: The use of intraoperative TOE is particularly emphasised in high-risk surgical interventions, guiding immediate surgical decisions by confirming the presence of vegetations or abscesses and assessing the outcomes of interventions like valve replacements (Delgado et al. 2023).

5.2 Cardiac CT: Definitive for Anatomical Assessment

Cardiac CT, specifically CT angiography (CTA), has become increasingly important in the context of IE, especially when echocardiography fails to provide sufficient clarity regarding complications such as abscesses or pseudoaneurysms (Gaudino et al. 2021).

- **Prosthetic Valve Endocarditis (PVE)**: The 2023 guidelines highlight CTA's role in PVE due to its excellent spatial resolution. CTA is particularly useful in detecting perivalvular complications such as abscesses, pseudoaneurysms, and fistulae, which may not be fully visualised on echocardiography. Additionally, CTA is preferred when detailed pre-surgical anatomical mapping is needed to evaluate the extent of valvular or paravalvular destruction (Delgado et al. 2023; Gaudino et al. 2021).
- **Coronary Artery Assessment**: In IE patients undergoing surgical intervention, CTA is also recommended to rule out coronary artery disease, especially in patients at high risk of ischemic heart disease. In situations where time allows, preoperative coronary assessment is vital for stratifying risk before surgery. This is particularly relevant when vegetations are located in proximity to the coronary ostia or in cases where aortic root abscesses are suspected, which may compromise coronary perfusion (Gaudino et al. 2021).

5.3 [18F]-FDG PET/CT: A Game-Changer for Complex Cases

One of the standout recommendations in the 2023 ESC guidelines is the growing reliance on [18F]-FDG PET/CT in the diagnostic workup for prosthetic valve endocarditis (PVE) and cardiovascular implantable electronic device (CIED) infections. This modality has high sensitivity for detecting both local infection around prosthetic material and systemic embolic complications (Pizzi et al. 2015).

- **Prosthetic Valve Endocarditis**: PET/CT is recommended in cases of suspected PVE where echocardiography is inconclusive. The guidelines highlight that PET/CT's ability to detect metabolic activity related to infection offers superior diagnostic accuracy in prosthetic valves where vegetations are often masked by the prosthetic material. The role of PET/CT is also underscored in situations where paravalvular abscesses are suspected but not visualised on standard echocardiography (Pizzi et al. 2015).
- **CIED-Related Endocarditis**: In cases of CIED infections, PET/CT is valuable for detecting lead vegetations, particularly when echocardiographic evidence is unclear. The guidelines suggest its use in combination with echocardiography to confirm the diagnosis and to rule out systemic involvement, such as septic emboli to other organs (Saby et al. 2013).
- **Systemic Embolism and Peripheral Lesions**: In IE patients with systemic symptoms, PET/CT's whole-body imaging capabilities are pivotal for detecting embolic lesions, which are often missed by other modalities. The sensitivity of PET/CT for detecting splenic, renal, and cerebral emboli makes it essential in patients with persistent bacteremia despite antibiotic therapy or those with unexplained systemic symptoms (Pizzi et al. 2015; Saby et al. 2013).

5.4 Magnetic Resonance Imaging (MRI): Brain and Cardiac Indications

MRI is particularly important in IE when there are neurological symptoms, with brain MRI being the imaging of choice for detecting embolic strokes or mycotic aneurysms. The guidelines strongly recommend brain MRI in symptomatic patients to evaluate the extent of ischemic or haemorrhagic lesions, as well as to detect abscesses and cerebritis in cases of septic emboli (Thuny et al. 2007).

- **Cardiac MRI**: Although less commonly used than echocardiography and CT, cardiac MRI can provide detailed information about myocardial involvement and perivalvular extension of infection in selected cases, especially when other imaging techniques are inconclusive. MRI's role is highlighted in complex presentations of perivalvular abscesses, particularly when CTA findings are indeterminate (Thuny et al. 2007).

6 Postoperative Care and Complication Management Following Surgery for Infective Endocarditis

Haemodynamic Monitoring In the immediate postoperative period following surgery for IE, vigilant haemodynamic monitoring is paramount to ensure optimal cardiac function and early detection of complications. Given the high-risk nature of these patients, who often present with preoperative heart failure or sepsis, advanced haemodynamic monitoring techniques are typically employed. This includes the use of pulmonary artery catheters for continuous measurement of cardiac output, systemic vascular resistance (SVR), and pulmonary artery pressures. These parameters are crucial for guiding fluid management and the administration of inotropes or vasopressors, particularly in cases of vasoplegic syndrome, a common complication following cardiopulmonary bypass (CPB) in IE patients (Baddour et al. 2015).

Vasoplegic syndrome, characterised by severe hypotension despite adequate cardiac output, often necessitates aggressive vasopressor therapy. Noradrenaline is the first-line agent due to its potent alpha-adrenergic effects, but adjunctive therapies such as vasopressin or methylene blue may be required in refractory cases. The use of continuous cardiac output monitors and transoesophageal echocardiography (TEE) is recommended to assess ventricular function and volume status, allowing for the timely adjustment of therapeutic interventions (Baddour et al. 2015).

Infection Control Postoperative management of infection is critical in patients who have undergone surgery for IE. Despite surgical intervention, there is a significant risk of residual infection, particularly in cases involving complex valve repairs or prosthetic valve endocarditis (PVE). Blood cultures should be routinely obtained 48–72 h postoperatively to monitor for persistent bacteremia. In cases where cultures remain positive, further investigation with imaging, such as CT scans, may be necessary to identify and manage extracardiac sources of infection, such as splenic or vertebral abscesses (Delgado et al. 2023; Gaudino et al. 2021).

Antibiotic therapy should be continued postoperatively, tailored to the pathogens identified preoperatively and intraoperatively. The duration of antibiotic therapy is typically guided by the intraoperative findings and the results of culture and sensitivity testing from surgical specimens. In general, a course of 4–6 weeks of intravenous antibiotics is recommended, though this may be extended in cases of prosthetic valve involvement or persistent bacteremia (Baddour et al. 2015).

6.1 Identification and Management of Complications

Bleeding and Tamponade Bleeding is a significant concern in the postoperative period, especially in patients with IE who often have coagulopathies related to sepsis or anticoagulation therapy. Early recognition of excessive bleeding is essential, as it can lead to cardiac tamponade, a life-threatening condition that requires prompt intervention. Management strategies include the use of point-of-care coagulation testing, such as thromboelastography (TEG) or rotational thromboelastometry (ROTEM), to guide the administration of blood products and coagulation factors (Baddour et al. 2015).

In cases of suspected tamponade, immediate bedside echocardiography should be performed to confirm the diagnosis. Surgical re-exploration may be required to evacuate the haematoma and achieve haemostasis. The decision to return to the operating room should be based on clinical judgement, considering the patient's haemodynamic stability and the amount of chest tube drainage (Baddour et al. 2015).

Conduction Abnormalities Postoperative conduction abnormalities, including complete heart block, are relatively common following IE surgery, particularly in cases involving aortic valve endocarditis or perivalvular abscesses. Continuous electrocardiographic monitoring is essential to detect these arrhythmias early. Temporary pacing may be required, and the decision to implant a permanent pacemaker should be based on the persistence of conduction disturbances beyond the immediate postoperative period (Baddour et al. 2015).

In patients with persistent heart block or significant bradyarrhythmias, early implantation of a permanent pacemaker is recommended. The timing of pacemaker implantation is critical, with some guidelines advocating for implantation within the first 5–7 days postoperatively if the conduction abnormality does not resolve (Baddour et al. 2015).

Recurrent Infection The risk of recurrent IE remains a significant concern, particularly in patients with prosthetic valves or those who had extensive debridement during surgery. To prevent recurrence, a strict protocol for monitoring and early intervention is necessary. This includes regular blood cultures, imaging studies to monitor for new or recurrent vegetations, and adherence to long-term antibiotic prophylaxis (Delgado et al. 2023).

Patient education is also crucial in preventing recurrent infections. Patients should be counseled on the importance of maintaining good oral hygiene and the need for antibiotic prophylaxis before dental or other invasive procedures. Regular follow-up with the endocarditis team is recommended to monitor for signs of recurrence and to manage any complications that may arise (Delgado et al. 2023).

7 Considerations in High-Risk Groups

(a) IV Drug Abusers

The global rise in intravenous drug use (IVDU) continues to contribute to a growing number of infective endocarditis (IE) cases, posing new challenges for cardiac surgeons. Despite efforts to reduce IVDU rates, patients who inject drugs are increasingly presenting with IE. These individuals tend to be younger and have fewer comorbidities compared to the broader cardiac surgical population. However, the mortality rate for IE in this group remains alarmingly high, nearing 40%, and 60–70% of these patients ultimately require surgical intervention. Clinical outcomes are further complicated by issues such as non-adherence to medical advice, ongoing drug use post-treatment, and infections caused by drug-resistant bacteria, which are often less responsive to conventional antibiotic regimens (Delgado et al. 2023; Baddour et al. 2015).

The 2023 guidelines emphasise that intravenous drug users (referred to as PWID—people who inject drugs) are particularly susceptible to right-sided IE, typically involving the tricuspid valve, with *Staphylococcus aureus* (including methicillin-resistant strains) being the most common pathogen. The high recurrence rate of IE, especially within the first 6 months post-surgery, is a significant concern, often due to persistent or resumed drug use. The guidelines recommend aggressive early treatment with antibiotics and, when indicated, surgery for large vegetations, persistent infection, or complications like severe tricuspid regurgitation or pulmonary emboli (Delgado et al. 2023).

Research has highlighted the complexity of managing IE in IVDU patients. For instance, a study by Zubarevich et al., which followed 24 IVDU patients who underwent valve surgery for IE, reported a 30-day survival rate of 88% and a 72% survival rate at 3 years. However, 20.8% were readmitted due to recurrent IE, and only 58% remained free from major complications such as recurrent endocarditis, reoperation, and stroke during the follow-up period (Zubarevich et al. 2020). Additionally, Bearpark et al. compared outcomes between IVDU and non-IVDU patients with IE who underwent surgery, finding that survival rates at 8 years post-surgery were significantly lower in IVDU patients (35%) compared to their non-IVDU counterparts (68%) (Bearpark et al. 2021).

The tricuspid valve is most frequently affected in IVDU-associated IE, with cases of complete valve destruction being relatively common. The choice and timing of surgical intervention are often challenging in these patients, with tricuspid valvectomy serving as a possible bridge to valve replacement, allowing time for infection control in cases of severe IE. The guidelines reinforce the need for early surgical intervention in these cases, combined with comprehensive antibiotic therapy and addiction support, to improve long-term outcomes, as the risk of recurrence and mortality remains high without sustained drug rehabilitation (Delgado et al. 2023).

(b) **Surgery in the Elderly**

The increasing aging population worldwide has led to a notable rise in the incidence of infective endocarditis (IE) among elderly individuals, making them a growing demographic that cardiac surgeons must assess and manage more frequently. Age and frailty are well-recognised prognostic factors for mortality in IE. However, the definition of "elderly" varies across studies, with some identifying individuals over 70 years old as elderly, while others consider those over 80 years old, contributing to heterogeneity in reported outcomes. A recent large-scale study in Japan, a country known for its rapidly aging population, analysed a national database of more than 20,000 IE patients. Kiriyama et al. reported a significant rise in IE cases among the very elderly (over 80 years old), with this group increasing from 19.1% to 29.7% over an 8-year period. Despite this surge, the study demonstrated that surgical intervention reduced in-hospital mortality even in this older population, though the rates of surgery remained lower than in younger patients, with less than 10% undergoing surgery (Kiriyama et al. 2022).

Another nationwide analysis from Sweden by Ragnarsson et al. confirmed these findings, showing that while the rates of surgery decreased with age, patients who underwent surgical intervention had significantly lower mortality compared to those treated with medical therapy alone. In fact, surgery was associated with better long-term outcomes, irrespective of age, although absolute mortality was predictably higher in the very elderly (Ragnarsson et al. 2022). These results highlight a general underuse of surgical options in elderly populations who could otherwise benefit from it. There remains a reluctance to offer surgery to older patients, which, as suggested by both studies, needs to be addressed through better patient selection and the involvement of a dedicated multidisciplinary endocarditis team (Ragnarsson et al. 2022).

The 2023 guidelines reinforce these observations, emphasising the importance of individualised assessment for elderly patients with IE. Age alone should not be a contraindication for surgery, especially when surgery can improve survival rates. The guidelines recommend careful evaluation of frailty, comorbidities, and overall patient resilience when making surgical decisions in the elderly population. The use of a dedicated "endocarditis team" is strongly advocated to ensure that elderly patients are not unnecessarily excluded from potentially life-saving interventions (Delgado et al. 2023). The guidelines also underline the need for a more proactive approach in offering surgery to elderly patients, as outcomes are shown to be favourable, particularly when compared to medical therapy alone (Delgado et al. 2023).

8 Conclusion

Infective endocarditis remains one of the most daunting challenges in cardiac surgery, requiring not only advanced surgical skills but also a deep understanding of the disease's complex pathophysiology. The urgency of surgical intervention in cases of IE, especially when complicated by heart failure, uncontrolled infection, or the risk of embolisation, cannot be overstated. Early surgical intervention has been consistently shown to improve patient outcomes, reducing mortality and preventing further complications. However, the decision to operate must be carefully balanced with the risks associated with surgery, particularly in the presence of active infection or recent cerebrovascular events.

Surgical management of IE is further complicated by the variety of scenarios surgeons may encounter, from isolated valve involvement to extensive periannular infection, and the presence of prosthetic devices. The choice between valve repair and replacement, the type of prosthesis, and the timing of surgery are all critical decisions that must be tailored to each individual patient.

Ultimately, the successful management of IE in emergency surgical settings hinges on a multidisciplinary approach, where close collaboration between cardiac surgeons, cardiologists, and infectious disease specialists ensures that each patient receives the optimal intervention at the right time. Continued advancements in surgical techniques and a deeper understanding of the disease will be essential in improving outcomes for this challenging patient population.

References

Arjomandi Rad A, Zubarevich A, Osswald A, Vardanyan R, Magouliotis DE, Ansaripour A, Kourliouros A, Sá MP, Rassaf T, Ruhparwar A, Sardari Nia P, Athanasiou T, Weymann A (2024) The surgical treatment of infective endocarditis: a comprehensive review. Diagnostics 14(5):464

Baddour LM, Wilson WR, Bayer AS et al (2015) Infective endocarditis in adults: diagnosis, antimicrobial therapy, and management of complications: a scientific statement for healthcare professionals from the American Heart Association. Circulation 132(15):1435–1486

Bearpark TC, Ragland AS, Wisely BL et al (2021) Outcomes of surgical treatment for infective endocarditis in intravenous drug users. J Thorac Cardiovasc Surg 161(1):190–196

Chirillo F, Scotto F, Rocco F et al (2010) Clinical predictors of prognosis in prosthetic valve endocarditis: the PALSUSE score. Circulation 121(8):892–898

Delahaye F, Lancellotti P, von Bardeleben RS et al (2023) Surgical management of infective endocarditis complicated by septic shock. Eur Heart J 44(8):1370–1377

Delgado V, Marsan NA, de Waha S, Bonaros N, Brida M, Burri H, Caselli S et al (2023) 2023 ESC Guidelines for the management of endocarditis: developed by the task force on the management of endocarditis of the European Society of Cardiology (ESC) Endorsed by the European Association for Cardio-Thoracic Surgery (EACTS) and the European Association of Nuclear Medicine (EANM). Eur Heart J 44(39):3948–4042

Durante-Mangoni E, Bradley S, Selton-Suty C et al (2022) Timing of surgery in infective endocarditis and outcome: a propensity analysis. Int J Cardiol 352:189–196

Eishi K, Watanabe G, Ishida M et al (2020) Timing of cardiac surgery in infective endocarditis complicated by stroke: early surgery and long-term results. J Thorac Cardiovasc Surg 159(2):705–713

Evangelista A, González-Alujas MT (2004) Echocardiography in infective endocarditis. Heart 90(6):614–617

Gammie JS, Chu VH, Griffith BP et al (2011) The Society of Thoracic Surgeons risk score for infective endocarditis surgery: contemporary outcomes from the STS Database. Ann Thorac Surg 92(5):1713–1720

Gammie JS, Chu VH, Griffith BP et al (2023) Surgical treatment of endocarditis: a clinical expert consensus statement of the European Association for Cardio-Thoracic Surgery. Eur J Cardiothorac Surg 64(4):832–846

Gaudino M, Rahouma M, Di Franco A et al (2021) Role of cardiac CT in the preoperative evaluation of infective endocarditis. Eur Heart J 42(7):742–749

Habib G, Erba PA, Iung B et al (2019) Clinical presentation, aetiology, and outcome of infective endocarditis. Results of the ESC-EORP EURO-ENDO (European Infective Endocarditis) Registry: a prospective cohort study. Eur Heart J 40(39):3222–3232

Kang DH, Kim YJ, Kim SH et al (2012) Early surgery versus conventional treatment for infective endocarditis. N Engl J Med 366(26):2466–2473

Kiriyama T, Okumura Y, Itoh M et al (2022) Clinical characteristics and outcomes of infective endocarditis in elderly patients in Japan: a retrospective cohort study. J Cardiol 80(5):510–517

Kowalski RL, Chu VH, Habib G et al (2022) Timing of cardiac surgery in patients with infective endocarditis complicated by stroke: a pooled analysis of observational data. Clin Neurol Neurosurg 214:107163

Liestøl K, Arnesen H, Guldvog I et al (1997) Predictive factors of mortality in patients undergoing surgery for infective endocarditis. Ann Thorac Surg 63(1):34–41

Moreillon P, Que YA (2004) Infective endocarditis. Lancet 363(9403):139–149

Nadji G, Remadi JP, Coveliers JP et al (2009) Superiority of early surgery versus medical therapy in patients with infective endocarditis complicated by heart failure: analysis of 259 cases. Eur J Cardiothorac Surg 35(5):903–911

Nashef SA, Roques F, Sharples LD et al (2012) EuroSCORE II: updated logistic risk model for cardiac surgery. Eur J Cardiothorac Surg 41(4):734–744

Pant S, Patel NJ, Deshmukh A et al (2015) Trends in infective endocarditis incidence, microbiology, and valve replacement in the United States from 2000 to 2011. J Am Coll Cardiol 65(19):2070–2076

Pizzi MN, Roque A, Fernández-Hidalgo N et al (2015) 18F-FDG PET/CT for the diagnosis of infective endocarditis in patients with prosthetic valves: a prospective cohort study. Lancet Infect Dis 15(8):983–991

Ragnarsson S, Björck S, Backlund E et al (2022) Outcomes of infective endocarditis surgery in the elderly: a nationwide study. Eur J Cardiothorac Surg 62(5):1028–1036

Revilla A, López J, Villacorta E et al (2007) Clinical and prognostic profile of patients with infective endocarditis complicated by heart failure: implications for timing of surgery. J Thorac Cardiovasc Surg 133(3):614–621

Saby L, Laas O, Habib G et al (2013) Positron emission tomography/computed tomography for diagnosis of prosthetic valve endocarditis: Increased accuracy compared to echocardiography. J Am Coll Cardiol 61(23):2374–2382

Sonne C, Bonow RO (2009) Role of echocardiography in the diagnosis and management of infective endocarditis. Curr Infect Dis Rep 11(5):322–329

Thuny F, Avierinos JF, Tribouilloy C et al (2007) Impact of cerebrovascular complications on mortality and neurologic outcome during infective endocarditis: a prospective multicenter study. Eur Heart J 28(9):1155–1161

Thuny F, Giorgi R, Habib G et al (2011a) The timing of surgery influences mortality and morbidity in adults with complicated left-sided native valve endocarditis: a propensity analysis. Eur Heart J 32(16):2027–2033

Thuny F, Giorgi R, Habib G et al (2011b) Risk score for infective endocarditis in-hospital mortality: a cohort study. Arch Cardiovasc Dis 104(12):613–620

Thuny F, Grisoli D, Habib G et al (2012) Management of infective endocarditis: challenges and perspectives. Lancet 379(9819):965–975

VIRSTA Study Group (2016) Predictors of outcome in Staphylococcus aureus infective endocarditis. JAMA Cardiol 1(5):455–463

Zubarevich A, Nagy A, Leontyev S et al (2020) Valve surgery in patients with infective endocarditis due to intravenous drug use: long-term outcomes. Ann Thorac Surg 109(5):1435–1443

Emergent Cardiac Surgery Following Transcatheter Aortic Valve Implantation

Rizwan Attia and Shakil Farid

Abstract Transcatheter aortic valve implantation (TAVI) is now a standard procedure for the treatment of symptomatic aortic valve stenosis. Complication rates have declined markedly from 5.5% to 2% over the last decade. This includes procedural complications such as device malpositioning, embolisation, coronary obstruction, annular/ aortic rupture, pericardial tamponade or severe paravalvular regurgitation needing surgery.

The complications, although rare, are clinically challenging and can be fatal if not dealt with expediently by experienced teams. The surgical mortality for these cases is high and can be up to 45–65%. This chapter deals with the commonest and most lethal complications that can occur following TAVI and how best to deal with those in an emergency setting.

Keywords Transcatheter aortic valve implantation (TAVI) · Periprocedural complications · Annular rupture · Free myocardial wall rupture · Left ventricular perforation · Coronary artery obstruction · Device embolisation · Cardiac tamponade · Vascular access complications · Paravalvular leak · Valve-in-valve procedures

1 Introduction

Overall, transcatheter aortic valve implantation (TAVI) is relatively safe with low periprocedural mortality rates, estimated to range between 1.1% and 4.2% (Leon et al. 2016). The risk profile of patients undergoing TAVI is well defined by the heart team and

R. Attia
Department of Cardiovascular Surgery, Minneapolis Heart Institute, Heart Hospital, Minneapolis, MN, USA

S. Farid (✉)
Department of Cardiothoracic Surgery, Royal Papworth Hospital NHS Foundation Trust, Cambridge, UK
e-mail: shakil.farid@nhs.net

A. Kourliouros (ed.), *Emergency Cardiac Surgery*,
https://doi.org/10.1007/978-3-032-15787-4_13

was typically of patients deemed as high-risk for surgery. More recently, TAVI is a non-inferior treatment compared to surgical valve replacement even in lower risk patients (Mack et al. 2023). The rate of periprocedural complications is low and usually stems from prosthetic valve deployment. Complications that occur periprocedurally are:

(i) Landing zone rupture
(ii) Free myocardial wall rupture
(iii) Coronary artery obstruction
(iv) Device embolisation
(v) Cardiac tamponade
(vi) Access site peripheral vascular complications
(vii) Severe paravalvular leak

There are further complications that can occur in the immediate post-procedure setting, which most commonly include cardiac arrhythmias and heart block, vascular access site bleeding, end-organ damage (stroke, acute kidney injury) and prosthetic valve complications.

We will deal with intra-procedural emergencies in the following section.

2 Device Landing Zone Rupture

The incidence of this devastating complication is below 1% and it carries a 50–75% mortality. It is more common with balloon-deployed devices when there is heavy asymmetric valve calcification (as in bicuspid valves), small annulus (<20 mm), calcified aortic root, oversized prosthesis (≥20%), when there is left ventricular outflow tract calcification or when calcific nodules (>5 mm) protrude into the aorta, low coronary height, severe sub annular left ventricle hypertrophy and small LV cavity in elderly patients. Injury can occur at time of balloon dilation, prosthetic valve deployment or re-dilatation for paravalvular leak (PVL).

The correct diagnosis of the condition is of paramount importance to expediently identify and treat it. Patients fail to recover haemodynamically post valve implantation with cardiovascular collapse. There is rapid development of pericardial effusion (identified on echocardiography) and contrast extravasation from the aorta (identified on aortography). The annular rupture can be sub-, intra-, supra-annular or combined.

Intra-annular: It is likely that small tears occur in the native annulus more frequently than recognised clinically. Usually, these are sealed by the prosthetic valve skirt. Small, localised tears are not clinically relevant. These might be recognised immediately post procedure as small area of contrast extravasation. These seal spontaneously and are not seen on subsequent echocardiographic and CT surveillance 48-h post procedure.

Sub-annular: This is rupture below the native valve annulus that can occur in the free myocardial wall of the LV, below the noncoronary sinus of Valsalva and the interventricular septum.

When the LV calcific nodules are presented into the myocardium during ballooning of the device, this causes the endocardial and myocardial tear. Systolic blood pressure then propagates this small tear into the posterolateral myocardium. This extends the whole thickness of the myocardium and proximal portions of left anterior descending and circumflex coronary arteries. It is stopped by the epicardium and it might lead to a subepicardial haematoma. This haematoma can spread to the LV apex. Where the epicardium ruptures, there is a remote bleeding point on the surface of the heart. This can lead to a misdiagnosis of an iatrogenic coronary artery injury.

Prompt diagnosis is usually made by having a clinical index of suspicion. Aortogram and echocardiography allow assessment of the aortic root. Presentation can be with pericardial tamponade with hypotension, pericardial effusion, subepicardial haematoma, intramural haematoma, haematoma between aorta and pulmonary artery, new regurgitation of atrioventricular valves, ventricular septal defect, aortic dissection, contrast extravasation and heart block.

Expedient initiation of cardiopulmonary bypass (CPB) using the already accessed femoral vessels is of paramount importance. This is followed by emergent sternotomy and surgical repair of the defect. This might include aortic root repair, valve replacement or root replacement. In rare cases when the rupture is under the non-coronary cusp extending into the anterior mitral valve leaflet, it might require a concomitant mitral valve replacement.

Generally, a second transcatheter valve to seal the tear is not recommended as a treatment strategy. In certain cases, with small effusion only, limited haematoma in a haemodynamically stable patient, a subxiphoid pericardial drain might help relieve pericardial constriction and judicious watchful waiting in critical care setting. The limited clinical data on this subset of patients show that there is a relatively high mortality in the hours to days and even months. Surgical mortality is higher than TAVI mortality. At least one half of all surgically treated patients will survive (Eggebrecht et al. 2013).

3 Free Myocardial Wall Rupture

This occurs most commonly below the left sinus at the point closest to the commissures of the aortic valve leaflets. The LVOT portion under the left sinus is protected by fibrous skeleton of the heart where the anterior mitral valve leaflet is attached. Another site is perforation of the left ventricle free wall with the introduction of the guidewire. This complication results in haemorrhage, leading to cardiac tamponade. In the first instance, a subxiphoid pericardial drain might help temporise the bleed and, in cases of small puncture, there might be spontaneous seal and resolution. In cases with ongoing blood loss, signs of cardiac tamponade or a large, undrained effusion on echocardiography, further intervention is warranted. Emergency CPB, sternotomy and repair of the free LV wall is required with pledgeted sutures. The heart usually requires a brief period of cardioplegic arrest to ensure a secure repair in a decompressed LV cavity. The authors routinely use an LV vent via the right superior pulmonary vein, for decompression to allow repair. Techniques to repair can vary from interrupted Teflon-pledgeted sutures to Teflon strips or bovine pericardial patch repair of the defect. In cases of occult trauma to the LV apex, patients can present with chronic pseudoaneurysm formation.

4 Obstruction of Coronary Arteries

The incidence is around 0.2% for native valves and 0.8% in valve-in-valve cases (Eggebrecht et al. 2013). This rare but serious complication is due to displacement of the leaflet most commonly in front of the left main coronary artery. This happens when the coronary height is low, for example, in patients with bicuspid valves where there can be coronary displacement. It occurs more commonly in women and carries a higher procedural and early morality rate. Percutaneous coronary intervention is feasible and the treatment of choice. Complete obstruction leads to cardiogenic shock with a high mortality. Mortality rate of delayed coronary obstruction was comparable to immediate obstruction. If percutaneous intervention cannot be carried out, then emergent surgery with CPB and IABP support may be required.

5 Device Embolisation

This is a rare complication occurring in less than 0.3% of cases. There is a nine-fold increase in mortality with this complication (Ibebuogu et al. 2015). Balloon-expandable valves were most commonly involved. Majority of the devices that embolise do so at the time of implantation (77%) with a much smaller percentage of early (<1 h 4%) remaining as late migration. Poor outcomes are associated with conservative management. Acute valve failure can be treated with valve in valve TAVI. This approach is associated with late valve failures. Device embolisation leads to leaflet malfunction and can lead to vascular occlusion of coronaries. The transvalvular AR is caused by inadequate valve expansion. Causes of embolisation include the following:

(i) very high calcium load (predicted by high calcium score on CT)
(ii) elongated leaflet morphology
(iii) post-dilation
(iv) low intra-procedural BP
(v) leaflets of the valve being stuck open
(vi) a tilted prosthesis

Pre-procedure echocardiographic variables associated with embolisation include the following:

(i) low peak velocity
(ii) poor LV function
(iii) large left ventricular cavity with a large end diastolic volume
(iv) large sinotubular junction
(v) moderate or greater mitral regurgitation

For patients treated with V-in-V therapy, the all-cause 30-day mortality is nearly 10% with occurrence of stroke, renal failure, vascular complications and need for open surgery.

In cases where there is haemodynamic collapse, there is failure of V-in-V therapy or where there is concomitant coronary occlusion, surgical aortic valve replacement is mandated. The patient is typically cannulated using femoral access for CPB. Then, a conventional aortic valve replacement is carried out following removal of the transcatheter prosthesis.

6 Cardiac Tamponade

The incidence of this complication varies from 0.2% to 4.3%. The causes are typically right ventricular perforation by temporary pacemaker, annular rupture or aortic dissection and tear in the left ventricular free wall caused by the stiff wire or catheter (Rezq et al. 2012). This complication is more likely to occur in older, shorter and female patients. Diagnosis is made promptly by having a high index of suspicion with patients' haemodynamic assessment and confirmation with transthoracic echocardiography. The treatment is dependent on the aetiology of the tamponade. In most cases of RV perforation, percutaneous pericardiocentesis and drain placement are all that might be required with judicious patient monitoring for 48-h and repeat imaging. In case of annular disruption, aortic dissection or LV perforation, patients usually require immediate resuscitation, placement on cardiopulmonary bypass and open surgical correction with LV repair, aortic root repair/ replacement and surgical treatment of dissection.

7 Access Site Peripheral Vascular Complications

These are amongst the most common complication of the procedure with an incidence between major (15.3%) and minor vascular complications (11.9%) as defined by VARC criteria (Généreux et al. 2012). Contemporary data suggest that the incidence has decreased to around 5%. Access site complications are strongly correlated morbidity and mortality.

Predictors of complication are female patients with peripheral vascular disease with small access vessels that are calcified, tortuous, when the sheath-to-femoral-artery ratio is <1.05 or when the sheath diameter that exceeds the minimal femoral diameter.

Most common site of injury is the common femoral artery (CFA) where complications include access site haematoma, vessel rupture, dissection and pseudoaneurysm formation. Management involves immediate blood volume substitution and medical resuscitation. Other possible causes for a haemodynamic compromise must be excluded (such as coronary artery obstruction or valve function impairment). Treatment involves vessel repair using either endovascular or surgical techniques. Wire access allows quick deployment of an occluding balloon to tamponade the bleeding and deploy a covered stent graft where feasible. Rapid crossover angiogram and early detection of the complication are important for successful outcome. In cases where endovascular treatment is not feasible, a groin cut down onto the vessels and open repair are carried out.

Access site haematomas are a relatively benign complication that has reduced due to increased operator experience and lower profile and size of sheaths. This can usually be corrected with correction of coagulation profile and manual compression. Retroperitoneal haemorrhage or haematoma can be due to injury to any groin or abdominal vessel. This can be a difficult as the symptoms are nonspecific, i.e. flank pain, back pain with or without haemodynamic changes. Once a diagnosis is made, treatment involves transfusion of blood and blood products to resuscitate the patient. The patient can have IR-guided site of bleeding localised and treated with coil embolisation or endograft placement. In large bleeds, surgery might be indicated.

8 Severe Paravalvular Leak

Severe paravalvular leak (PVL) is present between 0% and 24% of patients depending on the study analysed (COMMITTEE: et al. 2021; Matta et al. 2024). Greater than 2+ PVL is associated with higher short- and long-term mortality. These patients continue to have symptoms and usually do not respond to heart failure medications, with higher risk of heart failure admissions and death. Predictors of severe PVL include the following:

(i) Incomplete prosthesis apposition to the native annulus due to eccentric calcification
(ii) Annular eccentricity
(iii) Undersizing of the device
(iv) Malpositioning of the valve

Immediate post deployment, haemodynamics and angiogram provide indication of the PVL severity and this is confirmed on echocardiography. Once the diagnosis is made, it needs to be addressed immediately. Paravalvular regurgitant jets are typically eccentric and arise from irregularly shaped orifices. They originate between the annulus and the outer valve skirt, and unlike central jets, their size and length do not consistently reflect the true severity of regurgitation, making these measurements unreliable for grading its severity.

The treatment is guided by the cause of the PVL. In case of incomplete prosthesis apposition, balloon valvuloplasty can be performed to improve the PVL. An upsized balloon is used to expand the valve. This is a safe strategy to improve the degree of PVL, which is usually confirmed on echo. If there is no improvement, then the next strategy is a V-in-V procedure to improve the PVL. This is specifically indicated for patients in whom the valve was deployed too high or low. The final treatment if the above are not successful is surgical aortic valve replacement (Raffa et al. 2012).

References

COMMITTEE: V-3 W, Généreux P, Piazza N, Alu MC, Nazif T, Hahn RT, Pibarot P, Bax JJ, Leipsic JA, Blanke P, Blackstone EH, Finn MT, Kapadia S, Linke A, Mack MJ, Makkar R, Mehran R, Popma JJ, Reardon M, Rodes-Cabau J, Mieghem NMV, Webb JG, Cohen DJ, Leon MB (2021) Valve Academic Research Consortium 3: updated endpoint definitions for aortic valve clinical research. J Am Coll Cardiol 77(21):2717–2746. https://doi.org/10.1016/j.jacc.2021.02.038

Eggebrecht H, Schmermund A, Kahlert P, Erbel R, Voigtländer T, Mehta RH (2013) Emergent cardiac surgery during transcatheter aortic valve implantation (TAVI): a weighted meta-analysis of 9,251 patients from 46 studies. EuroIntervention 8(9):1072–1080. https://doi.org/10.4244/eijv8i9a164

Généreux P, Webb JG, Svensson LG, Kodali SK, Satler LF, Fearon WF, Davidson CJ, Eisenhauer AC, Makkar RR, Bergman GW, Babaliaros V, Bavaria JE, Velazquez OC, Williams MR, Hueter I, Xu K, Leon MB, Investigators PT (2012) Vascular complications after transcatheter aortic valve replacement insights from the PARTNER (Placement of AoRTic TraNscathetER Valve) trial. J Am Coll Cardiol 60(12):1043–1052. https://doi.org/10.1016/j.jacc.2012.07.003

Ibebuogu UN, Giri S, Bolorunduro O, Tartara P, Kar S, Holmes D, Alli O (2015) Review of reported causes of device embolization following trans-catheter aortic valve implantation. Am J Cardiol 115(12):1767–1772. https://doi.org/10.1016/j.amjcard.2015.03.024

Leon MB, Smith CR, Mack MJ, Makkar RR, Svensson LG, Kodali SK, Thourani VH, Tuzcu EM, Miller DC, Herrmann HC, Doshi D, Cohen DJ, Pichard AD, Kapadia S, Dewey T, Babaliaros V, Szeto WY, Williams MR, Kereiakes D, Zajarias A, Greason KL, Whisenant BK, Hodson RW, Moses JW, Trento A, Brown DL, Fearon WF, Pibarot P, Hahn RT, Jaber WA, Anderson WN, Alu MC, Webb JG, Investigators P2 (2016) Transcatheter or surgical aortic-valve replacement in intermediate-risk patients. N Engl J Med 374(17):1609–1620. https://doi.org/10.1056/nejmoa1514616

Mack MJ, Leon MB, Thourani VH, Pibarot P, Hahn RT, Genereux P, Kodali SK, Kapadia SR, Cohen DJ, Pocock SJ, Lu M, White R, Szerlip M, Ternacle J, Malaisrie SC, Herrmann HC, Szeto WY, Russo MJ, Babaliaros V, Smith CR, Blanke P, Webb JG, Makkar R, Investigators P3 (2023) Transcatheter aortic-valve replacement in low-risk patients at five years. N Engl J Med 389(21):1949–1960. https://doi.org/10.1056/nejmoa2307447

Matta A, Regueiro A, Urena-Alcazar M, Nombelo-Franco L, Riche M, Rodriguez-Gabella T, Santos IA, Chamandi C, Akiki T, Gabani R, Vera-Urquiza R, Lhermusier T, Bouisset F, Carrié D, Campelo-Parada F (2024) Comparison of paravalvular leak and 1-year survival after transcatheter aortic valve replacement with SAPIEN 3 versus EVOLUT PRO valves. Arch Cardiovasc Dis 117(1):S77–S78. https://doi.org/10.1016/j.acvd.2023.10.138

Raffa GM, Malvindi PG, Settepani F, Ornaghi D, Basciu A, Cappai A, Tarelli G (2012) Aortic valve replacement for paraprosthetic leak after transcatheter implantation. J Card Surg 27(1):47–51. https://doi.org/10.1111/j.1540-8191.2011.01351.x

Rezq A, Basavarajaiah S, Latib A, Takagi K, Hasegawa T, Figini F, Cioni M, Franco A, Montorfano M, Chieffo A, Maisano F, Corvaja N, Alfieri O, Colombo A (2012) Incidence, management, and outcomes of cardiac tamponade during transcatheter aortic valve implantation. JACC Cardiovasc Interv 5(12):1264–1272. https://doi.org/10.1016/j.jcin.2012.08.012

Emergency Cardiac Surgery Following Percutaneous Mitral Valve Intervention

Ranjit Deshpande, Nithiananthan Mayooran, Aaina Mittal, and Jonathan Byrne

Abstract Mitral valve disease is common in ageing populations, with mitral regurgitation (MR) being the most prevalent lesion. Surgical mitral valve repair or replacement remains the gold standard for most patients with severe symptomatic disease; however, nearly half are considered high-risk surgical candidates due to advanced age or significant comorbidities. Over the past decade, transcatheter interventions—including transcatheter edge-to-edge repair (TEER) and transcatheter mitral valve replacement (TMVR)—have expanded treatment options for patients who are inoperable or at prohibitive surgical risk. Procedural safety has improved markedly, with major complication rates after TEER falling to approximately 3%. Nonetheless, serious complications such as cardiac tamponade, clip embolisation, device detachment, severe residual MR, and persistent iatrogenic atrial septal defects may arise and necessitate urgent surgical intervention.

This chapter reviews current evidence and surgical considerations for managing patients who require cardiac surgery following percutaneous mitral valve procedures. Key aspects include strategies for cannulation, choice of sternotomy versus minimally invasive approach, and decision making on repair versus replacement—each tailored to patient suitability and case complexity. Although outcomes remain variable, reflecting the high-risk nature of this population, timely surgical intervention can be life-saving. Careful patient selection, multidisciplinary procedural planning, and readiness for immediate surgical conversion remain critical to optimising results.

Keywords Transcatheter edge-to-edge repair complications · TEER device detachment · TEER clip embolisation · persistent iatrogenic atrial septal defect · mitral surgery after failed TEER · cardiac tamponade · infective endocarditis of TEER device · TEER-induced mitral stenosis

---

R. Deshpande (✉) · N. Mayooran · A. Mittal · J. Byrne
Cardiac Department, King's College Hospital, London, UK
e-mail: ranjit.deshpande@nhs.net; jonathan.byrne@nhs.net

A. Kourliouros (ed.), *Emergency Cardiac Surgery*,
https://doi.org/10.1007/978-3-032-15787-4_14

1 Introduction

Mitral valve disease is prevalent across all age groups, with its incidence increasing with age; 5.1% of individuals aged 65 and over are affected by this condition (Harky et al. 2021). Patients with severe symptomatic or select asymptomatic mitral valve disease are typically best managed with surgical mitral valve repair or replacement. It is well documented that approximately 49% of mitral valve disease patients are considered high risk for surgical intervention due to significant comorbidities or advanced disease (Kargoli et al. 2021).

Mitral regurgitation is the most common type of mitral valve disease, affecting 10% of individuals aged 75 and older (Mazur et al. 2022). The underlying mechanism can be primary or secondary. Primary mitral regurgitation (PMR), also known as degenerative mitral regurgitation, results from deformity or damage to the mitral valve apparatus. Secondary mitral regurgitation (SMR), also known as functional mitral regurgitation, is due to dysfunction of the left atrium or left ventricle without any structural abnormalities of the valve itself.

The European Society of Cardiology/European Association for Cardiothoracic Surgery provides guidelines for the investigation and management of mitral valve disease based on the underlying mechanism. It recommends the use of echocardiography for investigation. Surgical mitral valve repair is the recommended standard of care in cases of symptomatic severe PMR with acceptable surgical risk or in asymptomatic patients with left ventricular dysfunction or atrial fibrillation, as well as in urgent cases of acute mitral regurgitation. In patients with contraindications to surgery or high operative risk, transcatheter mitral valve interventions, particularly transcatheter edge-to-edge repair (TEER), can be considered due to the most substantial evidence currently available supporting its efficacy. For SMR, intervention is recommended for patients with severe disease who remain symptomatic despite medical therapy. Surgery is recommended in the setting of significant coronary artery disease when deemed appropriate by the heart team, and TEER is recommended higher than surgery, provided certain anatomical criteria are met (Vahanian et al. 2021).

Although TEER (using devices such as MitraClip or Pascal systems) is widely used, certain anatomical requirements must be met before it can be considered. In high-risk patients with unsuitable mitral valve anatomy for TEER, those with previous mitral valve replacement or repair, transcatheter mitral valve implantation (TMVR) is a viable option. The presence of MAC is not a contraindication to TEER, but leaflet length and leaflet calcification may be.

TMVR is performed via the femoral vein with an atrial septostomy used to place an appropriately sized biological valve, pre-measured using cardiac computed tomography (CT) and transoesophageal echocardiography (TOE). There are specific devices to treat native mitral valve disease, e.g. Tendyne/Intrepid. The use of TAVI devices are to treat non-native disease—valve in valve/ring and rarely valve in mitral annular calcification.

Mitral stenosis has a prevalence of 0.2% and can be rheumatic or degenerative in aetiology (Chandrashekhar et al. 2009). Guidelines recommend percutaneous mitral commissurotomy for symptomatic patients without unfavourable characteristics or those with a contraindication or high risk for surgery. Surgery is recommended for symptomatic patients not suitable for percutaneous intervention (Vahanian et al. 2021).

Despite continuous improvements in delivery systems allowing effective treatment even in complex anatomies, complications can occur during or after transcatheter mitral interventions. Complications are categorised as procedure-related, device-related, and access-related. Significant procedure-related complications, such as pericardial tamponade, torrential mitral regurgitation (MR) due to damage or detachment of a leaflet, and device embolisation, require emergency mitral valve surgery. Emergency vascular access-related complications (dissection, perforation, rupture, or stenosis) are generally managed by vascular surgeons.

TEER registries report improvements in major adverse complications, decreasing from 15% in 2005 to less than 3% following such interventions (Schnitzler et al. 2021). Studies indicate that TMVR patients represent a comparatively high-risk population, with mortality rates ranging from 8% to 38% (Kargoli et al. 2021). TMVR patients are typically those not suitable for TEER procedures or those with prohibitive surgical risks for primary cardiac surgery.

2 Indications for Emergency Cardiac Surgery

The need for emergency cardiac surgery following transcatheter intervention depends on various factors. From a cardiac surgical perspective, these interventions can be categorised as emergent, urgent, or elective, based on the required time to intervene. The most common indications (though not limited to these) for surgical mitral valve intervention are listed in Table 1. These patients are often considered high-risk for surgical mitral valve procedures. When a complication arises, it presents a clinical challenge.

Table 1 illustrates the indications for mitral valve surgery after transcatheter MV interventions.

Indications for MV surgery after percutaneous mitral interventions
Cardiac tamponade
Device embolisation
Severe torrential MR
Recurrent MR
Residual MR
Single-leaflet device attachment
Partial detachment
Mitral stenosis
Mitral valve leaflet injury/tear/perforation
Endocarditis
Failed attempt
Persistent intra-atrial septal defect
Severe left ventricular outflow tract obstruction (LVOTO)

A multidisciplinary heart team meeting, including cardiologists, the interventional team, cardiac surgeons, anaesthetists, and intensivists, is often useful for obtaining a tailored assessment and consensus towards a management plan. At times, multidisciplinary team meetings are organised in an emergency informal setting (or through a virtual platform) to expedite decision making. We need to appreciate that not all the patients are suitable for salvage emergency mitral valve surgery. MDT's function is to triage the suitable patients for emergency cardiac surgery.

Patients requiring emergency cardiac surgery in a mitral valve intervention scenario typically fall into one of two categories. The first category involves acute injury to cardiac structures (left ventricle, mitral valve leaflets, atrial septal defect, and right ventricle), leading to either cardiac tamponade or severe mitral valve prolapse, which may cause cardiogenic shock. The second category involves the embolisation of a device or part of a damaged cardiac structure (e.g. ruptured leaflet or plaque of calcium).

Complications Requiring Emergency Cardiac Surgery

- **Cardiac Tamponade:** This complication has an incidence of 2.5–3% following TEER and can be caused by transseptal puncture (Flores et al. 2022). Small pericardial effusions are generally managed with a pericardial drain placed under echocardiographic guidance. Large effusions compressing heart chambers can cause significant haemodynamic instability. These patients require full sternotomy or, in selected cases, left-sided thoracotomy for release of tamponade and repair of the bleeding site. If the primary procedure (TEER/PMVR) is unsuccessful, surgical repair or valve replacement is necessary (Flores et al. 2022).
- **Clip Embolisation:** This can occur following complete detachment of a clip from both mitral valve leaflets, with an incidence of less than 1% (Flores et al. 2022). Surgical mitral valve repair is typically required following this complication.
- **Device Detachment:** Single-leaflet device attachment (SLDA) has an incidence of up to 4.8%, with most cases involving detachment from the posterior mitral valve leaflet. SLDA can be treated with repeat TEER procedure or medical therapy, and surgical repair/replacement is rarely required. Surgery is much more likely in cases of leaflet tear or perforation, and repeat percutaneous clip procedures tend to fail (Flores et al. 2022). While there are reported cases of mitral valve repair following device detachment, mitral valve replacement is commonly recommended for such complications (Elhmidi et al. 2016).
- **Severe Mitral Regurgitation:** Severe MR is a well-recognised complication following balloon mitral valvotomy (initially performed percutaneously for mitral stenosis). Severe or torrential MR can lead to pulmonary hypertension, right ventricular failure, and myocardial infarction (Bayya et al. 2014). In such situations, emergency mitral valve surgery is indicated to prevent end-organ damage. Factors predicting the need for emergency surgery in cases of this rare complication include right ventricular systolic pressure over 76 mmHg and the presence of non-commissural calcium on the mitral valve leaflet (Pande et al. 2012). These patients can quickly become unwell due to right ventricular failure and may rapidly progress to cardiogenic shock. Extracorporeal membrane oxygenation (ECMO) is a

useful adjunct to offload cardiopulmonary workload and plan definitive surgical management. Mitral valve repair attempts are generally not preferred in this patient group, as their perioperative mortality can be as high as 16% in reported series (Elhmidi et al. 2016). In the TEER population, severe MR due to leaflet damage is rare, but is an indication for surgery. In the TMVR population, severe paravalvular MR or LV OT obstruction involves more relevant risks.

- **Persistent Iatrogenic Atrial Septal Defect (iASD):** Following percutaneous intervention, another indication for surgery may arise, such as a persistent atrial septal defect resulting from transseptal puncture (Kargoli et al. 2021). Persistent iASDs one month after MitraClip deployment range from 43% to 82% (Shetty et al. 2021). Small, asymptomatic iASDs can be managed conservatively, using an Amplatzer device or being closed concomitantly if surgical re-intervention is indicated.

Complications Requiring Non-Emergent Cardiac Surgery

- **Mitral Stenosis:** The healing response to percutaneous intervention is not well understood. The literature hypothesises that extensive fibrosis around the site of TEER (e.g. MitraClip or Pascal) placement can lead to mitral stenosis in some patients following the procedure (Alozie et al. 2014). Mitral stenosis, which develops post TEER, is simply due to the reaction in valve area created by the devices. It is sometimes underestimated at the time of the procedure due to the blunted haemodynamics (particularly HR/BP) during the procedure. A mean transvalvular gradient pressure greater than 5 mmHg in patients with PMR has been associated with adverse clinical and functional outcomes (Flores et al. 2022). Patients with severe decompensated mitral stenosis may require emergency mitral valve replacement surgery, as the valves are often damaged beyond repair, making mitral valve replacement the ideal choice. In elective cases, there are some reports of repairing these valves, but the long-term results are awaited.
- **Infective Endocarditis (IE):** Patients who develop IE following a percutaneous mitral valve intervention are generally managed with antibiotics as a first-line therapy. Early surgery is recommended if there is an associated severe mitral valve lesion (MR, AR, etc.), large vegetations (>1 cm), or clinically progressive IE. Similar to prosthetic valve-related IE, post-TEER/TMVR carries a significantly higher rate of perioperative mortality, up to 42% (Asmarats et al. 2018).

3 Surgical Approach

The patient's haemodynamic status generally dictates when, where, and how the operation should be performed. Clinically unstable patients may require stabilisation with inotropes, with or without intra-aortic balloon pump (IABP) or extracorporeal membrane oxygenation (ECMO), and some may require emergency mitral valve (MV) surgery in a hybrid theatre.

Typically, TEER/TMVR procedures are performed in a hybrid theatre under general anaesthesia, intubated, ventilated with transoesophageal echocardiography (TOE), continuous arterial blood pressure monitoring, and a central venous line. These are essential adjuncts for escalating to open MV surgery if necessary.

(a) **Cannulation Strategy**

After a full dose of heparinisation, peripheral cannulation strategy is a quick and easy option for this cohort of patients, as femoral access is already established by the interventional team for TEER. Femoral cannulation is performed via the previously exposed femoral artery and vein, using a purse-string suture and the Seldinger technique under TOE guidance. This approach provides the surgeon with time and the patient with stability before planning the actual operation.

(b) **Sternotomy**

A standard median sternotomy is the preferred approach in emergencies such as tamponade, MV leaflet detachment, or device embolisation. Although there are isolated reports of successful minimally invasive approaches to mitral valves, the authors recommend a sternotomy for unstable patients with already complicated cardiac procedures. These patients often have additional complications, such as cardiac tamponade, or may require primary closure of an atrial septal defect (ASD) or repair of tricuspid valve regurgitation. Time and exposure are crucial in managing these patients, and a full sternotomy provides the surgeon with the best options for intervention.

(c) **Minimally Invasive Cardiac Surgery (MiCS)**

Utilising minimally invasive approach in an emergency depends on surgeon's experience, patient's body habitus, and comorbidities. Generally, sternotomy is a preferred approach; but the rationale for performing MiCS is to reduce to surgical trauma and bleeding. Patients with non-emergent indications can be planned to have an urgent in-house surgery using MiCS. There are reports of robotic-assisted and MiCS after TEER-related complications (Mitral valve repair after failed MitraClip therapy 2019).

At our centre, we have successfully operated through minimally invasive approach (MiCS) on five patients, who developed complications after TEER/ TMVR (AMVL tear, severe MR, tamponade, valve in ring complication, and embolisation).

(d) **Mitral Valve Repair vs. Replacement**

The aim of surgical intervention is to rescue the patient from life-threatening complications and provide a sustainable MV intervention that will last. Young patients with isolated leaflet injury due to MitraClip, and who have the potential for better repair outcomes, will benefit from repair by experienced surgeons. Elective mitral repairs after MitraClip interventions have been reported by specialised cardiac surgical centres (Mitral valve repair after failed MitraClip therapy 2019).

Decision making is critical in these emergency situations. The decision to perform, or at least have an idea of, the type of MV repair or replacement prior to initiating cardiopulmonary bypass (CPB) is pivotal in these emergency surgeries. This approach reduces CPB and cross-clamp times, which have been proven to improve outcomes in complicated patients (Chikwe et al. 2021).

In the United Kingdom, most TEER and TMVR patients are considered high risk for surgical interventions due to their comorbidities or history of previous cardiac surgeries. The primary objective is often to restore a competent mitral valve and repair any damage caused by the TEER/TMVR devices. Therefore, the debate between repair and replacement is generally of less concern.

4 Summary

In summary, despite the increasing prevalence of percutaneous mitral valve interventions, emergency cardiac surgery remains the gold standard procedure of choice for complicated emergency cases, regardless of their risk stratification. Suitable patients should receive minimally invasive approach, as this can reduce surgical trauma on a complicated patient.

References

Alozie A, Westphal B, Kische S, Kaminski A, Paranskaya L, Bozdag-Turan I et al (2014) Surgical revision after percutaneous mitral valve repair by edge-to-edge device: when the strategy fails in the highest risk surgical population. Eur J Cardiothorac Surg 46(1):55–60

Asmarats L, Rodriguez-Gabella T, Chamandi C, Bernier M, Beaudoin J, O'Connor K et al (2018) Infective endocarditis following transcatheter edge-to-edge mitral valve repair: a systematic review. Catheter Cardiovasc Interv 92(3):583–591

Bayya P, Varma P, Raman S, Neema P (2014) Emergency mitral valve replacement for acute severe mitral regurgitation following balloon mitral valvotomy: pathophysiology of hemodynamic collapse and peri-operative management issues. Ann Card Anaesth 17(1):52

Chandrashekhar Y, Westaby S, Narula J (2009) Mitral stenosis. Lancet 374(9697):1271–1283

Chikwe J, O'Gara P, Fremes S, Sundt TM, Habib RH, Gammie J et al (2021) Mitral surgery after transcatheter edge-to-edge repair. J Am Coll Cardiol 78(1):1–9

Elhmidi Y, Voss B, Lange R (2016) Surgical mitral valve intervention following a failed MitraClip procedure. EuroIntervention 12(Y):Y102–Y106

Flores G, Mesa D, Ojeda S, de Lezo JS, Gonzalez-Manzanares R, Dueñas G et al (2022) Complications of the percutaneous mitral valve edge-to-edge repair: role of transesophageal echocardiography. J Clin Med 11(16):4747

Harky A, Botezatu B, Kakar S, Ren M, Shirke MM, Pullan M (2021) Mitral valve diseases: pathophysiology and interventions. Prog Cardiovasc Dis 67:98–104

Kargoli F, Pagnesi M, Rahgozar K, Goldberg Y, Ho E, Chau M et al (2021) Current devices and complications related to transcatheter mitral valve replacement: the bumpy road to the top, vol 8, Frontiers in cardiovascular medicine. Frontiers Media SA

Mazur P, Arghami A, Zheng C, Alkhouli M, Schaff HV, Dearani J et al (2022) Mitral valve surgery after failed transcatheter edge-to-edge repair. JTCVS Tech 14:79–88

Mitral valve repair after failed MitraClip therapy. The Multimedia Manual for Cardio-Thoracic Surgery (2019)

Pande S, Agarwal SK, Kumar S, Shukla RK, Tripathy N, Singh RK et al (2012) Factors predicting emergency surgery in severe mitral regurgitation following mitral balloon valvotomy. J Heart Valve Dis 21(5):551–555

Schnitzler K, Hell M, Geyer M, Kreidel F, Münzel T, Stephan Von Bardeleben R (2021) Complications following MitraClip implantation. https://doi.org/10.1007/s11886-021-01553-9

Shetty M, Lampert MB, Levisay J, Erwin JP, Ricciardi MJ (2021) Iatrogenic atrial septal defect closure following mitral transcatheter edge-to-edge repair. JACC Case Rep 3(3):357–360

Vahanian A, Beyersdorf F, Praz F, Milojevic M, Baldus S, Bauersachs J et al (2021) 2021 ESC/EACTS Guidelines for the management of valvular heart disease. Eur Heart J

Emergency Interventions Following Percutaneous Closure of Atrial Septal Defect, Patent Foramen Ovale, and Left Atrial Appendage Occlusion

Ali Ansaripour and Tom J. Cahill

Abstract This chapter reviews the indications, techniques, and contemporary devices used for percutaneous closure of atrial septal defects (ASD), patent foramen ovale (PFO), and left atrial appendage occlusion (LAAO), with a particular focus on the recognition and management of complications requiring urgent intervention. While transcatheter closure has largely replaced surgery for most ASDs and PFOs, and LAAO is an established treatment options in selected patients with atrial fibrillation, these procedures carry risks including device embolisation, cardiac perforation and tamponade, vascular complications, residual shunts, peri-device leaks, and device-related thrombus. The chapter discusses patient selection, device sizing, and procedural planning as key factors in minimising complications. Management strategies are outlined in structured decision-making algorithms, prioritising percutaneous retrieval techniques such as gooseneck snare or bioptome-assisted methods, with surgical or hybrid approaches reserved for complex cases. Outcomes from reported case series demonstrate high success rates for both percutaneous and surgical retrieval when timely, multidisciplinary intervention is employed. Emphasis is placed on the importance of imaging guidance, operator expertise, and individualised treatment strategies to optimise patient safety and procedural success.

Keywords Atrial septal defect · Patent foramen ovale · Septal occluder · Left atrial appendage occlusion (LAAO) · Device embolisation · Cardiac perforation · Tamponade · Residual shunt after ASD closure · Peri-device leak LAAO · Closure device-related thrombus · Percutaneous closure device retrieval · Hybrid procedure for device retrieval

A. Ansaripour (✉) · T. J. Cahill
Heart Centre, John Radcliffe Hospital, Oxford, UK

University of Oxford, Oxford, UK
e-mail: Ali.Ansaripour@ouh.nhs.uk; Tom.Cahill@ouh.nhs.uk

A. Kourliouros (ed.), *Emergency Cardiac Surgery*,
https://doi.org/10.1007/978-3-032-15787-4_15

1 Percutaneous Atrial Septal Defect (ASD) and Patent Foreman Ovale (PFO) Closure

Atrial septal defects (ASDs) are congenital cardiac anomalies characterised by an abnormal opening in the interatrial septum, which permits abnormal blood flow between the left and right atria. With an incidence of 6–10 per 10,000 live births, ostium secundum atrial septal defects (ASD) are one of the most common forms of congenital heart disease (Hoffman and Kaplan 2002). ASDs typically cause a left to right shunt, leading to increased volume load on the right atrium and ventricle, resulting in right ventricular dilation, and, if untreated, pulmonary hypertension. Subtypes of ASDs include ostium secundum, ostium primum, and sinus venosus defects.

Patent foramen ovale (PFO) is a remnant of the foetal circulation that persists in about 25% of adults, making it the commonest congenital cardiac defect. A PFO occurs when the septum primum and septum secundum fail to close once the infant begins breathing (Bradley and Zaidi 2020). In the context of raised right atrial pressure (e.g. during straining or Valsalva), blood flow through a PFO allows shunting of blood from right to left atrium. In the presence of thrombus, this can cause paradoxical embolism and stroke. The commonest indication for closure of a PFO is cryptogenic stroke, where there has been presumed embolism of thrombus through the PFO.

1.1 Indications for ASD and PFO Closure

The indications for closure of ASDs and PFOs share some similarities but differ significantly in their underlying rationale and patient population focus. ASD closure is primarily indicated in patients with significant left-to-right shunting leading to right heart enlargement or volume overload (Butera et al. 2008; Warnes et al. 2008). In contrast, PFO closure is typically considered for patients with a history of paradoxical embolism, particularly those with a history of cryptogenic stroke or transient ischaemic attack (TIA) (Taramasso et al. 2016; Landzberg and Khairy 2004). PFO closure may also be considered in patients with associated conditions such as migraine with aura, decompression sickness, or platypnoea–orthodeoxia syndrome, where right-to-left shunting exacerbates symptoms.

The differences in indications are driven by the distinct pathophysiology of ASDs and PFOs. ASD closure is primarily driven by haemodynamic consequences, such as right heart overload and pulmonary hypertension, where early intervention prevents long-term complications like heart failure or arrhythmias (Fraisse et al. 2018). On the other hand, PFO closure is more focused on reducing the risk of embolic events. The decision for PFO closure often involves weighing the risks of recurrent stroke or systemic embolism against the procedural risks, especially in younger populations with fewer comorbidities.

1.2 Contemporary Devices for ASD/PFO Closure

Management of secundum ASDs and PFOs has evolved significantly from surgical repair to transcatheter device closure (Turner et al. 2022). Traditional surgical closure involves a sternotomy and cardiopulmonary bypass, which are associated with higher morbidity and longer recovery times. The advent of transcatheter closure techniques in the 1970s transformed ASD and PFO management, offering a less invasive option with comparable efficacy and fewer complications, and shorter length of hospital stay (King et al. 1976; Mullins 1998; Du et al. 2002). Surgery remains the mainstay of treatment for primum and most sinus venosus ASDs (Menillo et al. 2024).

In contemporary practice, two families of devices, the Amplatzer Septal Occluder (ASO; Abbott, St. Paul, MN, USA) and Gore Cardioform Septal Occluder (W.L. Gore & Associates, Flagstaff, AZ, USA), Fig. 1, have become preferred options for percutaneous closure of secundum ASDs and PFOs due to their high success rates, ease of use, and safety profiles.

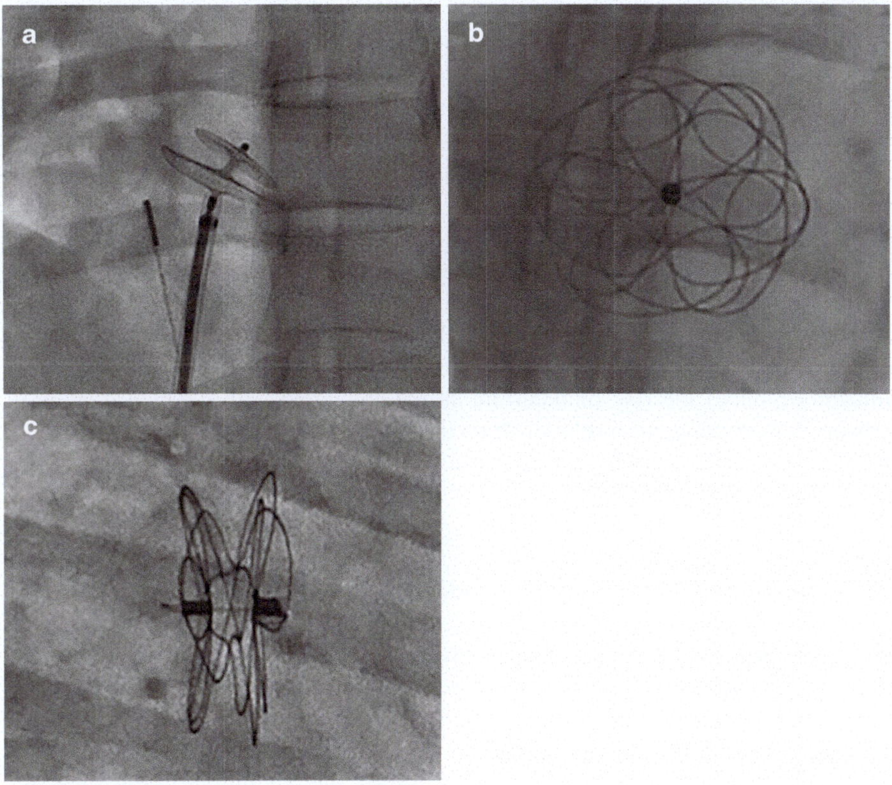

Fig. 1 Radiographic appearance of devices for transcatheter closure of ASD/PFO. (**a**) Amplatzer Talisman PFO occluder (Acquired by authors). (**b**) Gore Cardioform device en face view. (**c**) Gore Cardioform orthogonal views. (Courtesy of W.L. Gore and Associates Flagstaff, AZ; with permission)

1.2.1 Amplatzer Closure Devices

The Amplatzer Septal Occluder (ASO) is a double disc occluder with a central waist which is comprised of a nitinol mesh and polyester material. It is designed to anchor to the septal rims on each side of the defect and create a platform for tissue ingrowth after implantation. The ASO device is available in a range of sizes with the central waist of the device spanning from 4 mm to 38 mm. The Amplatzer Cribriform Occluder is a variant septal occluder device specifically designed for the closure of multi-fenestrated ASDs. This device features large, equal-sized right and left discs connected by a waist, providing a secure fit across the defect.

The ASO was the first device approved by the United States (US) Food and Drug Administration (FDA) in 2001 (Turner et al. 2022). Since its approval, numerous case series have reported excellent medium and long-term outcomes, and it is now used in 70–86% of ASD closures in US centres (Mullins 1998; Baumgartner et al. 2010; Liava'a and Kalfa 2018; Saver et al. 2017). Early trial data in the late 1990s highlighted the ASO's effectiveness, with a closure rate of 57% immediately post-procedure to 97% at 1 month (Masura et al. 1997). The ASO's safety and effectiveness have also been demonstrated in the Closure of Atrial Septal Defects With the Amplatzer Septal Occluder Post-Approval Study (ASD PMS II), a large prospective, nonrandomised, multicentric study of 1000 patients (Turner et al. 2017). This study showed a high success rate of ASD closure at 97.9%, with low rates of complication with haemodynamic compromise (0.65%) and device erosion (0.3%).

The Amplatzer PFO Occluder is a similar, self-expandable, double-disc device made from a nitinol wire mesh, available in multiple sizes. The 2 discs are linked together by a short connecting waist. The right atrial disc is larger than the left atrial disc, except for the smallest (18 mm) device, where the discs are of equal size. Several trials have now demonstrated the safety and efficacy of PFO closure in patients with cryptogenic stroke. The RESPECT, CLOSE, and REDUCE trials have shown that with careful patient selection, transcatheter PFO closure using ASO significantly reduces the risk of recurrent stroke compared with medical therapy in patients with cryptogenic stroke, with no increased risk of serious adverse events or influence on major bleeding (Saver et al. 2017; Mojadidi et al. 2018; Mas et al. 2017; Søndergaard et al. 2017).

1.2.2 Gore Cardioform Septal Occluders

The Gore Cardioform Septal Occluders are designed with a Nitinol wire frame covered by an expanded polytetrafluoroethylene (ePTFE) membrane, providing flexibility and biocompatibility for transcatheter closure of ASD and PFO, Figure 1. Although the early Helex devices, namely the Gore Helex Septal Occluder, demonstrated excellent safety and efficacy in both short- and medium-term outcomes for ASD closure (Vincent et al. 2003; Jones et al. 2007; Latson et al. 2006), their non-self-centring and size meant that its use was limited to smaller defects. The newer Cardioform models offer a larger central waist and an expanded size range to accommodate larger defects.

The efficacy of the Gore Cardioform Septal Occluder device was evaluated in the REDUCE trial, which compared PFO closure using the Helex or Cardioform devices combined with antiplatelet therapy against antiplatelet therapy alone (Søndergaard et al. 2017). In 664 patients with cryptogenic ischaemic stroke, recurrent stroke occurred in 1.4% of the PFO closure group versus 5.4% in the antiplatelet-only group. However, device closure was associated with a notable increase in atrial fibrillation or flutter (6.6% vs. 0.4%), highlighting the need to balance the benefits of stroke prevention with the risk of arrhythmias. The trial's findings, supported by consistent 5-year follow-up data, underscored the Cardioform's efficacy in reducing stroke recurrence, although the elevated arrhythmia rates warrant careful patient monitoring (Kasner et al. 2021).

The Gore Cardioform ASD Occluder (GCA) was later introduced, featuring a larger diameter central waist and an expanded range of diameters (8–35 mm defects), making it suitable for larger ASDs (Hribernik et al. 2023). It received FDA approval based on results from the ASSURED clinical study, which assessed its safety and efficacy in patients with secundum ASD (Sommer et al. 2020). The study included 125 patients across 22 US centres, with a focus on closure success at 6 months, defined by technical success, safety, and residual defect status. The device's performance, marked by high closure rates and low complication rates, validated its use across a wide range of patient demographics, including those with complex anatomical features such as deficient retro-aortic rims. It is important to note that wire frame fractures were observed in 31.7% of patients at 6 months, increasing to 56.8% of patients at 36 months. Despite the high frequency, no clinical sequelae were associated with these fractures throughout the trial period (Qureshi et al. 2024).

2 Left Atrial Appendage Occlusion (LAAO)

Percutaneous left atrial appendage occlusion (LAAO) has emerged as an alternative strategy to long-term anticoagulation for stroke prevention in selected patients with atrial fibrillation (AF) (Holmes et al. 2009, 2014). The intervention mechanically occludes the left atrial appendage, the primary site for thrombus formation in AF, thereby reducing stroke risk without the associated bleeding complications of anticoagulants.

2.1 *Evidence for LAAO*

Despite the initial promise demonstrated by early trials such as PROTECT-AF and PREVAIL, which showed that LAAO could reduce the risk of all-cause mortality and major bleeding compared to warfarin, concerns about procedural efficacy and safety—including rates of pericardial effusion, device embolisation, and stroke—initially tempered enthusiasm for LAAO as a mainstream stroke prevention strategy (Holmes et al. 2009, 2014).

The evidence supporting LAAO is still evolving. The primary trials comparing LAAO to anticoagulation, including PROTECT-AF, PREVAIL, and PRAGUE-17, have shown that LAAO is non-inferior to oral anticoagulation in carefully selected patients with non-valvular AF (Holmes et al. 2009, 2014; Osmancik et al. 2020, 2022). The 2020 PRAGUE-17 study, which compared LAAO with direct oral anticoagulants (DOACs), found that LAAO was non-inferior in preventing major AF-related cardiovascular, neurological, and bleeding events, further supporting its role as an alternative for patients at high risk for both stroke and bleeding. However, a key issue remains whether LAAO effectively eliminates the embolic source by excluding the LAA cavity from systemic circulation or whether its benefits are primarily due to mitigating bleeding risks associated with anticoagulation.

Current guidelines from both European and American professional societies recommend LAAO as an alternative strategy for patients who cannot tolerate anticoagulation (January et al. 2014; Kirchhof et al. 2017), with a class IIb recommendation from the European Society of Cardiology and a slightly stronger class IIa recommendation from the American Heart Association/American College of Cardiology (Joglar et al. 2024). LAAO still faces challenges, including device-related thrombus and peri-device leaks (PDL), which can compromise its effectiveness (Simard et al. 2022; Viles-Gonzalez et al. 2012). Regardless, following FDA approval, the utilisation rates of LAAO, particularly in the United States, has grown substantially, and the safety profile of the procedure remained excellent (Alkhouli et al. 2022; Freeman et al. 2020; Friedman et al. 2022).

2.2 *Patient Selection for LAAO*

Patient selection for LAAO requires careful clinical judgement, as the definitions of relative and absolute contraindications to oral anticoagulation can be ambiguous (van den Ham et al. 2021). Key candidates include those with prior intracranial haemorrhage (Osmancik et al. 2020; Nielsen-Kudsk et al. 2017), for whom ongoing anticoagulation poses a significant bleeding risk, and patients with major gastrointestinal bleeding, particularly from non-reversible sources (Joglar et al. 2024; Lempereur et al. 2017). Additionally, LAAO may be considered for individuals with end-stage renal disease or haemodialysis (Hindricks et al. 2021; Luani et al. 2019), where anticoagulation is challenging, and for those with haematological disorders or requiring prolonged antiplatelet therapy (Kramer et al. 2022). Non-compliant patients who struggle with regular medication adherence may also benefit. In all cases, a multidisciplinary, patient-centred approach is critical to align treatment with individual risk profiles.

2.3 Contemporary Devices

2.3.1 Watchman 2.5 and FLX Devices

The Watchman 2.5 device (Boston Scientific, Marlborough, MA, USA) received CE Mark approval in 2005 and FDA approval in 2015 (Bayard et al. 2010). It is a self-expandable, parachute-shaped nitinol device designed for endocardial LAA closure. The next-generation Watchman FLX includes improvements such as a closed-end nitinol structure and 24 J-shaped anchors, with enhanced sealing to reduce peri-device leakage. The Watchman FLX is associated with lower complication rates including mortality, pericardial effusion, and device embolisation, compared to the Watchman 2.5 (Reddy et al. 2014; Price et al. 2022; Kar et al. 2021). Its most recent iteration includes a fluoropolymer-coated membrane to increase thromboresistance and reduce the risk of device-related thrombosis (Saliba et al. 2023). The Watchman devices are extensively studied, with robust data supporting their safety and efficacy compared to oral anticoagulation from trials like PROTECT-AF and PREVAIL (Holmes et al. 2009, 2014).

2.3.2 Amplatzer Amulet Device

The Amplatzer Amulet device (Abbott) is an upgraded version of the Amplatzer Cardiac Plug, featuring a self-expanding nitinol structure with a lobe and disc connected by a central waist, incorporating polyester patches to facilitate occlusion. It is particularly effective for LAA anatomies with minimal implantation depth and complex orientations between the ostium and appendage body (Freeman et al. 2020; Asmarats and Rodés-Cabau 2017). In the Amulet IDE randomised trial ($n = 1878$), the Amulet was shown to be non-inferior to the Watchman in terms of safety and effectiveness for stroke prevention, with slightly higher occlusion rates (98.9% versus 96.8%) but also a higher rate of procedure-related complications (4.5% versus 2.5%) (Lakkireddy et al. 2021). The SWISS APERO trial, which randomised 221 patients between Watchman (2.5 or FLX) device and Amulet, also found that Amulet had lower PDL rates on transoesophageal echocardiography compared to Watchman, though it had a slightly higher incidence of pericardial effusion/tamponade (Galea et al. 2022).

2.3.3 Other LAAO Devices

Other LAAO devices include the Ultraseal, OMEGA, Lambre, and several new devices under development like the WaveCrest, SeaLA, and Laminar devices. The Ultraseal, a second-generation Cardia device, features a reduced radial force and flexible central waist, allowing adaptation to complex anatomies, although in-hospital complications remain notable at 5.8% (Pivato et al. 2022). The OMEGA device, distinct for its double-layer metal mesh coated with platinum, is suitable for very small LAA landing zones down to 10 mm. The Lambre device, with its hook-embedded umbrella and short central waist, is designed for LAA anatomies like the 'chicken wing', facilitating implantation in complex shapes (Huang et al. 2017). New devices continue to be explored, with several under clinical trials aimed at improving safety, occlusion rates, and reducing complications (Wong et al. 2023; Bavishi 2023).

3 Complications Associated with ASD, PFO, and LAAO Procedures

Despite the overall safety and efficacy of transcatheter ASD, PFO, and LAAO devices, a range of complications can arise, from minor issues to severe, life-threatening events, necessitating emergency interventions. Understanding these complications and strategies to mitigate them is crucial for optimising patient outcomes.

3.1 Device Embolisation

Device embolisation is a serious complication where the closure device dislodges and migrates within the heart or vascular system (Fig. 2). The incidence of device embolisation varies by device type and patient characteristics, with rates of less than 1% reported for ASD and PFO closures. It is important to note that the PFO device embolisation is less common than ASD devices. Contributing factors include inadequate device sizing, improper deployment techniques, and challenging anatomical features such as large or irregularly shaped defects. Butera et al. reported device embolisation in less than 1% of cases among 1013 patients with secundum ASD (Butera et al. 2008). Risk factors for embolisation include larger defects, floppy or deficient rims, thin atrial septal tissue, and excessive manipulation during deployment (Batta et al. 2021). The most common locations of the embolised ASD and PFO device were the main pulmonary artery, the right ventricular outflow tract, the right atrial cavity, and right pulmonary artery (Yetkin et al. 2014).

Similarly, device embolisation following LAAO is a significant complication. A systematic review and meta-analysis of 64 studies including 93 patients demonstrated an overall incidence of 2% (Murtaza et al. 2021). Embolisation predominantly occurs in the early post-procedural period. The most frequent sites of embolisation are the descending aorta and the left atrium, but devices can also migrate to the left ventricle or mitral apparatus, where the risk of severe outcomes is markedly increased (Eppinger et al. 2024).

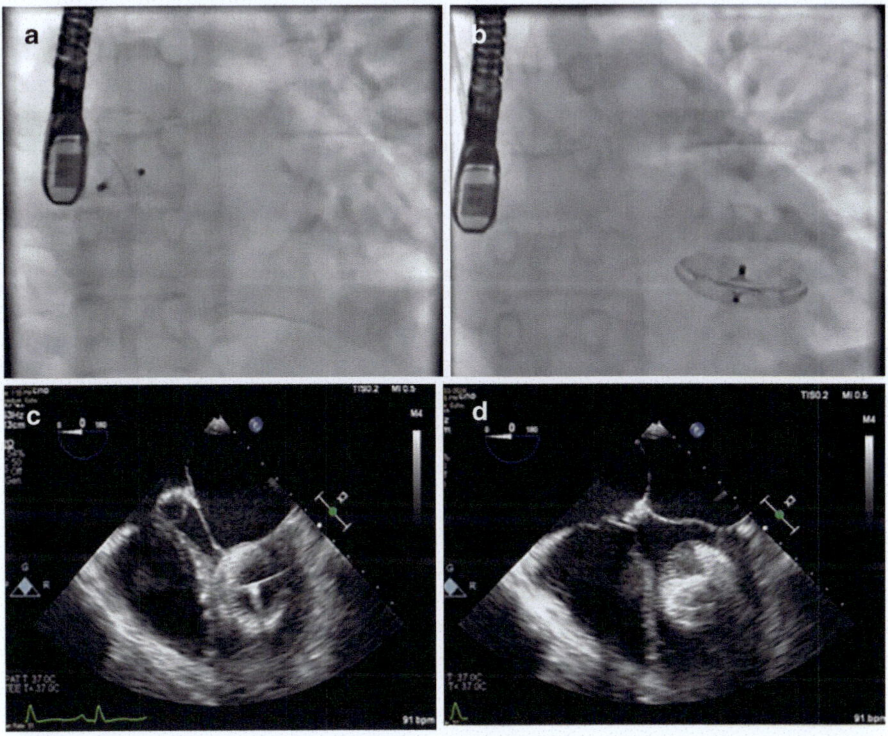

Fig. 2 Fluoroscopy and transoesophageal echocardiogram demonstrating appropriate position of ASD, (**a**), and its embolisation to the left ventricle (**b**–**d**)

Both studies identified device–appendage size mismatch and operator experience as key factors contributing to embolisation. Embolisation is more likely when there is a misalignment between the size of the device and the atrial appendage. Management of embolisation varies depending on the location of the device; most cases are managed percutaneously, but surgical retrieval is often necessary for devices that embolise to the left ventricle or mitral valve apparatus. This underscores the importance of careful procedural planning, the use of appropriate imaging modalities, and the need for ongoing operator training to minimise the risk of embolisation and improve patient outcomes in LAAO procedures.

3.2 Cardiac Perforation and Tamponade

Pericardial effusion and tamponade, which result from device-related trauma or erosion, are significant complications that can occur acutely or as delayed responses. These conditions occur in approximately 1–2% of cases and require immediate intervention, such as pericardiocentesis or surgical drainage (Amin et al. 2004).

Divekar et al. 2005 characterised cardiac perforation following ASD and PFO closures into two broad groups: first, technique-related often present early during the periprocedural period; second, delayed device-related perforation (Divekar et al. 2005). Device-related perforation typically occurs at the anterosuperior wall of the atria and may also extend to the aortic root (Divekar et al. 2005; Preventza et al. 2004). It has been hypothesised that the ASD closure devices transmit deformative forces at the point of contact between the device, the anterosuperior atrial wall, and the aorta, which may result in cardiac perforation. Factors that increase the risk of perforation include a deficient aortic or superior rim of the ostium secundum ASD, or both, and an oversized device.

The most common causes of pericardial effusion following LAAO include transseptal puncture, rigidity of the wires, guiding catheter, and device, damage to the cardiac wall by the device itself within the atrial appendage, and fragility of the appendage wall (Möbius-Winkler et al. 2015). Iatrogenic atrial septal defects from transseptal access usually resolve within 6 months and rarely cause haemodynamic issues.

Cardiac erosion is a rare late complication, which occurs when the device erodes through cardiac tissues, potentially leading to pericardial effusion and cardiac tamponade. This can occur with ASD, PFO, and LAAO devices. Risk factors include oversized devices, thin atrial walls, deficient septal rims, and excessive tension on the device (Amin et al. 2004).

3.3 *Vascular Complications*

Vascular complications at the femoral venous access site include haematomas, arteriovenous (AV) fistulas, femoral arterial pseudoaneurysms, vessel dissection, and retroperitoneal bleeding (Holmes et al. 2009; Cappato et al. 2005). These complications, although often manageable conservatively, underscore the importance of using proper access techniques, such as ultrasound-guided puncture and careful handling of vascular sheaths to minimise risks. Femoral AV fistulas are particularly rare, with reported rates ranging from 0.004% to 0.02% in moderate sample sizes (Schwerzmann et al. 2004; Jung et al. 2019).

3.4 *Residual Shunt and Peri-Device Leaks*

3.4.1 Residual Shunt Following ASD and PFO Closure

Residual shunts following ASD and PFO closure are not uncommon but carry different implications depending on the size and persistence of the shunt. After ASD closure with devices like the Amplatzer Septal Occluder (ASO), most residual shunts are detected early post-procedure, often as a result of flow through or around the device's waist, and tend to resolve over time due to endothelialisation (Zdradzinski et al. 2016; Kutty et al. 2012). However, persistent residual shunts are rare and may be associated with factors such as device oversizing, improper positioning, or incomplete coverage of the defect. In these cases, there is an increased risk of complications such as thromboembolism, and additional interventions may be necessary.

In the context of PFO closure, residual shunts occur in up to 25% of cases, with around 10% presenting as moderate or large shunts. A prospective cohort study of 1078 consecutive patients with PFO attributable cryptogenic stroke demonstrated that these larger residual shunts significantly increase the risk of recurrent stroke or TIA (2.32 events per 100 patient-years) compared to complete closure (0.75 events per 100 patient-years) over 11 years of follow-up (Deng et al. 2020).

3.4.2 Peri-Device Leak Following LAAO

Peri-device leaks (PDL) following LAAO are a relatively common finding, with variability in incidence depending on the device and study. For instance, in the PROTECT AF trial, a PDL was detected in 41% of patients, and larger leaks (>3 mm) were present in 13% of cases on 45-day transoesophageal echocardiography (Viles-Gonzalez et al. 2012). Similarly, in the Amulet IDE trial, PDLs were identified in 37% of Amulet device recipients and 54% of those with Watchman 2.5, with leaks larger than 3 mm occurring in 11% and 26%, respectively (Lakkireddy et al. 2021). Despite the higher incidence of PDL with the Watchman device, rates of ischaemic stroke or systemic embolism at 18 months were similar between both devices. Recent evidence has pointed towards an association between larger PDLs and increased risk of thromboembolic events. An analysis of the NCDR LAAO registry found that even small residual leaks (<5 mm) were linked to higher odds of stroke, transient ischaemic attack, and systemic embolisation (Khouli et al. 2022). Moreover, a long-term follow-up of patients in the PROTECT AF and PREVAIL trials revealed that leaks smaller than 5 mm were associated with a nearly two-fold increase in stroke or embolisation risk at 5 years (Holmes et al. 2009, 2014).

3.5 Device-Related Thrombus

Device-related thrombus (DRT) is a recognised complication following ASD and PFO closure, with incidence rates reported between 0.2% and 2% across studies (Krumsdorf et al. 2004; Chessa et al. 2002). A clinical study of 1,000 patients undergoing ASD or PFO closure demonstrated 2% incidence of DRT with higher rates in devices like CardioSEAL (7.1%) and StarFlex (5.7%) compared to the Amplatzer device, which had no recorded cases of DRT (Krumsdorf et al. 2004). DRT can manifest early post-procedure or, years after device implantation, potentially leading to serious outcomes such as cerebral emboli (Ruge et al. 2005).

Factors that increase the risk of DRT include incomplete endothelialisation, post-procedure atrial fibrillation, and the presence of a persistent atrial septal aneurysm (Khalil et al. 2024). Although dual antiplatelet therapy (DAPT) is commonly prescribed for 6 months following closure, the risk of late thrombus formation suggests that extended surveillance and, in some cases, prolonged anticoagulation may be necessary.

Following a LAAO procedure, DRT is more common, with an incidence of 3.9% reported in the Amulet IDE trial (Lakkireddy et al. 2021). A multicentre prospective study of 1088 patients undergoing LAAO observed that 61% of DRT events in the Amulet group occurred within the first 45 days, whereas most DRTs related to the Watchman device emerged after this period (Aminian et al. 2019). This difference in timing could be due to variations in endothelialisation or device design. Risk factors for DRT in LAAO include increasing age, female sex, and persistent atrial fibrillation. DRT significantly raises the risk of embolic stroke, up to a five-fold increase in stroke risk among patients with DRT (Dukkipati et al. 2018). Regular imaging, particularly transoesophageal echocardiography, is crucial for early detection, and prompt initiation of anticoagulation is recommended to prevent complications, even in patients initially considered unsuitable for long-term anticoagulation.

3.6 Other Complications

Other complications include new or worsening aortic regurgitation (AR), new-onset migraine, arrhythmias, thromboembolism, and left ventricular dysfunction. AR has been reported in 9–10% of patients following ASD or PFO closure at 12 months (Schoen et al. 2008). A potential cause for developing AR after percutaneous closure may be changes in septal geometry and traction on the root of the non-coronary aortic cusp. This traction on the aortic valve could be enhanced by endothelialisation and tissue overgrowing the device.

New-onset migraine, particularly with aura, has been observed in about 7% of patients undergoing ASD-PFO closure, predominantly in younger individuals, suggesting that factors beyond device composition contribute to this complication (Rodés-Cabau et al. 2008). Arrhythmias, including atrial fibrillation and supraventricular tachycardia, occur in approximately 3.9–10% of cases, due to mechanical irritation or stretching of the atrial tissue (Staubach et al. 2009). Thrombus formation on the closure device, especially on the left atrial side, poses a risk for embolic events, with a recurrence rate of 0–4.9% (Khairy et al. 2003). Ensuring stringent post-procedural anticoagulation protocols is essential, typically involving dual antiplatelet therapy or anticoagulation in high-risk patients, to mitigate this complication. Finally, left ventricular dysfunction, particularly in older patients, may arise from changes in atrial pressure and ventricular filling patterns following ASD closure, highlighting the decompressive effect of ASDs on the left ventricle in this population (Ewert et al. 2001).

4 Mitigating Complications

Mitigating the described complications associated with ASD, PFO closures, and LAAO involves careful patient selection, precise device sizing, and meticulous procedural techniques, with a multidisciplinary approach.

4.1 Patient Selection

Although the rate of major complications remains low, mitigating these complications begins with careful patient selection and comprehensive pre-procedural planning. Identifying patients who are most suitable for transcatheter closure involves evaluating anatomical and clinical factors. For ASD and PFO closures, this includes assessing defect size, shape, and location, as well as evaluating patient-specific factors such as age, comorbidities, and anatomical considerations like the size of the ASD and its associated rims for device anchoring. ASDs such as primum, sinus venosus, and unroofed coronary sinus defects are best treated surgically due to their complex anatomy and associated risks of percutaneous closure (Tanaka et al. 2022). Additionally, ASDs with significant rim deficiencies, particularly of the superior and anterior aortic rims, have a higher risk of complications like device embolisation and cardiac erosion, making surgical closure a safer option.

4.2 Procedural Planning and Execution

Choosing the optimal device type and size is equally critical. The device choice should be tailored to the ASD or PFO characteristics, guided by advanced imaging modalities such as transoesophageal echocardiography (TOE), and cardiac computed tomography (CT). Accurate sizing is crucial to minimise the risks of embolisation and erosion. For instance, oversized devices are more likely to cause cardiac erosion, while undersized devices may not anchor securely, increasing the likelihood of embolisation. During the procedure, intraprocedural echocardiography, such as TOE or intracardiac echocardiography (ICE), is essential for guiding device deployment and monitoring for complications (Rana 2018; van der Velde et al. 1994; Balzer 2014).

Procedural planning and execution of LAAO can be complex due to the high anatomical variability and structural intricacies of the atrial appendage. Classification systems, such as those categorising LAA into chicken wing, windsock, cactus, and broccoli morphologies, aid in managing this complexity (Yaghi et al. 2015); however, the inherent anatomical diversity often leads to significant overlap between these morphologies. Additional factors influencing the LAAO procedure include the presence of extensive trabeculation, multiple lobes, and the delicate thin-wall structure of the LAA, which increases the risk of complications like pericardial effusion. Moreover, anatomical variations in the interatrial septum and fossa ovalis pose challenges in achieving optimal transseptal puncture and coaxial alignment of the LAAO device with the LAA wall.

Imaging plays a critical role in both pre-procedural planning and intra-procedural guidance. TOE and cardiac CT are employed to assess LAA anatomy, exclude contraindications like LAA thrombosis, and guide decisions on device selection and positioning. TOE, particularly in its three-dimensional form, is widely regarded as the gold-standard modality for pre-procedural evaluation, offering detailed insights into LAA geometry and potential procedural pathways (Galea et al. 2021). Cardiac CT, on the other hand, provides high spatial resolution, facilitating precise assessment of LAA dimensions and enabling advanced applications such as 3D printing and computational modelling.

Technical expertise and procedural precision are also paramount to successful outcomes. The procedure should be performed by experienced operators who are proficient in utilising advanced imaging techniques to guide device deployment. Ensuring device stability and correct positioning before release significantly reduces the risk of embolisation and other placement-related complications. High levels of procedural skill and precision, supported by real-time imaging, are crucial in mitigating risks during deployment, especially in challenging anatomies or when deploying larger devices.

5 Management of Complications

The management of complications associated with transcatheter closure devices involves a structured decision-making algorithm, Figure 3, which prioritises percutaneous techniques as the first line of intervention. The algorithm for managing these complications begins with a comprehensive assessment of the patient's clinical stability, the nature of the complication, and the location and characteristics of the device involved. The goal is to resolve the complication effectively while minimising patient morbidity and avoiding the need for more invasive surgical procedures unless necessary.

5.1 Decision-Making Algorithms

The initial step in the decision-making process is to evaluate the urgency of the complication. Minor issues, such as small residual shunts or asymptomatic device malposition, may be managed conservatively. However, more severe complications, such as device embolisation, or significant malposition that impairs function

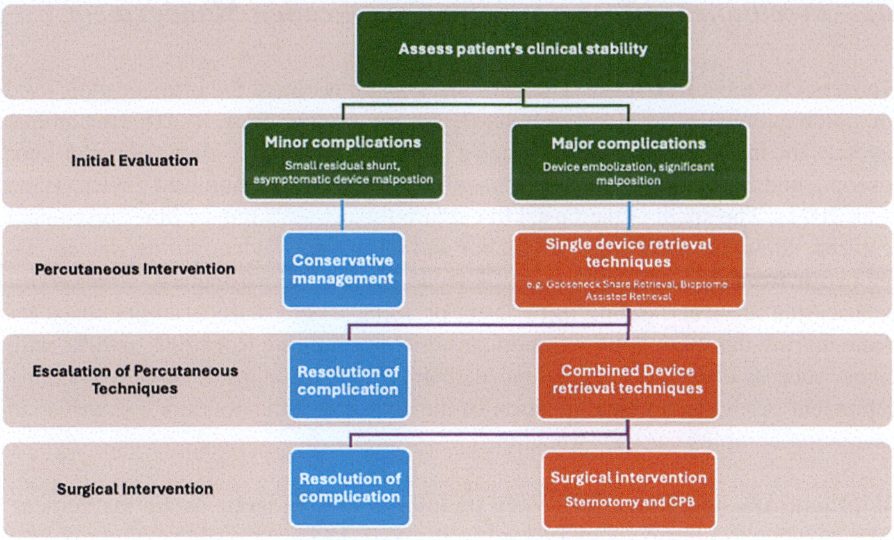

Fig. 3 Flow chart of decision-making algorithm for managing complications after catheter-based ASD, PFO, or LAAO interventions

necessitate prompt intervention. In such cases, percutaneous retrieval is the preferred approach given its minimally invasive nature and generally favourable outcomes.

The algorithm progresses based on the success or failure of initial percutaneous attempts. For example, if a device embolises but remains accessible within the left atrium, right atrium, or aorta, initial attempts typically involve basic snaring techniques using tools like the gooseneck snare. Should these basic attempts fail due to device orientation, structural challenges, or insufficient capture points, more advanced techniques, including bioptome-assisted retrieval or catheter-based snaring, are employed. Decisions to escalate to more complex retrieval methods are influenced by factors such as the device's location, the potential for causing additional harm during retrieval, and the availability of specialised equipment.

When percutaneous methods are deemed unsafe or unsuccessful, the algorithm dictates a transition to surgical intervention. Indications for surgical removal include embolisation into locations where percutaneous access may be challenging, such as the pulmonary arteries, entanglement with cardiac structures such as the mitral or tricuspid valve apparatus, and when the device poses a critical threat, such as obstructing major vascular structures. Multidisciplinary team discussions, incorporating input from interventional cardiologists, cardiac surgeons, and imaging specialists, are critical at this juncture to optimise patient outcomes and minimise the risks associated with surgery.

5.2 Percutaneous Techniques for Complication Management

Gooseneck Snare Retrieval The gooseneck snare is one of the primary tools used for percutaneous retrieval of embolised closure devices (Fig. 4). This technique involves the insertion of a snare through a large sheath, which is directed under fluoroscopic and echocardiographic guidance to the site of the embolised device (Batta et al. 2021). The snare is then used to capture the device's hub or other prominent features, allowing the operator to anchor and retract the device into the sheath and remove it from the patient. Gooseneck snare retrieval is particularly effective for devices that are free-floating in the atria or aorta, where there is ample space for manoeuvring the snare. Studies report success rates ranging from 70% to 90%, with higher success observed in experienced centres. This technique's efficacy is highly dependent on the anatomical location of the device and the operator's expertise in navigating complex cardiac structures.

Bioptome-Assisted Retrieval When traditional snaring methods are insufficient, such as when the device is embedded in tissue or lacks accessible capture points, bioptome-assisted retrieval offers a robust alternative (Ferraris et al. 2022). A bioptome, commonly used in endomyocardial biopsies, provides a firm grip on the device, facilitating secure retrieval. This technique is particularly beneficial for devices with complex shapes or those that have been partially endothelialised, making standard snaring ineffective. Bioptome-assisted retrieval has demonstrated a

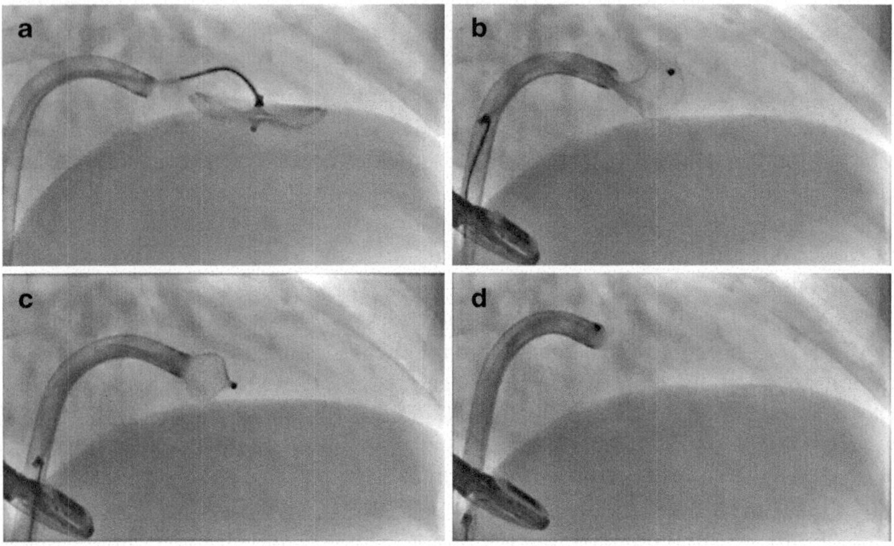

Fig. 4 Fluoroscopy demonstrating successful percutaneous retrieval of embolised ASD closure device from left ventricle via Pascal guide sheath. (**a**) ASD device is snared and retrieved back into the sheath (**b**–**d**)

success rate of over 80% in both ASD/PFO and LAAO embolised devices (Pala et al. 2010; Afzal et al. 2020).

Combined Device Retrieval Techniques In cases where a single tool, such as a snare or bioptome, is insufficient, the use of combined retrieval techniques employing two tools (e.g. snare and snare, snare and bioptome, snare and forceps, multiple loop snares, or coronary wire trap technique) has proven beneficial (Alkhouli et al. 2017). This approach enhances the safety of the retrieval process, shortens procedure time, and increases success rates, while reducing the risk of complications, such as cardiac injury or arrhythmias. Studies have demonstrated a 100% success rate for device retrieval without complications using this method in patients undergoing ASD/PFO closure or LAAO (Ha et al. 2018). Techniques such as the Waist Capture Technique, where the device's waist is secured using a looped guidewire, and the gooseneck snare method have also been successful (Her et al. 2018; O'Byrne and Levi 2019).

Hybrid Approaches In certain challenging cases, hybrid techniques that combine percutaneous and surgical elements may be considered. For instance, when a device is partially protruding from a cardiac structure, a controlled percutaneous approach may be used to reposition the device, followed by surgical reinforcement if necessary. Such approaches require a high level of coordination between interventional and surgical teams and are typically reserved for specialised centres with extensive experience in complex device management.

5.3 Surgical Techniques for Complication Management

Although percutaneous techniques are preferred as initial interventions due to their minimally invasive nature, surgical approaches become necessary when these methods fail or are deemed inappropriate. The transition to surgery is guided by the severity of the complication, device location, patient stability, and the potential for life-threatening outcomes. The decision to proceed with surgical management is highly individualised and involves careful consideration of the patient's clinical condition, the specific complication, and the anticipated risks of surgery versus continued percutaneous attempts. Ultimately, the goal of surgical management is to provide definitive resolution of the complication while minimising additional risks to the patient.

In dealing with both ASD/PFO closure and LAAO complications, surgical intervention is primarily indicated when percutaneous retrieval fails or when the complication poses an immediate and significant threat, such as device embolisation into critical structures such as the mitral valve, cardiac perforation, or obstruction of major vessels. Common complications necessitating surgery following ASD/PFO closure include device embolisation into the ventricles causing haemodynamic compromise, complex entanglement with valvular apparatus causing severe valvular dysfunction, or perforation leading to tamponade, and structural damage necessitating valve repair or replacement. Additionally, during LAAO, there is an extra risk of direct atrial appendage damage causing tamponade.

5.3.1 Sternotomy and Cardiopulmonary Bypass

Although all patients are routinely heparinised during the catheter-based procedures, upon the decision to proceed with surgical intervention, additional heparin is administered to achieve an activated coagulation time (ACT) of approximately 180 s. This step is critical to prevent clot formation on the device during surgical preparation and transfer to the operating theatre. Further heparinisation, typically at a dose of 300 units/kg, is required following sternotomy to maintain an ACT of 400 s before initiating cardiopulmonary bypass. Intraoperative TOE is essential for procedural guidance and must be used in all patients. The surgical approach is determined by the location of the embolised device and the nature of associated complications, with the primary objectives being device removal, closure of the ASD/PFO or surgical LAAO, and repair of any damaged cardiac structures. This may include closure of cardiac perforations and the repair or replacement of affected valves, such as the aortic, mitral, or tricuspid valves (Sarris et al. 2010).

In majority of cases, surgery is performed via median sternotomy with cardiopulmonary bypass established through cannulation of the aorta, superior vena cava, and inferior vena cava. The aorta is cross-clamped, and antegrade cold cardioplegia is administered into the aortic root to induce diastolic cardiac arrest.

The most common reported sites of embolisation for ASDs/PFOs include right ventricle, right ventricular outflow tract, pulmonary artery, left atrium, left ventricular outflow tract, arch of aorta, descending thoracic aorta, abdominal aorta, and common iliac artery (Lysitsas et al. 2009; Saha et al. 2018). The most common site of embolisation for LAAO devices is the left atrium, left ventricle, mitral valve apparatus, left ventricular outflow tracts, and descending/abdominal aorta. Devices embolised to the left ventricle and mitral valve apparatus are significantly more likely to require surgical intervention compared to the descending/abdominal aorta and the left atrium (Murtaza et al. 2021).

Surgical access to the most common embolised device locations may be achieved through the right or left atria, via the tricuspid or via ASD to mitral valves, or by performing an aortotomy and access through the aortic valve. Embolised devices are typically removed using forceps, either by folding two opposite edges of the device or by securing it with sutures for safe extraction, particularly in the ventricle, to minimise damage to the chordal apparatus (Yates and Anderson 2017). ASD/PFO closure must then be performed directly or with a pericardial patch, depending on the size of the defect followed by repair of any valvular injuries identified.

In cases of device embolisation into the ascending aorta or aortic arch, hypothermic circulatory arrest may be required to facilitate device retrieval. TOE is essential to confirm device position. Depending on the position of the device, the aortic access is via direct distal ascending aorta cannulation or femoral artery cannulation, to ensure that the device is not further embolised into the head and neck aortic branches or the descending aorta. Following hypothermic circulatory arrest, a distal ascending aortotomy is performed on to retrieve the embolised device, after which the aortotomy is closed following de-airing in the standard manner. During rewarming, secundum ASD closure can be completed via a right atriotomy.

5.3.2 Previous Sternotomy

Minimally invasive thoracoscopic surgery is an alternative to sternotomy for specific complications, such as embolised LAAO devices located in the left ventricular outflow tract or near the atrioventricular junction (Yilmaz et al. 2019). This is particularly useful in patients who have previously undergone cardiac surgery and the re-do sternotomy is high risk. With this technique, the patient is positioned in the supine position with a slightly elevated right side of the thorax. Venous cannulation is performed through the common femoral vein with or without additional internal jugular vein cannulation. The arterial cannulation site is the common femoral artery. A small 4-cm mini-thoracotomy is performed just below the right nipple, and the chest is entered through the right 4th intercostal space. Three additional 5-mm trocars are inserted into the right 3rd, 4th, and 5th intercostal space for the endoscopic instruments and the camera. The pericardium is opened and secured with stay sutures. Previous adhesions are carefully dissected. Purse-strings are placed for aortic root vent, and aortic cross clamp is applied. The cardioplegia is administered through the root vent to achieve diastolic cardiac arrest which would allow precise manipulation. The patient is then placed in the anti-Trendelenburg position, and the left atrium is opened allowing excellent access for retrieval of the embolised device. In cases of direct left atrial appendage injury, control can be achieved via a left mini thoracotomy allowing access to the left atrium and direct closure of the atrial appendage can be achieved.

5.3.3 Hybrid Procedure

In complex cases, hybrid techniques that combine elements of both percutaneous and surgical methods can be utilised. These approaches are particularly useful when initial percutaneous retrieval is partially successful but complete resolution requires surgical assistance. For example, partial percutaneous retrieval may stabilise an embolised device, allowing a less invasive surgical removal through a mini thoracotomy rather than a full sternotomy. These hybrid approaches are usually performed in specialised centres with access to advanced imaging and multidisciplinary teams capable of rapid transition between percutaneous and surgical techniques.

5.3.4 Outcomes

Surgical retrieval of embolised closure devices generally carries a high success rate, although it is associated with increased morbidity compared to primary device closure or initial percutaneous management. In a series of six patients requiring surgical intervention for embolised ASD devices, the overall success rate of surgical retrieval was reported to be nearly 100%, with no mortality observed among the patients (Yetkin et al. 2014). However, complications such as valve damage, which may necessitate valve repair or replacement, can extend the length of hospital stay and recovery time. Additionally, surgical retrieval carries inherent risks, including those associated with cardiopulmonary bypass, such as stroke, bleeding, and infection. In a retrospective study of 14 patients who underwent surgery for complications related to percutaneous ASD device closure, there was no operative mortality and minimal postoperative complications (Thingnam et al. 2018). The surgeries included device retrieval, ASD closure with patches, and, in one case, mitral valve replacement due to severe device-induced damage. These results underscore the efficacy of surgical intervention in resolving device-related complications when percutaneous methods are insufficient.

6 Summary

The chapter critically outlines the evolution and management of complications following percutaneous closure of ASD, PFO, and LAAO. While transcatheter procedures have largely replaced traditional surgical techniques due to their lower morbidity and quicker recovery times, these interventions are not without risks. Notably, device embolisation, cardiac erosion/tamponade, residual shunts, and device-related thrombus are the most significant complications, each with its unique risk factors.

Device embolisation is perhaps the most significant complication that could occur due to inadequate device sizing or challenging anatomical features. The management strategies following embolisation is dependent on the location of the embolisation and other intra-cardiac injuries. Percutaneous retrieval using snare techniques is preferred for device embolisation, with a high success rate, although surgery becomes necessary if embolisation occurs in areas like the ventricles or if the device is entangled with valvular structures. Furthermore, the importance of procedural planning and patient selection is critical and is guided by imaging studies.

References

Afzal MR, Ellis CR, Gabriels J, El-Chami M, Amin A, Fanari Z et al (2020) Percutaneous approaches for retrieval of an embolized or malpositioned left atrial appendage closure device: A multicenter experience. Heart Rhythm 17(9):1545–1553

Alkhouli M, Aljohani S, Kucera R, Moiduddin N, Hull R (2017) A double-snare technique for safe retrieval of embolized left atrial appendage occluders. JACC Cardiovasc Interv 10(5):e55–e56
Alkhouli M, Du C, Killu A, Simard T, Noseworthy PA, Friedman PA et al (2022) Clinical impact of residual leaks following left atrial appendage occlusion: insights from the NCDR LAAO registry. JACC Clin Electrophysiol 8(6):766–778
Amin Z, Hijazi ZM, Bass JL, Cheatham JP, Hellenbrand WE, Kleinman CS (2004) Erosion of Amplatzer septal occluder device after closure of secundum atrial septal defects: review of registry of complications and recommendations to minimize future risk. Catheter Cardiovasc Interv 63(4):496–502
Aminian A, Schmidt B, Mazzone P, Berti S, Fischer S, Montorfano M et al (2019) Incidence, characterization, and clinical impact of device-related thrombus following left atrial appendage occlusion in the prospective global AMPLATZER Amulet observational study. JACC Cardiovasc Interv 12(11):1003–1014
Asmarats L, Rodés-Cabau J (2017) Percutaneous left atrial appendage closure: current devices and clinical outcomes. Circ Cardiovasc Interv [Internet] 10(11). Available from: https://doi.org/10.1161/CIRCINTERVENTIONS.117.005359
Balzer D (2014) Intracardiac echocardiographic atrial septal defect closure. Methodist Debakey Cardiovasc J 10(2):88–92
Batta A, Naganur S, Rajan A, Ary KA, Gawalkar A, Barwad P (2021) Retrieval and repositioning of an embolized atrial septal defect closure device using a gooseneck snare. Egypt Heart J 73(1):51
Baumgartner H, Bonhoeffer P, De Groot NMS, de Haan F, Deanfield JE, Galie N et al (2010) ESC Guidelines for the management of grown-up congenital heart disease (new version 2010). Eur Heart J 31(23):2915–2957
Bavishi C (2023) Transcatheter left atrial appendage closure: devices available, pitfalls, advantages, and future directions. [cited 2024 Sep 2]. Available from: https://www.uscjournal.com/articles/transcatheter-left-atrial-appendage-closure-devices-available-pitfalls-advantages-and
Bayard YL, Omran H, Neuzil P, Thuesen L, Pichler M, Rowland E et al (2010) PLAATO (Percutaneous Left Atrial Appendage Transcatheter Occlusion) for prevention of cardioembolic stroke in non-anticoagulation eligible atrial fibrillation patients: results from the European PLAATO study. EuroIntervention 6(2):220–226
Bradley EA, Zaidi AN (2020) Atrial septal defect. Cardiol Clin 38(3):317–324
Butera G, Romagnoli E, Carminati M, Chessa M, Piazza L, Negura D et al (2008) Treatment of isolated secundum atrial septal defects: impact of age and defect morphology in 1,013 consecutive patients. Am Heart J 156(4):706–712
Cappato R, Calkins H, Chen SA, Davies W, Iesaka Y, Kalman J et al (2005) Worldwide survey on the methods, efficacy, and safety of catheter ablation for human atrial fibrillation. Circulation 111(9):1100–1105
Chessa M, Carminati M, Butera G, Bini RM, Drago M, Rosti L (2002) Early and late complications associated with transcatheter occlusion of secundum atrial septal defect. J Am Coll Cardiol 39(6):1711–1714
Deng W, Yin S, McMullin D, Inglessis-Azuaje I, Elmariah S, Hung J et al (2020) Residual shunt after patent foramen ovale closure and long-term stroke recurrence: A prospective cohort study: a prospective cohort study. Ann Intern Med 172(11):717–725
Divekar A, Gaamangwe T, Shaikh N, Raabe M, Ducas J (2005) Cardiac perforation after device closure of atrial septal defects with the Amplatzer septal occluder. J Am Coll Cardiol 45(8):1213–1218
Du ZD, Hijazi ZM, Kleinman CS, Silverman NH, Larntz K, Investigators A (2002) Comparison between transcatheter and surgical closure of secundum atrial septal defect in children and adults: results of a multicenter nonrandomized trial. J Am Coll Cardiol 39(11):1836–1844
Dukkipati SR, Kar S, Holmes DR, Doshi SK, Swarup V, Gibson DN et al (2018) Device-related thrombus after left atrial appendage closure: Incidence, predictors, and outcomes: Incidence, predictors, and outcomes. Circulation 138(9):874–885

Eppinger S, Piayda K, Galea R, Sandri M, Maarse M, Güner A et al (2024) Embolization of percutaneous left atrial appendage closure devices: timing, management and clinical outcomes. Cardiovasc Revasc Med 64:7–14

Ewert P, Berger F, Nagdyman N, Kretschmar O, Dittrich S, Abdul-Khaliq H et al (2001) Masked left ventricular restriction in elderly patients with atrial septal defects: a contraindication for closure? Catheter Cardiovasc Interv 52(2):177–180

Ferraris F, Millesimo M, Anselmino M, Castagno D, Vairo A, Alunni G et al (2022) Successful percutaneous retrieval of an embolized left atrial appendage occluder. JACC Case Rep 4(24):101689

Fraisse A, Latchman M, Sharma SR, Bayburt S, Amedro P, di Salvo G et al (2018) Atrial septal defect closure: indications and contra-indications. J Thorac Dis 10(Suppl 24):S2874–S2881

Freeman JV, Varosy P, Price MJ, Slotwiner D, Kusumoto FM, Rammohan C et al (2020) The NCDR left atrial appendage occlusion registry. J Am Coll Cardiol 75(13):1503–1518

Friedman DJ, Du C, Wang Y, Agarwal V, Varosy PD, Masoudi FA et al (2022) Patient-level analysis of watchman left atrial appendage occlusion in practice versus clinical trials. JACC Cardiovasc Interv 15(9):950–961

Galea R, Räber L, Fuerholz M, Häner JD, Siontis GCM, Brugger N et al (2021) Impact of echocardiographic guidance on safety and efficacy of left atrial appendage closure: an observational study. JACC Cardiovasc Interv 14(16):1815–1826

Galea R, De Marco F, Meneveau N, Aminian A, Anselme F, Gräni C et al (2022) Amulet or watchman device for percutaneous left atrial appendage closure: primary results of the SWISS-APERO randomized clinical trial. Circulation 145(10):724–738

Ha KS, Choi JY, Jung SY, Kim JS, Byun KH, Akagi T et al (2018) A novel double snare technique to retrieve embolized septal and left atrial appendage occluders. J Interv Cardiol 31(5):685–692

Her AY, Lim KH, Shin ES (2018) Transcatheter retrieval of embolized atrial septal defect occluder device by waist capture technique. Int Heart J 59(1):226–228

Hindricks G, Potpara T, Dagres N, Arbelo E, Bax JJ, Blomström-Lundqvist C et al (2021) Corrigendum to: 2020 ESC Guidelines for the diagnosis and management of atrial fibrillation developed in collaboration with the European Association for Cardio-Thoracic Surgery (EACTS): The Task Force for the diagnosis and management of atrial fibrillation of the European Society of Cardiology (ESC) Developed with the special contribution of the European Heart Rhythm Association (EHRA) of the ESC. Eur Heart J 42(40):4194

Hoffman JIE, Kaplan S (2002) The incidence of congenital heart disease. J Am Coll Cardiol 39(12):1890–1900

Holmes DR Jr, Kar S, Price MJ, Whisenant B, Sievert H, Doshi SK et al (2014) Prospective randomized evaluation of the Watchman Left Atrial Appendage Closure device in patients with atrial fibrillation versus long-term warfarin therapy: the PREVAIL trial. J Am Coll Cardiol 64(1):1–12

Holmes DR, Reddy VY, Turi ZG, Doshi SK, Sievert H, Buchbinder M et al (2009) Percutaneous closure of the left atrial appendage versus warfarin therapy for prevention of stroke in patients with atrial fibrillation: a randomised non-inferiority trial. Lancet 374(9689):534–542

Hribernik I, Thomson J, Bhan A, Mullen M, Noonan P, Smith B et al (2023) A novel device for atrial septal defect occlusion (GORE CARDIOFORM). EuroIntervention 19(9):782–788

Huang H, Liu Y, Xu Y, Wang Z, Li Y, Cao K et al (2017) Percutaneous left atrial appendage closure with the LAmbre device for stroke prevention in atrial fibrillation: a prospective, multicenter clinical study. JACC Cardiovasc Interv 10(21):2188–2194

January CT, Wann LS, Alpert JS, Calkins H, Cigarroa JE, Cleveland JC Jr et al (2014) 2014 AHA/ACC/HRS guideline for the management of patients with atrial fibrillation: a report of the American College of Cardiology/American Heart Association Task Force on practice guidelines and the Heart Rhythm Society. Circulation 130(23):e199–e267

Joglar JA, Chung MK, Armbruster AL, Benjamin EJ, Chyou JY, Cronin EM et al (2024) 2023 ACC/AHA/ACCP/HRS guideline for the diagnosis and management of atrial fibrillation: a report of the American College of Cardiology/American Heart Association Joint Committee on Clinical Practice Guidelines. Circulation 149(1):e1–e156

Jones TK, Latson LA, Zahn E, Fleishman CE, Jacobson J, Vincent R et al (2007) Results of the U.S. multicenter pivotal study of the HELEX septal occluder for percutaneous closure of secundum atrial septal defects. J Am Coll Cardiol 49(22):2215–2221

Jung SY, Kim AY, Jung JW, Choi JY (2019) Procedural, early and long-term outcomes after percutaneous closure of atrial septal defect: comparison between large and very large atrial septal defect groups. Korean Circ J 49(10):975–986

Kar S, Doshi SK, Sadhu A, Horton R, Osorio J, Ellis C et al (2021) Primary outcome evaluation of a next-generation left atrial appendage closure device: results from the PINNACLE FLX Trial. Circulation 143(18):1754–1762

Kasner SE, Rhodes JF, Andersen G, Iversen HK, Nielsen-Kudsk JE, Settergren M et al (2021) Five-year outcomes of PFO closure or antiplatelet therapy for cryptogenic stroke. N Engl J Med 384(10):970–971

Khairy P, O'Donnell CP, Landzberg MJ (2003) Transcatheter closure versus medical therapy of patent foramen ovale and presumed paradoxical thromboemboli: a systematic review. Ann Intern Med 139(9):753–760

Khalil MH, Haider M, Mehta S (2024) Late thrombosis of Gore Cardioform septal occluder device in a patient with history of patent foramen ovale closure. Radiol Case Rep 19(4):1386–1390

Khouli M, Du C, Killu A, Simard T, Noseworthy PA, Friedman PA (2022) Clinical impact of residual leaks following left atrial appendage occlusion: insights from the NCDR LAAO registry. JACC Clin Electrophysiol 8(6):766–778

King TD, Thompson SL, Steiner C, Mills NL (1976) Secundum atrial septal defect. Nonoperative closure during cardiac catheterization. JAMA 235(23):2506–2509

Kirchhof P, Benussi S, Kotecha D, Ahlsson A, Atar D, Casadei B et al (2017) 2016 ESC guidelines for the management of atrial fibrillation developed in collaboration with EACTS. Rev Esp Cardiol 70(1):50

Kramer AD, Korsholm K, Kristensen A, Poulsen LH, Nielsen-Kudsk JE (2022) Left atrial appendage occlusion in haemophilia patients with atrial fibrillation. J Interv Card Electrophysiol 64(1):95–102

Krumsdorf U, Ostermayer S, Billinger K, Trepels T, Zadan E, Horvath K et al (2004) Incidence and clinical course of thrombus formation on atrial septal defect and patient foramen ovale closure devices in 1,000 consecutive patients. J Am Coll Cardiol 43(2):302–309

Kutty S, Hazeem AA, Brown K, Danford CJ, Worley SE, Delaney JW et al (2012) Long-term (5- to 20-year) outcomes after transcatheter or surgical treatment of hemodynamically significant isolated secundum atrial septal defect. Am J Cardiol 109(9):1348–1352

Lakkireddy D, Thaler D, Ellis CR, Swarup V, Sondergaard L, Carroll J et al (2021) Amplatzer amulet left atrial appendage occluder versus watchman device for stroke prophylaxis (Amulet IDE): a randomized, controlled trial. Circulation 144(19):1543–1552

Landzberg MJ, Khairy P (2004) Indications for the closure of patent foramen ovale. Heart 90(2):219–224

Latson LA, Jones TK, Jacobson J, Zahn E, Rhodes JF (2006) Analysis of factors related to successful transcatheter closure of secundum atrial septal defects using the HELEX septal occluder. Am Heart J 151(5):1129.e7–1129.11

Lempereur M, Aminian A, Freixa X, Gafoor S, Shakir S, Omran H et al (2017) Left atrial appendage occlusion in patients with atrial fibrillation and previous major gastrointestinal bleeding (from the Amplatzer Cardiac Plug Multicenter Registry). Am J Cardiol 120(3):414–420

Liava'a M, Kalfa D (2018) Surgical closure of atrial septal defects. J Thorac Dis 10(Suppl 24):S2931–S2939

Luani B, Genz C, Herold J, Mitrasch A, Mitusch J, Wiemer M et al (2019) Cerebrovascular events, bleeding complications and device related thrombi in atrial fibrillation patients with chronic kidney disease and left atrial appendage closure with the WATCHMAN™ device. BMC Cardiovasc Disord 19(1):112

Lysitsas DN, Wrigley B, Banerjee P, Glennon PE, Parmar JM, Shiu MF et al (2009) Presentation of an embolised Amplatzer septal occluder to the main pulmonary artery 2 years after implantation. Int J Cardiol 131(3):e106–e107

Mas JL, Derumeaux G, Guillon B, Massardier E, Hosseini H, Mechtouff L et al (2017) Patent foramen ovale closure or anticoagulation vs. antiplatelets after stroke. N Engl J Med 377(11):1011–1021
Masura J, Gavora P, Formanek A, Hijazi ZM (1997) Transcatheter closure of secundum atrial septal defects using the new self-centering amplatzer septal occluder: initial human experience. Catheter Cardiovasc Diagn 42(4):388–393
Menillo AM, Lee LS, Pearson-Shaver AL (2024) Atrial septal defect. In: StatPearls. StatPearls Publishing, Treasure Island
Möbius-Winkler S, Majunke N, Sandri M, Mangner N, Linke A, Stone GW et al (2015) Percutaneous left atrial appendage closure: technical aspects and prevention of periprocedural complications with the watchman device. World J Cardiol 7(2):65–75
Mojadidi MK, Zaman MO, Elgendy IY, Mahmoud AN, Patel NK, Agarwal N et al (2018) Cryptogenic stroke and patent foramen ovale. J Am Coll Cardiol 71(9):1035–1043
Mullins C (1998) History of pediatric interventional catheterization: pediatric therapeutic cardiac catheterizations. Pediatr Cardiol 19:3–7
Murtaza G, Turagam K, Dar T, Akella K, Yarlagadda B, Gloekler S et al (2021) Left atrial appendage occlusion device embolization (the LAAODE study): understanding the timing and clinical consequences from a worldwide experience. J Atr Fibrillation 13(5):2516
Nielsen-Kudsk JE, Johnsen SP, Wester P, Damgaard D, Airaksinen J, Lund J et al (2017) Left atrial appendage occlusion versus standard medical care in patients with atrial fibrillation and intracerebral haemorrhage: a propensity score-matched follow-up study. EuroIntervention 13(3):371–378
O'Byrne ML, Levi DS (2019) State-of-the-art atrial septal defect closure devices for congenital heart. Interv Cardiol Clin 8(1):11–21
Osmancik P, Herman D, Neuzil P, Hala P, Taborsky M, Kala P et al (2020) Left atrial appendage closure versus direct oral anticoagulants in high-risk patients with atrial fibrillation. J Am Coll Cardiol 75(25):3122–3135
Osmancik P, Herman D, Neuzil P, Hala P, Taborsky M, Kala P et al (2022) 4-year outcomes after left atrial appendage closure versus nonwarfarin oral anticoagulation for atrial fibrillation. J Am Coll Cardiol 79(1):1–14
Pala S, Açar G, Tigen K, Kırma C (2010) Percutaneous retrieval of an interatrial septal occluder device embolized into the aortic arch. Turk Kardiyol Dern Ars 38(7):502–504
Pivato CA, Liccardo G, Sanz-Sanchez J, Pelloni E, Pujdak K, Xuareb RG et al (2022) Left atrial appendage closure with the II generation Ultraseal device: an international registry. The LIGATE study. Catheter Cardiovasc Interv 100(4):620–627
Preventza O, Sampath-Kumar S, Wasnick J, Gold JP (2004) Late cardiac perforation following transcatheter atrial septal defect closure. Ann Thorac Surg 77(4):1435–1437
Price MJ, Friedman DJ, Du C, Wang Y, Lin Z, Curtis JP et al (2022) Comparative safety of transcatheter LAAO with the first-generation watchman and next-generation watchman FLX devices. JACC Cardiovasc Interv 15(21):2115–2123
Qureshi AM, Sommer RJ, Morgan G, Paolillo JA, Gray RG, Love B et al (2024) Long-term results of the atrial septal defect Occluder ASSURED trial for combined pivotal/continued access cohorts. JACC Cardiovasc Interv 17(19):2274–2283
Rana BS (2018) Echocardiography guidance of atrial septal defect closure. J Thorac Dis 10(Suppl 24):S2899–S2908
Reddy VY, Sievert H, Halperin J, Doshi SK, Buchbinder M, Neuzil P et al (2014) Percutaneous left atrial appendage closure vs warfarin for atrial fibrillation: a randomized clinical trial. JAMA 312(19):1988–1998
Rodés-Cabau J, Mineau S, Marrero A, Houde C, Mackey A, Côté JM et al (2008) Incidence, timing, and predictive factors of new-onset migraine headache attack after transcatheter closure of atrial septal defect or patent foramen ovale. Am J Cardiol 101(5):688–692
Ruge H, Wildhirt SM, Libera P, Vogt M, Holper K, Lange R (2005) Images in cardiovascular medicine. Left atrial thrombus on atrial septal defect closure device as a source of cerebral emboli 3 years after implantation. Circulation 112(10):e130–e131

Saha S, Mondal T, Agarwal S, Geelani MA (2018) Surgical retrieval of atrial septal occluder device after late embolization in right ventricle. World J Cardiovasc Surg 08(12):233–238

Saliba WI, Kawai K, Sato Y, Kopesky E, Cheng Q, Ghosh SKB et al (2023) Enhanced thromboresistance and endothelialization of a novel fluoropolymer-coated left atrial appendage closure device. JACC Clin Electrophysiol 9(8 Pt 2):1555–1567

Sarris GE, Kirvassilis G, Zavaropoulos P, Belli E, Berggren H, Carrel T et al (2010) Surgery for complications of trans-catheter closure of atrial septal defects: a multi-institutional study from the European Congenital Heart Surgeons Association. Eur J Cardiothorac Surg 37(6):1285–1290

Saver JL, Carroll JD, Thaler DE, Smalling RW, MacDonald LA, Marks DS et al (2017) Long-term outcomes of patent foramen ovale closure or medical therapy after stroke. N Engl J Med 377(11):1022–1032

Schoen SP, Boscheri A, Lange SA, Braun MU, Fuhrmann J, Kappert U et al (2008) Incidence of aortic valve regurgitation and outcome after percutaneous closure of atrial septal defects and patent foramen ovale. Heart 94(7):844–847

Schwerzmann M, Windecker S, Wahl A, Mehta H, Nedeltchev K, Mattle H et al (2004) Percutaneous closure of patent foramen ovale: impact of device design on safety and efficacy. Heart 90(2):186–190

Simard TJ, Hibbert B, Alkhouli MA, Abraham NS, Holmes DR Jr (2022) Device-related thrombus following left atrial appendage occlusion. EuroIntervention 18(3):224–232

Sommer RJ, Love BA, Paolillo JA, Gray RG, Goldstein BH, Morgan GJ et al (2020) ASSURED clinical study: new GORE® CARDIOFORM ASD occluder for transcatheter closure of atrial septal defect. Catheter Cardiovasc Interv 95(7):1285–1295

Søndergaard L, Kasner SE, Rhodes JF, Andersen G, Iversen HK, Nielsen-Kudsk JE et al (2017) Patent foramen ovale closure or antiplatelet therapy for cryptogenic stroke. N Engl J Med 377(11):1033–1042

Staubach S, Steinberg DH, Zimmermann W, Wawra N, Wilson N, Wunderlich N et al (2009) New onset atrial fibrillation after patent foramen ovale closure. Catheter Cardiovasc Interv 74(6):889–895

Tanaka S, Imamura T, Narang N, Fukuda N, Ueno H, Kinugawa K (2022) Practical therapeutic management of percutaneous atrial septal defect closure. Intern Med 61(1):15–22

Taramasso M, Nietlispach F, Maisano F, Meier B (2016) Patent foramen ovale: indications for closure and techniques. EuroIntervention 12(Suppl X(X)):X7–X12

Thingnam SKS, Mahajan S, Kumar V (2018) Surgical perspective of percutaneous device closure of atrial septal defect. Asian Cardiovasc Thorac Ann 26(5):218492318776568

Turner DR, Owada CY, Sang CJ Jr, Khan M, Lim DS (2017) Closure of secundum atrial septal defects with the AMPLATZER septal occluder: a prospective, multicenter, post-approval study. Circ Cardiovasc Interv 10(8):e004212

Turner ME, Bouhout I, Petit CJ, Kalfa D (2022) Transcatheter closure of atrial and ventricular septal defects: JACC focus seminar. J Am Coll Cardiol 79(22):2247–2258

van den Ham HA, Souverein PC, Klungel OH, Platt RW, Ernst P, Dell'Aniello S et al (2021) Major bleeding in users of direct oral anticoagulants in atrial fibrillation: a pooled analysis of results from multiple population-based cohort studies. Pharmacoepidemiol Drug Saf 30(10):1339–1352

van der Velde ME, Sanders SP, Keane JF, Perry SB, Lock JE (1994) Transesophageal echocardiographic guidance of transcatheter ventricular septal defect closure. J Am Coll Cardiol 23(7):1660–1665

Viles-Gonzalez JF, Kar S, Douglas P, Dukkipati S, Feldman T, Horton R et al (2012) The clinical impact of incomplete left atrial appendage closure with the Watchman Device in patients with atrial fibrillation: a PROTECT AF (Percutaneous Closure of the Left Atrial Appendage Versus Warfarin Therapy for Prevention of Stroke in Patients With Atrial Fibrillation) substudy. J Am Coll Cardiol 59(10):923–929

Vincent RN, Raviele AA, Diehl HJ (2003) Single-center experience with the HELEX septal occluder for closure of atrial septal defects in children. J Interv Cardiol 16(1):79–82

Warnes CA, Williams RG, Bashore TM, Child JS, Connolly HM, Dearani JA et al (2008) ACC/AHA 2008 guidelines for the management of adults with congenital heart disease: a report of the American college of cardiology/American heart association task force on practice guidelines (writing committee to develop guidelines on the management of adults with congenital heart disease). Developed in collaboration with the American society of echocardiography, heart rhythm society, international society for adult congenital heart disease, society for cardiovascular angiography and interventions, and society of thoracic surgeons. J Am Coll Cardiol 52(23):e143–e263

Wong GX, Kar S, Smith TW, Spangler T, Bolling SF, Rogers JH (2023) Transcatheter left atrial appendage exclusion: preclinical and early clinical results with the laminar device. JACC Cardiovasc Interv 16(11):1347–1357

Yaghi S, Song C, Gray WA, Furie KL, Elkind MSV, Kamel H (2015) Left atrial appendage function and stroke risk. Stroke 46(12):3554–3559

Yates MT, Anderson DR (2017) Safe surgical retrieval of embolized atrial septal defect closure device. Ann Thorac Surg 103(2):e213–e214

Yetkin U, Yurekli I, Akyildiz ZI, Gokalp O, Tetik O, Lafci B et al (2014) Emergency surgical approach to device emboli due to migration of the atrial septal defect occluder. Arch Med Sci 10(3):464–469

Yilmaz A, Starinieri P, Antonic M (2019) Thoracoscopic retrieval of an atrial appendage occlusion device after embolization into the left ventricular outflow tract and damaging the mitral valve requiring replacement. Interact Cardiovasc Thorac Surg 28(4):650–651

Zdradzinski MJ, Elkin RL, Lee JM, Qureshi AM, El-Mallah W, Krasuski RA (2016) Contributors to and impact of residual shunting after device closure of atrial septal defects. Am Heart J 177:112–119

Emergency Cardiac Surgery During Ablation for Atrial Fibrillation and Ventricular Arrhythmias

Vivek Srivastava and Kim Rajappan

Abstract As the number and complexity of catheter ablation procedures being performed worldwide increase, the number of associated complications also become more frequent. Although uncommon, cardiac perforation is one of the most significant, as it can lead to pericardial effusion and tamponade that may require emergency surgical intervention. This chapter addresses diagnosis, investigations, and management of cardiac perforation during percutaneous ablation with particular focus on the surgical aspects of dealing with this potentially life-threatening complication. The chapter also discusses in brief atrio-oesophageal fistula, another severe complication with a significant mortality risk.

Keywords Atrial arrhythmias · Atrial fibrillation · Ventricular arrhythmias · Electrophysiology · Catheter ablation · Cardiac perforation · Pericardial effusion · Cardiac tamponade · Pericardiocentesis · Emergency sternotomy · Atrio-oesophageal fistula

1 Introduction

Catheter ablation is increasingly performed worldwide for atrial arrhythmias and ventricular arrhythmias. The number of ablations performed for the treatment of atrial fibrillation has particularly increased exponentially. The risk of serious complications from ablation procedures is generally low. Cardiac perforation is one of them with serious and even potentially life-threatening consequences. It is therefore important to be vigilant for this possibility during the procedure. Occasionally, bleeding can have a delayed presentation. There are various ways in which bleeding can be managed depending on the severity and timing of recognition. This chapter deals with management of bleeding during electrophysiological (EP) procedures,

V. Srivastava (✉) · K. Rajappan
John Radcliffe Hospital, Oxford, UK
e-mail: Vivek.Srivastava@ouh.nhs.uk; Kim.Rajappan@ouh.nhs.uk

A. Kourliouros (ed.), *Emergency Cardiac Surgery*,
https://doi.org/10.1007/978-3-032-15787-4_16

especially significant or catastrophic bleeding requiring emergency cardiac surgical intervention.

2 Incidence of the Problem

Cardiac perforation during ablation is an uncommon problem with a reported incidence of 1.2–1.7% (Wu et al. 2021a; Calkins et al. 2009; Cappato et al. 2010; Gupta et al. 2013) of all cases in the acute setting. That incidence is increased by the need for specific aspects of the ablation procedure such as the requirement for a trans-septal puncture to access the left atrium and/or left ventricle. There is a smaller incidence of delayed presentation of bleeding complications, reported variously up to 0.16% (Yetter et al. 2017; Siliato-Robles et al. 2019; Wolf et al. 2002; Xu et al. 2020; Cappato et al. 2011).

3 Diagnosis

The diagnosis of pericardial effusion and the possibility of tamponade clinically depends to some extent on the timing of presentation.

Close periprocedural monitoring usually identifies acute bleeding and the associated haemodynamic changes. Operators should be vigilant for subtle changes. Any concern should prompt immediate further imaging including fluoroscopy and echocardiography, which can identify new pericardial effusions indicating possible bleeding into the pericardium.

In contrast, a more insidious course can be seen with a slowly accumulating effusion, often related to an inflammatory reaction and therefore more serosanguinous collection. This may lead to development of symptoms through various mechanisms. Patients may present with any or a combination of breathlessness on exertion, orthopnoea or chest pain. Symptoms can arise from compression of surrounding structures due to an enlarging pericardial sac and can include nausea, dysphagia, hoarseness and hiccups. There may be tachycardia and hypotension at presentation (Roy et al. 2007).

4 Investigations

Echocardiography is usually the first mode of investigation and can identify haemopericardium, possibly with organisation of the effusion into haematoma. There may be accompanying echocardiographic evidence of pericardial tamponade. In the less acute setting, a CT scan of the chest can also identify pericardial effusions. It should be noted that in patients with previous cardiac surgery or pericarditis, there may be adhesions around the heart leaving pockets of space for collection of blood and therefore these effusions could be more localised rather than being global.

5 Management

Small perforations may result in only a small amount of bleeding. Such perforations can be self-limiting, and management can be conservative (Kim et al. 2010) with bleeding controlled by correction of anticoagulation. These can be followed up but do require close monitoring.

If, however, there is suggestion of large haemopericardium and evidence of pericardial tamponade with attendant haemodynamic compromise, expeditious management is vital. As a first measure, it is important to optimise oxygenation and haemodynamics and help from an anaesthetist is very valuable in this setting. The priority should be to evacuate the haemopericardium. Pericardiocentesis with insertion of a pericardial drain is usually the first intervention (Mentzer et al. 2024). A subcostal approach is often the chosen route with use of echocardiographic with or without fluoroscopic guidance. The pericardial drain can be used to aspirate blood from the pericardium to relieve tamponade while any coagulation derangement is corrected. The rate of drainage and serial echocardiographic guidance can be used to assess control of bleeding.

Other measures which are often effective at control of bleeding source are use of protamine and antidotes to DOACs (Mentzer et al. 2024), although the latter appears to be a less common practice (Mentzer et al. 2023). Any blood aspirated from the pericardial drain can be reinfused to the patient (Mentzer et al. 2023), preferentially with the use of a cell saver as reinfusing blood directly after aspiration from the pericardial space can lead to disturbance in coagulation itself. In many cases of pericardial effusion in the setting of catheter ablation, the pericardial drain can be removed once the bleeding has stopped and there is no residual significant collection.

However, the surgical team should be alerted regarding the event so arrangements can be made for an emergency surgical procedure if needed. This is especially important if the cardiac surgical service is not located in the immediate vicinity of the cardiology catheter lab area, or in some cases, cardiac surgery services may even be on another site. In the latter case, consideration should be given to the best location for the ongoing management of the patient.

Based on large surveys (Mentzer et al. 2023, 2024) including multinational ones and individual centre experience (Wu et al. 2021b; Hamaya et al. 2018), emergent surgical intervention is generally considered for the following indications:

- Continued bleeding for more than 60–80 min
- Large volume of drainage, varying between 1000 and 3000 ml
- No reduction in rate of drainage
- Continued haemodynamic instability
- Suspicion of a left atrial or a left ventricular perforation

In the authors' experience, there should also be consideration for surgical intervention if a pericardial drain is ineffective or insufficient to cope with the volume of bleeding, or there is incomplete relief of cardiac tamponade, for example, with thrombus formation in the pericardium. The possibility of requiring emergency cardiac surgery is potentially less in a patient with previous cardiac surgery, where the pericardium is likely to be adherent to the heart and any localised collections are likely to be controlled spontaneously and less likely to give rise to haemodynamic compromise.

Surgical intervention is much more common during left atrial procedures or ablation of ventricular tachycardia compared to ablation of supraventricular tachycardia (Fink et al. 2020; Bollmann et al. 2018).

The decision to proceed with emergency cardiac surgery should take into account the general condition of the patient including age, frailty, etc., which may have impact on a patient's ability to recover from emergency cardiac surgery. However, in general, most patients should be considered for emergency surgery, given this can be lifesaving in this scenario.

6 Emergency Cardiac Surgery for Bleeding and Tamponade

6.1 Approach

The most common approach for dealing with significant bleeding following ablation procedures is via median sternotomy. There is possibility of requirement for support with use of cardiopulmonary bypass and therefore the location for conduct of these procedures is an important consideration. If the patient has unstable haemodynamics with requirement for continuous resuscitative measures, transferring the patient to a cardiac surgical theatre may not be possible and procedure should be performed in the catheter lab setting. In such a situation, arrangements should be made for surgical personnel and equipment including cardiopulmonary bypass machine to be transferred to the cath lab urgently.

If there is the possibility of moving the patient safely to a fully equipped cardiac surgical operating theatre, this should be considered preferentially. Cell salvage is an important adjunct, which should be utilised in both settings, catheter lab and cardiac surgical theatre. Any blood aspirated from a pericardial drain can be returned to the patient following processing with the cell salvage system. Similarly, blood suctioned from the pericardial cavity at surgery can be processed and returned to the patient.

6.2 Incision

A median sternotomy is rapidly performed and provides the best access to the likely locations for bleeding, namely the pulmonary veins, left atrium, right ventricle and the left ventricle.

6.3 *Procedure*

Following sternotomy and pericardiotomy, any blood and clot should be suctioned out using the cell salvage sucker. Careful systematic exploration should be made to identify the site of injury. Attention should be focussed on area of highest suspicion, which will depend on the procedure being performed and discussion with the EP operator can be very helpful to guide this. Occasionally, bleeding may have stopped, making it difficult to find the source of bleeding. In this case, monitoring and correction of any coagulation defects are appropriate. Adjunct measures, e.g. topical haemostatic agents, can be added on to the suspected 'culprit' areas.

Certain areas may be accessible more easily, e.g. the right-sided pulmonary veins and anterior or inferior surface of the right ventricle. Left-sided pulmonary veins or posterior structures are difficult to access and cardiopulmonary bypass may be essential to maintain control over haemodynamics with cardiac manipulation or if bleeding is ongoing.

If an area is identified as bleeding, management will depend on the size of injury. It may be possible to control small perforations with packing and use of topical haemostatic agents. However, larger defects will usually require control with a suture, which can be pledgeted or without pledgets, depending on the quality of tissue as judged by the surgeon.

Once bleeding is controlled, the chest is closed over drains as per usual preference of the surgeon. Further management depends on the usual preference of the surgeon.

7 Atrio-oesophageal Fistula

An atrio-oesophageal fistula is another rare complication of percutaneous AF ablation procedure. The incidence is reported to be 0.03–0.08% (Han et al. 2017), although the true incidence may be underrecognised. The typical time to presentation appears to be around 20–21 days from procedure (Han et al. 2017; Chavez et al. 2015; Della Rocca et al. 2021). The most common symptoms at presentation appear to be fever and neurological deficits followed by gastrointestinal symptoms including haematemesis (Chavez et al. 2015; Della Rocca et al. 2021; Pappone et al. 2013). A CT chest with contrast is the optimal investigation and may demonstrate pneumomediastinum or air in the left atrium (Pappone et al. 2013) or left ventricle (Fig. 1). Invasive oesophageal investigations and procedures are contraindicated as they contribute to deterioration and death. Emergent surgery improves survival compared to non-operative management (Chavez et al. 2015).

Surgical Procedure

These are uncommon procedures with small individual experiences only. Surgery is technically challenging with inflammation causing loss of usual tissue planes and friability of left atrial wall. Access is also difficult due to the location of these lesions, being deep in the posterior mediastinum.

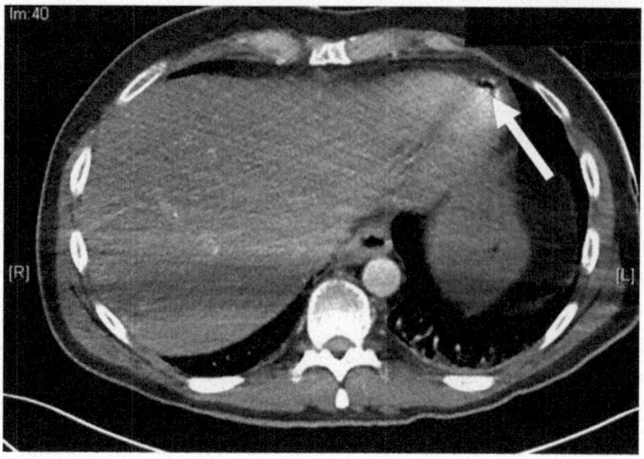

Fig. 1 CT scan showing air in tip of left ventricle (indicated by the white arrow). This has entered the systemic circulation through an atrio-oesophageal fistula

Various procedures have been described with different approaches including sternotomy, left thoracotomy (Khandhar et al. 2010) and right thoracotomy (Raja et al. 2018; Duda et al. 2022). Procedures have been described with use of cardiopulmonary bypass (Raja et al. 2018) (femoral artery (Raja et al. 2018) or descending aorta (Duda et al. 2022) for arterial return and right atrial or bicaval cannulation for venous drainage). There is also counter argument to avoid cardiopulmonary bypass (Khandhar et al. 2010) to reduce the risk of further cerebral bleeds in the setting of recent stroke.

In general, the principles in such operative approaches include control of the fistula, layered closure of the oesophagus (Raja et al. 2018; Duda et al. 2022), closure of the left atrial defect (Khandhar et al. 2010; Raja et al. 2018; Duda et al. 2022) and use of an intercostal muscle flap (Khandhar et al. 2010; Raja et al. 2018; Duda et al. 2022) interposed between the repaired oesophagus and left atrium or use of omentum (Hartman et al. 2012). (Figs. 2 and 3)

8 Conclusion

Although uncommon, there are potentially life-threatening complications with cardiac catheter ablation procedures. The increasing number of complex left atrial and left ventricular ablations being performed worldwide means more of these complications are encountered. The need for surgical intervention should always be considered amongst treatment options when planning any arrhythmia procedure for the management of acute procedural complications such as cardiac perforation and tamponade or delayed complications like atrio-oesophageal fistula.

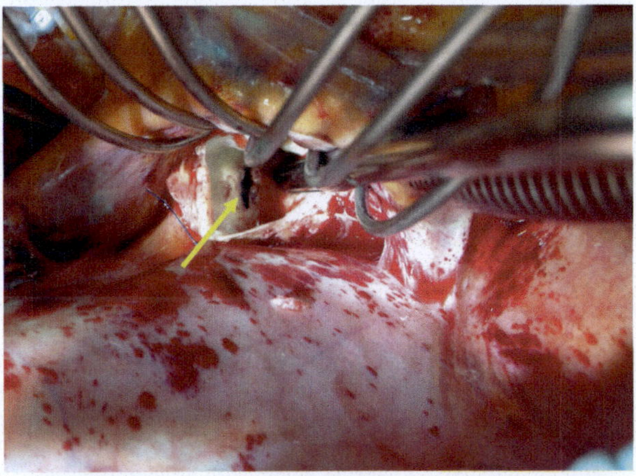

Fig. 2 Intraoperative photo showing the inside of the left atrium and a perforation in the atrium (indicated by the yellow arrow) where the atrial wall has broken down and led to the creation of a fistula with the oesophagus

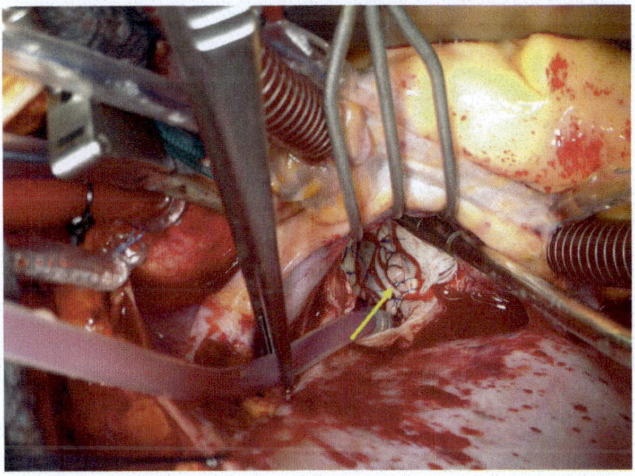

Fig. 3 Intraoperative photo showing the inside of the left atrium after repair of the perforation seen in Fig. 2 (indicated by the yellow arrow)

References

Bollmann A, Ueberham L, Schuler E et al (2018) Cardiac tamponade in catheter ablation of atrial fibrillation: German-wide analysis of 21 141 procedures in the Helios atrial fibrillation ablation registry (SAFER). Europace 20:1944–1951

Calkins H, Reynolds MR, Spector P et al (2009) Treatment of atrial fibrillation with antiarrhythmic drugs or radiofrequency ablation: two systematic literature reviews and meta-analyses. Circ Arrhythm Electrophysiol 2:349–361

Cappato R, Calkins H, Chen SA et al (2010) Updated worldwide survey on the methods, efficacy, and safety of catheter ablation for human atrial fibrillation. Circ Arrhythm Electrophysiol 3:32–38

Cappato R, Calkins H, Chen SA et al (2011) Delayed cardiac tamponade after radiofrequency catheter ablation of atrial fibrillation: a worldwide report. J Am Coll Cardiol 58:2696–2697

Chavez P, Messerli FH, Casso Dominguez A et al (2015) Atrioesophageal fistula following ablation procedures for atrial fibrillation: systematic review of case reports. Open Heart 2:e000257. https://doi.org/10.1136/openhrt-2015-000257

Della Rocca DG, Magnocavallo M, Natale VN et al (2021) Clinical presentation, diagnosis, and treatment of atrioesophageal fistula resulting from atrial fibrillation ablation. J Cardiovasc Electrophysiol 32(9):2441–2450. https://doi.org/10.1111/jce.15168

Duda A, Beers K, Mitiek M (2022) Surgical management of atrial-esophageal fistula as a complication of atrial fibrillation ablation. J Surg Case Rep 2022(1):rjab497

Fink T, Sciacca V, Feickert S et al (2020) Outcome of cardiac tamponades in interventional electrophysiology. Europace 22:1240–1251

Gupta A, Perera T, Ganesan A et al (2013) Complications of catheter ablation of atrial fibrillation: a systematic review. Circ Arrhythm Electrophysiol 6:1082–1088

Hamaya R, Miyazaki S, Taniguchi H et al (2018) Management of cardiac tamponade in catheter ablation of atrial fibrillation: single-centre 15 year experience on 5222 procedures. Europace 20:1776–1782

Han HC, Ha FJ, Sanders P et al (2017) Atrioesophageal fistula: clinical presentation, procedural characteristics, diagnostic investigations, and treatment outcomes. Circ Arrhythm Electrophysiol 10(11):e005579. https://doi.org/10.1161/CIRCEP.117.005579

Hartman AR, Glassman L, Stanley K et al (2012) Surgical repair of a left atrial-esophageal fistula after radiofrequency catheter ablation for atrial fibrillation. Ann Thorac Surg 94(4):e91–e93

Khandhar S, Nitzschke S, Niv A (2010) Left atrioesophageal fistula following catheter ablation for atrial fibrillation: off-bypass, primary repair using an extrapericardial approach. J Thorac Cardiovasc Surg 139(2):507–509

Kim RJ, Siouffi S, Silberstein TA et al (2010) Management and clinical outcomes of acute cardiac tamponade complicating electrophysiologic procedures: a single center case series. Pacing Clin Electrophysiol 33:667–674

Mentzer A, Reubold SD, Schönhofer S et al (2023) Management of pericardial tamponade in the electrophysiology laboratory: results from a national survey. Clin Res Cardiol 112:1727–1737

Mentzer A, Sultan A, Futyma P et al (2024) Prevention and treatment of pericardial tamponade in the electrophysiology laboratory: a European Heart Rhythm Association survey. Europace 26:1–8

Pappone C, Vicedomini G, Santinelli V (2013) Atrio-esophageal fistula after AF ablation: pathophysiology, prevention & treatment. J Atr Fibrillation 6(3):860. https://doi.org/10.4022/jafib.860

Raja S, Shraufnagel D, Roselli E et al (2018) When atrial ablation leads to atrio-esophageal fistula: how to save the day. https://consultqd.clevelandclinic.org/when-atrial-ablation-leads-to-atrio-esophageal-fistula-how-to-save-the-day. Accessed 2 July 2024

Roy CL, Minor MA, Brookhart MA et al (2007) Does this patient with a pericardial effusion have cardiac tamponade? JAMA 297(16):1810–1818. https://doi.org/10.1001/jama.297.16.1810

Siliato-Robles MS, Gracia-Baena JM, Sureda-Barbosa JC et al (2019) Delayed cardiac tamponade after catheter ablation therapy due to a valsalva manoeuvre. Eur J Cardiothorac Surg 55:369–370

Wolf DA, Burke AP, Patterson KV et al (2002) Sudden death following rupture of a right ventricular aneurysm 9 months after ablation therapy of the right ventricular outflow tract. Pacing Clin Electrophysiol 25:1135–1137

Wu S-J, Fan Y-F, Chien C-Y (2021a) Surgical strategies for cardiac perforation after catheter ablation or electrophysiology study: a systemic review. Int Heart J 62:1257–1264

Wu N, Wu F, Yang G et al (2021b) Surgical intervention for cardiac tamponade during atrial fibrillation ablation: who and when? A single-center experience. J Interv Card Electrophysiol 62(2):373–380. https://doi.org/10.1007/s10840-020-00907-7

Xu X, Meng X, Ma F (2020) Delayed cardiac tamponade following catheter ablation of frequent premature ventricular complexes: a case report. BMC Cardiovasc Disord 20:359

Yetter E, Brazg J, Del Valle DD et al (2017) Delayed cardiac tamponade: a rare but life-threatening complication of catheter ablation. Am J Emerg Med 35:803.e1–803.e3

Emergency Cardiac Surgery for Cardiac Device Lead Extraction

Rohan Wijesurendra, Antonios Kourliouros, and Matthew Ginks

Abstract Cardiovascular implanted electronic devices (CIEDs) are widely used in the management of heart rhythm disorders, and include bradycardia pacemakers, biventricular pacemakers, and implantable cardioverter–defibrillators (ICDs). Removal of a CIED lead (with or without the entire system) that has been in situ for more than 1 year requires a lead extraction procedure, which should be done in a specialist centre with cardiac surgical capabilities.

Lead extraction is an integral part of holistic CIED management and is most commonly indicated due to infection, lead dysfunction, or redundancy. An initial percutaneous transvenous lead extraction (TLE) technique is used initially in most cases, with a wide spectrum of tools and techniques available for this purpose, but in specific situations, an initial open extraction with sternotomy and cardiopulmonary bypass may be preferred. Risk stratification and procedure planning are a critical part of any TLE procedure. The anticipated procedural risk will vary considerably from case to case, depending on various clinical features; the dwell time and type of lead are most critical.

All percutaneous TLE cases will require a multidisciplinary team including a device extraction operator (usually a cardiologist trained in TLE) and a cardiac anaesthetist, and in higher risk cases, a cardiac surgeon, perfusionist, and surgical scrub team may be required to be physically present on standby during the procedure. The objective of TLE is to remove the implanted leads in their entirety without causing damage to surrounding structures. The main safety concerns include vascular tear, cardiac perforation, or valvular damage. Emergency cardiac surgery during TLE is required in up to 3% of cases. The surgical principles that govern emergency surgery for TLE complications are access and provision of haemodynamic stability

R. Wijesurendra (✉) · A. Kourliouros · M. Ginks
John Radcliffe Hospital, Oxford, UK
e-mail: Rohan.Wijesurendra@ouh.nhs.uk; a.kourliouros@gmail.com; Matthew.Ginks@ouh.nhs.uk

A. Kourliouros (ed.), *Emergency Cardiac Surgery*,
https://doi.org/10.1007/978-3-032-15787-4_17

followed by the definitive surgical correction of the cardiac or vascular injury. Each of these aspects is discussed in detail in this chapter. With appropriate pre-procedural risk stratification and patient selection, and a dedicated multidisciplinary team approach, TLE complications can be mitigated, and outcomes optimised even in cases when emergency cardiac surgery is required.

Keywords Cardiovascular implanted electronic devices (CIED) · Pacemaker · Defibrillator · Transvenous lead extraction (TLE) · Risk stratification for TLE · TLE techniques · Complications of TLE · Endovascular occlusion balloon · Emergency cardiac surgery during TLE

1 Introduction

Cardiovascular implanted electronic devices (CIEDs) are widely used in the management of heart rhythm disorders, with over 400,000 implanted each year in the United States (Al-Khatib and Leopold 2024). They include bradycardia pacemakers (conventional or conduction system), biventricular pacemakers, and implantable cardioverter–defibrillators (ICDs).

Revision or removal of CIED leads within a year of the initial implant is usually straightforward and can be undertaken at the same site as the index procedure. In contrast, removal of a CIED lead (with or without the entire system) that has been in situ for more than 1 year requires a lead extraction procedure (Kusumoto et al. 2017; Bongiorni et al. 2018), done in a specialist centre with cardiac surgical capabilities. Lead extraction is an integral part of holistic CIED management and is most commonly indicated due to infection, lead dysfunction, or redundancy. Each year, approximately 20,000 lead extraction procedures are undertaken worldwide (Wazni and Wilkoff 2016). An initial percutaneous transvenous lead extraction (TLE) technique is used initially in most cases, with a wide spectrum of tools and techniques available for this purpose. In specific situations, an initial open extraction with sternotomy and cardiopulmonary bypass may be preferred. A hybrid approach that combines TLE with minimally invasive surgery or thoracoscopy may also be advocated in certain centres and/or clinical scenarios. Irrespective of the initial approach chosen, any extraction procedure may require emergency cardiac surgical intervention with a thoracotomy or sternotomy within minutes in the event of a major complication (Kusumoto et al. 2017; Bongiorni et al. 2018). It is therefore vital that cardiologists trained in device extraction, cardiac surgeons, and the wider multiprofessional team all work closely together when listing and undertaking these cases.

2 Indications for Lead Extraction

2.1 *Infection*

CIED infection is the commonest indication for TLE (just over 50% of all TLE cases in a large European Registry) (Bongiorni et al. 2017). The infection rate following a new device implant is around 0.5%, but is higher following reinterventions such as generator change, lead revision or upgrade procedures. Factors known to increase infection rates include comorbidities such as diabetes, renal failure and heart failure, procedure duration, device complexity, antiplatelet or anticoagulant therapy, and number of reinterventions (Blomström-Lundqvist et al. 2020).

CIED infection can be in the form of a localised pocket infection, bacteraemia, endocarditis or a combination of the above. Pocket infection may be obvious in the event of wound dehiscence, purulent discharge or device erosion. The clinical findings may be more subtle and include pain, erythema or tethering of the skin over the device, which is often a precursor to erosion. Bacteraemia may be accompanied by signs of sepsis but may be more insidious and is suggestive of device infection, especially when it recurs following an initial course of antibiotics.

CIED infection increases mortality threefold (Wilkoff et al. 2020) and TLE is recommended in all CIED-related infections other than superficial wound infection (Blomström-Lundqvist et al. 2020) because recurrence rates are high when attempts are made to manage CIED infection with antibiotics alone or without full system extraction (Le et al. 2011). Diagnosis is made on clinical grounds, incorporating microbiology and imaging, typically with transthoracic echocardiography initially, with consideration of the need for transoesophageal echocardiography. Occasionally, further assessment with FDG-PET/CT or radiolabelled white blood cell SPECT/CT may be required (Wilkoff et al. 2020).

In cases of established CIED infection, TLE should be performed without delay and is associated with superior outcomes when compared with conservative management (Blomström-Lundqvist et al. 2020; Pokorney et al. 2023). Most extractions can be performed with relatively low risk using a percutaneous TLE approach, but the presence of large (>30 mm) vegetations, abscess, severe valvular regurgitation causing haemodynamic compromise or prosthetic valve dehiscence necessitate consideration of surgical LE. Whichever approach is used, device and lead extraction are performed alongside ongoing antimicrobial therapy.

2.2 *Redundant Hardware*

Implanted leads can develop insulation defects, lead fracture and issues with displacement or fibrosis at the interface with the myocardium, resulting in poor sensing or loss of capture. Lead failure occurs in up to 20% of leads at 10 years (Kleemann et al. 2007). Implanted leads, as well as devices, can also be subject to manufacturer advisories or recalls that can result in the need for extraction or replacement. Management of patients with non-infective lead issues is more controversial. Commonly, this involves weighing the up-front risks of a TLE procedure (discussed below) against the long-term downsides of leaving non-functioning hardware in situ. The latter approach may avoid the risks of TLE now but can potentially store them up for a later stage, at which point, the dwell time will be longer and the associated risks of TLE are likely to be higher. There is a class IIa indication to extract according to the HRS consensus guidelines if lead implantation is going to result in more than 4 leads from one side or more than 5 leads through the superior vena cava (SVC) or if existing hardware is likely to impact device function (Kusumoto et al. 2017). The threshold for extraction is lower in experienced centres and is lower in younger patients in order to avoid problems in the future with abandoned leads.

2.3 *Vascular Issues*

Lead-related venous stenosis is not uncommon (Czajkowski et al. 2022), but typically venous collaterals develop to avoid symptoms developing due to subclavian venous obstruction. Obstruction of the SVC causes unpleasant symptoms but is rare (Czajkowski et al. 2022), and usually necessitates LE with or without stenting (Mekary et al. 2024). TLE is more commonly needed to maintain vascular access when the subclavian vein is found to be occluded at the time of device upgrade.

2.4 *Mechanical Issues*

Less common issues requiring TLE include pain, arrhythmia, cardiac perforation, tricuspid regurgitation, need for radiotherapy to be delivered to the area (more of a concern in a patient who is pacing dependent), or the need for magnetic resonance imaging (MRI) in a patient with a non-MRI conditional device. The latter scenario can now commonly be managed in an experienced centre who may well be happy to perform MRI (the risk of which is typically much lower than the risk of TLE).

3 Risk Stratification and Procedure Planning

3.1 *Rationale*

Risk stratification and procedure planning is a critical part of any TLE procedure. The anticipated procedural risk will vary very considerably from case to case, depending on various clinical features (as discussed in more detail below). This risk profile will affect all aspects of the management of the case, beginning with whether TLE is indeed the recommended option. This will in turn depend on the indication for TLE and any alternative management strategies that may be available. In cases where the risk/benefit of TLE is in doubt, or where there are various potentially viable treatment options, careful discussion in a multidisciplinary team meeting is recommended to review the details and the possible options. Clearly, the patient and his or her family members should also usually be involved using a shared decision-making approach. In rare circumstances (including very large vegetations, abscess, another indication for cardiac surgery, or jailed leads), a primary surgical extraction may be recommended following multidisciplinary team discussion; the technical aspects of primary surgical extraction do not fall within the scope of this chapter and are not discussed further here.

Once a decision is made to go ahead with TLE, the risk stratification remains highly relevant in then directing various aspects of the procedural planning, including personnel, location (catheterisation lab versus surgical operating theatre or hybrid facility), timing, necessary pre-procedure investigations, anaesthetic and surgical preparations, extraction equipment, and postoperative care. If urgent inpatient TLE is required, for example in cases of septic shock related to CIED endocarditis, it is recommended that the same pre-procedural planning is undertaken, but on an expedited basis.

3.2 *Clinical Features Predicting Risk of TLE*

Indwelling leads become attached to the heart and vessels due to the development of a fibrotic reaction, which can become extremely intense over longer durations (Epstein et al. 1998). For this reason, the number and type of indwelling leads and the dwell time are the most important features to consider when stratifying the risk of TLE. ICD leads are higher risk than pacing leads, due to the presence of one or two shock coils, which are frequently strongly adherent (to cardiac tissue in the case of single-coil leads, and additionally to the SVC in the case of dual-coil leads). The incidence of mechanical complications during TLE increases proportionately with increasing dwell time; there does not seem to be an upper bound beyond which risk does not increase, based on published data of TLE of leads in situ for over 20 or 30 years (Kutarski et al. 2022; Issa 2021; Ząbek et al. 2019).

The ELECTRa Registry Outcome Score (EROS) (Sidhu et al. 2021) has recently been developed and applied in the large-scale ELECTRa registry, which includes over 3500 procedures undertaken in 73 European centres. Overall, 57.5% of patients were classified as EROS 1, 31.8% as EROS 2, and 10.7% as EROS 3. Patients with EROS 2 or 3 were more likely to need powered sheaths and a femoral approach to achieve successful TLE. Patients with EROS 3 were more likely to experience major complications from TLE, including procedure-related death (5.1% vs. 1.3% for EROS 1 and 2 combined, $p < 0.0001$), cardiac avulsion or tear (3.8% vs. 0.5%, $p < 0.0001$), and cardiovascular lesions requiring pericardiocentesis, chest tube, or surgical repair (4.6% vs. 1.0%, $p < 0.0001$). The EROS classification scheme is shown in Table 1.

Our local practice in Oxford is to use an alternative classification scheme, which was first introduced in 2019 and has recently been updated following audit (Table 2). It has the advantage over EROS that it only routinely requires information on lead type and dwell time.

In addition to the clinical features discussed above and in the EROS and Oxford schemes, the ELECTRa prospective TLE registry also showed that TLE procedures undertaken in high-volume centres (those that undertake at least 30 TLE procedures annually) have a higher success rate with lower all-cause complication and mortality rates when compared to those procedures done in low-volume centres (those that undertake fewer than 30 TLE procedures annually) (Bongiorni et al. 2017).

3.3 *Pre-Procedure Investigations*

Careful pre-procedure investigation and workup are critical in all patients where TLE is being considered; the results of relevant investigations should ideally be available at the time of any multidisciplinary discussion undertaken to decide amongst the available options for management. The relevant investigations, split into those that are mandatory in all cases, and those that need to be considered on a case-by-case basis are outlined in Table 3. The purpose of these investigations is to determine whether percutaneous TLE is feasible and the associated risk, the need for temporary pacing during the procedure, and whether ongoing device therapy will be needed in the longer term after TLE, and if so the possible prescription(s), and to guide emergent cardiac surgery in the event of a complication.

Table 1 EROS classification scheme

EROS 1	EROS 2	EROS 3
Pacemaker lead ≤15 years from implant *or* ICD lead ≤10 years from implant *and* No other features that would increase risk to EROS 2	Pacemaker lead ≤15 years from implant *or* ICD lead ≤10 years from implant *and one of:* 1. Congenital heart disease 2. Initial implant at age <15 years 3. Chronic kidney disease and serum creatinine >2 mg/dL 4. Infectious indication for extraction and any of the following: (a) White cell count > 12×10^9/L (b) Positive blood culture (c) Vegetation on transoesophageal echocardiogram 5. Chronic heart failure and NYHA class IV	Pacemaker lead >15 years from implant *or* ICD lead >10 years from implant

Table 2 Oxford risk classification scheme

Low risk (green)	Medium risk (amber)	High risk (red)*
Pacemaker lead <10 years from implant *or* Single-coil ICD lead ≤2 years from implant	Pacemaker lead 10–20 years from implant *or* Single-coil ICD lead 2–15 years from implant *or* Dual-coil ICD lead 2–10 years from implant	Pacemaker lead >20 years from implant *or* Single-coil ICD lead >15 years from implant *or* Dual-coil ICD lead >10 years from implant

*Operator discretion can be used for any case considered to be higher risk on the basis of patient factors (e.g. low body mass index, extremes of age, low LVEF, comorbidities, specific lead types (e.g. starfix)
*Leads with dwell times >20 years and patients with vegetations >3 cm require MDT discussion

Table 3 Pre-procedure investigations

Mandatory	Consider on a case-by-case basis
Full blood count Renal function CRP 12-lead ECG Chest radiograph Transthoracic echocardiogram Device check (underlying rhythm, pacing burden, any therapies delivered from devices with a defibrillator function)	Group and screen or crossmatch blood (depending on risk stratification) Transoesophageal echocardiogram (if uncertainty regarding presence/size of—vegetations on transthoracic echocardiogram) CT chest (if previous cardiac surgery/ sternotomy)

3.4 Procedure Planning

After a decision to undertake percutaneous TLE has been made, the results of the risk stratification process outlined above will also impact the procedural planning.

The first decision to be made is the location of the procedure—i.e. cardiac catheterisation or device laboratory versus cardiac theatres. Low- and medium-risk procedures, and most high-risk cases, would usually be undertaken in the cardiac catheterisation or device laboratory, but selected high-risk cases may be better done in cardiac theatres. Hybrid laboratories, when available, are ideally suited for higher risk TLE cases. Following on from this, personnel required for the procedure should be considered. All percutaneous TLE cases will require a device extraction operator (usually a cardiologist trained in TLE), a cardiac anaesthetist and operating department practitioner, cardiac physiologist, radiographer, and at least two nursing staff. In higher risk cases, a cardiac surgeon, perfusionist, and surgical scrub team may be required to be physically present on standby during the procedure, ready to step in immediately in the event of a complication requiring emergent cardiac surgery. A post-procedure high dependency or intensive care bed may be required, at least on standby. In all cases, specialised percutaneous device extraction equipment should be available (e.g. locking stylets, mechanical cutting sheaths, and snares).

Table 4 Oxford pre-extraction procedure planning

Low risk (green)	Medium risk (amber)	High risk (red)
No requirement to discuss with surgical team	Surgical theatre coordinator aware Group and screen blood Drape for sternotomy Peri-procedural transoesophageal echocardiography Arterial line and femoral venous sheath Post-procedure monitored bed	Cardiac surgeon physically present during procedure Consider location of procedure (catheterisation lab versus cardiac theatres) Perfusion team physically present and prepare pump Crossmatch 2–4 units of blood Femoral access obtained Other preparation as for medium-risk cases

The Oxford protocol for procedural planning is outlined in Table 4.

4 Techniques for Lead Extraction

The objective of TLE is to remove the implanted leads in their entirety without causing damage to surrounding structures. The main safety concerns include vascular tear, cardiac perforation, or valvular damage, due to the fibrosis which causes tethering of the leads at points of contact.

The standard approach for TLE is to remove the leads from the site where they were originally implanted (typically in the pre-pectoral region) and are connected to the pulse generator. An incision is made with the location chosen to allow access to both the generator and lead collars. The generator and leads are freed up with dissection and electrocautery (diathermy or PlasmaBlade™, Medtronic). Further debridement is performed to remove non-viable or infected tissue. Stylets are passed down the lumen of each lead in order to confirm patency, and to retract the helix of active fixation leads. If the dwell time is short, it may be possible to remove the lead with manual traction alone. However, most extractions will require a locking stylet to be passed down the lead. This is deployed when positioned as far down the lead as possible. The locking stylet allows traction to be delivered along the length of the lead, and is less likely to jeopardise the lead integrity. Assuming that traction on the lead with the locking stylet alone does not result in the lead to be removed easily, an extraction sheath will be required. The extraction sheath is then passed over the lead and traction applied on the lead with counter traction from the tip of the extraction sheath.

Extraction sheaths may be unpowered—a relatively simple polypropylene dilator (Cook Vascular, USA), reliant on the operator to lyse adhesions with mechanical rotation (Byrd et al. 2007; Gaubert et al. 2016)—or powered. The latter type is more commonly used for leads with a longer dwell time. Powered sheaths include the Laser sheath (Spectranetics, Phillips Medical) which uses a Xenon gas laser to break down tissue within a few microns of the sheath (Epstein et al. 1999; Wazni et al. 2010), and mechanical sheaths such as the Evolution™ (Cook Vascular, USA) or Tightrail™ (Spectranetics, Phillips Medical) sheaths, which incorporate a rotational mechanical cutting mechanism within the tip of the sheath to cut through fibrotic attachments and calcified lesions (Mazzone et al. 2018; Aytemir et al. 2016). The technique of traction on the lead and counter-traction on the tip of the sheath allows co-axial deployment of force to overcome areas of adhesion and minimise the risk of trauma to vascular structures. The extraction sheath is passed to the distal end of the lead, at the interface with the myocardium, in order to free it up and remove it in its entirety. If necessary to maintain venous access for lead reimplantation, a guide wire can be passed down the sheath once the lead has been removed.

In the scenario where the lead integrity fails, or it does not prove possible to complete the extraction from above, it is necessary to use a different approach (typically from the femoral vein) in order to snare the lead from below and extract via that route. Some centres advocate a femoral approach up front, but this is usually only required for leads with a much longer dwell time.

Safety considerations are discussed above. In all but low-risk extraction procedures, we position a guide wire in the SVC at the start of the procedure using femoral venous access, in case an SVC tear should occur and the Bridge Occlusion Balloon ™ (Spectranetics, Phillips Medical) can then be deployed in order to stabilise the situation prior to emergency surgery (Azarrafiy et al. 2019).

Transoesophageal echocardiography is valuable in identifying pericardial effusion at an early stage in the event of haemodynamic instability. Should pericardial tamponade develop, this would initially be drained using emergency pericardiocentesis (typically using a subxiphoid or apical approach) but if haemostasis is not achieved promptly, then emergency cardiac surgery should be undertaken.

5 Technical Aspects of Emergency Cardiac Surgery in Cardiac Device Lead Extraction Cases

Emergency cardiac surgery during TLE is required in up to 3% of unselected cases depending on patient characteristics and operator experience (Bashir et al. 2016). Risk stratification tools have discriminatory power to detect high-risk groups for cardiovascular injuries allowing for appropriate procedural planning including for emergency sternotomy or thoracotomy (Sidhu et al. 2021). The surgical principles that govern emergency surgery for TLE complications are access (into the chest and circulation), provision of haemodynamic stability, and definitive surgical correction of the cardiac or vascular injury.

5.1 Access

It is essential that the surgical team is present for the huddle prior to any high-risk TLE procedure, with emphasis on discussing the underlying cardiac pathology, previous surgery, and availability of vascular access. Previous cardiac or thoracic surgery has implications for the immediate access to the chest should this become necessary. Performing emergency re-sternotomy safely requires knowledge of the proximity of the aorta and right ventricle to the sternum, and careful review of the CT is required in all TLE extractions with previous sternotomy. For those identified as high-risk TLE procedures, the presence of a scrub theatre team and perfusionist (with a primed cardiopulmonary bypass machine) in the room is required. Antiseptic skin preparation and chest draping are similar to that of a cardiac surgical procedure allowing for access both to the subclavian area and to the midline for a possible emergency sternotomy. In those less common cases where a thoracotomy would be the preferred emergency incision strategy (e.g. presence of previous sternotomy), skin preparation and draping should include the lateral aspect of the chest, as much as this is allowed with the patient in a supine position. In medium-risk cases and, more importantly, in low-risk ones where the surgical team are not physically present in the laboratory, access to the chest could be obtained through an all-in-one adhesive drape with a transparent film over the centre. There is no need for antiseptic skin preparation (with its requirement to dry) in an emergency situation while CPR is taking place and where definitive management can only be delivered by sternotomy. We favour the use of a battery-operated sternal saw, ensuring charged batteries, against the pneumatic one that may take more time to connect. For redo sternotomy where an oscillating saw is required, we would aim to establish haemodynamic stability through percutaneous drainage of the collection with or without auto-transfusion and/or establishment of peripheral cardiopulmonary bypass, rather than carrying one out in haste and risking more damage. In this group, we would selectively insert both arterial and venous femoral sheaths in the groin at the beginning of the TLE procedure, to allow for quick percutaneous cannulation if needed, and this strategy is discussed at the pre-procedural huddle. In those redo cases, where the provision for swift peripheral cannulation is not in place and patients are rapidly losing output, a right supine anterolateral thoracotomy is a more preferable approach, as it allows for pericardial drainage but also establishment of central cardiopulmonary bypass by accessing the right atrium and the ascending aorta through the right chest.

5.2 Provision of Haemodynamic Stability

For contained cardiac or intrathoracic vascular injuries with significant haemodynamic effect due to blood collection and where percutaneous drainage has not been able to provide stability, the release of tamponade through expeditious sternotomy may be the only intervention necessary. The use of cell salvage and careful packing of the pericardial space will buy time in small and in a few moderate injuries, to allow for resuscitative transfusion, identification of the bleeding point, and decision whether cardiopulmonary bypass should be utilised. A form of manual control of significant bleeding, if possible, takes precedence over the establishment of cardiopulmonary bypass; maintaining circulating volume is critical even when definitive management necessitates its use. As the majority of injuries during TLE occur to the right heart and venous system, areas which are not subjected to systemic pressures, the aforementioned step of packing and manual compression could provide the stability required for definitive management to almost 80% of those with small injuries, and 66% of those with moderate ones (Bashir et al. 2016). It should be emphasised that cardiopulmonary bypass cannot provide adequate tissue perfusion in the absence of essential circulating volume, and its use in providing haemodynamic stability in excessive bleeding is through the use of cardiotomy suction. At this point, it is also worth highlighting the following regarding cannulation and cardiopulmonary bypass in an 'empty' circulation: aortic cannulation can be challenging as the aorta is flaccid and there is little or no blood filling the aortic cannula retrogradely for a connection without air entrapment. One needs to have appropriate solution (e.g. Hartmann's) at hand to ensure filling of the aortic cannula and a 'wet' connection to the pump outflow tubing. If there is an extensive right atrial or SVC tear, one must be mindful of the potential for an 'air lock' and the need to control it, or at least reduce it, to allow for safe cardiopulmonary bypass. This can be achieved with temporarily clamping or snaring the proximal aspect of the SVC (for injuries, more cephalad), or with a snare around the IVC (for RA injuries) assuming a single-stage venous drainage cannula.

Finally, we have found two temporising measures that can occasionally provide haemodynamic stability until definitive management, one before sternotomy and the other one after. Endovascular occlusion balloon can be a very useful adjunct when there is an SVC tear (identified in almost 50% of all TLE-related injuries). It can be deployed quickly through a femoral venous sheath (often in less than 2 min), and can play a significant role in reducing blood loss and allow for a more planned surgical rescue protocol (Azarrafiy et al. 2019). In our practice, patients undergoing medium- and high-risk TLE, especially in the presence of previous sternotomy, will usually receive a purpose-specific venous femoral sheath and a stiff guide wire advanced to the SVC before commencing any lead extraction. Along the same principles, SVC and right atrial tears identified upon emergency sternotomy can be temporised with the use of a Foley catheter advanced through the defect. The balloon is then inflated and the catheter withdrawn until resistance is felt, 'plugging' the defect until definitive repair is performed. It is essential that the drainage port of the catheter is clamped or spigotted to prevent blood coming out, and that any stitching around the defect (in the form of 'purse-string' for instance) to repair it has to be done cautiously; otherwise, it can inadvertently puncture the balloon and deflate it.

5.3 *Definitive Surgical Correction of Injuries*

In terms of frequency, approximately 50% of lacerations are identified in the SVC, the majority of which are located in its body (Arora et al. 2022). These can be caused by the advancement of the extraction sheath against the SVC wall, in the attempt to direct it caudally into the right atrium. Very small defects can sometimes be controlled with simple suturing and without cardiopulmonary bypass, but definitive correction of more complex SVC injuries can be challenging. Cardiopulmonary bypass with aortic return and caval cannulation to the IVC with a two-stage cannula could provide stability, but there is the risk of air entrapment through the SVC defect. Also, if needed to isolate the SVC in cases where extensive reconstruction is necessary, the head and neck venous system must be adequately drained, and one has to be confident with high SVC cannulation if feasible, or alternative cannulation sites, such as the brachiocephalic vein (directly with a small angled venous cannula) or the right jugular vein percutaneously, in addition to the IVC inflow cannula. Snaring of the cavae could help prevent air entrapment into the cardiopulmonary bypass circuit and provide a field free of excessive blood from venous return.

Whichever surgical repair method is going to be utilised in an SVC tear, it is important not to cause SVC stenosis that can subsequently lead to SVC syndrome. Patch reconstruction with bovine pericardium is often preferable to repair long tears where over-and-over direct suturing could cause significant luminal stenosis. In extensive circumferential tears or in those cases where the integrity of the SVC wall is compromised, part or all of the SVC can be replaced with a tubularised bovine pericardial conduit that the surgeon can construct using a 20-ml syringe as a temporary scaffold. The pericardium is wrapped around it and its edges approximated with a running 4/0 prolene suture. Once again, as such reconstructive procedures ideally require a bloodless operating field with haemodynamic stability and head and neck drainage, cardiopulmonary bypass with appropriate inflow configuration, as described above, should be considered. Of note, such right-sided cardiac surgery will not require aortic clamping in the majority of cases, allowing for myocardial perfusion and 'beating heart' reconstruction while on cardiopulmonary bypass and with more liberal time constraints.

While management of right atrial injuries, especially of the free wall, is often achieved with direct suturing (as there is no significant risk of causing chamber narrowing as with SVC tears), right ventricular wall perforation needs special consideration. These tears are often small and can be fixed directly using Teflon pledgets for better tension distribution, but the requirement to lift the heart in case they are apically located or where the right ventricular wall is very thin and friable may still necessitate the use of cardiopulmonary bypass.

Injury to the coronary sinus from extraction of active fixation leads causing bleeding will need immediate sternotomy in the majority of cases, to allow repair of the coronary sinus with the use of cardiopulmonary bypass. Direct suturing of the coronary sinus from the diaphragmatic surface of the heart can cause significant stenosis, compromising coronary venous drainage and leading to haemodynamic instability and arrhythmias. For this reason, we propose establishment of standard aorto-caval cardiopulmonary bypass and aortic cross clamping, and an on-lay pericardial patch repair to cover the injury in the coronary sinus, secured circumferentially into the surrounding epicardium with a running prolene suture (Aigner et al. 2006). Finally, tricuspid valve dysfunction can occur in up to 9.6% of patients after TLE, but the requirement for immediate repair is very rare (<0.1%) (Polewczyk et al. 2022). When emergency tricuspid surgery is indicated, repair techniques addressing the defect or valve replacement can be performed as per standard principles.

Mortality rates for patients requiring emergency surgery due to cardiovascular injuries during TLE vary from 12% in selected series (Bashir et al. 2016) to 34% in a large registry analysis (Sood et al. 2018). The high mortality rate found in this latter real-world unselected cohort is likely the reflection of large variability in TLE practice and support arrangements, including surgical availability and expertise.

In conclusion, we advocate that best outcomes are achieved through experienced and dedicated TLE teams that can identify high-risk cases and provide a holistic approach, including standardised percutaneous stabilisation and open surgical repairs, should complications occur. Data collection and audit can further inform best practice and aid in establishing standard operating procedures, to achieve optimal outcomes in this growing cohort of patients.

References

Aigner C, Wolner E, Mohl W (2006) Management of central coronary sinus ruptures using the pericardial patch repair technique. Ann Thorac Surg 81:1275–1278. https://doi.org/10.1016/j.athoracsur.2005.11.037

Al-Khatib SM, Leopold JA (2024) Cardiac implantable electronic devices. N Engl J Med 390:442–454. https://doi.org/10.1056/NEJMra2308353

Arora Y, D'Angelo L, Azarrafiy R, Bashir J, Kennergren C, Carrillo R (2022) Location of superior vena cava tears in transvenous lead extraction. Ann Thorac Surg 113:1165–1171. https://doi.org/10.1016/j.athoracsur.2021.04.068

Aytemir K, Yorgun H, Canpolat U, Şahiner ML, Kaya EB, Evranos B, Özer N (2016) Initial experience with the TightRail™ Rotating Mechanical Dilator Sheath for transvenous lead extraction. Europace 18:1043–1048. https://doi.org/10.1093/europace/euv245

Azarrafiy R, Tsang DC, Wilkoff BL, Carrillo RG (2019) Endovascular occlusion balloon for treatment of superior vena cava tears during transvenous lead extraction. Circ Arrhythm Electrophysiol 12. https://doi.org/10.1161/circep.119.007266

Bashir J, Fedoruk LM, Ofiesh J, Karim SS, Tyers GFO (2016) Classification and surgical repair of injuries sustained during transvenous lead extraction. Circ Arrhythm Electrophysiol 9. https://doi.org/10.1161/circep.115.003741

Blomström-Lundqvist C, Traykov V, Erba PA, Burri H, Nielsen JC, Bongiorni MG, Poole J, Boriani G, Costa R, Deharo J-C et al (2020) European Heart Rhythm Association (EHRA) international consensus document on how to prevent, diagnose, and treat cardiac implantable electronic device infections—endorsed by the Heart Rhythm Society (HRS), the Asia Pacific Heart Rhythm Society (APHRS), the Latin American Heart Rhythm Society (LAHRS), International Society for Cardiovascular Infectious Diseases (ISCVID), and the European Society of Clinical Microbiology and Infectious Diseases (ESCMID) in collaboration with the European Association for Cardio-Thoracic Surgery (EACTS). Eur Heart J 41:2012–2032. https://doi.org/10.1093/eurheartj/ehaa010

Bongiorni MG, Kennergren C, Butter C, Deharo JC, Kutarski A, Rinaldi CA, Romano SL, Maggioni AP, Andarala M, Auricchio A et al (2017) The European Lead Extraction ConTRolled (ELECTRa) study: a European Heart Rhythm Association (EHRA) Registry of Transvenous Lead Extraction Outcomes. Eur Heart J 38:2995–3005. https://doi.org/10.1093/eurheartj/ehx080

Bongiorni MG, Burri H, Deharo JC, Starck C, Kennergren C, Saghy L, Rao A, Tascini C, Lever N, Kutarski A et al (2018) 2018 EHRA expert consensus statement on lead extraction: recommendations on definitions, endpoints, research trial design, and data collection requirements for clinical scientific studies and registries: endorsed by APHRS/HRS/LAHRS. EP Europace 20:1217–1217. https://doi.org/10.1093/europace/euy050

Byrd CL, Schwartz SJ, Hedin NB, Goode LB, Fearnot NE, Smith HJ (2007) Intravascular lead extraction using locking stylets and sheaths. Pacing Clin Electrophysiol 13:1871–1875. https://doi.org/10.1111/j.1540-8159.1990.tb06906.x

Czajkowski M, Jacheć W, Polewczyk A, Kosior J, Nowosielecka D, Tułecki Ł, Stefańczyk P, Kutarski A (2022) Severity and extent of lead-related venous obstruction in more than 3000 patients undergoing transvenous lead extraction. Vasc Health Risk Manag 18:629–642. https://doi.org/10.2147/vhrm.S369342

Epstein AE, Kay GN, Plumb VJ, Dailey SM, Anderson PG (1998) Gross and microscopic pathological changes associated with nonthoracotomy implantable defibrillator leads. Circulation 98:1517–1524. https://doi.org/10.1161/01.Cir.98.15.1517

Epstein LM, Byrd CL, Wilkoff BL, Love CJ, Sellers TD, Hayes DL, Reiser C (1999) Initial experience with larger laser sheaths for the removal of transvenous pacemaker and implantable defibrillator leads. Circulation 100:516–525. https://doi.org/10.1161/01.Cir.100.5.516

Gaubert M, Giorgi R, Franceschi F, Koutbi-Franceschi L, Gitenay E, Maille B, Deharo J-C (2016) Outcomes and costs associated with two different lead-extraction approaches: a single-centre study. Europace. https://doi.org/10.1093/europace/euw254

Issa ZF (2021) Outcome of transvenous lead extraction of leads older than 20 years. J Cardiovasc Electrophysiol 32:3042–3048. https://doi.org/10.1111/jce.15229

Kleemann T, Becker T, Doenges K, Vater M, Senges J, Schneider S, Saggau W, Weisse U, Seidl K (2007) Annual rate of transvenous defibrillation lead defects in implantable cardioverter-defibrillators over a period of >10 years. Circulation 115:2474–2480. https://doi.org/10.1161/circulationaha.106.663807

Kusumoto FM, Schoenfeld MH, Wilkoff BL, Berul CI, Birgersdotter-Green UM, Carrillo R, Cha Y-M, Clancy J, Deharo J-C, Ellenbogen KA et al (2017) 2017 HRS expert consensus statement on cardiovascular implantable electronic device lead management and extraction. Heart Rhythm 14:e503–e551. https://doi.org/10.1016/j.hrthm.2017.09.001

Kutarski A, Głowniak A, Kosior J, Jacheć W, Nowosielecka D, Czajkowski M, Polewczyk A (2022) Outcomes of transvenous extraction of leads older than 20 and 30 years—a large cohort study. Int J Environ Res Public Health 19. https://doi.org/10.3390/ijerph192114184

Le KY, Sohail MR, Friedman PA, Uslan DZ, Cha SS, Hayes DL, Wilson WR, Steckelberg JM, Baddour LM (2011) Impact of timing of device removal on mortality in patients with cardiovascular implantable electronic device infections. Heart Rhythm 8:1678–1685. https://doi.org/10.1016/j.hrthm.2011.05.015

Mazzone P, Migliore F, Bertaglia E, Facchin D, Daleffe E, Calzolari V, Crosato M, Melillo F, Peruzza F, Marzi A et al (2018) Safety and efficacy of the new bidirectional rotational Evolution® mechanical lead extraction sheath: results from a multicentre Italian registry. EP Europace 20:829–834. https://doi.org/10.1093/europace/eux020

Mekary W, Hebbo E, Shah A, Westerman S, Bhatia N, Byku I, Babaliaros V, Greenbaum A, Merchant FM, El-Chami MF (2024) Managing superior vena cava syndrome in patients with cardiac implantable electronic device leads: strategies and considerations. Heart Rhythm. https://doi.org/10.1016/j.hrthm.2024.06.060

Pokorney SD, Zepel L, Greiner MA, Fowler VG, Black-Maier E, Lewis RK, Hegland DD, Granger CB, Epstein LM, Carrillo RG et al (2023) Lead extraction and mortality among patients with cardiac implanted electronic device infection. JAMA Cardiol 8. https://doi.org/10.1001/jamacardio.2023.3379

Polewczyk A, Jacheć W, Nowosielecka D, Tomaszewski A, Brzozowski W, Szczęśniak-Stańczyk D, Duda K, Kutarski A (2022) Tricuspid valve damage related to transvenous lead extraction. Int J Environ Res Public Health 19. https://doi.org/10.3390/ijerph191912279

Sidhu BS, Ayis S, Gould J, Elliott MK, Mehta V, Kennergren C, Butter C, Deharo J-C, Kutarski A, Maggioni AP et al (2021) Risk stratification of patients undergoing transvenous lead extraction with the ELECTRa Registry Outcome Score (EROS): an ESC EHRA EORP European lead extraction ConTRolled ELECTRa registry analysis. EP Europace 23:1462–1471. https://doi.org/10.1093/europace/euab037

Sood N, Martin DT, Lampert R, Curtis JP, Parzynski C, Clancy J (2018) Incidence and predictors of perioperative complications with transvenous lead extractions. Circ Arrhythm Electrophysiol 11. https://doi.org/10.1161/circep.116.004768

Wazni O, Wilkoff BL (2016) Considerations for cardiac device lead extraction. Nat Rev Cardiol 13:221–229. https://doi.org/10.1038/nrcardio.2015.207

Wazni O, Epstein LM, Carrillo RG, Love C, Adler SW, Riggio DW, Karim SS, Bashir J, Greenspon AJ, DiMarco JP et al (2010) Lead extraction in the contemporary setting: the LExICon study. J Am Coll Cardiol 55:579–586. https://doi.org/10.1016/j.jacc.2009.08.070

Wilkoff BL, Boriani G, Mittal S, Poole JE, Kennergren C, Corey GR, Krahn AD, Schloss EJ, Gallastegui JL, Pickett RA et al (2020) Cost-effectiveness of an antibacterial envelope for cardiac implantable electronic device infection prevention in the us healthcare system from the WRAP-IT trial. Circ Arrhythm Electrophysiol 13. https://doi.org/10.1161/circep.120.008503

Ząbek A, Boczar K, Dębski M, Matusik PT, Pfitzner R, Ulman M, Musiał R, Lelakowski J, Małecka B (2019) Transvenous extraction of very old (over 20-year-old) pacemaker leads using mechanical systems: effectiveness and safety. Pacing Clin Electrophysiol 42:998–1005. https://doi.org/10.1111/pace.13714

Mechanical Circulatory Support in Perioperative Cardiogenic Shock

Antonios Kourliouros

Abstract The primary aim of this chapter is to elucidate the utilisation of extracorporeal life support (ECLS) in both the immediate management of patients failing to separate from cardiopulmonary bypass (CPB) during cardiac surgery, and those presenting with poor cardiac output postcardiotomy despite pharmacological support. The application of ECLS in the presentation of cardiogenic shock prior to cardiac surgery as a means of patient optimisation and improving post-surgical outcomes will also be explored. Various forms of temporary mechanical circulatory support (MCS) are available in such contexts including veno-arterial extracorporeal membrane oxygenation (VA ECMO), left ventricular assist devices (LVAD), right ventricular assist devices (RVAD) and biventricular assist devices (BiVAD). The differential characteristics of such variations of MCS are an important consideration in the treatment strategy of postcardiotomy failure, with various configurations offered depending upon patient physiology. Through appropriate patient selection, ECLS type and adherence to certain clinical management strategies, satisfactory outcomes can be achieved in this otherwise very high-risk patient cohort.

Keywords Extracorporeal life support (ECLS) · Mechanical circulatory support (MCS) · Veno-arterial extracorporeal membrane oxygenation (VA ECMO) · Left ventricular assist device (LVAD) · Right ventricular assist device (RVAD) · Biventricular assist device (BiVAD) · Microaxial pump/Impella · Cardiogenic shock · Postcardiotomy ECLS · Peripheral cannulation for VA ECMO · Central VA ECMO · Outcomes MCS

A. Kourliouros (✉)
Cardiothoracic Surgery, John Radcliffe Hospital, Oxford, UK
e-mail: a.kourliouros@gmail.com

A. Kourliouros (ed.), *Emergency Cardiac Surgery*,
https://doi.org/10.1007/978-3-032-15787-4_18

1 Description of Different Types of ECLS

Extracorporeal life support (ECLS) encompasses several components, including a combination of vascular grafts or cannulae, connecting tubing and centrifugal pump, which together encourage haemodynamic stability and adequate tissue perfusion whilst bypassing the heart and lungs. ECLS devices are temporary by definition, allowing for cardiac recovery, the delivery of definitive treatments and interventions, and can be upgraded to durable MCS devices or transplantation.

The type of temporary support utilised is determined by expertise and the area of the cardiopulmonary circulation involved which needs to be bypassed. As such, there is non-selective CPB in the form of VA ECMO, RVAD to bypass the right ventricle (RV), and LVAD to bypass the left ventricle (LV). A defining feature across such devices is that VA ECMO always requires an oxygenator, whilst VADs do not, though an oxygenator can be incorporated into the VAD circuit to provide respiratory support should the lungs be unable to provide adequate oxygenation. Finally, the aforementioned two VAD systems can operate in parallel creating a BiVAD which delivers selective right and left ventricle bypass, alongside respiratory support if connected to an oxygenator. In this chapter, we will not describe the use of ECLS for isolated respiratory indications (veno-venous ECMO), but will concentrate on its role in predominant circulatory support.

Any ECLS circuit can be broken down into three major components: the cannulae, centrifugal pump, and polyvinyl chloride (PVC) tubing connecting the circuit. The cannulae are attached to different areas of the heart or major vessels to provide blood inflow into the ECLS circuit, and outflow via the return line to deliver support where required. A non-occlusive centrifugal pump (with or without an oxygenator) controls the rate of blood flow and is preferred over an occlusive one as it induces less haemolysis and heat when in long-term use. Centrifugal pumps are also preload dependent and afterload sensitive allowing blood flow rate to respond to situations of hypovolaemia and increased systemic vascular resistance, respectively. Finally, PVC tubing connects the access cannula to the pump, which is the inflow component (away from the patient and into the pump) and the tubing that returns blood to the patient, which is the outflow component.

- VA ECMO is an extracorporeal configuration with a cannula draining blood from the venous system, more frequently peripherally from the common femoral vein, into the centrifugal pump with an oxygenator, and returning this oxygenated blood into the arterial component of the circulation through a large peripheral artery such as the common femoral or subclavian artery. In the postcardiotomy setting, which will be discussed in the relevant section, there is the option to establish ECMO centrally through the open chest (Fig. 1). It is therefore, essentially a ‘closed CPB circuit’, able to provide full cardiorespiratory support.
- An RVAD is an extracorporeal system that bypasses the RV. This can be achieved with an open or percutaneous technique. In the open technique, mainly reserved for the postcardiotomy cases, a cannula drains the right atrium (RA) directly and

Fig. 1 Central VA ECMO

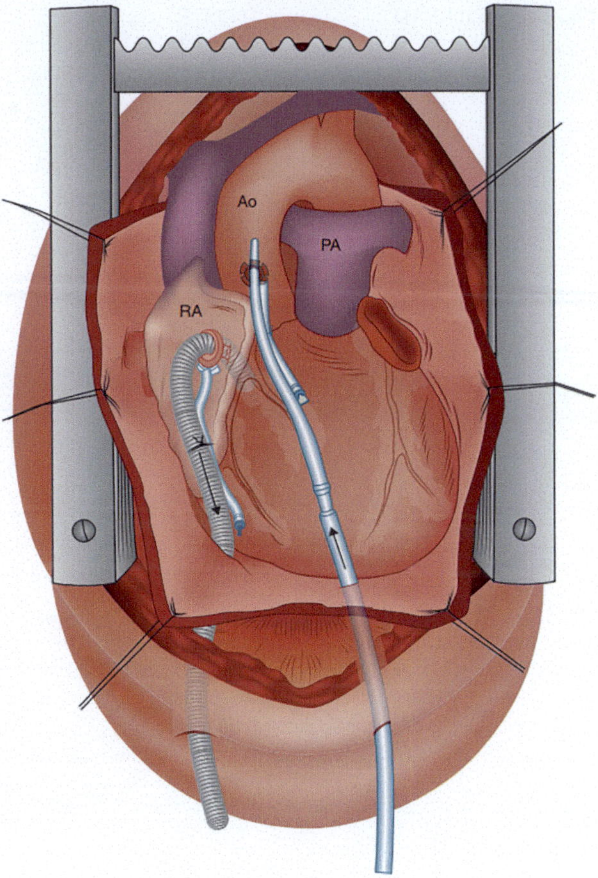

with the assistance of the centrifugal pump, blood is returned into the pulmonary artery (PA) via a vascular graft or an arterial cannula (Fig. 2). The percutaneous approach would entail two separate insertion points into large veins. The access cannula is often a multistage cannula introduced through the common femoral vein, whilst the return cannula is placed through the right jugular or subclavian vein, with the tip sitting in the main PA in a direction not dissimilar to a Swan catheter. However, percutaneous RVAD configuration may also be achieved with a single dual lumen cannula such as the ProtekDuo (LivaNova, London, UK). This technique only requires one insertion point into the right jugular or subclavian veins; the tip of the cannula is advanced into the PA whilst the more proximal aspect sits within the RA. Blood is drained into the external lumen at the level of the RA into the pump and returned from within the internal lumen into the PA via the distal opening. Any RVAD (open or percutaneous) circuit can have an oxygenator incorporated into it, thus providing oxy-RVAD support.

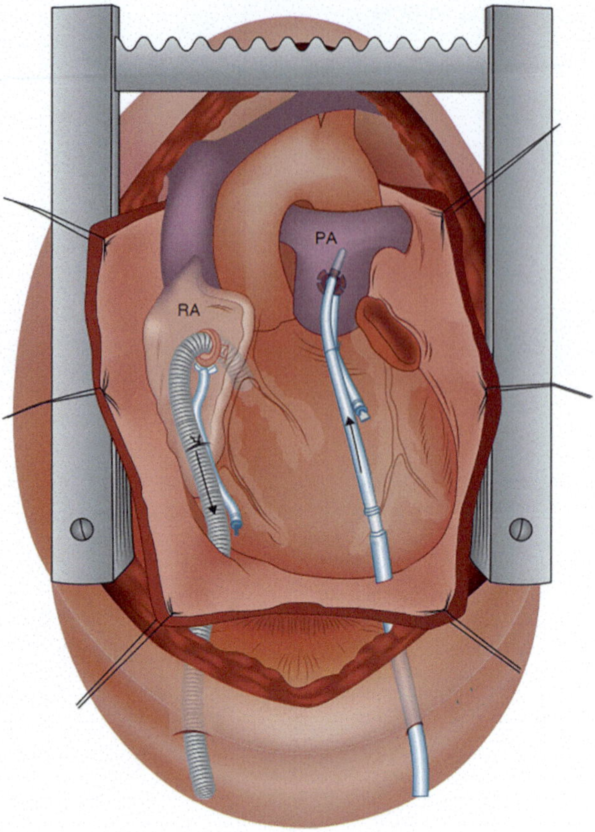

Fig. 2 Central RVAD

- An extracorporeal LVAD is a system that drains blood from the LA [through the right superior pulmonary vein (RSPV)] or directly from the apex of the LV into the centrifugal pump, returning it to the systemic circulation often via the aorta (Fig. 3). Therefore, the LVAD therapy can fully bypass the LV. In addition, blood entering the LA is pre-oxygenated by the lungs, provided that respiratory function remains intact, and therefore, an oxygenator may not be necessary. This is almost always performed as an open (surgical) procedure.
- BiVAD is a combination of the RVAD and LVAD. Blood is drained from the RA and returned into the PA on the right side of the heart, and from the LA (via the RSPV) or the left ventricular apex to the aorta on the left with the use of 2 centrifugal pumps configured in parallel (Fig. 4).

ECLS is part of a wider MCS strategy as, by definition, MCS also incorporates long-term durable devices such as the HeartMate 3 (Abbott, Chicago, IL), but more

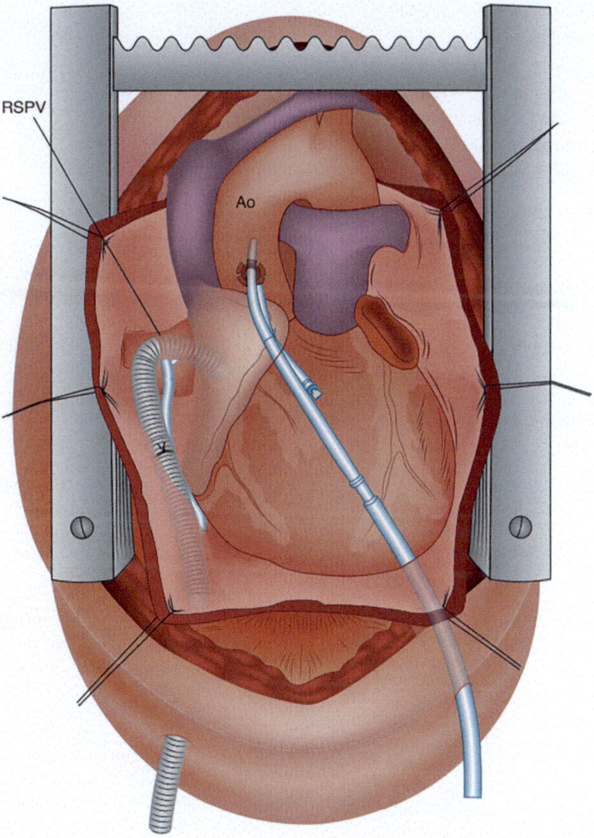

Fig. 3 Central LVAD

importantly for this topic, percutaneously placed pumps that are temporary yet not extracorporeal. The Impella (Abiomed, Danvers, MA) is a microaxial pump with the inflow located in the left ventricle and the outflow into the aorta just above the aortic valve. Impella pumps possess the capacity to provide forward flow up to 5.5 l/min, depending on the type of Impella and site of implantation, with its use gaining in popularity. The requirement for fluoroscopy for safe positioning makes it less attractive as a simultaneous procedure in the postcardiotomy setting, especially in the absence of a hybrid operating theatre, however, remains feasible with acceptable outcomes despite the early experience (Sommer et al. 2023). The Impella will herein be referenced as a means of LVAD or venting strategy; however, the mainstay of postcardiotomy temporary MCS remains the aforementioned extracorporeal systems.

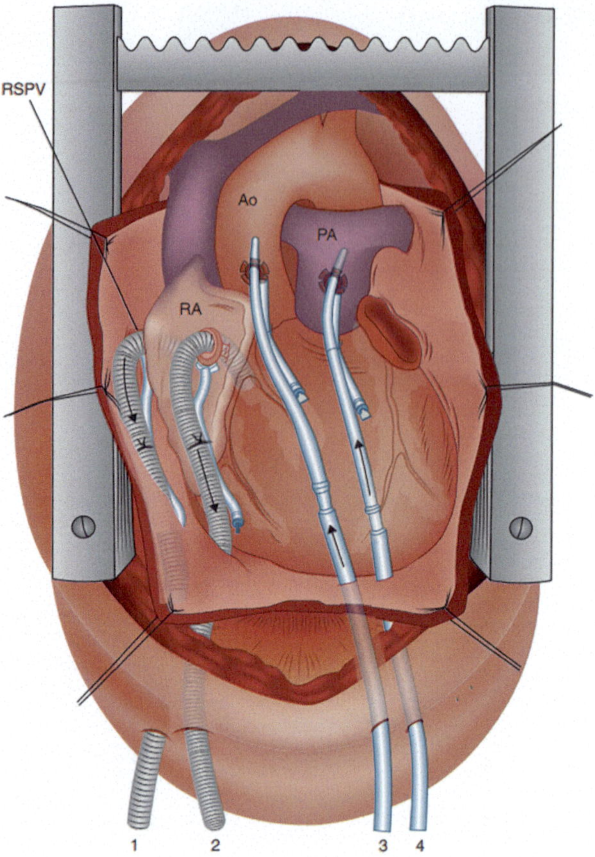

Fig. 4 Central BiVAD. It consists of an RVAD (access cannula 2 and return cannula 4) and an LVAD (access cannula 1 and return cannula 3) configured in parallel

2 Management of Perioperative Cardiogenic Shock with ECLS

Cardiogenic shock in the cardiac surgical patient can ensue before a procedure has taken place, and is often observed if the procedure is required as an emergency, e.g. postinfarct ventricular septal defect repair. However, cardiogenic shock may also present intraoperatively as postcardiotomy failure, or later in the early postoperative course.

2.1 Preoperative Optimisation with ECLS

Myocardial infarction, with or without mechanical complications, or other acute cardiovascular pathologies can occasionally lead to a rapidly evolving cardiogenic shock. For those cases where definitive management is surgical, there is observational data to suggest that haemodynamic and metabolic optimisation with MCS can yield better postoperative outcomes compared to intra- or postoperative institution of MCS (Minhas et al. 2022). Peripheral VA ECMO with or without the use of an Impella device is the configuration of choice (Fig. 5). At this point, it is pertinent to discuss the role of the Impella in VA ECMO as it can be a useful adjunct, one that is more likely to be utilised in the preoperative setting.

As previously mentioned, the objective of ECLS is to provide adequate tissue perfusion while the heart is 'rested', by offloading the function of the left or right ventricle, to allow for myocardial recovery in cases where when the condition is potentially reversible. In order for this to be achieved, the LV should not distend. In addition to aortic regurgitation, which must be assessed before commencing someone on VA ECMO, the physiological shunt of the bronchial circulation adds a reasonable amount of volume to the LA and subsequently the LV. Assuming one puts a perfectly normal heart on ECMO, once the volume of blood in the LV reaches a specific level, contraction is induced and blood ejected as per the Frank-Starling Law. However, the sick heart does not exhibit the same characteristics, hence the blood accumulates and distends the LV. Not only does this defeat the purpose of VA ECMO, which is to rest the heart, but also congests the lungs and hinders respiratory recovery. It is therefore appreciated that LV distention must be avoided, whilst evidence supports the use of an Impella to offer more effective and/or safe LV unloading compared to alternative methods such as inotropes, IABP and atrial septostomy.

The Impella has been used both in isolation pre-emptively for protected high-risk cardiac surgery, and also as a stabilisation method in patients in cardiogenic shock requiring emergency cardiac surgery (Pieri et al. 2024). The latter strategy, which is

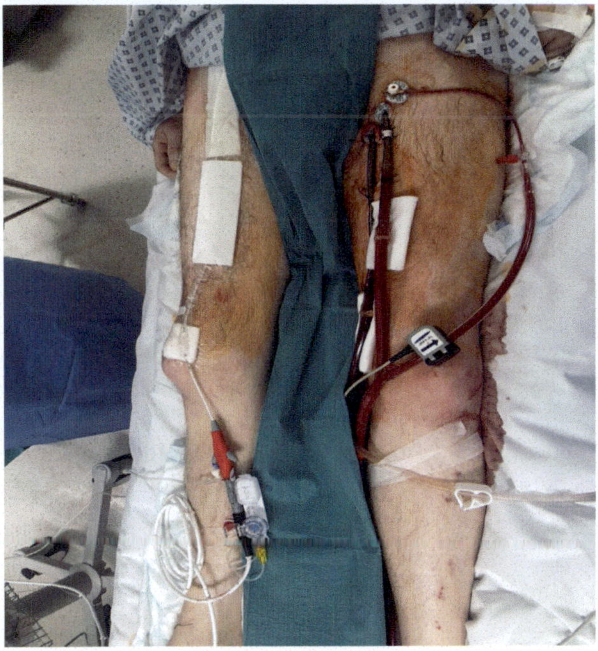

Fig. 5 Combination of peripheral VA ECMO (left of the patient) and Impella (right). Note the limb antegrade perfusion cannula

of relevance to this topic, appears to offer superior outcomes to the combination of VA ECMO and Impella based on results from observational studies (Marin-Cuartas et al. 2022). One has to be aware, however, that there is inherent selection bias in such studies, as patients receiving Impella device implantation are more likely to have isolated LV failure (rather than biventricular failure with respiratory impairment), and therefore be of a more favourable risk profile to their VA ECMO counterparts.

2.2 *Postcardiotomy ECLS*

The use of ECLS in the postacardiotomy setting is not a novel therapy; however, it has historically been delivered infrequently and only in a few select centres possessing the relevant expertise, mainly in heart transplantation. Even less than 10 years ago, there was an attempt by the author and other groups to gather evidence in the United Kingdom, quite sparse at the time, to reinforce its further adoption. It is now not only a more widespread and accepted means for the management of cardiogenic shock but also recommended in the postcardiotomy setting, endorsed by leading organisations in the field of cardiac surgery and critical care (Lorusso et al. 2020). Identifying the patients who would benefit the most from this therapy has also evolved. There are no universally accepted criteria for patient selection for VA ECMO or the other more selective forms of ECLS, and the decision-making is based on the survival probability with VA ECMO against the natural history of the disease progression. The use of survival prediction models in VA ECMO, such as the SAVE score can be useful tools, although, similar to other risk models, they have many limitations including the fact that they are not validated in the postcardiotomy setting (Schmidt et al. 2015; Erdoğan et al. 2024). The expert consensus published by EACTS/ELSO/STS/AATS on postcardiotomy ECLS is a very useful tool in the decision-making and its safe delivery (Lorusso et al. 2020). With regard to decision-making, there are two overarching principles, namely timing and recoverability, summarised as follows:

- Initiation of postcardiotomy ECLS must occur before the establishment of end-organ injury and anaerobic metabolism, as indicated by a lactate of <4 mmol/l. For the patient with postcardiotomy syndrome (i.e. inability to separate from CPB or persistent cardiogenic shock despite inotropes) and wherein IABP therapy with optimal medical management has failed to provide stability, early initiation of ECLS is required. There is evidence to suggest that establishing this therapy in the operating theatre provides superior outcomes to a staged procedure, taking place after a few hours following chest closure and a persistent low cardiac output state.
- The possibility of myocardial recovery is crucial. Should there be high likelihood for recovery, then the threshold for postcardiotomy ECLS initiation is lower.

However, if the possibility of myocardial recovery is low, then the candidacy of the patient for advanced MCS therapies (durable LVAD) or transplantation must be assessed and agreed prior to initiating ECLS. The list is not exhaustive though the following are considered as favourable criteria for transplantation and therefore for postcardiotomy ECLS if myocardial recovery is unlikely: age < 70, absence of secondary pulmonary hypertension (i.e. transpulmonary gradient <15 mmHg, PVR < 5 Wood units), BMI < 35 kg/m^2, no known neoplastic–metastatic disease, no end-organ dysfunction because of diabetes or peripheral arteriopathy or presence of irreversible renal dysfunction (cardiorenal syndrome), no current substance abuse, compliance with previous treatments and appointments, no evidence of frailty or severe cognitive-behavioural disabilities. The latter has to include the possibility of significant neurological injury due to persistent low-flow states during cardiogenic shock or arrest.

Another practical yet important consideration in the postcardiotomy ECLS setting is surgical bleeding. Conversion from CPB to VA ECMO whilst the patient is fully heparinised is challenging because, in the absence of cardiotomy suction, haemostasis must be achieved in the coagulopathic patient without the option of reversing the anticoagulatory effect of heparin. Heparin may not be reversed with protamine sulphate as the semi-porous membrane oxygenator present in the ECMO circuit may become laden with clots, preventing blood flow across the membrane of the oxygenator and back into the systemic circulation. For this reason, surgical causes of bleeding must be addressed fully before deciding to commence VA ECMO or any other types of ECLS involving an oxygenator.

The underlying pathology and the type of surgical procedure performed are also of paramount importance. With uncontrollable bleeding currently being the only absolute contraindication, other marginal conditions were ECLS was not considered a priori (e.g. post aortic dissection repair) have now become relative contraindications and determined both case by case and based on institutional expertise. In patients requiring post-CABG support, which represent the largest group in the postcardiotomy ECLS recipients, incompleteness of revascularisation and/or established infarct could determine candidacy. For example, significant myocardial damage that is unlikely to recover means that the patient will ideally need to meet transplant criteria before being considered for short-term ECLS. Equally, a valve condition that has not been fully corrected during surgery or exhibiting a complication/malfunction (e.g. a severe periprosthetic leak), which cannot be addressed further with surgical or percutaneous intervention, also increases the threshold to ECLS. Finally, VA ECMO and RVAD are useful adjuncts to address primary graft failure immediately after heart transplantation and acute RV dysfunction at durable LVAD implantation, respectively. As such treatments fall within the more specialist area of transplantation/heart failure surgery, perioperative ECLS indications and management will not be elucidated further.

3 Selection of ECLS Mode and Technical Aspects

As previously mentioned, the majority of patients presenting with cardiogenic shock requiring ECLS prior to cardiac surgery would receive a percutaneous device in the form of VA ECMO and/or Impella. This section is going to provide some insights and practical considerations in the postcardiotomy setting, including presentation of a clinical case as an example.

3.1 Selection of ECLS

Four primary means of ECLS have been identified and discussed, namely VA ECMO, RVAD, LVAD and BiVAD. The decision on which system is to be utilised in the postcardiotomy setting is taken by the dominant pathology, team expertise and equipment availability. Postcardiotomy RV dysfunction (pre-existing or new) is the most common pathology requiring ECLS, often in the form of an RVAD. The benefit of an isolated RVAD is that it can be delivered fully percutaneously allowing for chest closure and mitigating the associated bleeding complications of an open chest. Especially in the absence of an oxygenator, one can be more liberal with regard to temporary cessation of anticoagulation in this context. However, in the acutely charged emotional state that failure to wean from CPB could induce to the team, it is very difficult to accurately assess isolated ventricular function and oxygenation capacity of the lungs. It is also not uncommon that a well-functioning LV placed under ischaemia and prolonged CPB duration may develop signs of strain when preloaded with full RV output provided by an RVAD. Additionally, for the benefit of deploying a percutaneous RVAD, there will have to be capacity for fluoroscopy in the operating theatres or the option of transferring the patient to the interventional suite (mainly for the insertion and correct positioning of the return cannula), which is not ideal in this setting. For these reasons and for most cases at institutions that do not have an established advanced MCS programme, initiation of VA ECMO is preferred even when the dominant culprit for postcardiotomy failure is the RV. Similarly, there would be very few conditions where only the LV needs to be supported in isolation and native right ventricular function would be adequate to provide the preload necessary for an open LVAD. It requires expertise, and in the presence of efficient fully percutaneous MCS systems such as the Impella, the author would once again recommend establishment of VA ECMO first, provision of stability and transition to left-sided Impella later, if still indicated. In situations of biventricular failure leading to postcardiotomy syndrome, then VA ECMO should be the first choice of ECLS used. As VA ECMO provides nonselective CPB, the following principal conditions must be met in order to successfully and timely wean the patient from extracorporeal support to avoid unnecessary prolongation of ECMO and associated complications. Such conditions include recovery of RV function, recovery of the LV function and ability of the lungs to oxygenate adequately.

However, in acute biventricular failure, the rates of recovery can often be differential, presenting a physiology that does not favour complete discontinuation from VA ECMO altogether; instead, a staged transition to a more selective (and likely less invasive) ECLS system should be contemplated. The specific parameters and process for weaning from VA ECMO or other forms of ECLS are outside the scope of this chapter.

An open BiVAD is rarely recommended outside the cohort of heart transplant candidates who suffered deterioration and need to be stabilised for super urgent re-listing, and has therefore very little role in the postcardiotomy setting. If one, however, has elected to establish univentricular support and this is still not adequate to provide appropriate tissue perfusion and heart 'resting', a second VAD system can be inserted as a staged procedure, ultimately providing BiVAD support, e.g. percutaneous RVAD requiring left-sided Impella, or the opposite.

3.2 Technical Aspects

Certain technical aspects in the establishment and delivery of ECLS are important in complication mitigation; however, this consideration can also influence the type of ECLS to be utilised in different settings.

Arterial cannulation for peripheral VA ECMO: The average common femoral artery diameter is around 10 mm in adult males and 8 mm in females. As an example, a 20 Fr EOPA™ cannula (Medtronic) has a diameter of almost 7 mm, leaving little space within the artery for antegrade blood flow to the distal limb. Other than carrying out an open cut down with an end-to side vascular graft attachment, one can place an additional antegrade flow cannula into the superficial femoral artery at the time of VA ECMO cannulation providing distal limb perfusion (see Fig. 5). Improved limb arterial perfusion has a significant positive impact on limb viability and avoidance of complications. The authors also advocate for a carefully performed common femoral artery reconstruction upon decannulation as opposed to the mere tightening of pre-existing purse-strings.

Central (vs. peripheral) cannulation: Central VA ECMO cannulation provides the benefit of antegrade blood flow, which may limit the occurrence of LV distension as well as the appearance of differential oxygenation termed 'Harlequin' syndrome, especially if the lungs are not in a position to adequately oxygenate. The detailed physiology behind left ventricular distension (aortic regurgitation being an obvious reason), or 'Harlequin' is outside the scope of this chapter. Exchange of central aortocaval CPB to VA ECMO is straightforward; other than the short interruption of perfusion for the establishment of new connections, the conversion of standard half inch venous CPB tubing into 3/8 inch ECMO inflow cannula tubing will require a connector to the venous cannula. Surgeons should endeavour to approximate the sternum and close temporarily the skin by exteriorising the central cannulae through the upper anterior abdominal wall, or at least approximate the skin over the stented sternum to reduce bleeding complications, infection risk, and achieve more optimal chest tube management (compared to the fully opened chest covered by a membrane). Evidence is inconclusive with regard to optimal outcomes and mode of VA ECMO delivery (central vs. peripheral). We advocate central cannulation if the probability of left ventricular distention is high, such as in instances of minimal native ejection, when there is poor lung function, and in the presence of small or calcified peripheral vessels. Peripheral cannulation has a place if antegrade limb perfusion can be established, there is some natural unloading of the ventricle and less likelihood to require additional venting, and a 'hostile' chest where definitive chest closure at the time of original surgery is favoured. More technical aspects of cannulation (e.g. use of vascular grafts to facilitate outflow, exteriorisation techniques and sites for the tubing, and adjuncts to cannulation like pledgeted purse-strings and spigots) vary among surgeons and institutional preference and therefore will not be discussed further.

Other conditions could also influence the mode of ECLS used and type of cannulation. The presence of mechanical valves (most commonly aortic and mitral) can complicate VA ECMO with valve thrombosis or disproportionate left ventricular distension if there is no preload due to full flow ECMO, and heart ejection is minimal. For this reason, an isolated RVAD could be preferable if the main postcardiotomy issue is RV failure, or even pre-emptively decide to implant a bioprosthesis if there is a high probability that the patient would require ECLS as a bridge to postoperative recovery. This is also pertinent to the use of the Impella, which cannot be delivered through an aortic mechanical prosthesis, and can also cause issues with valve thrombosis in cases with a mechanical mitral valve in situ.

3.3 Clinical Case

We herein present a case, which culminates some of the aforementioned principles for decision making and techniques. A patient underwent a difficult redo aortic valve replacement with a mechanical prosthesis and suffered cardiac arrest while in hospital secondary to transient ostial right coronary occlusion. They had immediate chest reopening but acute right ventricular failure was apparent with bleeding of the left lung during mobilisation of adhesions. The patient was haemodynamically unstable and central CPB was initiated until a specialist team was called to manage the patient and possibly retrieve to the nearest MCS hub centre. VA ECMO was contemplated initially but the presence of a mechanical aortic prosthesis was in relative competition (for thrombosis) with the requirement of full flow for oxygenation and CO_2 removal, and resting of the RV. The heart was not fully mobilised previously from pericardial adhesions, as it was not deemed necessary, and access to the main pulmonary artery was difficult. It was therefore decided to establish percutaneous oxy-RVAD by accessing the right common femoral vein for drainage and return was obtained through the right subclavian vein with the use of a C-Arm fluoroscopy machine (Fig. 6) with concurrent separation from CPB. Patient transfer to the hub unit was completed and underwent percutaneous intervention of the main

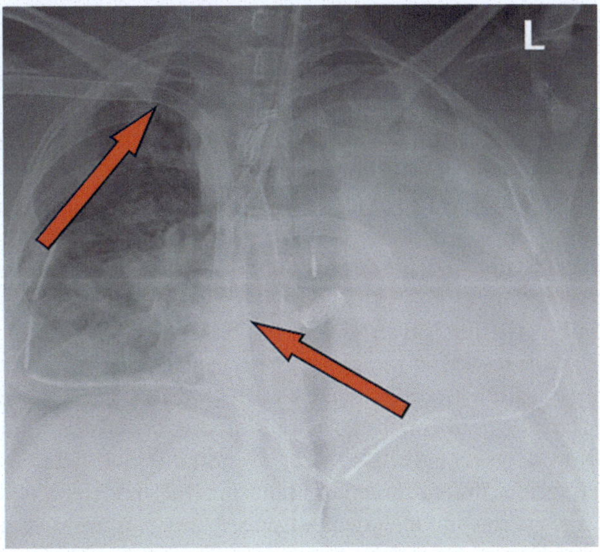

Fig. 6 Postcardiotomy percutaneous RVAD. Red arrows demonstrate the inflow (centre of the chest) and outflow (right of the chest) cannulae through the right common femoral and right subclavian veins, respectively

right coronary artery. The right ventricular function recovered eventually following a few days of support. Of note, one of the great benefits of RVAD with an oxygenator is that once right ventricular recovery has been obtained but lungs may still be affected, one can withdraw both venous cannulae appropriately and establish veno-venous ECMO for respiratory support only, as performed in this case.

4 Outcomes of Postcardiotomy ECLS

Postcardiotomy syndrome is highly lethal due to the vicious cycle of shock and irreversible organ damage as a result of pump failure, vasoplegia and metabolic disturbance. The outcomes of postcardiotomy ECLS have to be viewed against the almost certainty of rapid deterioration and death without it. There are no randomised controlled trials to compare ECLS against optimal medical management or other forms of short-term univentricular support in this setting. However, the use of observational data from large registries provides important insights into the complications and outcomes of postcardiotomy ECLS, the vast majority of which refers to VA ECMO. Once again, these are patients who tend to have worse outcomes post ECLS (against myocarditides, cardiomyopathies, or other causes) because they often have undergone prolonged or very complex procedures and more commonly than not have had a complication, corrected or uncorrected, that led to failure from separation from CPB.

Robust complication outcomes come from the PELS-1 multicentre cohort study of 2058 patients who received postcardiotomy VA ECMO (Mariani et al. 2023). Postoperative bleeding occurred in 57% of this cohort and was strongly associated with mortality. As previously discussed, the combination of coagulopathy from prolonged cardiopulmonary bypass, anticoagulation requirement for the VA ECMO, and open chest (42% in the study population), creates the substrate for bleeding, re-explorations (up to 40%), massive transfusion and transfusion-related complications. Stroke and leg ischaemia account for 10% of the complications each. Specifically for leg ischaemia, its incidence is less than some other reports (Bonicolini et al. 2019), likely because of the more widespread adoption of distal limb perfusion (66%) seen in PELS-1.

With regard to mortality, the recent report from the extracorporeal life support organisation (ELSO), which is the world's largest registry, demonstrated a 42% survival to hospital discharge of adult postcardiotomy VA ECMO recipients (Kowalewski et al. 2021). Similar mortality rates were reported in the PELS-1 study, alongside the observation that survival has remained unchanged over the last 20 years despite technical advancements and improvements in care protocols. It is extrapolated from data, however, and reinforced by our personal observations, that higher risk patients are nowadays offered the option of postcardiotomy ECLS as part of a standard escalation pathway. It has to be reiterated that this vulnerable group of patients would incur an almost always fatal outcome without initiation of some form of ECLS upon failure to separate from CPB. As such, survival rates in the 40% have to be viewed with optimism and positivity, as it is a testament to the commitment and tirelessness of a wider group responsible for the care of these patients.

5 Conclusions

Postcardiotomy ECLS is an efficient way to halt and reverse the spiral of cardiogenic shock whilst supporting the heart to regain its function, or bridge to an additional intervention including durable mechanical support and transplantation. VA ECMO is the most commonly utilised form of MCS, although depending on patient characteristics and team expertise, more selective temporary VAD support can be utilised. The rate of complications remains high but can be mitigated to an extent by certain practices (e.g. careful haemostasis and anticoagulation management, and distal limb perfusion), whilst mortality rates are acceptable for this very precarious pathology. Other percutaneous MCS devices in the form of microaxial pumps are being increasingly utilised which could potentially exhibit a more favourable risk profile, and further improve outcomes in patients suffering postcardiotomy failure.

References

Bonicolini E, Martucci G, Simons J, Raffa GM, Spina C, Lo CV et al (2019) Limb ischemia in peripheral veno-arterial extracorporeal membrane oxygenation: a narrative review of incidence, prevention, monitoring, and treatment. Crit Care 23. https://doi.org/10.1186/s13054-019-2541-3

Erdoğan SB, Bastopcu M, Usca MK, Çakmak AY, Sargın M, Aka S (2024) The utility of risk scores in postcardiotomy extracorporeal membrane oxygenation. Perfusion (United Kingdom) 39. https://doi.org/10.1177/02676591231154741

Kowalewski M, Zieliński K, Brodie D, Maclaren G, Whitman G, Raffa GM et al (2021) Venoarterial extracorporeal membrane oxygenation for postcardiotomy shock—analysis of the extracorporeal life support organization registry∗. Crit Care Med 49. https://doi.org/10.1097/CCM.0000000000004922

Lorusso R, Whitman G, Milojevic M, Raffa G, Mcmullan DM, Boeken U et al (2020) EACTS/ELSO/STS/AATS expert consensus on post-cardiotomy extracorporeal life support in adult patients. Eur J Cardiothorac Surg 2021, 59. https://doi.org/10.1093/ejcts/ezaa283

Mariani S, Heuts S, Van Bussel BCT, Di Mauro M, Wiedemann D, Saeed D et al (2023) Patient and management variables associated with survival after postcardiotomy extracorporeal membrane oxygenation in adults: the PELS-1 multicenter cohort study. J Am Heart Assoc 12. https://doi.org/10.1161/JAHA.123.029609

Marin-Cuartas M, Wehrmann K, Hobartner M, Lehmann S, Etz CD, Saeed D et al (2022) Perioperative temporary mechanical circulatory support with Impella in cardiac surgery patients. J Cardiovasc Surg 63. https://doi.org/10.23736/S0021-9509.22.12173-7

Minhas AMK, Abramov D, Chung JS, Patel J, Mamas MA, Zieroth S et al (2022) Current status of perioperative temporary mechanical circulatory support during cardiac surgery. J Card Surg 37. https://doi.org/10.1111/jocs.17020

Pieri M, D'Andria Ursoleo J, Nardelli P, Ortalda A, Ajello S, Delrio S et al (2024) Temporary mechanical circulatory support with Impella in cardiac surgery: a systematic review. Int J Cardiol 396. https://doi.org/10.1016/j.ijcard.2023.131418

Schmidt M, Burrell A, Roberts L, Bailey M, Sheldrake J, Rycus PT et al (2015) Predicting survival after ECMO for refractory cardiogenic shock: the survival after veno-arterial-ECMO (SAVE)-score. Eur Heart J 36. https://doi.org/10.1093/eurheartj/ehv194

Sommer W, Arif R, Kremer J, Al Maisary S, Verch M, Tochtermann U et al (2023) Temporary circulatory support with surgically implanted microaxial pumps in postcardiotomy cardiogenic shock following coronary artery bypass surgery. JTCVS Open 15. https://doi.org/10.1016/j.xjon.2023.06.015

Donor Heart Allocation Systems for Adult Recipients Incorporating Clinical Urgency—An International Comparison

William John Jenner, Stephen Pettit, and Steven Tsui

Abstract Heart transplantation remains the definitive treatment for advanced heart failure, but continues to be constrained by a global shortage of suitable donor organs. In response, national heart transplant allocation systems have evolved to determine the prioritisation of recipients based on clinical urgency, anticipated outcomes and equity of access.

This chapter provides an international comparative analysis of adult donor heart allocation frameworks, focusing on high-volume transplant systems including the United Kingdom, United States, France and Eurotransplant. It outlines the assessment of clinical urgency in advanced heart failure, including the role of inotropic dependence and mechanical circulatory support.

Key differences in allocation methodologies are identified, determining clinical urgency and other important factors within the frameworks. The chapter further explores the ethical foundations of organ allocation, considering the application of distributive justice and equity in contemporary practice.

Finally, the implications of allocation policy on waiting lists, transplant outcomes and system behaviours are discussed, together with future developments in donor heart distribution, including data-driven models and technological innovation. Insights from international allocation frameworks can guide clinicians and policymakers in developing fairer, evidence-based approaches to prioritising patients with advanced heart failure.

Keywords Heart transplant allocation systems · Donor heart allocation · Clinical urgency in heart transplantation · Global organ allocation policies · International heart transplant allocation · International transplant systems · Ethical allocation of organs · Advanced heart failure · Mechanical circulatory support · Heart transplantation

---

W. J. Jenner (✉) · S. Pettit · S. Tsui
Royal Papworth Hospital, Cambridge, UK
e-mail: william.jenner@nhs.net; stephen.pettit@nhs.net; steven.tsui@nhs.net

A. Kourliouros (ed.), *Emergency Cardiac Surgery*,
https://doi.org/10.1007/978-3-032-15787-4_19

Abbreviations

ACHD	Adult Congenital Heart Disease
CTAG	Cardiothoracic Advisory Group
DBD	Donation after Brain Death
DCD	Donation after Circulatory-Determined Death
ECMO	Extracorporeal Membrane Oxygenation
IABP	Intra-aortic Balloon Pump
MCS	Mechanical Circulatory Support
NUHAS	Non-Urgent Heart Allocation System
OPTN	Organ Procurement and Transplant Network
SUHAS	Super-Urgent Heart Allocation System
UHAS	Urgent Heart Allocation System
UNOS	United Network for Organ Sharing

1 Introduction

Heart transplantation is an excellent treatment for carefully selected patients with advanced heart failure, leading to median survival of around 15 years and good quality of life for most recipients. Improved recipient selection, donor optimisation, surgical techniques and post-transplant care have led to improved survival in successive eras (Javier et al. 2021). However, heart transplantation remains limited by a shortage of suitable donor hearts. For example, in 2022, there were only 3.53 heart transplants per million population performed in Europe, a lower rate than kidney (36.7) and liver (14.2) transplants (Global Observatory on Donation and Transplantation 2024). As a result of mismatch between demand for heart transplantation and supply of donor hearts, the median waiting time in the United Kingdom for patients who were registered on the non-urgent heart transplant waiting list between 1 April 2017 and 31 March 2020 was 867 days (95% confidence interval 631–1103 days), i.e. 2.4 years (NHS Blood and Transplant 2024).

Countries must allocate donor hearts in a manner that is acceptable to the public to maintain support for organ donation and transplantation. Many competing interests exist in organ allocation and most allocation systems have evolved to minimise waiting list mortality by prioritisation of patients in greatest need of transplantation, whilst trying to ensure acceptable survival and quality of life after heart transplantation.

This chapter will review international donor heart transplant allocation systems. It will focus on how clinical urgency is determined and incorporated into allocation policies. It will discuss how justice is maintained for patients awaiting heart transplantation. Finally, it will explore the consequences of allocation policies and consider the future of donor heart allocation.

2 How to Allocate a Donor Heart?

There is no universal approach to donor heart allocation. Each country determines its own method of allocating donor hearts to potential recipients. Firstly, careful assessment is required to determine whether a patient should be offered a place on the heart transplant waiting list. Key considerations are:

1. Does the patient have advanced heart failure despite optimal conventional treatment?
2. Does the patient have cardiac or non-cardiac issues that confer an unacceptably high risk of early death or poor long-term outcome after heart transplantation?

Once a patient is accepted for heart transplant, they will be assigned to a 'waiting list' of potential recipients. Waiting lists are typically managed by an individual transplant centre but are often shared with organ allocation networks. Multiple factors are considered in the decision to allocate a donor heart to a specific recipient, including donor-recipient matching factors such as blood group compatibility and donor–recipient predicted heart mass ratio and recipient factors such as the severity of heart failure and waiting time (NHS Blood and Transplant 2023a). In addition, logistical issues such as transplant centre availability, transport time for the donor organ and the expected total ischaemic times are important.

All patients waiting for heart transplantation are at risk of death or deterioration which may mean that heart transplantation is no longer possible. Minimising patient removal from the waiting list due to death or deterioration is a key consideration in many allocation systems. The principle of 'sickest first' is important in most allocation policies and waiting lists tend to be categorised by clinical urgency. This is challenging because tools to predict death or deterioration on the waiting list are imperfect. Furthermore, the sickest patients may also be at the greatest risk of death after transplantation and there is a risk of strategic futility. Heart transplantation in critical cardiogenic shock is associated with worse outcomes than in patients who have been stabilised (Barge-Caballero et al. 2013).

3 How to Assess Clinical Urgency in Advanced Heart Failure?

Prognostication in advanced heart failure is challenging. There are many causes of heart failure and these differ in clinical features, trajectory and impact on quality of life. Certain clinical features, biomarkers or objective measures of cardiovascular performance are associated with a higher likelihood of death, but there is inadequate precision to predict mortality at the level of a single individual. Multiple variables may be combined in statistical models of mortality prediction such as the Seattle Heart Failure Model (Levy et al. 2006) or the Meta-analysis Global Group in

Chronic Heart Failure (MAGGIC) score (Pocock et al. 2013), but these models are also insensitive, imperfectly calibrated and lack precision at the individual level.

As patients deteriorate whilst waiting for heart transplantation, they may be commenced on intravenous inotropes and mechanical circulatory support (MCS) to preserve end-organ function or sustain life. These interventions are frequently used as surrogates of clinical status.

3.1 Inotropic Support as a Surrogate for Clinical Urgency

Inotropic drugs may be used in patients with advanced heart failure when there is hypoperfusion and hypotension leading to cardiogenic shock or secondary end-organ dysfunction. Inotropes increase myocardial oxygen demand, increase the risk of arrhythmias and have generally been found to increase mortality in randomised placebo-controlled trials. As such, the need for inotropic support suggests that a patient is in urgent clinical need of heart transplantation. Use of inotropes as a surrogate for clinical urgency is common but imperfect because they are used at the discretion of clinicians. Furthermore, inotropic support may be inappropriate for certain advanced heart failure patients with deteriorating haemodynamics, such as those with frequent ventricular arrhythmias.

3.2 Mechanical Circulatory Support as a Surrogate for Clinical Urgency

Temporary MCS includes intra-aortic balloon pumps (IABP), veno-arterial extracorporeal membrane oxygenation (VA-ECMO), percutaneous ventricular assist devices and surgically implanted ventricular assist devices (Kar et al. 2012). Temporary MCS may be used for days, weeks or months, but patients must remain in an intensive care unit, and they are at high risk of adverse events such as infection, bleeding, thrombosis or device failure. Given this limited time-window, unless being used as a bridge to recovery, use of temporary MCS suggests that the patient is in urgent clinical need of heart transplantation.

Devices such as implantable left ventricular assist devices (LVAD) and total artificial hearts may be used for longer periods of support. These devices were historically limited by adverse events including bleeding, stroke, pump thrombosis, infection and device failure (Phan et al. 2023). However, magnetically levitated, centrifugal, continuous flow LVAD such as the HeartMate 3 (Abbott, Illinois, USA) have lower rates of adverse event and can be used to support patients at home for many years with good quality of life (Mehra et al. 2022). However, if adverse events do occur during implantable LVAD support, then these are associated with very high mortality.

Many allocation policies prioritise patients with temporary MCS or those with implantable LVAD who have developed certain device-related adverse events. However, prioritising patients with MCS may disadvantage patients who are unsuitable for such devices due to their underlying cardiac condition, including those with adult congenital heart disease (ACHD) and specific cardiomyopathies with a small left ventricular cavity. As such, these patients may require a specific priority status.

4 International Donor Heart Allocation Policies

Clinicians, centres and regulatory bodies have a responsibility to ensure fair allocation of any scarce and valuable resource. This section reviews international allocation policies, identified through search of literature and regulatory body websites. The focus is on countries with high-volume heart transplant programmes performing greater than fifty transplants per year and with transparent allocation policies.

4.1 United Kingdom

In the United Kingdom, donor heart allocation is regulated by the National Health Service Blood and Transplant (NHSBT) (NHS Blood and Transplant 2023a). Guidelines and policies relevant to heart transplant are overseen by the Cardiothoracic Advisory Group, which is a forum for clinicians and other parties to improve the number and quality of organs donated and transplanted, and to improve outcomes for patients awaiting and following transplant (ODT Clinical—NHS Blood and Transplant 2024).

The UK policy uses a tier-based system according to clinical urgency (Table 1). There are three tiers: the non-urgent heart allocation scheme (NUHAS), the urgent heart allocation scheme (UHAS) and the super-urgent heart allocation scheme (SUHAS) (NHS Blood and Transplant 2023b). The UHAS offers an intermediate level of prioritisation to patients who must satisfy one of a range of specific criteria, each of which is associated with a poor short-term prognosis. The SUHAS offers the highest level of prioritisation for patients who are receiving temporary MCS (Rushton et al. 2020).

All UK adult heart transplant centres have a regional allocation zone that are regularly adjusted to balance a centres' demand for heart transplantation (assessed by registrations on transplant waiting list) and supply of donor hearts (assessed by heart donation rates within zone). The purpose of regional allocation is to minimise donor organ travel time and therefore total ischaemic time. A donor heart is offered in the sequence shown in Figure 1.

Organs are allocated according to blood group to reduce the disadvantage experienced by blood group O recipients. Otherwise, patients within tiers are ordered by

Table 1 Listing criteria for UK adult urgent and super-urgent heart transplant allocation criteria

Category	Urgent heart allocation system	
21	Adult inpatient with advanced heart failure requiring continuous inotrope therapy and/or IABP support **AND** with a cardiac index of <2.0 L/min/m^2 **AND** at least one of the following sub-categories:	1. Cardiogenic shock: blood lactate >2.0 mmol/L **AND** clinical evidence of hypoperfusion 2. Cardiorenal or hepatic indication: eGFR <40 ml/min/1.73 m^2 **AND/OR** bilirubin >2× upper limit of normal (40 μmol/L) 3. Adverse pulmonary haemodynamics: TPG >12 mmHg **AND/OR** PVR >4 WU at baseline, despite conventional medical therapy, leading to the use of inotropes and resulting in improvement in TPG and PVR, in patients where durable LVAD therapy is not preferred
22	Adult long-term VAD or TAH patient, agreed by CTAG Adjudication Panel and evidence of agreement emailed to NHSBT, with one of the following complications:	1. Right ventricular failure dependent on inotropes 2. Recurrent systemic infection related to VAD/TAH 3. Other VAD/TAH issues including recurrent or refractory VAD/TAH thrombosis
23	Exceptionally sick adult patient—high risk of dying or having an irreversible complication but does not meet urgent listing criteria Patient registration must be agreed by CTAG Adjudication Panel and evidence of agreement emailed to NHSBT	
31	ACHD arrhythmia patients. Refractory arrhythmia (>1 hospital admission over last 3 months with haemodynamic instability or associated with kidney or liver dysfunction) Refractory arrhythmia (>1 hospital admission over last 3 months with haemodynamic instability or associated with kidney or liver dysfunction)	
32	ACHD patients with no option for conventional escalation of therapy. Inpatients unsuitable for inotropes and/or VAD with one of the following:	1. Bilirubin and transaminases >2× normal 2. Deteriorating renal function (eGFR <50 ml/min/1.73 m, or 20% reduction from baseline) 3. Requirement for dialysis/CVVH for fluid or electrolyte management 4. Recurrent admissions (>3 in preceding 3 months) with episodes of right heart failure or protein-losing enteropathy requiring ascites drainage
Category	**Super-urgent heart allocation system**	
11	Adult or small adult patient on temporary VAD or VA-ECMO support	
12	Agreed by CTAG (Heart) Adjudication Panel and evidence of agreement emailed to NHSBT, and either:	1. On IABP support 2. At imminent risk of dying or irreversible complications. Meets criteria for urgent listing but is not suitable for long-term VAD and/or other exceptional circumstances

From NHSBT Pol 229/11 Heart Transplantation: Selection Criteria and Recipient Registration, date 02/10/2023

Abbreviations: *IABP* intra-aortic balloon pump, *eGFR* estimated glomerular filtration rate, *VAD* ventricular assist device, *TAH* total artificial heart, *CTAG* cardiothoracic advisory group, *NHSBT* NHS Blood and transplant, *ACHD* adult congenital heart disease, *CVVH* continuous veno-venous haemofiltration, *VA-ECMO* veno-arterial extra-corporeal membrane oxygenation, *TPG* transpulmonary gradient, *PVR* pulmonary vascular resistance, *WU* woods units

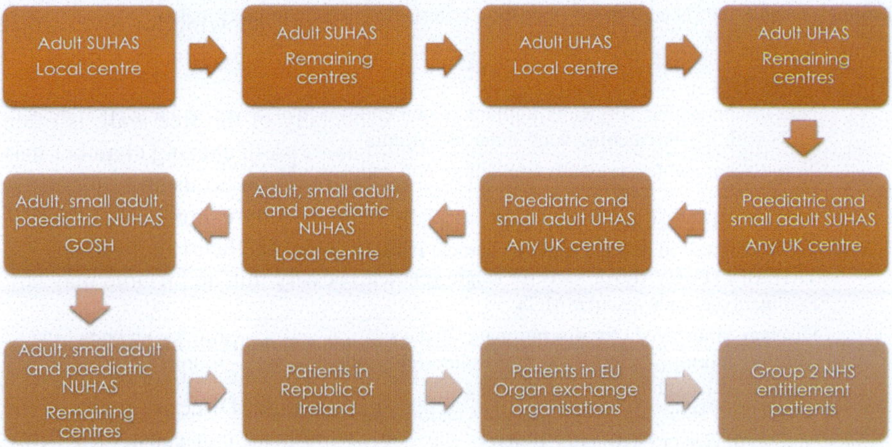

Fig. 1 The UK allocation of adult deceased brainstem death donor hearts. Donors ≥16 years old. (Adapted from POL 228/16—Heart Transplantation: Organ Allocation, NHS Blood and Transplant, Dec 2023)Abbreviations: *SUHAS* Super-urgent Heart Allocation Scheme, *UHAS* Urgent Heart Allocation Scheme, *NUHAS* Non-Urgent Heart Allocation Scheme, *GOSH* Great Ormond Street Hospital for Children, *EU* European Union

waiting time, but centres will consider size-matching, logistics and any other recipient characteristics that may be important.

4.2 United States

In the United States, the United Network for Organ Sharing (UNOS) regulates the network of transplant centres through the Organ Procurement and Transplantation Network (OPTN). The current OPTN adult heart allocation system was implemented in 2018, with allocation based on clinical urgency, blood type matching and geographical distance (Organ Procurement and Transplantation Network 2024). Clinical urgency status, like the United Kingdom, is based predominantly upon presence or absence of MCS, but has six statuses, rather than three tiers, from the most to least urgent (Table 2).

4.3 France

France has a points-based, rather than a tier-based, allocation system (Agence de la biomedicine 2021). Potential recipients receive a Candidate Risk Score, calculated using a regularly updated set of established biological variables, whilst also incorporating donor–recipient matching (Dorent et al. 2020). This system stratifies risk

Table 2 The US OPTN adult heart allocation criteria for medical urgency status

Status	Adult heart allocation, criteria for medical urgency status	
1	VA-ECMO Non-dischargeable, surgically implanted, non-endovascular biventricular support device MCS with life-threatening ventricular arrhythmia	
2	Non-dischargeable, surgically implanted, non-endovascular LVAD IABP V-tach/V-fib, mechanical support not required MCS with device malfunction/mechanical failure TAH, BiVAD, RVAD, or VAD for single ventricle patients Percutaneous endovascular MCS	
3	Dischargeable LVAD for discretionary 30 days Multiple inotropes or single high-dose inotrope with continuous haemodynamic monitoring VA-ECMO after 7 days; percutaneous endovascular circulatory support device or IABP after 14 days Non-dischargeable, surgically implanted, non-endovascular LVAD after 14 days	MCS with one of the following: device infection haemolysis pump thrombosis right heart failure mucosal bleeding aortic insufficiency
4	Dischargeable LVAD without discretionary 30 days Inotropes without haemodynamic monitoring Retransplant Diagnosis of one of the following: ACHD ischaemic heart disease with intractable angina hypertrophic cardiomyopathy restrictive cardiomyopathy amyloidosis	
5	On the waitlist for at least one other organ at the same hospital	
6	All remaining candidates	

Adapted from OPTN criteria for medical urgency status infographic (2/2018)
Abbreviations: *MCS* mechanical support, *IABP* intra-aortic balloon pump, *eGFR* estimated glomerular filtration rate, *LVAD* left ventricular assist device, *TAH* total artificial heart, *CTAG* cardiothoracic advisory group, *ACHD* adult congenital heart disease, *CVVH* continuous veno-venous haemofiltration, *VA-ECMO* veno-arterial extra-corporeal membrane oxygenation, *RVAD* right ventricular assist device, *BiVAD* biventricular assist device, *VAD* ventricular assist device

of mortality whilst awaiting transplantation (Agence de la biomedicine 2017). The calculation incorporates two factors related to severity of heart failure (use of VA-ECMO and concentrations of natriuretic peptides) and two factors related to end-organ dysfunction (GFR and bilirubin), which are each multiplied by a coefficient and summed to give an overall score. Exceptions to the scoring system can be requested where the score does not reflect certain high-risk situations.

Uniquely, the French allocation system also assigns a Transplant Risk Score to a donor–recipient pair, which is an estimate of graft loss following transplantation (Jasseron et al. 2019). This incorporates seven recipient variables (previous cardiac surgery, diabetes, ACHD and valvular heart disease, mechanical ventilation at transplantation, renal dysfunction, total bilirubin and age >50) and two donor variables (age and sex mismatch). If the estimate of graft loss at 1 year is greater than 50%, then this is deemed unacceptably high, and the recipient would not be eligible for that donor heart (Daniel et al. 2023). There is also a score attributed to the geography between donor and recipient, combining level of priority and travel time between the procurement and the transplant centres.

4.4 Eurotransplant

Eurotransplant is an organ-sharing system that involves eight central European countries (Austria, Belgium, Croatia, Germany, Hungary, Luxembourg, the Netherlands and Slovenia) and serves 137 million people (Moris et al. 2021). Eurotransplant has set goals of ensuring optimal use of available donated organs, having an objective and fair allocation system, supporting donor procurement, improving outcomes of transplantation and promoting, supporting and coordinating organ donation and transplant.

To achieve these goals, Eurotransplant holds a central database of listed potential recipients. Upon donor availability, the regional tissue typing laboratory determines the donor blood group and tissue typing, following which a matching list is created. It incorporates expected outcome criteria, clinical urgency, national organ balance and recipient waiting time into the allocation algorithm (Eurotransplant 2023). For clinical urgency, Eurotransplant has an international high-urgency (HU) status, below which, individual countries may have their own national HU status, which gives some flexibility to individual nations to modify their allocation process. In the Netherlands, for example, the HU status is split broadly into a 1A unstable tier and then a 1B stable but inotrope-dependent tier. Belgium includes residency status in allocation, whilst Germany incorporates recipient immunisation. Furthermore, Austria, Belgium and the Netherlands have active donation after circulatory-determined death (DCD) heart transplant programmes, which are accommodated into their national allocation systems.

4.5 Scandiatransplant

Scandiatransplant is a northern European organ-sharing programme spanning six countries, including Iceland, Norway, Sweden, Denmark, Finland and Estonia, and serving a population of 29 million people. It operates a common list process and stratifies patients into either Priority 0 or Priority 2 (Scandiatransplant 2023). Priority 0 includes patients on short-term MCS and long-term MCS with complications. Available organs are first offered to local priority 0 recipients, then nationally and then across the Scandiatransplant area. If there is no suitable priority 0 patient, then the organ is offered locally or nationally to priority 2 patients.

4.6 *Spain, Italy, Poland and the EU*

Spain updated their national heart allocation criteria in 2023, and stratifies potential recipients into four tiers from the highest urgency including MCS with biventricular support, down to regional urgency, and then prioritises patients based on sensitisation (González-Costello et al. 2024). In Italy, there are three tiers, urgent 1, urgent 2 and standard, which are linked to geographical availability of donors. Patients in urgent 1 can be matched with any of the national pool of donors, patients in urgent 2 have access to a macro-area (either the north or south of Italy) and the standard listing can only receive a donor heart from the local centre (Iacoviello et al. 2022). Poland, like France, has a point-based system, although this is based on treatments, rather than on biochemical markers (Poltransplant 2023).

Beyond the organ-sharing programmes, since 2010, a EU directive has provided legislation to encourage uniformity of standards and shared organ practice across the EU, and as such, 16 other European transplant programmes have arranged collaborative organ sharing with Eurotransplant (Directive 2010/53/EU of the European Parliament and of the Council of 7 July 2010 on standards of quality and safety of human organs intended for transplantation 2010).

4.7 *Canada, Japan and Australia*

Canada and Japan operate tier-based systems which are mostly according to therapy (Canadian Cardiac Transplant Network 2021; Fukushima 2023). However, in Canada, there are additional specific considerations when there may be multiple potential recipients for a donor, and that includes age, recipient sensitisation, duration on the waiting list and whether the patient and donor are in the same Canadian province (Chih et al. 2020). These differ from Australia, which prioritises donor hearts going to local recipients within the same state, before offering to recipients in other states on a rotational basis (The Transplantation Society of Australia and New Zealand 2024).

5 Comparison of International Allocation Policies

5.1 Allocation According to Mechanical Circulatory Support

The level of prioritisation given to patients with different forms of MCS differs between allocation systems. In the United Kingdom, United States, Canada, Spain and Italy, use of temporary MCS affords the highest priority. In the United Kingdom, the introduction of a highest priority tier for patients with temporary MCS was associated with a reduction in waiting time from 108 days (2014–2016) to 23 days (2017–2018) for these patients (Rushton et al. 2020). Eurotransplant has a single high-urgency status and does not differentiate between use of temporary MCS or inotropes. Since 2023, Spain has prioritised patients with temporary biventricular MCS above patients with temporary univentricular MCS. There are also differences between allocation systems in prioritisation of patients with adverse events during implantable LVAD support. For example, thrombotic adverse events fall into the highest-priority tier in Spain, Italy, Canada, Eurotransplant and South Korea, but an intermediate priority tier in the United States and United Kingdom.

5.2 Allocation According to Other Determinants of Clinical Urgency

With the exception of France, all allocation systems use current treatments, such as use of intravenous inotropic agents or use of MCS, as surrogate marker of clinical urgency. The French system is noteworthy because it uses some non-therapy-based biological parameters to identify patients who should be prioritised. This system may promote greater equity of access to organs between potential transplant recipients and reduce clinician bias. However, the French system has limited ability to discriminate patients with life-threatening arrhythmias, device-related complications and those supported with MCS apart from VA-ECMO. In the experience of one French centre, over 10% of listed candidates required exceptions to increase their priority on the waiting list, predominantly due to implantable MCS-related complications or arrhythmia (Daniel et al. 2023).

5.3 Other Allocation Priorities

Some countries try to prioritise patients who are less likely to receive transplants due to an immutable characteristic, such as their blood group or if highly sensitised to human leucocyte antigen (HLA) in the donor pool. In Canada, patients with high levels of anti-HLA antibodies (≥80% calculated reaction frequency) are allocated organs on a national basis, rather than on a regional basis (Canadian Cardiac Transplant Network 2021). In Spain, patients with greater than 50% calculated reaction frequency are given priority in organ allocation (González-Costello et al. 2024).

Some countries incorporate geographical logistics into their considerations. Canada and Australia are both vast countries but with contrasting approaches. In Canada, donor hearts are offered nationally to any patient on the highest tier of urgency. However, in Australia, organs are first offered within their state, and only if there is no potential recipient, are the organs offered to other Australian states.

6 Justice on the Waiting List

Transplant candidates, relatives and the wider population expect open and fair systems, and rely on overseeing organisations to implement this. Indeed, the first US heart transplant allocation policy from 1988 considered guidance in the 1984 National Organ Transplant Act that allocations should be equitable and based on specific criteria (Colvin-Adams et al. 2012). The US Code of Medical ethics expects that allocation of organs is based on 'likelihood of benefit, urgency of need, change in quality of life' and not non-medical criteria such as 'age, social worth, ability to pay, or the role of patients' lifestyle and behaviour in contributing to their illnesses' (Crigger 2016).

The OPTN assesses access to transplant against a framework of factors that have previously shown to contribute to health disparities (NIMHD Research Framework 2017). These include biological factors (blood group, immune sensitisation, body mass index and diagnosis), as well as sociocultural factors (age, citizenship, educational level, gender and ethnicity) and then healthcare system and environmental factors (insurance type, community risk score, rural vs. urban, distance to transplant centre and donation service area) (United Network for Organ Sharing 2016).

It is a challenge to create allocation policies based on clinical decision making that do not inadvertently contribute to health disparities. It may be challenging for a clinician to balance their responsibility to an individual patient with that of other potential recipients on the transplant waiting list. Whilst treatments such as continuous inotropic support or MCS are associated with a very poor prognosis, it must be acknowledged that these treatments are selected by clinicians for individual patients. As such, it is difficult to avoid clinician bias. This issue may be even more pronounced in countries where urgent listing is at the discretion of the local Transplant Unit Director, such as in Australia and New Zealand (The Transplantation Society of Australia and New Zealand 2023).

An example where non-clinical decisions influence waiting list position is the Israeli 2012 transplant allocation system, which awarded additional priority points based on a patient or their families' contribution to either being organ donors themselves, or being on the organ donor register (Berzon 2018). This was introduced due to a markedly low number of organ donors in a population with religious and cultural barriers to transplantation, which had driven a practice of potential recipients going abroad for organ transplantation, i.e. transplant tourism. Whilst incentivising the population may increase the donor pool to the waiting list cohort, the practical delivery of lowering the priority of candidates who had not signed up to be organ donors themselves is controversial and complicated to implement.

7 Consequences of Allocation Policies

7.1 Mortality on the Transplant Waiting List

One aim of integrating recipient clinical urgency into donor organ allocation is to reduce mortality on the waiting list. In the United Kingdom, following the 2016 policy change, an overall reduction in waiting list mortality was seen, from 5% to 2% (Rushton et al. 2020). This supported prioritising patients requiring temporary MCS above other urgent candidates. In the United States, introducing six tiers of clinical urgency in the 2018 system contributed to a significant overall improvement in time on the transplant waiting list, which was reduced from 112 to 39 days (Goff et al. 2020; Gong and Hall 2023). Patients with certain heart failure aetiologies have reported improved waiting list times, including patients with restrictive cardiomyopathy, hypertrophic cardiomyopathy and ACHD (Trivedi and Slaughter 2020). However, there was no difference in survival on the waiting list (OPTN Thoracic Committee 2020).

7.2 *Survival Following Heart Transplant*

Some countries have assessed whether implementation of a new allocation system has changed post-transplant survival. In the United States, once ischaemic time was accounted for, there were no differences in 30-day and 1-year mortality post-transplant following implementation of the 2018 system (Siddiqi et al. 2022). In the United Kingdom, prior to the new allocation system (2014–2016), 1-year post heart transplant survival was 80.6%, compared to 81.9% following the change in allocation (2017–2018) (Rushton et al. 2020). A 2017 change in the Spanish allocation system also did not result in overall change in post-transplant mortality (González-Costello et al. 2024).

The French system incorporates a transplant risk score to avoid futile transplants. In an analysis of the impact of the transplant risk score in one centre, only 3 of 257 candidates were excluded based on this score; however, more candidates were excluded from specific donor categories. For example, 12.4% of candidates were excluded from donors who were sex-mismatched and more than 55 years old (Daniel et al. 2023).

7.3 *Bias in Choice of Advanced Heart Failure Therapy*

Dependence on MCS is often used as a proxy for clinical urgency in allocation policies. However, decisions about timing and type of MCS vary from unit to unit and from country to country. A further consideration is whether to use temporary or implantable MCS, knowing that this influences donor allocation tier, and ultimately, the likelihood of whether a patient will receive a transplant (Gong and Hall 2023). For example, in the United States, initiating a potential recipient on temporary MCS could lead to status 2 priority, whilst an implantable LVAD could be status 4. Prior to 2018, implantable LVAD used to confer a discretionary 30 days of Status 1 in the United States, but this provision was removed when the UNOS allocation system was revised in 2018.

To promote appropriate treatment decisions in patients waiting for heart transplantation, the UNOS set haemodynamic criteria for initiating inotropic support or MCS. Despite this, use of implantable LVAD decreased and use of IABP and ECMO increased after the UNOS allocation system changed in 2018 (Parker et al. 2020; Mullan et al. 2021). Accordingly, transplant centres listed more high-priority status patients than expected after the UNOS allocation system changed, even with adjustment for candidate characteristics (Ran et al. 2021). A similar study compared management of 384 patients with cardiogenic shock before and after the change in the UNOS allocation system, and compared practice in US centres against Canadian and US non-transplant centres. The proportion of patients being treated with temporary MCS increased from 25% to 43% in US transplant centres, but did not change in non-US centres (Varshney et al. 2020).

A potential explanation for these observations is that patients want to receive a heart transplant and centres are financially incentivised to perform heart transplants. Patients and clinicians may therefore favour a form of MCS that affords prioritisation for heart transplantation. All allocation systems are vulnerable to bias, as clinicians attempt to increase the likelihood of their patient receiving a heart transplant. Centres competing in delivering a transplant must be carefully managed by overseeing bodies to ensure that national allocation systems maintain equity of access to organs for the whole population.

7.4 *Other Issues with Policy Changes*

Policy changes can sometimes result in unintended consequences. After the change in the UNOS allocation system in 2018, average organ travel distance increased from 82 miles to 243 miles and the resulting total ischaemic time also increased (Trivedi and Slaughter 2020). With increased travel came a doubling of procurement cost from $6,812.07 to $12,383.64 (Lampert et al. 2020). Furthermore, the increased use of temporary MCS since the implementation of the 2018 UNOS policy contributed to an additional cost of $40,000 per heart transplant in 2019 (Abramov et al. 2022).

Allocation systems can also change regional practice. A change in the Korean allocation system in 2018 led to regional disparities in duration on the waiting list and number of LVAD implants (Kim 2023). This was attributed to disproportionate regional numbers of brain deaths compared to transplant-performing hospitals, as well as regional transportation logistics.

7.5 *International Collaborations or National Allocation Systems*

Collaborative organ-sharing programmes rely on common goals that will be beneficial for the whole population. These networks appear to be particularly favourable for smaller countries, with the Eurotransplant programme assisting Croatia and Slovenia to deliver some of the highest rates of heart transplant per million population, whilst maintaining a balance of donor organs allocated across the members states (Miličić 2023).

Organ-sharing systems also support collaboration of expertise and services. As such, Eurotransplant has developed a more liberal approach to accepting donors with a higher prevalence of cardiovascular risk factors including smoking and hypertension, more donors aged 56–64 and more donations after circulatory-determined death (Wayda et al. 2023). This has been associated with a steady reduction in the Eurotransplant heart waiting list mortality, from 22.1% in 2009 to 11.3%

in 2018, despite an increasing proportion of patients being on the waiting list for more than 12 months (Moris et al. 2021).

However, coordinating an international organ-sharing programme relies on collaborations that may need to overcome cultural, ethical and economic differences, organ travel distances, language barriers and legal obstacles. Scandiatransplant recently assessed these factors when reviewing whether to integrate Lithuania and Latvia. A working group considered each country's current transplant programmes, potential impact on the existing organ sharing within Scandinavia, potential benefits to the populations of Lithuania and Latvia and each state's ethical and legal approach to transplantation (Scandiatransplant work group 2022).

8 Future Considerations for Donor Heart Allocation

Future allocation policies need to balance technological and ethical developments in heart transplantation. International heart allocation policies may be shaped by better predictive models for pre- and post-transplant survival, as seen in other organs (Loupy et al. 2019). Artificial intelligence may improve risk prediction in advanced heart failure and heart transplantation (Grzyb et al. 2024). Machine learning methods have improved prediction of LVAD and transplant failure (Kampaktsis et al. 2021). Based on the French models, a candidate risk score was developed for 16,905 US heart transplant candidates (Zhang et al. 2024). This score predicted waiting list mortality more accurately than the current 6-tiered UNOS allocation system. Automated systems such as candidate risk scores may also reduce treatment bias introduced by clinicians. However, systems will continue to need a clinician exception where scoring does not reflect certain high-risk situations and there is always a need for human scrutiny of allocation decisions (Palmieri et al. 2023).

The potential pool of donor hearts has increased over the past decade with development of DCD heart transplantation and machine perfusion technology that can enable longer periods of organ transport. Approximately one-third of heart transplants in the United Kingdom now result from DCD donors (Messer et al. 2016, 2020). Organs may now be transported across distances that would previously have been impossible (Lebreton and Leprince 2024). As such, countries with DCD heart programmes must decide how to include these organs within their allocation policies and whether to adopt machine perfusion technology.

9 Conclusion

The chapter has reviewed the justifications for heart transplant allocation policies and compared policies in countries with large transplant programmes. Clinical urgency is the most important factor in organ allocation, but the definition of clinical urgency is variable and subject to bias. Allocation policies should improve equity of access to organs and improve outcomes for patients waiting for heart transplantation, but may have unintended consequences. Future donor heart allocation policies will need to consider real-world data, technological advances and population expectations to ensure that they remain just and fair to the population who donate organs.

References

Abramov D et al (2022) Impact of the heart transplant allocation policy change on inpatient cost of index hospitalization. Clin Transpl 36(7):e14692. https://doi.org/10.1111/ctr.14692

Agence de la biomedicine (2017) Guide du Score Coeur. Available at: https://www.agence-biomedecine.fr/IMG/pdf/guide_score_coeur_2018.pdf. Accessed 8 June 2024

Agence de la biomedicine (2024) Organes—Greffe cardiaque. Available at: https://rams.agence-biomedecine.fr/greffe-cardiaque-0. Accessed 8 June 2024

Barge-Caballero E et al (2013) Preoperative INTERMACS profiles determine postoperative outcomes in critically ill patients undergoing emergency heart transplantation: analysis of the Spanish National Heart Transplant Registry. Circ Heart Fail 6(4):763–772. https://doi.org/10.1161/CIRCHEARTFAILURE.112.000237

Berzon C (2018) Israel's 2008 Organ Transplant Law: continued ethical challenges to the priority points model. Isr J Health Policy Res 7:11. https://doi.org/10.1186/s13584-018-0203-6

Canadian Cardiac Transplant Network (2021) Heart Status Listing Revision. Available at: https://ccs.ca/wp-content/uploads/2022/01/StatusListingRevision_November9_2021.pdf. Accessed 17 Sept 2024

Chih S et al (2020) Canadian Cardiovascular Society/Canadian Cardiac Transplant Network Position Statement on Heart Transplantation: patient eligibility, selection, and post-transplantation care. Can J Cardiol 36(3):335–356. https://doi.org/10.1016/j.cjca.2019.12.025

Colvin-Adams M et al (2012) Lung and heart allocation in the United States. Am J Transplant 12(12):3213–3234. https://doi.org/10.1111/j.1600-6143.2012.04258.x

Crigger B-J (2016) AMA Code of Medical Ethics' opinions relevant to organ transplantation and procurement. AMA J Ethics 18(2):122–125. https://doi.org/10.1001/journalofethics.2016.18.2.coet1-1602

Daniel L et al (2023) Practical application of the French two-score heart allocation scheme: insights from a high-volume heart transplantation centre. Arch Cardiovasc Dis 116(4):210–218. https://doi.org/10.1016/j.acvd.2023.02.004

Directive 2010/53/EU of the European Parliament and of the Council of 7 July 2010 on standards of quality and safety of human organs intended for transplantation (2010). Available at: http://data.europa.eu/eli/dir/2010/53/2010-08-06/eng. Accessed 10 June 2024

Dorent R et al (2020) New French heart allocation system: comparison with Eurotransplant and US allocation systems. Am J Transplant 20(5):1236–1243. https://doi.org/10.1111/ajt.15816

Fukushima N (2023) Heart transplantation and mechanical circulatory support in Japan—past, current and future aspects. In: End stage therapy and heart transplantation. IntechOpen. Available at: https://doi.org/10.5772/intechopen.113730

Global Observatory on Donation and Transplantation (2024) GODT Data charts and tables, GODT. Available at: https://www.transplant-observatory.org/data-charts-and-tables/. Accessed 11 June 2024

Goff RR et al (2020) A change of heart: preliminary results of the US 2018 adult heart allocation revision. Am J Transplant 20(10):2781–2790. https://doi.org/10.1111/ajt.16010

Gong TA, Hall SA (2023) Challenges with the current United Network for Organ Sharing heart allocation system. Curr Opin Organ Transpl 28(5):355. https://doi.org/10.1097/MOT.0000000000001092

González-Costello J et al (2024) Review of the allocation criteria for heart transplant in Spain in 2023. SEC-Heart Failure Association/ONT/SECCE consensus document. Rev Esp Cardiol (English Edition) 77(1):69–78. https://doi.org/10.1016/j.rec.2023.11.001

Grzyb C, Du D, Nair N (2024) Artificial intelligence approaches for predicting the risks of durable mechanical circulatory support therapy and cardiac transplantation. J Clin Med 13(7):2076. https://doi.org/10.3390/jcm13072076

Iacoviello M et al (2022) Position paper ANMCO: Percorso assistenziale del paziente con insufficienza cardiaca avanzata candidabile a trapianto/assistenza ventricolare meccanica. G Ital Cardiol 23(5):340–378

Jasseron C et al (2019) Optimization of heart allocation: the transplant risk score. Am J Transplant 19(5):1507–1517. https://doi.org/10.1111/ajt.15201

Javier MFVM, Javier Delmo EM, Hetzer R (2021) Evolution of heart transplantation since Barnard's first. Cardiovasc Diagn Ther 11(1):171–182. https://doi.org/10.21037/cdt-20-289

Kampaktsis PN et al (2021) State-of-the-art machine learning algorithms for the prediction of outcomes after contemporary heart transplantation: results from the UNOS database. Clin Transpl 35(8):e14388. https://doi.org/10.1111/ctr.14388

Kar B et al (2012) Percutaneous circulatory support in cardiogenic shock. Circulation 125(14):1809–1817. https://doi.org/10.1161/CIRCULATIONAHA.111.040220

Kim K-H (2023) Optimizing outcomes for post-ECMO heart transplant patients in South Korea: addressing multi-organ failure and allocation challenges. Int J Heart Failure 5(2):100–101. https://doi.org/10.36628/ijhf.2023.0023

Lampert BC et al (2020) More money and more miles: the hidden costs of donor procurement with the new heart allocation system. J Heart Lung Transplant 39(4):S175. https://doi.org/10.1016/j.healun.2020.01.745

Lebreton G, Leprince P (2024) Successful heart transplant after 12 h preservation aboard a commercial flight. Lancet 403(10431):1019. https://doi.org/10.1016/S0140-6736(24)00258-7

Levy WC et al (2006) The Seattle Heart Failure Model: prediction of survival in heart failure. Circulation 113(11):1424–1433. https://doi.org/10.1161/CIRCULATIONAHA.105.584102

Loupy A et al (2019) Prediction system for risk of allograft loss in patients receiving kidney transplants: international derivation and validation study. BMJ 366:l4923. https://doi.org/10.1136/bmj.l4923

Mehra MR et al (2022) Five-year outcomes in patients with fully magnetically levitated vs axial-flow left ventricular assist devices in the MOMENTUM 3 randomized trial. JAMA 328(12):1233–1242. https://doi.org/10.1001/jama.2022.16197

Messer SJ et al (2016) Functional assessment and transplantation of the donor heart after circulatory death. J Heart Lung Transplant 35(12):1443–1452. https://doi.org/10.1016/j.healun.2016.07.004

Messer S et al (2020) A 5-year single-center early experience of heart transplantation from donation after circulatory-determined death donors. J Heart Lung Transplant 39(12):1463–1475. https://doi.org/10.1016/j.healun.2020.10.001

Miličić D (2023) Thirty-five years of heart transplantation in Croatia. Medicus 32(2. Transplantacija):265–269

Moris D et al (2021) Decreasing wait list mortality for heart transplantation in the Eurotransplant Network. Exp Clin Transplant 19(5):508–509. https://doi.org/10.6002/ect.2020.0420

Mullan CW et al (2021) Changes in use of left ventricular assist devices as bridge to transplantation with new heart allocation policy. JACC Heart Failure 9(6):420–429. https://doi.org/10.1016/j.jchf.2021.01.010

NHS Blood and Transplant (2023a) Heart Allocation Policy—POL228. Available at: https://www.odt.nhs.uk/transplantation/tools-policies-and-guidance/policies-and-guidance/. Accessed 8 June 2024

NHS Blood and Transplant (2023b) Heart Selection Policy—POL229. Available at: https://www.odt.nhs.uk/transplantation/tools-policies-and-guidance/policies-and-guidance/. Accessed 8 June 2024

NHS Blood and Transplant (2024) Transplant activity report, Section 7—Cardiothoracic activity. NHS Blood and Transplant. Available at: https://www.organdonation.nhs.uk/helping-you-to-decide/about-organ-donation/statistics-about-organ-donation/transplant-activity-report/. Accessed 6 Sept 2024

NIMHD Research Framework (2017) National Institute on Minority Health and Health Disparities. Available at: https://www.nimhd.nih.gov/researchFramework. Accessed 7 July 2024

ODT Clinical—NHS Blood and Transplant (2024) Cardiothoracic Advisory Group, ODT Clinical—NHS Blood and Transplant. Available at: https://www.odt.nhs.uk/transplantation/cardiothoracic/cardiothoracic-advisory-group/. Accessed 1 July 2024

OPTN Thoracic Committee (2020) One-year monitoring of heart allocation proposal to modify the heart allocation system. Final Report. Available at: https://www.google.com/url?sa=t&source=web&rct=j&opi=89978449&url=https://optn.transplant.hrsa.gov/media/3701/data_report_thoracic_committee_heart_subcommittee_20200227_rpt1_revised_508_compliant.pdf&ved=2ahUKEwinmuzQ8MyGAxUQT0EAHWyNBDoQFnoECBMQAQ&usg=AOvVaw23xqWbXxyiEAH0wW26mD1f. Accessed 8 June 2024

Organ Procurement and Transplantation Network (2024) OPTN Organ Procurement and Transplantation Network Policy 6: allocation of hearts and heart-lungs. Available at: https://optn.transplant.hrsa.gov/professionals/by-organ/heart-lung/. Accessed 8 June 2024

Palmieri V et al (2023) Artificial intelligence, big data and heart transplantation: actualities. Int J Med Inform 176:105110. https://doi.org/10.1016/j.ijmedinf.2023.105110

Parker WF et al (2020) Practice changes at U.S. transplant centers after the new adult heart allocation policy. J Am Coll Cardiol 75(23):2906–2916. https://doi.org/10.1016/j.jacc.2020.01.066

Phan J et al (2023) Thrombotic and hemorrhagic complications following left ventricular assist device placement: an emphasis on gastrointestinal bleeding, stroke, and pump thrombosis. Cureus 15(12):e51160. https://doi.org/10.7759/cureus.51160

Pocock SJ et al (2013) Predicting survival in heart failure: a risk score based on 39 372 patients from 30 studies. Eur Heart J 34(19):1404–1413. https://doi.org/10.1093/eurheartj/ehs337

Poltransplant (2023) Zasady alokacji i dystrybucji pobrań serc uwzględniające wielonarządowe przeszczepy serca i płuc

Ran G et al (2021) Between-center variation in high-priority listing status under the new heart allocation policy. Am J Transplant 21(11):3684–3693. https://doi.org/10.1111/ajt.16614

Rushton S et al (2020) The introduction of a super-urgent heart allocation scheme in the UK: a 2-year review. J Heart Lung Transplant 39(10):1109–1117. https://doi.org/10.1016/j.healun.2020.06.013

Scandiatransplant (2023) Guidelines for Thoracic Organ Exchange in the Scandiatransplant Area (April 2023). Available at: https://www.scandiatransplant.org/organ-allocation/Guideline_SHLG_april_2023.pdf. Accessed 10 June 2024

Scandiatransplant work group (2022) Report from the Scandiatransplant Work Group on Evaluation of Membership for organ transplant hospitals in Riga (Latvia) and Kaunas and Vilnius (Lithuania). Available at: http://www.scandiatransplant.org/about-scandiatransplant/organisation/working-group-on-latvia-lithuania. Accessed 10 June 2024

Siddiqi U et al (2022) Ischemic time and patient outcomes after the 2018 UNOS donor heart allocation system change. J Card Surg 37(9):2685–2690. https://doi.org/10.1111/jocs.16668

The Transplantation Society of Australia and New Zealand (2023) Clinical guidelines for organ transplantation from deceased donors V1.11

The Transplantation Society of Australia and New Zealand (2024) National SOP: organ allocation organ rotation urgent listing version 4.1. ATCA-OTA-TSANZ Standard Operating Procedures (SOPs)

Trivedi JR, Slaughter MS (2020) "Unintended" consequences of changes in heart transplant allocation policy: impact on practice patterns. ASAIO J 66(2):125. https://doi.org/10.1097/MAT.0000000000001128

United Network for Organ Sharing (2016) Organ transplantation, report on equity in access. Available at: https://insights.unos.org/equity-in-access/. Accessed 7 July 2024

Varshney AS et al (2020) Use of temporary mechanical circulatory support for management of cardiogenic shock before and after the united network for organ sharing donor heart allocation system changes. JAMA Cardiol 5(6):1–6. https://doi.org/10.1001/jamacardio.2020.0692

Wayda B et al (2023) Disparities in donor heart acceptance between the USA and Europe: clinical implications. Eur Heart J 44(44):4665–4674. https://doi.org/10.1093/eurheartj/ehad684

Zhang KC et al (2024) Development and validation of a risk score predicting death without transplant in adult heart transplant candidates. JAMA 331(6):500–509. https://doi.org/10.1001/jama.2023.27029

Emergency Surgery in Patients with Left Ventricular Assist Devices

Aris Karatasakis, Dominik Steck, and Ioannis Dimarakis

Abstract Durable left ventricular assist devices (LVADs) have transformed care for patients with end-stage heart failure, functioning as both a bridge to transplantation and destination therapy. Advances in device technology, particularly magnetically levitated pumps, have improved survival and reduced complications. However, LVAD recipients remain prone to surgical emergencies related to device failure, anticoagulation, altered haemodynamics, and comorbidities. This chapter discusses the incidence, presentation, and management of urgent surgical scenarios in this population.

Keywords Heart-assist devices · Heart failure · Ventricular assist device (VAD) · Left ventricular assist device (LVAD) · VAD postoperative complications · LVAD emergencies · LVAD outflow graft obstruction · LVAD driveline damage · LVAD pump thrombosis · LVAD exchange · Heart transplantation

1 Introduction

Durable mechanical circulatory support with left ventricular assist devices (LVADs) has markedly advanced the management of patients with end-stage heart failure over the past decades. Two major indications for LVAD

A. Karatasakis
Section of Advanced Heart Failure and Transplant, Division of Cardiology, Department of Medicine, University of Washington, Seattle, WA, USA

D. Steck
Department of Anesthesiology & Pain Medicine, University of Washington, Seattle, WA, USA

I. Dimarakis (✉)
Division of Cardiothoracic Surgery, Department of Surgery, University of Washington, Seattle, WA, USA
e-mail: ijd22@uw.edu

A. Kourliouros (ed.), *Emergency Cardiac Surgery*,
https://doi.org/10.1007/978-3-032-15787-4_20

implantation are currently recognised: bridge to heart transplantation (BTT) and permanent destination therapy in refractory heart failure patients not planned for transplantation at the time of implant (destination therapy, DT). In the United States alone, more than 25,000 patients have received a durable LVAD in the 10-year period spanning 2013–2022 (Jorde et al. 2024). Technological developments, including the increasing use of magnetically levitated devices with improved haemocompatibility outcomes (thrombosis, stroke, bleeding) have contributed to ongoing improvement in survival (86% at 1 year and 64% at 5 years in a real-world setting) (Jorde et al. 2024; Mehra et al. 2019, 2022). Despite these advancements, patients with durable LVADs remain vulnerable to a variety of complications that may constitute surgical emergencies relating to device components, need for indefinite therapeutic anticoagulation, altered haemodynamics with non-pulsatile blood-flow, and a constellation of comorbidities that often accompany advanced heart failure. The purpose of this chapter is to address the incidence, presentation, and management of common urgent/emergent surgical scenarios encountered in this population.

2 Basics of LVAD Function

LVADs encountered in contemporary clinical practice are continuous-flow pumps, as opposed to the prior generation pulsatile-flow devices, consisting of a combination of fundamental components including: (i) the pump itself, (ii) an inflow cannula draining the left ventricle (LV), (iii) an outflow graft connecting the pump to the ascending aorta (rarely to the descending aorta or subclavian artery (Dorken Gallastegi et al. 2022; Bedi et al. 2022)), (iv) an extracorporeal controller, (v) a driveline cable connecting the controller and pump, and (vi) a power source connected to the controller (Figure 1). Key characteristics of the three most prevalent devices in the United States are shown in Table 1. The HeartMate II (Abbott, Lake County, Illinois) was the latest iteration of an *axial*-flow device. Newer *centrifugal* flow devices include the HeartWare HVAD System (Medtronic, Minneapolis, Minnesota) and the HeartMate 3 (Abbott, Lake County, Illinois). The HVAD is no longer commercially available since a Class I recall in June 2021 due to unexpected pump stoppage with failed or delayed restart, as well as accumulating data about increased mortality and cerebrovascular events compared with the other latest-generation devices (FDA 2024; Cho et al. 2021). The HeartMate 3 succeeded HeartMate II device following publication of the MOMENTUM 3 trial showing superior outcomes, and is the only device currently available for de novo implantation in the United States (Mehra et al. 2022). All of these devices require long-term therapeutic anticoagulation for safe operation, typically with warfarin to achieve an international normalised ratio of 2 to 3, and often antiplatelet agent as adjuncts.

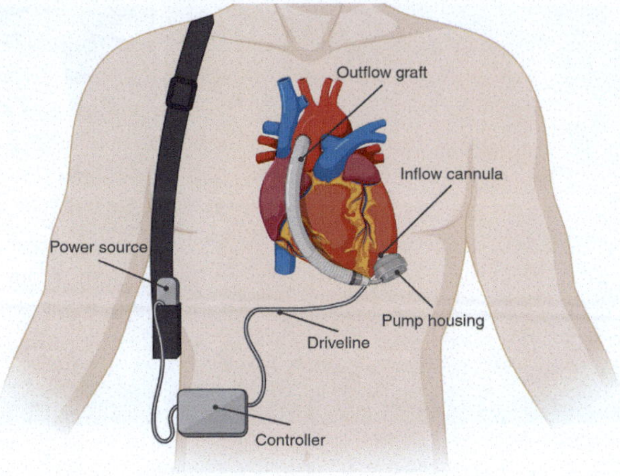

Fig. 1 Contemporary left ventricular assist device components. (Created in BioRender. Karatasakis, A. (2024) BioRender.com/l01s679)

Table 1 Key features of LVAD systems encountered in contemporary practice

Device name	HeartMate 3	HeartWare HVAD	HeartMate II
Pump type	Centrifugal - fully magnetically levitated	Centrifugal, hybrid	Axial
Pump position	Intrathoracic	Intrathoracic	Extrathoracic (pre--peritoneal/ intra-abdominal)
Pump speed (RPM); usual range (full range)	5000–6000 (3000–9000)	2800–3200 (1800–4000)	8000–10,000 (6000–15,000)
Pump flow[a] (L/min)	4–6	4–6	4–7
Pulsatility index[a] (flow pulsatility)	3.5–5.5	2–4	5–8
Pump power[a] (W)	4.5–6.5	3–7	5–8
Outflow graft diameter (mm)	14	10	14

[a]Typical clinical operating range

3 Surgical Anatomy

An appreciation of contemporary surgical implantation techniques is required to comprehend the anatomic location of LVAD components and avoid potential pitfalls during surgical dissection. Implantation can be performed either via median sternotomy or sternum-sparing approaches combining a limited left anterior thoracotomy with a right upper parasternal rib sparing incision. Main determinants of choice

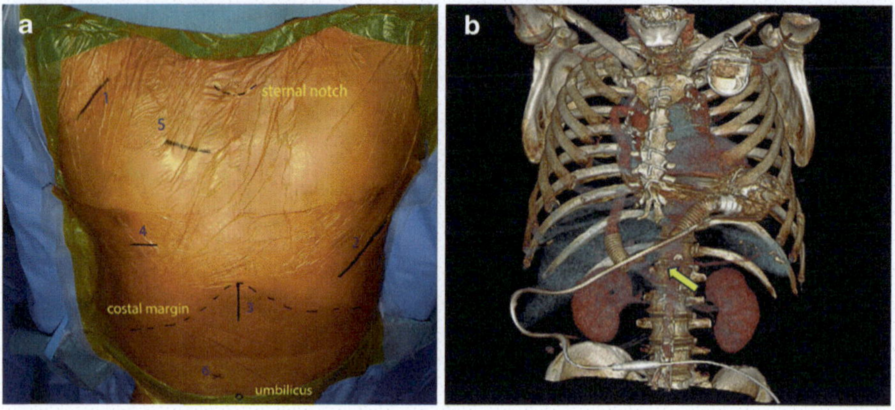

Fig. 2 (**a**) Representative preoperative planning for sternal-sparing LVAD implantation in a patient with previous coronary artery bypass graft surgery. (**b**) Postoperative CT reconstruction of the same patient with the arrow indicating both outflow graft as well as driveline lying within the upper abdominal wall. Any upper abdominal incision may put at risk the integrity of these LVAD components

of approach encompass the need for any concomitant procedures at the time of implantation, as well as reducing the burden of mediastinal adhesions prior to subsequent transplantation. A number of accessory incisions may be utilised such as in the case of previous heart surgery with mediastinal adhesions (Figure 2a).

Knowledge of the course of travel of the outflow graft may be of paramount importance as inadvertent damage may lead to uncontrollable bleeding with life--threatening consequences. With regard to the course of the driveline, this may be variable depending on patient body habitus, hand dominance, and surgeon preference. Once again, inadvertent damage or even interruption of the driveline can lead to abrupt stoppage of the device with circulatory collapse. It is worth mentioning that in patients with in situ HeartMate II devices, attention should be paid to pump location, as pump pockets have a tendency to shrink over time causing distortion to the original surgical positioning (Adamson et al. 2015).

Preoperative evaluation of patient surface anatomy, available operative notes, in addition to high-quality contrast-enhanced (if not contraindicated) imaging must always guide subsequent surgical incision placement or other intervention (Figure 2b).

4 Anaesthesia and Other Perioperative Considerations

Patients undergoing LVAD implantation for left ventricular decompensation often present with several comorbidities, such as obesity, renal and hepatic dysfunction, and pulmonary hypertension (Lander et al. 2022). Assessment of right ventricular function is pertinent not only in the selection of eligible patients and in the period around implantation of the device but also at later stages. Since these patients are often on diuretics and vasodilators, even slight haemodynamic changes caused by anaesthetics, such as vasodilation and myocardial depression, or positive pressure ventilation (decreased preload), as well as increased afterload caused by surgical stimuli or vasoconstriction secondary to hypothermia, can lead to situations that are challenging to manage (Min et al. 2024).

The same holds true for acute hypovolemia, for example, caused by vomiting or diarrhoea, or gastrointestinal bleeding, promoted by anticoagulation (Leebeek and Muslem 2019). Managing acute, relative, or absolute hypovolemia is imperative to allow for continued adequate functioning of the device, and, in the acute situation, may make a temporary reduction in pump speed necessary. During volume resuscitation, it should always be kept in mind that the patient's right ventricular function may be marginal, and "over doing" it could have deleterious effects as well (Rodenas-Alesina et al. 2022). Maintaining or improving right ventricular function acutely can prove to be difficult, and besides inotropic support, pulmonary vasodilators could be considered. Due to increased right ventricular afterload in the setting of positive pressure ventilation, if feasible, early extubation has also been recommended (Rodenas-Alesina et al. 2022).

Being able to quickly respond to these potential haemodynamic changes requires a high degree of vigilance and appropriate monitoring modalities. Due to the operating principle of generating continuous, rather than pulsatile, flow, non-invasive blood pressure measurement with an oscillometric modality is usually not feasible. Two alternatives are commonly used instead: non-invasive, intermittent measurement with a blood pressure cuff and a Doppler device, or invasive blood pressure measurement through arterial cannulation. While other modern non-invasive devices are in existence, their availability may be limited (Castagna et al. 2017; Lankheet et al. 2022). Pulse oximetry can also be affected by the absence of pulsatile flow and may warrant the use other oximetric devices, such as NIRS (Maldonado et al. 2014). Another unique monitoring entity is usually a console that tracks the function of the device itself, allowing to quickly respond to sudden changes in power (Min et al. 2024).

The required anticoagulation can confront the perioperative physician with unique challenges. Balancing the risk of device thrombosis, against acute bleeding risks, may require a tailored approach. Should reversal of the anticoagulation be required, one should keep in mind that that patient ultimately will require anticoagulation again, and this may warrant only a partial reversal of the anticoagulation or withholding replacement of vitamin K to facilitate a rapid reinstatement of vitamin K antagonists (Leebeek and Muslem 2019; Stevenson et al. 2024).

Lastly, it is common for patients with LVADs to have implanted cardioverter--defibrillators (ICDs) and implanted pacemakers. Depending on the body area, a surgery involving the use of monopolar cautery, particularly above the diaphragm, may require the temporary deactivation of such a device, either by reprogramming or application of a magnet (Min et al. 2024).

5 LVAD-Specific Emergencies

5.1 Outflow Graft Obstruction

Outflow graft obstruction can occur via a variety of mechanisms, including a kink, twist, or extrinsic compression. The clinical presentation is usually related to failure to unload the LV with signs and symptoms of worsening heart failure; persistent low-flow alarms may ensue as flow through the device decreases (<2.5 l/min for HeartMate 3), and in extreme cases, the device may thrombose. Without attendant pump thrombosis, there is usually no significant haemolysis. Echocardiography may reveal a dilated LV with septal shift towards the RV, more systolic aortic valve opening and mitral regurgitation; outflow graft systolic Doppler velocity may increase above typical values (up to ~2.5 m/s for the HeartMate 3) as the lumen progressively narrows (Hacket 2020; Stainback et al. 2015). Review of the system log files often reveals insidious decrease in estimated pump flow. Ultimately, CT angiography with multiplanar reconstruction is the key test to distinguish outflow graft issues from other causes of low flow. Diagnostic algorithms for troubleshooting frequent/persistent low flow alarms have been previously described (Mehra et al. 2018; Goldstein et al. 2024).

Outflow graft twist can notably occur in the HeartMate 3 device, in which the connection between the graft and the pump body has a swivel joint to facilitate rotation of the graft intraoperatively for optimal orientation; in vivo preferential rotation of this connection in one or the other direction may result in twisting and occlusion (Mehra et al. 2018). This was addressed by the manufacturer in October 2018, with the implementation of a clip that prevents untoward rotation of the assembly, and later by a pump design change (November 2019). As prophylactic surgical intervention to add the clip was not recommended for patients implanted prior to those dates who did not have evidence of graft obstruction, patients at risk for outflow graft twist by this mechanism are still present in the community.

An increasingly apparent mode of outflow graft failure is external compression of the graft. Acellular "biodebris" can accumulate over time in the space between the outflow graft portion covered by the bend relief, as the graft is constructed of gelatin-impregnated woven polyester, which has porosity, and the bend relief of impermeable reinforced polymer; Figures 3 and 4) (Venkateswaran and Dimarakis 2021). This phenomenon, which occurs with increasing frequency after 1 year (incidence up to 5.2% and 9.1% at 4 and 5 years, respectively (Wert et al. 2024)), has been the subject of device recall and the manufacturer is updating the design to prevent this complication (Abbott/Thoratec Corp 2024). Similarly, some surgeons wrap the outflow graft with an additional layer (Dacron™, Gore-Tex™, or bovine pericardium) aiming to protect the graft during chest re-entry; biodebris can also accumulate between these covers and the outflow graft, and their use is not recommended in the current guidelines (2023 ISHLT, Class III recommendation, level of evidence [LOE] C) (Saeed et al. 2023). Finally, in vivo disconnection of the bend relief has been reported to occur in up to one-third of patients with the HeartMate II

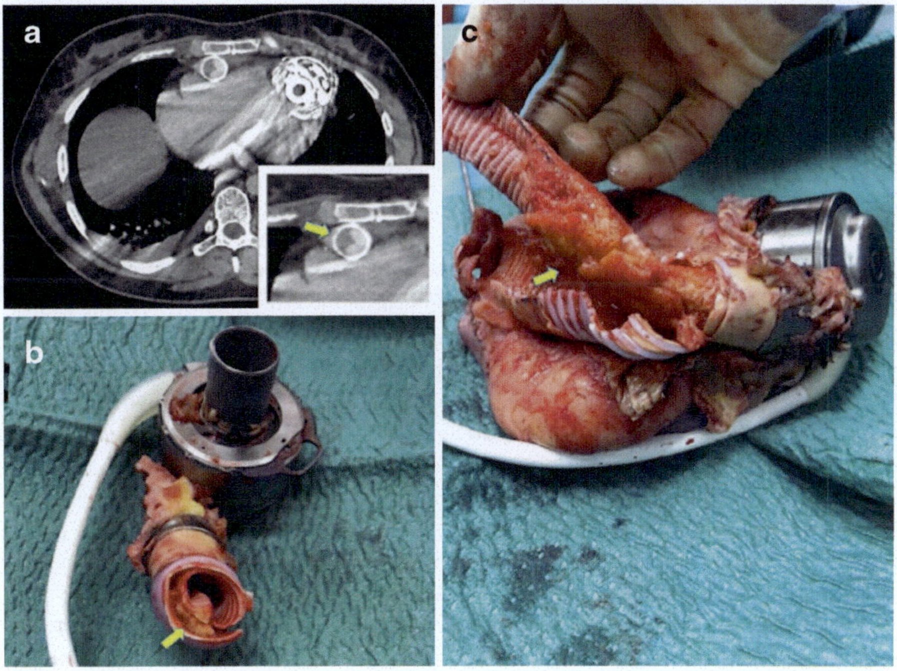

Fig. 3 Computed tomographic angiography (upper left) and intraoperative images of extrinsic outflow graft obstruction within the bend relief from accumulated biodebris (arrows). (Venkateswaran and Dimarakis 2021. © The Author(s) 2021. Reprinted by Permission of Sage Publications)

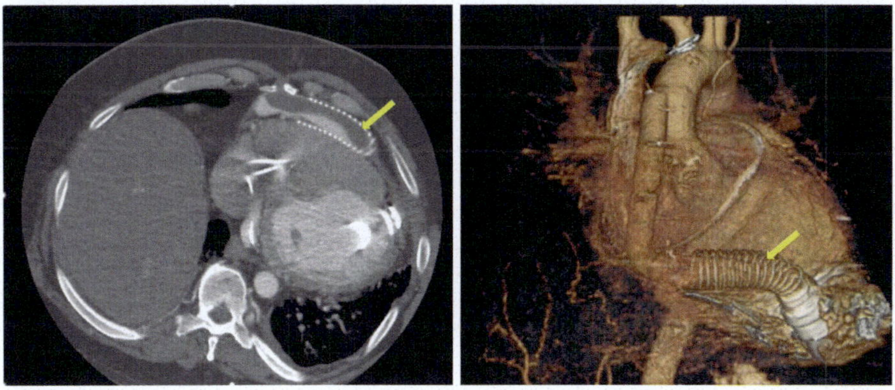

Fig. 4 Computed tomographic angiographic imaging (left) and 3D reconstruction (right) of extrinsic outflow graft obstruction by accumulated acellular biodebris (arrows)

device, and appears to be less frequent with the HeartMate 3; this can result in obstruction or even laceration of the outflow graft, which can constitute a surgical emergency due to heart failure, haemolysis, or bleeding (Waller et al. 2014; Donato et al. 2024; Yuzefpolskaya et al. 2013).

5.1.1 Management

Emergency management of outflow graft obstruction varies depending on patient stability and mode of obstruction. Graft kinks, anastomotic strictures, twists, and biodebris causing extrinsic compression can all be addressed surgically. The approach may vary depending on the location of the obstruction; issues near the pump body and bend relief can typically be addressed with left anterior thoracotomy, whereas more distal obstructions along the outflow graft and near the aortic anastomosis may require right thoracotomy (Goldstein et al. 2024). In complex cases where optimal exposure is needed, a full sternotomy may be required. Cases that require temporary pump stoppage must be performed under therapeutic anticoagulation to prevent pump thrombosis. Cardiopulmonary bypass support may be needed in scenarios or haemodynamic instability during periods of LVAD pump stoppage.

Surgical revision for outflow graft kinks may require shortening/resection of excess graft with graft-to-graft anastomosis, or graft repositioning. An alternative approach in which the right pleura is opened and the excess outflow graft is allowed to reside in the intrapleural space has been described (Goldstein et al. 2024). While not widely described in the literature, percutaneous stenting for anastomotic kinks has been successfully performed. Graft twist will also typically require surgical correction, including pre-November 2019 HeartMate 3 devices that may require addition of the aforementioned clip.

Various treatment (and prevention, e.g. a priori fenestrating the bend relief) (Farber et al. 2022) approaches have been developed for extrinsic outflow graft obstruction at the bend relief. Surgical resolution involves splitting the bend relief open and evacuation of the biodebris, while excising an adequate portion (or the entirety) of the bend relief to prevent reaccumulation. Careful clinical and imaging assessment for concurrent pump thrombosis should be undertaken, which can be a consequence of chronic low flow in the outflow graft and require pump exchange or urgent cardiac transplantation. While surgical intervention has the strongest recommendation in the most recent guidelines (2023 ISHLT, Class I, LOE C), percutaneous treatment with stenting of the outflow graft has become a common first-line treatment (2023 ISHLT, Class IIb, LOE B) (Saeed et al. 2023). Key technical caveats include (i) appropriate stent sizing, typically utilising 14/16 mm peripheral stents to match the outflow graft size; (ii) landing the distal end of the stent in the pump house to prevent untreated areas, and (iii) covering the entirety of the bend relief is preferred to prevent merely "shifting" the biodebris within the bend relief with persistent obstruction. Outflow graft stenting has a high success rate and can result in dramatic improvement in haemodynamic gradients across the obstruction (Figure 5) (Goldstein et al. 2024; Agrawal et al. 2021).

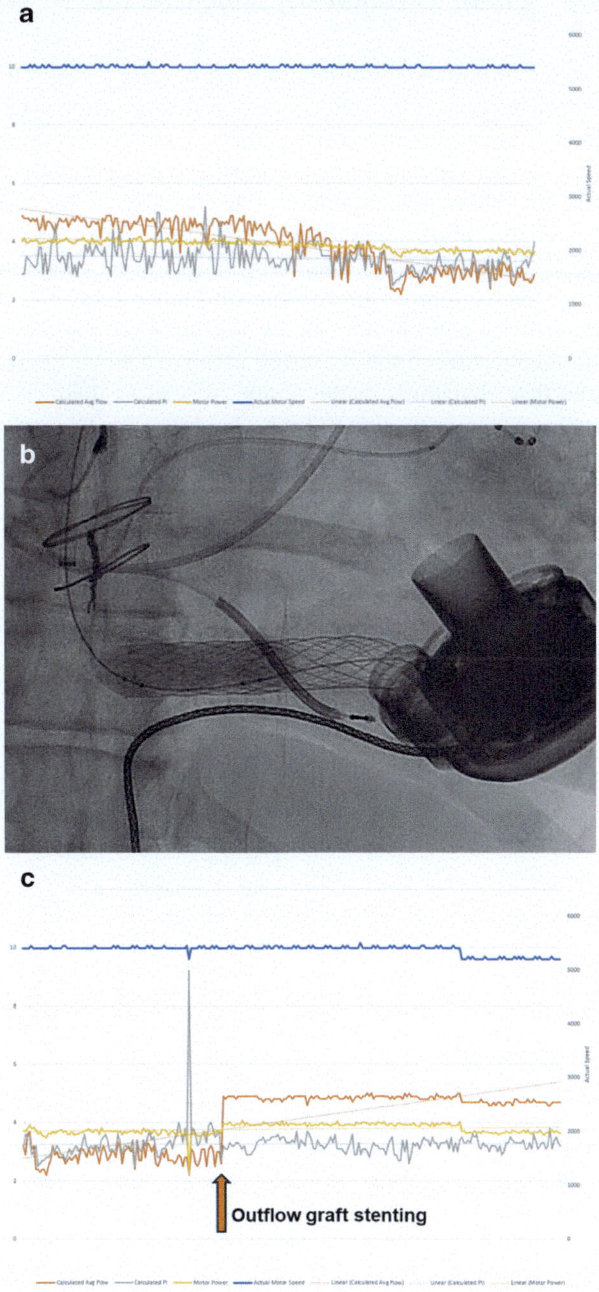

Fig. 5 (**a**) Gradual decline in motor power consumption (yellow) and calculated flow (orange) over several days in a patient diagnosed with extrinsic outflow graft obstruction; (**b**) successful stenting of the outflow graft within the bend relief; peak-to-peak gradient between the proximal outflow graft and aorta was reduced from 95 mmHg to 3 mmHg; (**c**) motor power consumption and calculated flow sharply increase and stabilise after stenting

5.2 Pump Thrombosis, Stoppage, and System Exchange

Device thrombosis encompasses the development of in situ thrombus in the pump inflow portion, rotor housing, or outflow graft, as well as thrombus ingestion via the left ventricle (Saeed et al. 2023). A variety of pump- (e.g. inflow cannula position, device type, and low pump speed) and patient-related (e.g. infection, hypertension, and hypercoagulable state) factors are associated with augmented risk of device thrombosis (Goldstein et al. 2013). The clinical presentation is dependent on an array of factors including native heart function and clot burden/location, from the asymptomatic patient with laboratory evidence of mild haemolysis, to progressive heart failure, shock, and stroke or systemic embolism. There are often attendant power (and therefore estimated flow) aberrations that may not reflect true flow dynamics in the pump, as well as distinctive imaging, laboratory, and haemodynamic findings (Table 2; Figure 6). Diagnostic algorithms were developed in an era of increasing recognition of device thrombosis (in the range of up to 7–12% per year with the prior generation devices), and the most recent guidelines make several recommendations for the diagnosis and treatment of this complication (Table 3) (Saeed et al. 2023; Goldstein et al. 2013; Kirklin et al. 2014, 2015). Recent data indicates that the HeartMate 3 device may have significantly lower haemocompatibility-related events, including pump thrombosis (0.01 events/patient-years) (Mehra et al. 2022).

In addition to thrombosis, pump stoppage may occur due to major malfunction of any of the critical device components. While such malfunction has become

Table 2 Diagnostics and possible findings in suspected LVAD thrombosis

Echocardiography	↓LV unloading
	  ↑LV size
	  ↑Mitral regurgitation
	  ↑AV opening
	  ↑RV systolic pressure
	  Septum bowing towards RV
	↓inflow/outflow cannula Doppler velocities
	Ramp study: inability to unload LV with increased pump speed

Laboratory testing	Haemolysis markers
	  LDH > 3× ULN
	  Plasma free haemoglobin >40 mg/dL
	  Haemoglobinuria
	↓End-organ function

LVAD alarm and log-file review	Inflow: ↓ power Rotor/impeller: ↑↑ power Outflow: ↓ power
CT angiogram	Contrast defect in location of thrombus, particularly if within outflow graft

AV aortic valve, *CT* computed tomography, *LDH* lactate dehydrogenase, *LV* left ventricle, *LVAD* left ventricle assist device, *RV* right ventricle

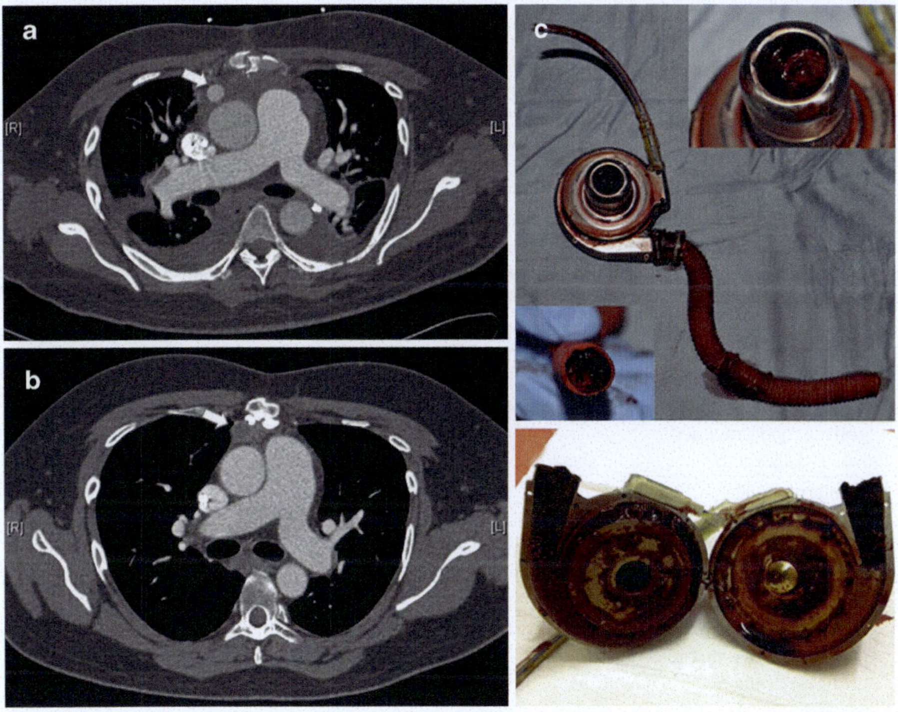

Fig. 6 A case of pump thrombosis involving the outflow graft. Left: computed tomography angiographic imaging showing baseline appearance of the outflow graft (panel A, arrow) and after thrombosis (panel B, arrow). Right: intraoperative images of the LVAD showing thrombus inside the pump and outflow graft (panel C). (Reprinted from Dimarakis et al. 2014, Copyright © 2014 The American Association for Thoracic Surgery, with permission from Elsevier)

increasingly rare due to evolving LVAD technology, modern continuous-flow devices have no mechanism to manually actuate the device in the event of pump stoppage, which therefore constitutes a critical emergency. A common cause of non-thrombosis power failure is driveline fracture or damage, which in turn occurs in up to 10–15% of LVAD patients (Merzah et al. 2023; Kalavrouziotis et al. 2014; D'Antonio et al. 2021). If this is suspected, all connections along the device and the driveline should be inspected for signs of damage, corrosion, or unsecured connections (Saeed et al. 2023). The entire driveline should be imaged with X-ray. Depending on the extent and location of damage (in the internal vs. externalised portion of the driveline), it may be feasible to repair the driveline; the HeartMate 3 has a modular driveline component that can be exchanged non-operatively if damage is limited to that portion (Merzah et al. 2023). In cases of driveline transection, splicing the color-coded internal wires of the driveline with haemostats or alligator clips as a temporising measure has been described (Cubillo et al. 2014; Ziegler et al. 2021). If the damage is not repairable, pump exchange, device explant/decommissioning, or urgent transplantation may be undertaken.

Table 3 2023 ISHLT key guideline recommendations for device thrombosis and device exchange (Saeed et al. 2023)

Class I
Diagnosis
The initial evaluation of suspected device thrombosis should include device interrogation with manufacturer log file analysis to assess pump parameter changes over time
Level of evidence B
The initial evaluation of suspected device thrombosis should include laboratory tests (lactate dehydrogenase, haemoglobin, and plasma free haemoglobin) to assist in the diagnosis of intravascular haemolysis and haemoglobinuria (urinalysis) and to detect end-organ dysfunction
Level of evidence B
The initial evaluation of suspected device thrombosis should include an echocardiogram to assess for LV unloading with and without speed adjustment (i.e. RAMP study)
Level of evidence B
In patients with a high suspicion of device thrombosis, CT angiogram to evaluate the outflow graft is recommended
Level of evidence B
Management
Class I
Initial management of patients with confirmed device thrombosis should include intravenous systemic anticoagulation with heparin
Level of evidence C
In patients with confirmed device thrombosis who are candidates for surgery, pump exchange is the definitive therapy
Level of evidence B
Class IIa
Pump exchange may be accomplished by minimal incisions (subcostal, thoracotomy), or full sternotomy depending on the component(s) to be exchanged and extent of infection, and/or thrombus
Level of evidence C
Early LVAD exchange should be considered in patients with pump thrombosis who progress despite initial management
Level of evidence C
In patients with confirmed device thrombosis who are haemodynamically stable and expected wait time for heart transplant is short, it may be reasonable to defer the pump exchange for urgent transplantation
Level of evidence C
In carefully selected patients supported by a hydrodynamic centrifugal pump with confirmed device thrombosis, systemic or intraventricular thrombolytic therapy can be considered as an initial management strategy over device exchange
Level of evidence C
Class IIb
In the heightened thrombotic proclivity of patients with recurrent pump thrombosis, exchange to HeartMate 3 from prior device may be reasonable
Level of evidence C
LVAD exchange for infection may be performed with distinct operative field/planes to avoid contamination of the new pump
Level of evidence C
It might be reasonable to choose bivalirudin over heparin as an initial agent for intravenous systemic anticoagulation
Level of evidence C

ISHLT International Society for Heart & Lung Transplantation, *LVAD* left ventricular assist device

5.2.1 Management

The cornerstone of medical management for pump thrombosis is intravenous therapeutic anticoagulation. Most commonly, unfractionated heparin is employed; direct thrombin inhibitors (such as bivalirudin) have also been utilised and may have the added benefit of anti-platelet properties and activity on thrombin that is already clot-bound (Saeed et al. 2023; Weeks et al. 2018; Hollis et al. 2024). For patients in whom this resolves the thrombus, transition back to warfarin with or without augmentation of the INR goal is reasonable. Addition of adjuvant antiplatelet agents is sometimes employed, but there is no high-level evidence to guide this practice (Goldstein et al. 2013; Baumann Kreuziger et al. 2015). GP2B3A inhibitors have not been shown to improve outcomes in this setting and are not recommended (Tellor et al. 2014). In patients who do not respond to optimised anticoagulation or who are clinically unstable, thrombolysis, urgent cardiac transplantation, or system exchange are options. Thrombolytics including catheter-instilled therapy directly in the left ventricle have been used but with high complication rates (Schlendorf et al. 2014). In general, early system exchange should be considered in patients with thrombosis who progress efforts at initial medical management (ISHLT 2023; Class IIa, LOE C) (Saeed et al. 2023).

Pump exchange can be achieved by various surgical approaches depending on the exposure required; factors affecting this choice include: (i) the presence of concomitant infection, (ii) the type of device in situ including plan for exchange to a different device, (iii) the extent of LVAD components involved, especially the outflow graft. The modular nature of contemporary devices means that exchange of both individual components and the entire system is generally feasible. Full system exchange including pump and outflow graft (such as in the case of extensive thrombosis) is best achieved by median sternotomy with cardiopulmonary bypass, which also enables lower LVAD flows and thus minimises the risk of air embolism. A limited exchange (pump only) can be achieved via limited incisions including subcostal, small left thoracotomy, and occasionally without the use of cardiopulmonary bypass (Levin et al. 2015; Hanke 2018; Osho and D'Alessandro 2022). Contrast-enhanced CT angiography is routinely employed to study the anatomy and location of the pump components and to anticipate high-risk portions of the operation. In cases of hostile chest, peripheral cardiopulmonary bypass cannulation may be necessary. Regardless of approach, LVAD flows should typically be reduced to the lowest rate to maintain perfusion and minimise risk of air embolism in the event of outflow graft injury (Osho and D'Alessandro 2022).

Data suggests that the intermediate term risk of re-thrombosis after exchange for thrombosis of HeartMate II is as high as 31–51% (Levin et al. 2015; Urban et al. 2020). Replacement with swapping to the latest generation HeartMate 3 system may be considered when recurrent thrombosis occurs (ISHLT Class IIb, LOE C). Pump exchange with or without model swap may carry significant risk, such as RV failure and stroke in up to 20%; exchange to a HeartMate 3 may have lower risk of 30-day mortality based on a recent meta-analysis (13% with HVAD vs. 5% with HeartMate3, $p = 0.03$) (Austin et al. 2021). Key factors to consider when planning a system swap to a different model include differences in sewing ring size (HVAD: 43 mm vs. HeartMate 3: 39.9 or 50 mm), inflow cannular external diameter (HVAD: 20.6 mm vs. HeartMate 3: 20.5 mm), and outflow graft size. In exchanging from HVAD/HeartMate II to HeartMate 3, closest adherence to the manufacturer's recommendations would dictate that the previous sewing ring should be removed and a new HeartMate 3 apical connector utilised. However, if a full sternotomy or complete replacement of the sewing ring and/ or outflow graft is felt to be of unacceptable risk due to patient factors, modifications have been described including (i) implantation of the HeartMate 3 apical connector *over* the existing HVAD sewing ring (which may present challenges with haemostasis and positions the HeartMate 3 inflow cannula slightly less deep into the LV); (ii) implantation of the HeartMate3 inflow cannula *within* the HVAD sewing ring (with a diameter mismatch of 0.1 mm) with the addition of a 0.1 mm rubber seal for haemostasis, or within the HeartMate II sewing ring with a sterile cable tie and ligatures (Hanke et al. 2017).

6 Non-Cardiac Surgery

Urgent or emergent non-cardiac surgery in LVAD patients is a common occurrence associated with significant morbidity and mortality (Bhat et al. 2012; Morgan et al. 2012; Mentias et al. 2020; Arnaoutakis et al. 2014). In a contemporary analysis of 8118 LVAD patients from a US administrative database, approximately one in six patients (16.3%) underwent non-cardiac surgery over a period of 6 years (excluding the index hospitalisation) (Mentias et al. 2020). The majority (75.4%) of these procedures were urgent or emergent and included, in order of decreasing frequency, general surgeries (most frequently hernia repairs, cholecystectomy, and colorectal resection), followed by thoracic, orthopedic, and genitourinary procedures. Urgent or emergent non-cardiac surgery was associated with a significant risk of major adverse cardiovascular events in this study (up to 16.9%), and a 10.2% 30-day mortality.

Key considerations in the operative management of these patients are: (i) anaesthesia and haemodynamic monitoring, (ii) management of anticoagulation, and (iii) careful surgical planning to avoid LVAD components, especially injuring the driveline and outflow graft or violating the pump pocket (Givertz et al. 2019). Depending on the procedure (and for most emergent surgeries), multidisciplinary involvement including ideally a cardiac anaesthetist with experience with MCS patients, a person able to manage LVAD function intraoperatively (e.g. an LVAD coordinator, ICU nurse, or perfusionist), heart failure cardiologist, and an LVAD surgeon is recommended for optimal preoperative planning (Givertz et al. 2019). Therefore, if possible, major surgical procedures should be performed at LVAD centres. Appropriate imaging should be obtained, and the pump position, outflow graft, and driveline course should be noted. LVAD flow is fundamentally "preload-dependent, and afterload-sensitive". Several surgical factors, such as blood volume resuscitation, patient positioning, and pneumoperitoneum for laparoscopic procedures affect venous return/cardiac preload, on which LVAD flow is directly dependent, and often require active management with fluids and pump speed adjustments. Accurate blood pressure monitoring that allows maintenance of a stable mean arterial pressure of 70–90 mmHg is key to ensure optimised flow; for most procedures with risk of haemodynamic instability, this should be performed with an arterial catheter (ISHLT 2023 guidelines, Class II, LOE C) (Saeed et al. 2023). In patients requiring thoracic surgery, it is pertinent that a balance between protective lung ventilation and right heart protection is maintained (Hayes et al. 2020). The main objectives of RV-protective ventilation strategies include reduction of plateau and driving pressures, while avoiding hypoxia, hypercapnia, and acidemia (Rana et al. 2019).

Patients on LVAD support are at particularly high risk for bleeding spontaneously or perioperatively above and beyond what is expected in the typical anticoagulated patient (Wever-Pinzon et al. 2013). This is due to a variety of factors including non-pulsatile flow, platelet dysfunction, acquired von Willebrand syndrome, and often hepatic congestion and dysfunction in the setting of RV failure (Givertz et al. 2019; Uriel et al. 2010; Sparrow et al. 2015). More recently, monotherapy with a vitamin K antagonist (VKA) has been shown to be non-inferior to dual therapy including VKA and aspirin with respect to thromboembolic events, and to reduce bleeding events (Mehra et al. 2023). For procedures associated with a low bleeding risk—typically not classified as urgent/emergent—VKA and antiplatelet therapy may occasionally be continued. If interrupted, therapeutic anticoagulation should be recommenced as soon as possible, and typically within 24–28 h with bridging (Hollis et al. 2024; Ben Gal et al. 2021). For emergency procedures, VKA reversal with fresh frozen plasma (FFP), prothrombin protein concentrate (PCC), or vitamin K may be necessary (2023 ISHLT guidelines, Class I, LOE B) (Stevenson et al. 2024; Saeed et al. 2023). This is especially pertinent in patient with haemorrhagic stroke or other neurosurgical bleeding emergencies. Procedural antibiotic prophylaxis has not been studied in this population; current MCS guidelines align with recommendations for the highest infectious risk patients, and do not recommend antibiotics for routine respiratory tract, gastrointestinal, and urogenital procedures; high-risk dental procedures and any surgery that routinely mandates antibiotics in a non-LVAD patient should be performed with antibiotic prophylaxis (Saeed et al. 2023).

In case of inadvertent damage to LVAD components during surgical dissection, it is pertinent that the respective surgical team is prepared to react accordingly. The most "vulnerable" component to iatrogenic injury is the outflow graft, especially in the uncovered portion outside the bend relief. In many instances, a simple laceration if access is adequate can be primarily repaired under an ultra-brief period of reduced LVAD flow. In cases where access is limited and bleeding is uncontrollable, one may have to initiate peripheral extracorporeal membrane oxygenation (ECMO) or even full cardiopulmonary bypass with or without a brief period of deep hypothermic circulatory arrest in order to proceed with further tissue dissection and definitive repair. In any case, it is advisable to secure femoral venous as well as arterial access once the patient is anaesthetised.

7 Trauma

Management of LVAD patients sustaining blunt or penetrating trauma should be carried out in line with advanced trauma life support protocols including trauma sonography and simultaneous LVAD interrogation, especially if LVAD-trained personnel are available. Additional information for mechanical component damage including drive line fracture can be obtained by targeted plain X-rays. In the case of driveline fractures, even though these can be repaired by manufacturer engineers with good long-term repair durability (Stulak et al. 2017), device exchange may be required.

Overall, management is guided by the interaction between haemodynamic stability and LVAD function. The ultimate goal remains transfer of the patient to a centre with an LVAD program once haemodynamic stability has been achieved. If the patient remains haemodynamically unstable with a well-functioning LVAD, the treating surgical team should proceed to surgery as for any non-cardiac surgery situation. In the scenario of haemodynamic instability alongside LVAD malfunction (having failed to restore LVAD function), and the patient is deemed salvageable, temporary mechanical circulatory support in the form of peripheral ECMO should be initiated and the patient reassessed for candidacy for further treatment.

8 Closing Remarks

An increasing prevalence of patients with durable LVADs effectively translates to an increasing number of these patients presenting with LVAD-related as well as non-related surgical pathology. In carefully selected patients with appropriate preoperative workup and perioperative management, outcomes can be safeguarded. In the event of major intervention, especially if general anaesthesia is required, it is preferable that this is carried out in an implanting centre with cardiothoracic anaesthetic availability and LVAD specialist support.

References

Abbott/Thoratec Corp (2024) Recalls HeartMate II and HeartMate 3 Left Ventricular Assist System (LVAS) due to Long-term buildup causing an obstruction. https://www.fda.gov/medical-devices/medical-device-recalls/abbottthoratec-corp-recalls-heartmate-ii-and-heartmate-3-left-ventricular-assist-system-lvas-due

Adamson RM, Mangi AA, Kormos RL, Farrar DJ, Dembitsky WP (2015) Principles of HeartMate II implantation to avoid pump malposition and migration. J Card Surg 30:296–299. https://doi.org/10.1111/jocs.12478

Agrawal A, Alexy T, Kamioka N, Shafi T, Stowe J, Morris AA, Vega JD, Babaliaros V, Burke MA (2021) Outflow graft obstruction after left ventricular assist device implantation: a retrospective, single-centre case series. ESC Heart Fail 8:2349–2353. https://doi.org/10.1002/ehf2.13333

Arnaoutakis GJ, Bittle GJ, Allen JG, Weiss ES, Alejo J, Baumgartner WA, Shah AS, Wolfgang CL, Efron DT, Conte JV (2014) General and acute care surgical procedures in patients with left ventricular assist devices. World J Surg 38:765–773. https://doi.org/10.1007/s00268-013-2403-0

Austin MA, Maynes EJ, Gadda MN, O'Malley TJ, Morris RJ, Shah MK, Pirlamarla PR, Alvarez RJ, Entwistle JW, Massey HT et al (2021) Continuous-flow LVAD exchange to a different pump model: systematic review and meta-analysis of the outcomes. Artif Organs 45:696–705. https://doi.org/10.1111/aor.13893

Baumann Kreuziger LM, Kim B, Wieselthaler GM (2015) Antithrombotic therapy for left ventricular assist devices in adults: a systematic review. J Thromb Haemost 13:946–955. https://doi.org/10.1111/jth.12948

Bedi R, Vu T, Bansal A (2022) Left ventricular assist device implantation to the left subclavian artery with distal banding: a novel technique for hostile chest. Ann Thorac Surg 113:e381–e383. https://doi.org/10.1016/j.athoracsur.2021.08.010

Ben Gal T, Ben Avraham B, Milicic D, Crespo-Leiro MG, Coats AJS, Rosano G, Seferovic P, Ruschitzka F, Metra M, Anker S et al (2021) Guidance on the management of left ventricular assist device (LVAD) supported patients for the non-LVAD specialist healthcare provider: executive summary. Eur J Heart Fail 23:1597–1609. https://doi.org/10.1002/ejhf.2327

Bhat G, Kumar S, Aggarwal A, Pauwaa S, Rossell G, Kurien S, Kumar A, Pappas PS, Tatooles A (2012) Experience with noncardiac surgery in destination therapy left ventricular assist devices patients. ASAIO J 58:396–401. https://doi.org/10.1097/MAT.0b013e31825b8d36

Castagna F, Stohr EJ, Pinsino A, Cockcroft JR, Willey J, Reshad Garan A, Topkara VK, Colombo PC, Yuzefpolskaya M, McDonnell BJ (2017) The unique blood pressures and pulsatility of LVAD patients: current challenges and future opportunities. Curr Hypertens Rep 19:85. https://doi.org/10.1007/s11906-017-0782-6

Cho SM, Mehaffey JH, Meyers SL, Cantor RS, Starling RC, Kirklin JK, Jacobs JP, Kern J, Uchino K, Yarboro LT (2021) Cerebrovascular events in patients with centrifugal-flow left ventricular assist devices: propensity score-matched analysis from the Intermacs registry. Circulation 144:763–772. https://doi.org/10.1161/CIRCULATIONAHA.121.055716

Cubillo E, Weis RA, Ramakrishna H (2014) Emergent reconnection of a transected left ventricular assist device driveline. J Emerg Med 47:546–551. https://doi.org/10.1016/j.jemermed.2014.07.028

D'Antonio ND, Maynes EJ, Tatum RT, Prochno KW, Saxena A, Maltais S, Samuels LE, Morris RJ, Massey HT, Tchantchaleishvili V (2021) Driveline damage and repair in continuous-flow left ventricular assist devices: a systematic review. Artif Organs 45:819–826. https://doi.org/10.1111/aor.13901

Dimarakis I, Shaw S, Venkateswaran R (2014) HeartWare left ventricular assist device thrombosis including outflow graft. J Thorac Cardiovasc Surg 148:1746–1747. https://doi.org/10.1016/j.jtcvs.2014.01.049

Donato BB, Seadler BD, Mohammed BW, Zdanovec A, Ubert HA, Durham LA 3rd. (2024) Heartmate 3 left ventricular assist device bend relief disconnection causing laceration of the outflow graft. ASAIO J. https://doi.org/10.1097/MAT.0000000000002287

Dorken Gallastegi A, Hoscoskun EB, Kahraman U, Yagmur B, Nalbantgil S, Engin C, Yagdi T, Ozbaran M (2022) Long-term outcomes in ventricular assist device outflow cannula anastomosis to the descending aorta. Ann Thorac Surg 114:1377–1385. https://doi.org/10.1016/j.athoracsur.2021.08.071

Farber G, Kirov H, Schwan I, Grager S, Diab M, Tkebuchava S, Doenst T (2022) Bend relief fenestration might prevent outflow graft obstruction in patients with left ventricular assist device. Interact Cardiovasc Thorac Surg 35. https://doi.org/10.1093/icvts/ivac149

FDA (2024) Stop new implants of the medtronic HVAD system—letter to health care providers. https://public4.pagefreezer.com/content/FDA/21-02-2024T12:58/https://www.fda.gov/medical-devices/letters-health-care-providers/stop-new-implants-medtronic-hvad-system-letter-health-care-providers

Givertz MM, DeFilippis EM, Colvin M, Darling CE, Elliott T, Hamad E, Hiestand BC, Martindale JL, Pinney SP, Shah KB et al (2019) HFSA/SAEM/ISHLT clinical expert consensus document on the emergency management of patients with ventricular assist devices. J Heart Lung Transplant 38:677–698. https://doi.org/10.1016/j.healun.2019.05.004

Goldstein DJ, John R, Salerno C, Silvestry S, Moazami N, Horstmanshof D, Adamson R, Boyle A, Zucker M, Rogers J et al (2013) Algorithm for the diagnosis and management of suspected pump thrombus. J Heart Lung Transplant 32:667–670. https://doi.org/10.1016/j.healun.2013.05.002

Goldstein DJ, Kanwar M, Cowger J, Patel S, Meyer DM, Molina E, Salerno C, Elmer A, Schettle S, Teuteberg J et al (2024) Extrinsic outflow graft obstruction of the HeartMate 3 LVAD: A state-of-the-art review. J Heart Lung Transplant. https://doi.org/10.1016/j.healun.2024.07.005

Hacket IS (2020) Redefining normal outflow cannula velocity reference values for each left ventricular assist device. J Heart Lung Transplant 39:S416

Hanke JS (2018) Exchange of a HeartMate 3 left ventricular assist device through thoracotomy. Oper Tech Thorac Cardiovasc Surg 23:62–75

Hanke JS, Rojas SV, Dogan G, Feldmann C, Beckmann E, Deniz E, Wiegmann B, Michaelis JE, Napp LC, Berliner D et al (2017) First series of left ventricular assist device exchanges to HeartMate 3. Eur J Cardiothorac Surg 51:887–892. https://doi.org/10.1093/ejcts/ezx010

Hayes T, Charlesworth M, Garcia M (2020) Patients with left ventricle assist devices presenting for thoracic surgery and lung resection: tips, tricks and evidence. Curr Opin Anaesthesiol 33:17–26. https://doi.org/10.1097/ACO.0000000000000817

Hollis IB, Jennings DL, Krim S, Ton VK, Ducharme A, Cowger J, Looby M, Eulert-Green JJ, Bansal N, Horn E et al (2024) An ISHLT consensus statement on strategies to prevent and manage hemocompatibility related adverse events in patients with a durable, continuous-flow ventricular assist device. J Heart Lung Transplant 43:1199–1234. https://doi.org/10.1016/j.healun.2024.04.065

Jorde UP, Saeed O, Koehl D, Morris AA, Wood KL, Meyer DM, Cantor R, Jacobs JP, Kirklin JK, Pagani FD et al (2024) The Society of Thoracic Surgeons Intermacs 2023 annual report: focus on magnetically levitated devices. Ann Thorac Surg 117:33–44. https://doi.org/10.1016/j.athoracsur.2023.11.004

Kalavrouziotis D, Tong MZ, Starling RC, Massiello A, Soltesz E, Smedira NG, Fryc R, Heatley G, Farrar DJ, Moazami N (2014) Percutaneous lead dysfunction in the HeartMate II left ventricular assist device. Ann Thorac Surg 97:1373–1378. https://doi.org/10.1016/j.athoracsur.2013.11.039

Kirklin JK, Naftel DC, Kormos RL, Pagani FD, Myers SL, Stevenson LW, Acker MA, Goldstein DL, Silvestry SC, Milano CA et al (2014) Interagency Registry for Mechanically Assisted Circulatory Support (INTERMACS) analysis of pump thrombosis in the HeartMate II left ventricular assist device. J Heart Lung Transplant 33:12–22. https://doi.org/10.1016/j.healun.2013.11.001

Kirklin JK, Naftel DC, Pagani FD, Kormos RL, Myers S, Acker MA, Rogers J, Slaughter MS, Stevenson LW (2015) Pump thrombosis in the Thoratec HeartMate II device: an update analysis of the INTERMACS Registry. J Heart Lung Transplant 34:1515–1526. https://doi.org/10.1016/j.healun.2015.10.024

Lander M, Bhardwaj A, Kanwar M (2022) Selection and management considerations to enhance outcomes in patients supported by left ventricular assist devices. Curr Opin Cardiol 37:502–510. https://doi.org/10.1097/HCO.0000000000000996

Lankheet S, Pieterse MM, Rijnhout R, Tuerlings E, Oppelaar AC, van Laake LW, Ramjankhan FZ, Westerhof BE, Oerlemans M (2022) Validity and success rate of noninvasive mean arterial blood pressure measurements in cf-LVAD patients: a technical review. Artif Organs 46:2361–2370. https://doi.org/10.1111/aor.14367

Leebeek FWG, Muslem R (2019) Bleeding in critical care associated with left ventricular assist devices: pathophysiology, symptoms, and management. Hematology Am Soc Hematol Educ Program 2019:88–96. https://doi.org/10.1182/hematology.2019000067

Levin AP, Uriel N, Takayama H, Mody KP, Ota T, Yuzefpolskaya M, Colombo PC, Garan AR, Dionizovik-Dimanovski M, Sladen RN et al (2015) Device exchange in HeartMate II recipients: long-term outcomes and risk of thrombosis recurrence. ASAIO J 61:144–149. https://doi.org/10.1097/MAT.0000000000000170

Maldonado Y, Singh S, Taylor MA (2014) Cerebral near-infrared spectroscopy in perioperative management of left ventricular assist device and extracorporeal membrane oxygenation patients. Curr Opin Anaesthesiol 27:81–88. https://doi.org/10.1097/ACO.0000000000000035

Mehra MR, Salerno C, Naka Y, Uriel N, Cleveland JC, Horstmanshof D, Goldstein DJ, Investigators M (2018) A tale of the twist in the outflow graft: an analysis from the MOMENTUM 3 trial. J Heart Lung Transplant 37:1281–1284. https://doi.org/10.1016/j.healun.2018.08.011

Mehra MR, Uriel N, Naka Y, Cleveland JC Jr, Yuzefpolskaya M, Salerno CT, Walsh MN, Milano CA, Patel CB, Hutchins SW et al (2019) A fully magnetically levitated left ventricular assist device—final report. N Engl J Med 380:1618–1627. https://doi.org/10.1056/NEJMoa1900486

Mehra MR, Goldstein DJ, Cleveland JC, Cowger JA, Hall S, Salerno CT, Naka Y, Horstmanshof D, Chuang J, Wang A et al (2022) Five-year outcomes in patients with fully magnetically levitated vs axial-flow left ventricular assist devices in the MOMENTUM 3 randomized trial. JAMA 328:1233–1242. https://doi.org/10.1001/jama.2022.16197

Mehra MR, Netuka I, Uriel N, Katz JN, Pagani FD, Jorde UP, Gustafsson F, Connors JM, Ivak P, Cowger J et al (2023) Aspirin and hemocompatibility events with a left ventricular assist device in advanced heart failure: the ARIES-HM3 randomized clinical trial. JAMA 330:2171–2181. https://doi.org/10.1001/jama.2023.23204

Mentias A, Briasoulis A, Vaughan Sarrazin MS, Alvarez PA (2020) Trends, perioperative adverse events, and survival of patients with left ventricular assist devices undergoing noncardiac surgery. JAMA Netw Open 3:e2025118. https://doi.org/10.1001/jamanetworkopen.2020.25118

Merzah AS, Hanke JS, Li T, Saad Merzah FA, Gabriel M, Derda AA, Homann K, Haverich A, Schmitto JD, Dogan G (2023) Outcomes of modular cable exchange in HeartMate 3 patients versus conventional driveline repair in HeartMate II patients. Artif Organs 47:380–386. https://doi.org/10.1111/aor.14413

Min JJ, Cho YH, Lee SM, Lee JH (2024) Anesthetic management for non-cardiac surgery in patients with left ventricular assist devices. Korean J Anesthesiol 77:175–184. https://doi.org/10.4097/kja.23169

Morgan JA, Paone G, Nemeh HW, Henry SE, Gerlach B, Williams CT, Lanfear DE, Tita C, Brewer RJ (2012) Non-cardiac surgery in patients on long-term left ventricular assist device support. J Heart Lung Transplant 31:757–763. https://doi.org/10.1016/j.healun.2012.02.023

Osho AA, D'Alessandro DA (2022) Approaches to ventricular assist device exchange: resternotomy versus limited incisions. JTCVS Tech 12:94–99. https://doi.org/10.1016/j.xjtc.2021.10.062

Rana M, Yusuff H, Zochios V (2019) The right ventricle during selective lung ventilation for thoracic surgery. J Cardiothorac Vasc Anesth 33:2007–2016. https://doi.org/10.1053/j.jvca.2018.11.030

Rodenas-Alesina E, Brahmbhatt DH, Rao V, Salvatori M, Billia F (2022) Prediction, prevention, and management of right ventricular failure after left ventricular assist device implantation: a comprehensive review. Front Cardiovasc Med 9:1040251. https://doi.org/10.3389/fcvm.2022.1040251

Saeed D, Feldman D, Banayosy AE, Birks E, Blume E, Cowger J, Hayward C, Jorde U, Kremer J, MacGowan G et al (2023) The 2023 International Society for Heart and Lung Transplantation guidelines for mechanical circulatory support: a 10- year update. J Heart Lung Transplant 42:e1–e222. https://doi.org/10.1016/j.healun.2022.12.004

Schlendorf K, Patel CB, Gehrig T, Kiefer TL, Felker GM, Hernandez AF, Blue LJ, Milano CA, Rogers JG (2014) Thrombolytic therapy for thrombosis of continuous flow ventricular assist devices. J Card Fail 20:91–97. https://doi.org/10.1016/j.cardfail.2013.12.011

Sparrow CT, Nassif ME, Raymer DS, Novak E, LaRue SJ, Schilling JD (2015) Pre-operative right ventricular dysfunction is associated with gastrointestinal bleeding in patients supported with continuous-flow left ventricular assist devices. JACC Heart Fail 3:956–964. https://doi.org/10.1016/j.jchf.2015.09.009

Stainback RF, Estep JD, Agler DA, Birks EJ, Bremer M, Hung J, Kirkpatrick JN, Rogers JG, Shah NR, American Society of E (2015) Echocardiography in the management of patients with left ventricular assist devices: recommendations from the American Society of Echocardiography. J Am Soc Echocardiogr 28:853–909. https://doi.org/10.1016/j.echo.2015.05.008

Stevenson B, Roberts AJ, Dager WE (2024) Temporarily reversing warfarin with low-dose 4-factor prothrombin complex concentrate in left ventricular assist device patients undergoing an invasive procedure. Ann Pharmacother:10600280241248172. https://doi.org/10.1177/10600280241248172

Stulak JM, Schettle S, Haglund N, Dunlay S, Cowger J, Shah P, Aaronson KD, Pagani FD, Maltais S (2017) Percutaneous driveline fracture after implantation of the HeartMate II left ventricular assist device: how durable is driveline repair? ASAIO J 63:542–545. https://doi.org/10.1097/MAT.0000000000000531

Tellor BR, Smith JR, Prasad SM, Joseph SM, Silvestry SC (2014) The use of eptifibatide for suspected pump thrombus or thrombosis in patients with left ventricular assist devices. J Heart Lung Transplant 33:94–101. https://doi.org/10.1016/j.healun.2013.11.002

Urban M, Um J, Moulton M, Stoller D, Zolty R, Lowes B, Macdonald C, McCain N, Siddique A (2020) Recurrent pump thrombosis is common after axial continuous-flow left ventricular assist device exchange. Int J Artif Organs 43:109–118. https://doi.org/10.1177/0391398819876293

Uriel N, Pak SW, Jorde UP, Jude B, Susen S, Vincentelli A, Ennezat PV, Cappleman S, Naka Y, Mancini D (2010) Acquired von Willebrand syndrome after continuous-flow mechanical device support contributes to a high prevalence of bleeding during long-term support and at the time of transplantation. J Am Coll Cardiol 56:1207–1213. https://doi.org/10.1016/j.jacc.2010.05.016

Venkateswaran R, Dimarakis I (2021) A tale of two grafts. Perfusion 36:643–644. https://doi.org/10.1177/0267659120957179

Waller AH, Dunne R, Stewart GC, Ghosh N, Gosev I, Rybicki FJ, Blankstein R, Couper GS, Steigner M (2014) Evaluation of bend relief disconnection in patients supported by a HeartMate II left ventricular assist device. Circ Cardiovasc Imaging 7:844–848. https://doi.org/10.1161/CIRCIMAGING.114.001736

Weeks P, Sieg A, Rajapreyar I, Nathan S, Jumean M, Patel M, Radovancevic R, Kar B, Gregoric I (2018) Bivalirudin for left ventricular assist device thrombosis. J Thromb Thrombolysis 46:496–501. https://doi.org/10.1007/s11239-018-1725-z

Wert L, Stewart GC, Mehra MR, Milwidsky A, Jorde UP, Goldstein DJ, Selzman CH, Stehlik J, Alshamdin FD, Khaliel FH et al (2024) A multicenter evaluation of external outflow graft obstruction with a fully magnetically levitated left ventricular assist device. J Thorac Cardiovasc Surg 167:1322–1330 e1326. https://doi.org/10.1016/j.jtcvs.2022.09.051

Wever-Pinzon O, Selzman CH, Drakos SG, Saidi A, Stoddard GJ, Gilbert EM, Labedi M, Reid BB, Davis ES, Kfoury AG et al (2013) Pulsatility and the risk of nonsurgical bleeding in patients supported with the continuous-flow left ventricular assist device HeartMate II. Circ Heart Fail 6:517–526. https://doi.org/10.1161/CIRCHEARTFAILURE.112.000206

Yuzefpolskaya M, Uriel N, Chow DS, Restaino SW, Mancini DM, Flannery M, Te-Frey R, Chichetti J, Ota T, Kim H et al (2013) Prevalence and timing of bend relief disconnection in patients supported by the late version HeartMate II left ventricular assist device. J Heart Lung Transplant 32:320–325. https://doi.org/10.1016/j.healun.2012.11.016

Ziegler LA, Pousatis S, Kaczorowski DJ, Madathil RJ (2021) Emergency splicing of transected ventricular assist device driveline. Ann Thorac Surg 111:e329–e331. https://doi.org/10.1016/j.athoracsur.2020.07.073

Emergency Neonatal and Paediatric Cardiac Surgery

Michael Murphy

Abstract Emergency neonatal and paediatric cardiac surgery, although infrequent, remains among the most demanding areas of congenital cardiac care. This chapter reviews the principal indications and operative strategies for emergent intervention, focusing on conditions such as obstructed total anomalous pulmonary venous drainage, critical coarctation of the aorta refractory to prostaglandin therapy, simple transposition of the great arteries with inadequate mixing and anomalous left coronary artery from the pulmonary artery. The application of extra-corporeal membrane oxygenation is examined as a vital adjunct in perioperative stabilisation and postoperative support. The chapter also considers the evolving role of immediate post-natal surgery, facilitated by advances in foetal cardiac imaging and multidisciplinary perinatal planning. Emphasis is placed on the integration of timely diagnosis, surgical decision making and critical care optimisation in improving survival and functional outcomes. While these interventions are associated with substantial physiological and technical challenges, continuing progress in surgical technique, mechanical circulatory support and perioperative management has led to significant improvements in morbidity and mortality across this high-risk patient population.

Keywords Emergency neonatal cardiac surgery · Emergency paediatric cardiac surgery · ECMO in neonatal/paediatric cardiac surgery · Total anomalous pulmonary venous drainage · Coarctation of the aorta · Simple transposition of the great arteries · Arterial switch operation · Anomalous left coronary artery from the pulmonary artery (ALCAPA) · Immediate post-natal cardiac surgery · Atrial septostomy

---

M. Murphy (✉)
Royal Brompton Hospital, London, UK

A. Kourliouros (ed.), *Emergency Cardiac Surgery*,
https://doi.org/10.1007/978-3-032-15787-4_21

1 Introduction

Whilst semi-elective or urgent surgery is a common feature of contemporary paediatric, and in particular neonatal cardiac surgery, emergent surgery necessitating intervention prior to the next available elective list is less common. Device embolisation or other complications after catheter laboratory interventions are described in Chapter 'Emergency Cardiac Surgery Following Paediatric and Adult Congenital Percutaneous Interventions'. So-called palliative operations such as the modified Blalock–Thomas–Taussig shunt or pulmonary artery banding are usually performed as urgencies to augment pulmonary blood flow or limit pulmonary over-circulation respectively. Similarly with endocarditis, surgery is often performed on an urgent basis, but emergency surgery for cardiovascular infection is vanishingly rare.

Post-natal diagnosis of severe lesions or more critical post-partum presentation than expected can lead to emergency surgery in the neonatal period, but even in these situations, most patients can be stabilised with escalating care to the cardiac ICU, normally complemented by maintaining or re-establishing ductal patency with prostaglandins.

A group of patients where emergency surgery is frequently performed is the establishment of peripheral or central extra-corporeal membrane oxygenation. In neonates, this is most commonly veno-arterial, as veno-venous can be challenging to establish safely in this age group (Lillie et al. 2021). Mechanical support can be necessary in postoperative patients, new presentations of severe cardiac lesions, arrhythmias unresponsive to medical management and acute deterioration in patients with cardiomyopathies.

Other situations that may require emergency surgery can be broadly broken down into obstructed total anomalous pulmonary venous drainage, coarctation of the aorta where there is limited distal perfusion despite high-dose prostaglandins, simple transposition with hypoxia or low cardiac output and patients with severe left ventricular dysfunction with or without severe mitral regurgitation due to anomalous left coronary artery form the pulmonary artery. Emergency pacemaker insertion can be required in severe bradycardias or complete heart block where cardiac output is compromised and is unresponsive to pharmacological stabilisation. Safe implantation of a permanent epicardial system can be extremely challenging below 3 kg and so, in this situation, many units will initially implant a temporary epicardial system to facilitate growth (Kato et al. 2024). De novo pericardial effusions causing compromise due to tamponade are frequently dealt with percutaneous drainage, whereas for postoperative patients, loculated collections or collections unresponsive to percutaneous drainage typically require emergency surgical drainage.

2 Extra-Corporeal Membrane Oxygenation (ECMO)

Extra-corporeal support makes up a sizeable proportion of emergent surgical management in neonatal and paediatric patients and is utilised in a range of distinct situations and conditions. Post cardiotomy haemodynamic instability is usually supported by central cannulation with right atrial drainage and arterial return to the aorta or innominate artery via a chimney graft with or without a left-sided vent, depending on the circumstance.

Establishing ECMO preoperatively or in an emergency due to critically low perfusion is normally done peripherally via the right neck in neonates, infants and young children, but in older patients, we can also utilise a femoral drainage via a multistage cannula with arterial return to the femoral or axillary artery, often via a chimney graft. Achieving satisfactory venous drainage can require adjustment of both the filling status and repositioning of the venous cannula. In general, when venous return is initially satisfactory with good right atrial drainage and minimal ejection through the aortic valve seen on the arterial line tracing, the cannula should not require repositioning. Similarly, arterial return that produces good flows, without a high pressure reading and is reasonably far away from the aortic valve does not reward repositioning, which can be a risky procedure out of hours or in inexperienced hands.

Coagulopathy is a particularly challenging issue in maintaining a safe 'pump run' with ECMO and can be precipitated by consumption of endogenous clotting products by the extra-corporeal circuit or overzealous anticoagulation. Regular surveillance for coagulation abnormalities or increase in D-dimers should stimulate rapid correction before manifesting by bleeding from cannulation sites that were previously haemostatic. Once a cascade of coagulopathy commences, it can take a sizeable transfusion to correct and can require surgical exploration of peripheral or central cannulation sites. Regular examination of the circuit for clot or fibrin and surveillance of the trans-membrane pressure ensure that the circuit is healthy or detect when the circuit needs to be changed or support weaned.

3 Total Anomalous Pulmonary Venous Drainage (TAPVD)

TAPVD is characterised by an absence of the normal connection between the pulmonary veins and the left atrium. The pulmonary veins characteristically coalesce to a confluence which drains to the systemic venous system, directly in the case of cardiac type TAPVD (25%) or via a connecting vein in supra- (45%) or infra-cardiac type TAPVD (20%). The remainder are mixed type (10%), but these patients seldom present as an emergency. In cardiac type, the pulmonary veins commonly come together at or near the coronary sinus and restriction to left-sided filling is at the inter-atrial communication with surgery usually performed electively.

In infra-cardiac and supra-cardiac TAPVD, the confluence connects to the systemic veins via a connecting vein. In supra-cardiac, this is generally to the innominate vein and obstruction typically occurs as the connector vein courses between the pulmonary artery and the bronchus. In infra-cardiac TAPVD, the connecting vein becomes obstructed as it descends through the diaphragm or by connecting to a high resistance venous system.

Patients with obstructed TAPVD often present critically unwell in a low cardiac output state with cyanosis and a clinical picture of pulmonary venous congestion. Though some centres have described trans-catheter temporisation of the situation by relieving obstruction, maintaining patency of the ductus venosus with prostaglandins or using ECMO, these measures seldom postpone surgery in a meaningful way and so most centres will perform emergency surgery for obstructed TAPVD. Repair of infra- or supra-cardiac TAPVD consists of surgical connection of the confluence to the back of the left atrium. Though this can be performed as a simple circumferential anastomosis, some centres prefer a wider incision in the back of the left atrium that is sutured to the adjacent pericardium around a widely opened confluence, rather than to the confluence tissue itself, the so-called sutureless repair (Yanagawa et al. 2011). Though true obstruction of cardiac TAPVD is rare, repair is by unroofing the coronary sinus that receives the pulmonary veins and relocating the atrial septum to above the coronary sinus, committing all veins to the left side.

Though mortality rates are low in elective repair of unobstructed TAPVD, emergency repair, particularly in the setting of coexistent pulmonary hypertension, is considerable. It is common to use pulmonary vasodilators such as nitric oxide and avoid using adrenaline in the management of these patients, but some patients can require postoperative extra-corporeal membrane oxygenation (ECMO) to support their recovery. The haemodynamic compromise seen after TAPVD repair can relate to the massive increase in preload to an underdeveloped and possibly non-compliant left ventricle with consequent high left atrial pressure. This can be further compounded by a reactive pulmonary vascular bed and it can sometimes be useful to monitor the left atrial or pulmonary artery pressure in the first few days after repair.

Survivors of surgery tend to have an excellent prognosis, but patients with pulmonary vein stenosis tend to develop progressive pulmonary hypertension and do poorly despite progresses in surgical, interventional and pharmacological treatment (Feins et al. 2022).

4 Coarctation

Coarctation of the aorta is characterised by narrowing of the aortic lumen in the isthmic region between the left subclavian and the insertion of the ductus arteriosus. The aortic blood flow is comprised not only of the narrowing of the vessel lumen, with or without more proximal aortic arch hypoplasia, but is further compromised in neonates and infants by discrete or circumferential aortic ductal tissue that contracts as the duct closes, further reducing or even completely obstructing peripheral flow.

Foetuses with suspicion for coarctation detected on ante-natal scans will often be delivered near a cardiac centre with ready access to post-natal echocardiographic assessment of aortic narrowing. In unwell neonates with a clinical suspicion or proven coarctation, prostaglandins will frequently be commenced with a view to maintaining or re-establishing ductal patency and distal perfusion. Once stable, these patients can be investigated for coexisting lesions, particularly associated arch hypoplasia and adequacy of left-sided structures. These patients are usually discussed in a multidisciplinary team meeting and have semi-elective treatment of their coarctation.

Occasionally, new-borns or young infants without ante-natal suspicion of congenital cardiac disease will present unwell in heart failure with poor distal perfusion and metabolic derangement. Once the diagnosis of coarctation is established, these patients are commenced on prostaglandins to improve or re-establish ductal and aortic luminal patency, with high doses often required to achieve a satisfactory response (Desai et al. 2013). In those patients who remain unwell and do not respond to prostaglandins, emergency treatment is required to relieve obstruction in the aortic isthmus. Although some centres would advocate for balloon angioplasty in the setting of severe left ventricular dysfunction (Hysko et al. 2023), emergency surgery is often required. If the aortic arch is adequate, the procedure can be performed by thoracotomy where, during a brief period of aortic cross clamping, the narrowed segment of aorta and any remanent ductal tissue is resected and the aorta is reconstructed to provide unobstructed blood flow to the descending aorta. Reperfusion of the lower body after a period of ischaemia can result in a temporary haemodynamic instability that requires a short period of escalated support as the metabolic picture improves and any ventricular dysfunction resolves. In patients where the aortic arch is deemed to be inadequate, the coarctation is repaired via sternotomy with measures to improve the lumen size of the arch after resection of the coarctation segment. This procedure is performed on cardio-pulmonary bypass utilising circulatory arrest, with or without antegrade cerebral perfusion to augment the arch, often utilising a patch of pulmonary homograft.

5 Simple Transposition

One of the most common indications for cardiac surgery in the neonatal period is simple transposition. In this condition, the right ventricle gives rise to the aorta and left ventricle gives rise to the pulmonary artery, producing circulations that are in parallel rather than in sequence. Oxygenation is entirely dependent on shunting at atrial, ventricular or ductal level. In patients with intact ventricular septum, mixing at atrial septal level can be inadequate and mixing at ductal level is seldom sufficient. In situations where saturation or cardiac output is inadequate, due to suboptimal mixing, the arterial switch operation can be deferred for a time with a transcatheter balloon atrial septostomy. Once oxygenation has stabilised, the prostaglandins are often stopped and the duct is allowed to close allowing for relatively elective surgery off prostaglandins.

A small percentage of patients with simple transposition will continue to be desaturated or in a low cardiac output state despite atrial septostomy and maintenance of ductal patency. These patients can be metabolically quite unwell and present the team with a difficult choice between ECMO, further transcatheter attempts to improve mixing or emergency arterial switch operation. Preoperative ECMO or further transcatheter attempts to improve mixing in this setting can be high risk, particularly for systemic thromboembolism and so the majority of centres will manage this situation with emergency surgery with outcomes that are not dissimilar to semi-elective surgery (Anderson et al. 2013). At arterial switch, the coronaries are resected from the aorta and transferred to the pulmonary or neo-aortic root, which is then connected to the ascending aorta. The neo-pulmonary root is reconstructed with patch material, replacing the defect where the coronary buttons were harvested and right ventricle to pulmonary artery continuity restored after anterior relocation of the pulmonary arteries (Le-Compte manoeuvre). Any atrial communications are closed such that the left atrium fills the left ventricle and ejects into the aorta. Although emergency surgery for simple transposition is infrequently encountered, outcomes remain similar to urgent or semi-electively performed arterial switch operation (Hussey et al. 2023).

6 Anomalous Left Coronary Artery from the Pulmonary Artery (ALCAPA)

ALCAPA is a rare condition that is seldom diagnosed antenatally. Although some patients will have incidental diagnosis in early life, it is more common for infants to be increasingly unwell for a period of time and at presentation to have severely depressed left ventricular function with or without mitral regurgitation. Less than a third of all cases occur outside infancy (Cashen et al. 2021). The presence of severely depressed left ventricular function in an infant with an inability on echo to trace the left main back to the aorta will usually raise suspicion of ALCAPA, which is frequently confirmed on emergent CT angiography or cardiac catheterisation. Though some patients can be stable, it is not uncommon for patients to deteriorate requiring progressive escalation in support that may even include preoperative ECMO. The underlying lesion of the left main coronary artery arising from the pulmonary root is associated with enlargement of the right coronary system. As the pulmonary vascular resistance drops postnatally, the flow is reversed in the left coronary system and the flow and volumes through the right compensate to provide coronary blood supply to the whole heart as well as the runoff into the pulmonary vascular bed. Because of this physiology, the electrocardiogram is often grossly abnormal with evidence of ischaemia and/or infarction. The mitral regurgitation associated with the dilated and poorly functioning left ventricle is almost always due to annular dilatation though there can also be restriction of the posterior leaflet due to necrosis or fibrosis of the subvalvar apparatus.

With the threat of ongoing ischaemia/infarction and the possibility of arrest, surgical repair is often performed emergently but can occasionally be postponed until the next morning. It is important to anticipate the need for ECMO postoperatively and counsel the parents appropriately. Initial repair is by extensive epicardial mobilisation of the excised left main coronary button, translocation to the aorta with closure of the defect in the pulmonary root with a patch of pericardium, similar to the translocation performed at arterial switch operation. In most centres, the mitral valve is not approached at this stage and long-term studies seem to indicate that this procedure is sufficient to achieve long-term stabilisation of ventricular function and gradual normalisation of mitral valve function, though a proportion will have mitral intervention for mitral regurgitation (Cashen et al. 2021).

Central VA ECMO is frequently used postoperatively, though LVAD support can also be considered, as the issue is often purely left ventricular function, rather than right ventricular dysfunction or oxygenation. Either way, left atrial pressure monitoring is helpful for weaning, and support beyond a week is not uncommon (Kwiatkowski et al. 2021).

7 Immediate Post-Natal Surgery

With progress in antenatal diagnosis in the foetus by echocardiogram or more recently by MRI (Moray et al. 2024), certain situations have been managed by emergency surgery immediately after birth. In these rare cases, invariably after prolonged discussion and planning, the foetus is delivered in an operating room in a cardiac centre with a full team ready in an adjacent operating room for an immediate post-natal procedure. Situations where this is deemed to be beneficial are atrial septectomy in hypoplastic left heart syndrome with restrictive atrial septum unsuitable for balloon atrial septostomy, tumours compromising the cardiovascular or respiratory system and patients with critical aortic stenosis and extremely poor ventricular function.

References

Anderson BR, Ciarleglio AJ, Hayes DA, Friedman R, Bacha E (2013) A prompt arterial switch operation improves outcomes and reduces costs for neonates with transposition of the great arteries. J Am Coll Cardiol 61(10):E504. https://doi.org/10.1016/s0735-1097(13)60504-5

Cashen K, Kwiatkowski DM, Riley CM et al (2021) Anomalous origin of the left coronary artery from the pulmonary artery: a retrospective multicenter study. Pediatr Crit Care Med 22(12):e626–e635. https://doi.org/10.1097/pcc.0000000000002820

Desai AR, Maiya S, Inwald D, Slavik Z (2013) Prostaglandin in aortic coarctation and closed arterial duct—treatment beyond ductal re-opening. Cor Vasa 55(5):e460–e462. https://doi.org/10.1016/j.crvasa.2013.04.004

Feins EN, Ireland C, Gauvreau K et al (2022) Pulmonary vein stenosis: anatomic considerations, surgical management, and outcomes. J Thorac Cardiovasc Surg 163(6):2198–2207.e3. https://doi.org/10.1016/j.jtcvs.2021.10.022

Hussey AD, Gentles TL, Perelini F, Beca J, Finucane K (2023) Emergency arterial switch: rescue therapy for life-threatening hypoxemia in infants with transposition of great arteries with intact intraventricular septum. J Thorac Cardiovasc Surg 166(1):183–190. https://doi.org/10.1016/j.jtcvs.2022.11.014

Hysko K, Hohmann D, Bobylev D et al (2023) Recovery of biventricular function after catheter intervention or surgery for neonatal coarctation of the aorta. JACC Adv 2(3):100326. https://doi.org/10.1016/j.jacadv.2023.100326

Kato A, Kitano M, Shimabukuro A, Sato S, Nishioka M (2024) Successful pacemaker implantation for congenital complete heart block with pulmonary valve stenosis in an extremely low birth weight infant. J Pediatr Cardiol Card Surg 8(2):92–95. https://doi.org/10.24509/jpccs.23-017

Kwiatkowski DM, Mastropietro CW, Cashen K et al (2021) Characteristics and surgical outcomes of patients with late presentation of anomalous left coronary artery from the pulmonary artery: a multicenter study. Semin Thorac Cardiovasc Surg 33(1):141–150. https://doi.org/10.1053/j.semtcvs.2020.08.014

Lillie J, Pienaar A, Budd J et al (2021) Multisite veno-venous cannulation for neonates and nonambulatory children*. Pediatr Crit Care Med 22(8):692–700. https://doi.org/10.1097/pcc.0000000000002753

Moray A, Mugaba PM, Joynt C et al (2024) Predicting high-risk fetal cardiac disease anticipated to need immediate postnatal stabilization and intervention with planned pediatric cardiac operating room delivery. J Am Heart Assoc Cardiovasc Cerebrovasc Dis 13(6):e031184. https://doi.org/10.1161/jaha.123.031184

Yanagawa B, Alghamdi AA, Dragulescu A et al (2011) Primary sutureless repair for "simple" total anomalous pulmonary venous connection: midterm results in a single institution. J Thorac Cardiovasc Surg 141(6):1346–1354. https://doi.org/10.1016/j.jtcvs.2010.10.056

Emergency Adult Congenital Cardiac Surgery

Michael Murphy, Jared Beller, and Alex Stockenhuber

Abstract Emergency surgery in adults with congenital heart disease (ACHD) is uncommon, but presents exceptional complexity due to diverse anatomy, prior interventions and comorbid conditions. This chapter reviews the principal indications, surgical strategies and perioperative considerations in the emergent management of ACHD patients. Key clinical scenarios include fulminant infective endocarditis with haemodynamic instability, aortic emergencies, acute decompensated heart failure and complications arising from percutaneous interventions. Additional sections address the challenges of emergency re-sternotomy, pacing in complex anatomy and surgery during pregnancy. The chapter highlights the importance of meticulous preoperative assessment, multidisciplinary decision making and tailored use of mechanical circulatory support, including extra-corporeal membrane oxygenation and ventricular assist devices. Risk prediction models such as the PEACH score are discussed within the context of perioperative mortality and comorbidity burden. Despite high procedural risk, outcomes continue to improve through advances in imaging, surgical technique and postoperative care. Ultimately, successful emergency surgery in ACHD relies on collaboration across the disciplines to deliver safe, individualised and timely interventions in this high-risk patient population.

Keywords Adult congenital heart disease (ACHD) · Emergency cardiac surgery in ACHD · Cardiac surgery risk stratification in ACHD · PEACH score · Re-sternotomy in ACHD · Infective endocarditis in ACHD · Aortic emergencies in ACHD · Conotruncal abnormalities · Aortic dissection in ACHD · Sinus of Valsalva rupture · Acute decompensation of heart failure in ACHD · Mechanical

M. Murphy (✉)
Royal Brompton Hospital, London, UK

J. Beller
University of Virginia Heath, Charlottesville, VA, USA

A. Stockenhuber
John Radcliffe Hospital, Oxford, UK
e-mail: Alexander.Stockenhuber@ouh.nhs.uk

A. Kourliouros (ed.), *Emergency Cardiac Surgery*,
https://doi.org/10.1007/978-3-032-15787-4_22

circulatory support in ACHD · Emergency surgery after percutaneous intervention in ACHD · Emergency cardiac surgery in pregnant ACHD patients · Surgical emergency pacing in ACHD

1 Introduction

Adult congenital heart disease (ACHD) encompasses a broad spectrum of diagnoses and conditions. The vast majority of presentations allow for medical stabilisation prior to surgical intervention and so emergency surgery is infrequent. However, there are a number of select circumstances where urgent or emergent intervention is required. Broadly, these can be categorised into four main groups: (1) fulminant endocarditis with ongoing emboli or haemodynamic instability, (2) aortic emergencies, (3) acute decompensation of heart failure and (4) complications of percutaneous interventions, which are more broadly covered in Chapter 'Emergency Cardiac Surgery Following Paediatric and Adult Congenital Percutaneous Interventions'.

Many patients with ACHD will have had previous interventions, which often confound their acute presentation. Review of previous operative notes, transcatheter interventions and diagnostic reports is critical to operative planning in ACHD surgery. In the emergent setting, this is not always available but any recent imaging should be reviewed to obtain as much information on prior interventions and altered anatomy as possible. In addition, previous implantation of prosthetic material and valves places this population at elevated risk of infective endocarditis, which is a frequent and recurrent theme of urgent and emergent surgery in this population. End-stage heart failure and cardiogenic shock are increasingly prevalent in the ACHD population where several distinct forms of heart failure may be encountered including the consequences of long-standing valvular dysfunction, coronary insufficiency, the failing single ventricle and conditions where there is a systemic right ventricle. After surgical correction of congenital heart disease, lifelong follow-up is recommended for a large proportion of patients (Bedzra et al. 2022). However, ACHD patients are often lost to follow-up either because they do not connect with adult services after transition or routine surveillance discontinues to the extent that over half of patients are not seen in the specialised clinics recommended by guidelines (Moons et al. 2021). As such, these patients may present precipitously with advanced disease requiring emergent intervention.

The diverse pathologies of varying severity seen in patients with ACHD, often in the context of previous surgical or transcatheter procedures, oblige careful consideration prior to emergency surgical intervention. Altered anatomy, prior interventions and at times incomplete information are hallmarks of the contemporary management of ACHD patients. In this population, nowhere are the challenges greater than when emergency surgery is required.

ACHD patients represent a cohort that massively benefits from carefully considered multidisciplinary care, but the usual scrutiny by the broader team of ACHD cardiologists, surgeons, radiologists and intensive care physicians can often be unfeasible in the setting of an acute presentation requiring emergency surgery. In every domain, there are critical nuances that may be overlooked when these patients are cared for outside of a collaborative, specialised multidisciplinary team.

Ensuring expeditious availability of up-to-date diagnostic tests is an essential step towards selecting and executing the emergency management strategy. Surgical planning begins with appropriate risk stratification and several different risk models have been proposed with a range of comorbidities and presentations being accounted for (Constantine et al. 2021; Abdelrehim et al. 2023). Given the heterogeneity of diagnoses and presentations, a uniform model has not been widely accepted. Urgent or emergent surgery has consistently been shown to be associated with increased mortality in most forms of cardiovascular procedures and patients with ACHD represent a group at elevated risk from non-elective surgery. In addition to complex congenital cardiac disease, coexistent heart failure, kidney disease and multiple prior surgeries are prevalent in this patient group, all of which have been shown to be predictive of worse outcomes (Table 1).

Table 1 Perioperative mortality risk in ACHD patients undergoing cardiac surgery—the PEACH score (Constantine et al. 2021)

Factors for calculation of the PEACH score	
	Score
NYHA functional class	
I/II	0
III/IV	1
Procedural urgency	
Non-urgent	0
Urgent	1
Renal function (eGFR), ml/min/1.73 m^2	
≥60	0
<60	1
Active endocarditis	
No	0
Yes	1
Multiple previous sternotomies	
<2	0
≥2	1
ACHS score	
0.1–1.5	0
1.6–3.0	1
Haemoglobin level, g/L	
100–200	0
<100 or >200	1

2 Sternal Re-Entry During Emergency Cardiac Surgery

The optimal operative approach in emergency surgery in patients with ACHD requires in-depth understanding of not only of the underlying cardiac anatomy but how that anatomy has been altered by previous interventions and the acute pathology. Prior to surgery, evaluation of peripheral vasculature either with computed tomography angiography or ultrasound is helpful to plan for peripheral cardiopulmonary bypass, as a primary intention or should it be required after sternotomy. It is important to appreciate that patients with ACHD can have peripheral vessels that are unsuitable or sub-optimal to establish full-flow peripheral bypass. The combination of thrombosis or scarring from prior surgical or transcatheter interventions in vessels that may be congenitally hypoplastic, absent or aberrant can make achieving sufficient flow on bypass challenging, particularly when systemic cooling is required. In addition, many patients with ACHD have a long-standing low cardiac output state, such that the peripheral arteries are poorly developed and so smaller than would be expected in an age- and sex-matched population.

Mediastinal adhesions from previous surgery may delay institution of central cannulation and proximity of critical vascular structures to the posterior table of the sternum can all add to the complexity and risk of emergency surgery. The anterior free wall of the right ventricle is often closely associated with, but only rarely adherent to, the posterior table of the sternum and so can usually be dissected out safely if care is taken to divide adhesions prior to spreading the sternal halves. Preoperative axial imaging when available can inform the operative teams of the proximity of the innominate vein, atria, ventricles or great vessels to the posterior sternal table but can also be falsely reassuring that sternal re-entry will be straightforward. Differing philosophies to sternal re-entry abound within the specialty, ranging from routine use of peripheral bypass prior to re-sternotomy to a more expectant approach of dissecting as much of the mediastinal structures away from the sternum prior to reopening, with the primary intention of central cannulation. Using either strategy, avoidance of major injury to the cardiac structures is a central component to delivering a safe outcome. Uncontrolled bleeding, entraining air into cardiac chambers or damage to the ventricle can have as sizeable an impact on patient outcomes as the cardiac procedure performed. The presence of transcatheter pulmonary valves or right ventricular outflow tract stents may also result in dense adhesions to the back of the sternum, making mobilising the structures on the left-hand side of the mediastinum even more hazardous. Systemic cooling in preparation for circulatory arrest, with or without carotid/innominate artery cannulation, to allow for antegrade cerebral perfusion, is helpful in cases where major cardiac structures are at high risk for injury. Careful assessment of intracardiac shunting on echocardiogram, frequently complemented by a bubble study, is important in these scenarios, keeping in mind that completely excluding the possibility of a residual shunt by preoperative imaging is challenging. Entrainment of air, particularly into the left side of the heart, puts the patient at extremely high risk of a neurological event and may require complete arrest of the circulation to safely dissect out the cardiac structures prior to aortic cross-clamping.

1. Fulminant Endocarditis with Ongoing Emboli or Haemodynamic Instability

Patients with ACHD are at greatly elevated risk of endocarditis compared with the general population (Windsor et al. 2022; 2023 ESC Guidelines for the management of endocarditis 2023). Right-sided endocarditis is particularly common in this population, due in part to the prevalence of right heart disease but also to the frequency of prior transcatheter or surgical interventions and consequent infection of prosthetic material. Given the complex anatomy and lifetime risk of multiple interventions, attempts to avoid surgery in patients with endocarditis through the use of carefully considered antibiotic therapy is more common than in acquired cardiac disease. This allows for temporisation of the infective process in the hope of sterilising the field and to allow for a period of recovery prior to surgical treatment.

Emergency surgery for infective endocarditis has traditionally been reserved for cases of severe haemodynamic compromise due to valvular or ventricular dysfunction, but more contemporary guidelines also suggest local complications suggestive of uncontrolled infections such as abscesses, false aneurysms, fistulas and the presence of emboli with large vegetations (>10 mm) as indications for urgent surgery (Fig. 1). Most recently, acute neurological injury due to embolism from infective endocarditis is considered an indication for urgent or emergency surgery (2023 ESC Guidelines for the management of endocarditis 2023). It is worth considering that the momentum behind these guidelines and recommendations are often extrapolated from the data on left-sided infective endocarditis and generalisability towards ACHD patients is not well established. Emboli are better tolerated in right-sided infective endocarditis and so the guidelines use a larger cut-off for right-sided

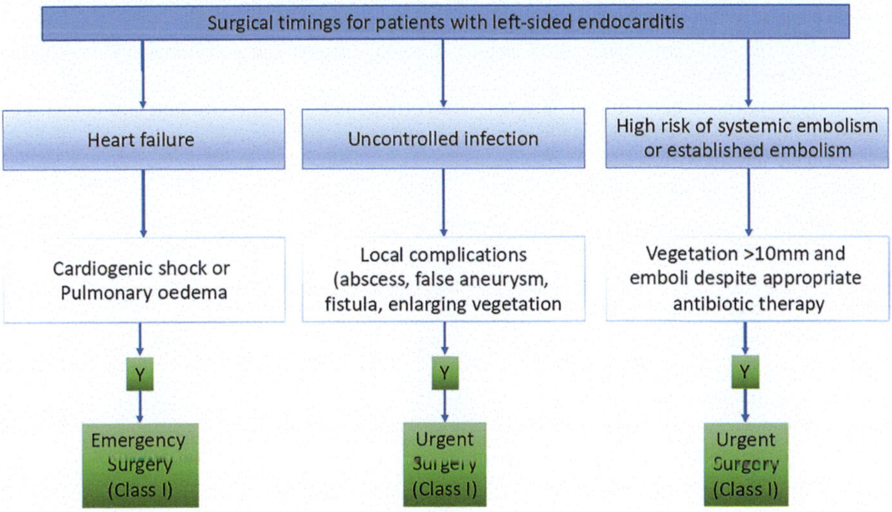

Fig. 1 Clinical urgency of cardiac surgery in patients with left-sided infective endocarditis

vegetations (>20 mm) and require repeated pulmonary emboli or respiratory compromise to recommend emergency or urgent surgical intervention (Table 2).

The emphasis of surgical management for infective endocarditis in ACHD is the radical debridement of infected or devitalised tissue with particular attention to prosthetic material as a potential nidus for residual and recurrent infection followed by reconstruction. These procedures can be particularly problematic, as complete removal of prosthetic material is not always feasible, as these can be heavily embedded within the heart or can be heavily calcified and reconstruction in this setting can be challenging and is often facilitated by using homograft material.

Table 2 The indication for emergent and urgent cardiac surgery in infective endocarditis modified from the ESC guidelines

Indication for emergency/urgent surgery in infective endocarditis	Timing	Class
Left-sided infective endocarditis		
Heart failure with cardiogenic shock or pulmonary oedema	Emergency	Class I
Uncontrolled infection with local complications (abscess, fistulas, pseudoaneurysms)	Urgent	Class I
Vegetation >10 mm and emboli despite appropriate antibiotic therapy	Urgent	Class I
Heart failure with poor haemodynamic tolerance	Urgent	Class I
Persistent positive blood cultures	Urgent	Class IIa
Vegetation >10 mm and other reason for surgery	Urgent	Class I
Vegetation >10 mm without evidence of embolism	Urgent	Class IIb
Infective endocarditis with stroke		
Ischaemic stroke and cardiogenic shock as long as coma is absent and a meaningful recovery Is possible	Emergency	Class I
Ischaemic stroke and heart failure, uncontrolled infection, abscess, or persistent high embolic risk, as long as coma is absent and a cerebral haemorrhage has been excluded	Urgent	Class I
Right-sided infective endocarditis		
Right-sided heart failure not responding to diuretics	Emergency/ Urgent	Class I
Persistent vegetation with respiratory insufficiency requiring respiratory support after recurrent pulmonary emboli	Urgent	Class I
Vegetation >20 mm after recurrent septic pulmonary emboli	Urgent	Class I
Simultaneous involvement of left heart structures	Urgent	Class I
Persistent positive blood cultures	Urgent	Class IIa

Table describing the indications for emergency or urgent surgical intervention in infective endocarditis. Adapted from the 2023 ESC guidelines for the management of infective endocarditis (2023)

2. Aortic Emergencies

Dilation of the aortic root, ascending aorta and, to a lesser extent, aortic arch are common in patients with ACHD. The challenge lies in separating expected or physiologic dilation, which is often long-standing on serial imaging, from pathologic progressive dilation. In all cases, a balance can be hard to achieve where the risk of dissection or rupture outweighs the risk of what is often high-risk surgery. It is likely that these difficult decisions will remain individualised, as it is hard to apply guidelines based on adult populations to those with ACHD. A basic understanding of the underlying pathology is critical. Patients with cono-truncal abnormalities such as transposition of the great arteries, truncus arteriosus or tetralogy of Fallot will develop some degree of aortic dilation over time. While there is an association between cono-truncal abnormalities and aortic dilation, it appears that the risk of aortic dissection or rupture is not significantly increased compared to the general population (Frischhertz et al. 2015).

Single-institution studies demonstrate that at medium- to long-term follow-up after the arterial switch, no aortic dissection or rupture is seen, but reoperative aortic root surgery is relatively common, usually for progressive aortic incompetence associated with root dilatation (van der Palen et al. 2021). However, many centres advocate for prophylactic replacement of the aortic root for diameters greater than 55 mm, rapidly progressing enlargement or if there is significant neo-aortic valve regurgitation. Given the small patient numbers that have long-term follow-up, there is insufficient data to make definitive recommendations. The lack of aortic emergencies reported in the ACHD population would seem to indicate that the risk of rupture or dissection is lower than would be expected, but aortic diameter remains an important risk factor for dissection in this population.

Emergency aortic operations for decompensation of severe aortic regurgitations in ACHD patients are rare but have significant risk associated. Safe sternal re-entry can be a challenge. Root replacement with preservation of the native semi-lunar valve has been described in transposition and variants tetralogy of Fallot, though the valve is seldom retained if the root requires replacement in truncus arteriosus. In the acute setting, a second bypass run on a sick ventricle is not advisable and so composite root replacement is often preferentially performed. Although mechanical prostheses are often chosen by patients and clinicians because of improved durability, in the emergent situation, bioprosthetic valves are sometime preferable as management of postoperative mechanical support is often easier with tissue valves. As the dilated root generally allows for a larger size valve implantation, along with the improved contemporary outcomes of valve-in-valve transcatheter valve implantation, it can often be a difficult decision to make as to which prosthesis to implant. Replacement of the ascending aorta is often necessary in cono-truncal abnormalities, but arch intervention is unusual. When required, axillary cannulation or innominate artery cannulation in the chest can facilitate antegrade cerebral perfusion, which can be very useful in scenarios where the amount of arch needing to be replaced can be difficult to anticipate and the anatomy can be unconventional.

Procedures that involve arch replacement often involve aortic surgeons in conjunction with ACHD surgeons.

Emergency surgery for rupture or dissection warrants involvement of aortic surgeons to help decide on the amount of aorta to replace in what are usually relatively young patients, where resection of the tear site is important and where leaving a dissected arch will almost always lead to the need for redo arch replacement in the future. In the setting of an acute symptomatic presentation with dissection on axial imaging, it is difficult to manage these situations conservatively, but if the symptoms are less acute and there is a possibility of a more sub-acute presentation, delayed treatment can sometimes be a safer approach.

Another situation where emergency aortic surgery can be required is rupture of a sinus of Valsalva. The condition has often yet to be diagnosed on presentation and can present to the ECMO services for mechanical support, when the diagnosis is finally made. These patients have abnormalities of their aortic roots such that the sinus dilates into a sinus of Valsalva aneurysm that enlarges caudally towards the right ventricle, left ventricle or atria. When the aneurysm ruptures, the presentation is often with a sudden onset of severe aortic regurgitation with pressure and volume overload of the affected chamber. Surgical repair usually involves patching both ends of the defect as well as any ventricular septal defects and despite successful repair, patients may need mechanical support with ECMO postoperatively. As the entire aortic root can be abnormal in this situation, root replacement may also be required, but given that patients often present to the operative theatre in extremis with profound shock, an expeditious operation is often prudent.

3. Acute Decompensation of Heart Failure

Cardiac failure is a frequent feature amongst patients with ACHD for a myriad of differing and frequently overlapping aetiologies. Deterioration of systolic or diastolic ventricular function can occur at any stage of life and chronic volume and/or pressure loading from aortic narrowing, valvular disease, and ventricular disease or as a consequence of aortopulmonary collaterals. These conditions can exist alone or in combination with cardiomyopathies associated with single ventricle physiology, systemic right ventricle or abnormalities of the outflow tracts. Chronic management of cardiac failure in ACHD patients is challenging and many will ultimately require the difficult decision to either perform high-risk surgery to optimise symptoms and improve cardiac function or to refer for consideration for a durable ventricular assist device or transplantation. Acute presentation can occasionally require emergency surgery, which is almost always based on introducing mechanical support in the form of ECMO or LVAD+/−RVAD rather than acute transplantation or reoperative surgery. However, at times, temporary mechanical circulatory support as a bridge to surgical intervention may be considered. Involvement of the heart failure team will be essential if ventricular assist device implantation is the preferred approach, even as an emergency or after stabilisation with ECMO. Veno-arterial ECMO, with the intent of recovery and decannulation or as a bridge to durable device should not be prolonged, as there is a high rate of complications when this invasive therapy is used for more than a few days (Malik et al. 2024). The use of durable ventricular assist devices has been steadily on the rise as has the population of single ventricle patients over recent years (Cedars et al. 2021). In particular, the population of single ventricle patients with systemic right ventricles after Norwood procedure and Fontan completion is increasing in numbers.

Short-term and intermediate survival on ventricular assist devices is generally good with 76% survival at 6 months. A crucial factor for the successful outcome of ventricular assist devices is patient selection and understanding systolic and diastolic ventricular dysfunction is critically important. The presence of elevated pulmonary vascular resistance can complicate ventricular assist device function. While elective implantation is generally preferable and associated with better outcomes, improvement of end-organ function after implantation of ventricular assist devices in emergency situations is increasingly described.

4. Emergency Cardiac Surgery After Percutaneous Intervention

With the advances in percutaneous techniques, more and more ACHD pathologies are treated by interventional cardiologists. It is imperative that the surgeon stay abreast of these developments and understand how these procedures are performed which will help inform management strategies of complications. In general, transcatheter techniques are safe and effective with an overall favourable risk profile and more rapid recovery than surgical intervention, and thus, their broad adoption.

Commonly, occlusion devices are used to close atrial and ventricular septal defects with excellent outcomes. The risk of device embolisation is less than 1% and while many devices can be retrieved percutaneously, there are situations that will require emergent cardiac surgery (Kamla et al. 2021). Devices can embolise into the right and left side of the heart with the potential to cause a range of complications including left or right ventricular outflow tract obstruction, acute valvular regurgitation, cardiac arrhythmia or frank perforation. In addition to acute embolisation, late erosions related to occlusion devices can occur with haemopericardium or tamponade having been reported to require emergency surgery. The close proximity of the atrial septum and the non-coronary sinus of the aortic root puts this area in jeopardy from erosions, especially in cases of root aneurysms.

In patients with repaired Tetralogy of Fallot with pulmonary valve insufficiency or other abnormalities of the right ventricular outflow tract, transcatheter pulmonary valve implantation has become a commonly performed intervention to restore valvular competency. Similar to transcatheter closure of intracardiac shunts, this procedure has an excellent safety profile and procedural volumes continue to grow. A number of distinct complications can occur after percutaneous pulmonary valve insertions that have the potential to require emergent surgery. In cases of calcified conduits, there is the potential for frank rupture, which is commonly managed with covered stents. If it is not feasible to cover the site of rupture with a stent or haemodynamic compromise persists, surgical repair is required. This situation is frequently in the setting of redo surgery and peripheral bypass is often instituted prior to re-sternotomy for replacement of the ruptured right ventricular to pulmonary artery conduit. Coronary artery compression with consequent myocardial ischaemia is also encountered during percutaneous pulmonary valve implantation, but often resolves with deflation of the expanding balloons or coronary artery intervention in the catheter laboratory. In cases where myocardial ischaemia persists frequently with impaired ventricular function, it is necessary to emergently operate on these patients to relieve ischaemia. These operations can range from surgical replacement of the conduit with the transcatheter valve inside, to dissecting out the affected coronary territory to relieve local pressure to coronary artery bypass when relief of ischaemia is not possible.

In all cases, a deliberate and carefully considered operative approach is required. For cases where there has been device embolisation that mandates surgical removal, it should be clear prior to surgery if the original pathology that led to the intervention should be addressed at the same time as device retrieval and as valvular compromise can occur due to the device or as a consequence of its removal, careful consideration is needed as to the need for valve repair during the device extraction. Should coronary compromise exist prior to emergency surgery, it is important to appreciate the relationship of the coronaries to existing structures and appreciate the cause of the ischaemia, be it external compression after intervention, damage or internal occlusion of the coronary itself during intervention or an event related to native coronary artery disease. Plans to perform percutaneous coronary intervention or coronary artery bypass at the end of procedure should be in place prior to the emergency surgery should the ischaemia not resolve from device retrieval. Coronary compromise due to a balloon dilation or stenting of the right ventricular outflow tract or a right ventricular to pulmonary artery conduit will often require careful removal of the occluding tissue and right ventricular outflow tract or pulmonary trunk replacement to relieve the obstruction. Removal of recently sited transcatheter devices lodged within vessels or the heart can often be quite straightforward. When the device is embedded, retrieval can be assisted by engaging the device with a large calibre suture and drawing the suture and so the device through a large bore snugger, such as that used for caval snaring. This will allow reduction in size and crimping of the device, which can make retrieval of a lodged device easier and safer.

3 Emergency Cardiac Surgery in Pregnant ACHD Patients

An infrequent but challenging situation is patients with ACHD who have deteriorating cardiac function during pregnancy present in cardiac failure, either due to a severe valvular lesion or ventricular dysfunction or both. Volume overload confounds the haemodynamic effects of cardiac disease in pregnancy. Although good clinical management centres around avoiding pregnancy until any gross haemodynamic issues are optimised and avoidance of surgery until the patient is a number of weeks postpartum, occasionally life-saving surgery is required during the pregnancy. Although a number of techniques are described to try to avoid foetal demise, operations that involve cardiopulmonary bypass are very frequently associated with in utero death. General considerations for emergency cardiac surgery during pregnancy in the non-ACHD population are discussed in greater detail in Chapter 'Emergency Cardiac Surgery During Pregnancy'.

4 Surgical Emergency Pacing in Complex Congenital Patients

Patients with complex congenital heart disease have a high incidence of permanent pacing indications including for atrioventricular nodal block and sinus node disease. In both cases, ACHD patients can present with haemodynamic instability or syncope requiring emergency pacemaker implantation. Transvenous pacing, while the preferred option in many circumstances, should be avoided in situations where there is stenosis within the systemic veins, after cavopulmonary connection, after complex atrial surgery, following tricuspid valve surgery or where there are congenital abnormalities within the systemic venous abnormalities (Chubb et al. 2016). In such circumstances, urgent surgical epicardial pacing might be necessary, which can involve extensive dissection by repeat sternotomy. Coexisting ventricular dysfunction or ventricular dyssynchrony are common in this patient group and so siting the ventricular lead close to the LV apex or arranging for bi-ventricular pacing should be considered. In situation where repeat sternotomy is not advisable or feasible, epicardial systems can usually be safely implanted via left thoracotomy, which gives access to the ventricular mass, as well as the left atrial appendage for dual chamber pacing. This technique can be particularly useful in patients after prior Fontan procedure. Removal of infected pacemaker material can occasionally be necessary as part of endocarditis surgery, though this is often in coordination with electrophysiology teams.

Surgical teams can be required to respond with emergency surgery to deal with the complications of laser lead extraction such as injury to a major venous or atrial structure and resolve any tamponade (see Chapter 'Emergency Cardiac Surgery for Cardiac Device Lead Extraction' for more details). These situations often benefit from a tailored approach but peripheral bypass and cooling prior to re-sternotomy are frequently necessary. Once the heart is dissected out from the mediastinal adhesions, it may be necessary to repair the tricuspid valve and site an epicardial system.

5 Summary

Adult congenital heart disease is a heterogenous patient group with unique and often unanticipated challenges. Emergency surgery in this cohort could be more intricate and surgical treatment in the acute setting should be approached thoughtfully and carefully. With a multidisciplinary approach and appropriate diagnostics to aid careful planning, emergency surgery in the ACHD population can be performed safely with excellent results.

References

2023 ESC Guidelines for the management of endocarditis: Developed by the task force on the management of endocarditis of the European Society of Cardiology (ESC) Endorsed by the European Association for Cardio-Thoracic Surgery (EACTS) and the European Association of Nuclear Medicine (EANM). Eur Heart J 44(39):3948–4042 (2023). https://doi.org/10.1093/eurheartj/ehad193

Abdelrehim AA, Dearani JA, Holst KA, Miranda WR, Connolly HM, Todd AL, Burchill LJ, Schaff HV, Pochettino A, Stephens EH (2023) Risk factors and early outcomes of repeat sternotomy in 1960 adults with congenital heart disease: a 30-year, single-center study. J Thorac Cardiovasc Surg S0022-5223(23):01090–01095

Bedzra EKS, Adachi I, Peng DM, Amdani S, Jacobs JP, Koehl D, Cedars A, Morales DL, Society of Thoracic Surgeons Fontan VAD Group (2022) Systemic ventricular assist device support of the Fontan circulation yields promising outcomes: an analysis of The Society of Thoracic Surgeons Pedimacs and Intermacs Databases. J Thorac Cardiovasc Surg 164(2):353–364. Wray J, Frigiola A, Bull C, Adult Congenital Heart disease Research Network (ACoRN) (2013) Loss to specialist follow-up in congenital heart disease; out of sight, out of mind. Heart 99(7):485–490. https://doi.org/10.1136/heartjnl-2012-302831. Epub 2012 Dec 20. PMID: 23257171; PMCID: PMC3595142

Cedars A, Kutty S, Danford D, Schumacher K, Auerbach SR, Bearl D et al (2021) Systemic ventricular assist device support in Fontan patients: a report by ACTION. J Heart Lung Transplant 40:368–376. https://doi.org/10.1016/j.healun.2021.01.011

Chubb H, O'Neill M, Rosenthal E (2016) Pacing and defibrillators in complex congenital heart disease. Arrhythmia Electrophysiol Rev 5(1):57–64. https://doi.org/10.15420/aer.2016.2.3

Constantine A, Costola G, Bianchi P, Chessa M, Giamberti A, Kempny A, Rafiq I, Babu-Narayan SV, Gatzoulis MA, Hoschtitzky A, Shore D, Aw TC, Ranucci M, Dimopoulos K (2021) Enhanced assessment of perioperative mortality risk in adults with congenital heart disease. J Am Coll Cardiol 78(3):234–242

Frischhertz BP, Shamszad P, Pedroza C, Milewicz DM, Morris SA (2015) Thoracic aortic dissection and rupture in conotruncal cardiac defects: a population-based study. Int J Cardiol 184:521–527. https://doi.org/10.1016/j.ijcard.2015.03.061. Epub 2015 Mar 4. PMID: 25767008

Kamla CE, Buech J, Doldi PM, Hagl C, Juchem G, Dashkevich A (2021) Atrio-aortic erosion caused by Amplatzer Atrial Septal Occluder—a case report. J Cardiothorac Surg 16(1):36. https://doi.org/10.1186/s13019-021-01411-3. PMID: 33743762; PMCID: PMC7981898

Malik MI, Fakim D, Drullinksy D, Nagpal AD (2024) Indication for ECMO predicts time to first actionable bleeding complication. Indian J Thorac Cardiovasc Surg 40(2):177–183. https://doi.org/10.1007/s12055-023-01601-9. Epub 2023 Oct 19. PMID: 38389766; PMCID: PMC10879057

Moons P, Skogby S, Bratt EL, Zühlke L, Marelli A, Goossens E (2021) Discontinuity of cardiac follow-up in young people with congenital heart disease transitioning to adulthood: a systematic review and meta-analysis. J Am Heart Assoc 10(6):e019552

van der Palen RLF, Blom NA, Kuipers IM, Rammeloo LAJ, Jongbloed MRM, Konings TC, Bouma BJ, Koolbergen DR, Hazekamp MG (2021) Long-term outcome after the arterial switch operation: 43 years of experience. Eur J Cardiothorac Surg 59(5):968–977. https://doi.org/10.1093/ejcts/ezab006. PMID: 33942860; PMCID: PMC8106945

Windsor J, Mukundan C, Stopak J, Ramakrishna H (2022) Analysis of the 2020 European Society of Cardiology (ESC) Guidelines for the Management of Adults With Congenital Heart Disease (ACHD). J Cardiothorac Vasc Anesth 36(8 Pt A):2738–2757

Emergency Cardiac Surgery Following Paediatric and Adult Congenital Percutaneous Interventions

Michael Murphy, Katia Librandi, Lisa Bianco, and Alain Fraisse

Abstract Although percutaneous interventions are integral to the management of congenital heart disease, they carry an inherent risk of major complications that may necessitate emergency cardiac surgery. This chapter reviews the aetiology, recognition and management of such complications in both paediatric and adult congenital populations. Common indications for emergent surgical intervention include vascular injury, cardiac perforation with tamponade, device malposition or embolisation and structural or valvular damage. The chapter discusses the role of established risk stratification tools such as C3PO, CHARM, CRISP, IMPACT and the recently developed PREDIC3T score, in predicting adverse events and facilitating timely rescue. It also highlights the significance of multidisciplinary preparedness, real-time imaging and the availability of surgical and mechanical support, including extracorporeal membrane oxygenation. Particular emphasis is placed on early detection, coordinated response and the collaborative interface between interventional cardiology, surgery, anaesthesia and intensive care. Despite the low incidence of catastrophic events, proactive risk assessment, adherence to procedural protocols and robust institutional preparedness remain essential in ensuring optimal outcomes following congenital cardiac catheterisation.

Keywords Congenital heart disease percutaneous intervention · Emergency cardiac surgery following congenital heart disease percutaneous intervention · Risk prediction scores for congenital heart disease percutaneous intervention · Vascular complications of percutaneous interventions (congenital heart disease) · Cardiac perforation in percutaneous interventions congenital heart disease · Cardiac tamponade · Valve injuries during percutaneous interventions for congenital heart disease · Device malposition/embolisation · Complications during percutaneous pulmonary valve implantation

---

M. Murphy (✉) · K. Librandi · L. Bianco · A. Fraisse
Royal Brompton Hospital, London, UK

A. Kourliouros (ed.), *Emergency Cardiac Surgery*,
https://doi.org/10.1007/978-3-032-15787-4_23

1 Background

Despite advancements in techniques and equipment, complications that can potentially require emergency surgery remain a significant concern of percutaneous catheterisation for congenital heart disease. There is a relative paucity of publications specifically related to emergency surgery following paediatric and adult congenital percutaneous interventions. Despite the increased complexity and spectrum of diagnostic studies and interventional procedures, the incidence of major complications related to paediatric cardiac catheterisation has continued to decrease (Cassidy et al. 1992). However, variable data collection criteria used across different studies hamper our ability to fully appreciate the precise mortality rate related to cardiac catheterisation. All catheterisation procedures, regardless of their acuity or complexity, involve definite risks with potentially serious consequences. These interventions can occur at any stage of the procedural process and can affect multiple organ systems, as well as the cardiovascular system. The youngest patients are at highest risk of adverse events related to catheterisation, with young age and small patient size independent risk factors for most complications' categories (Vitiello et al. 1998; Mehta et al. 2008; Yilmazer et al. 2012). Both the joint American College of Cardiology/American Heart Association and the British Paediatric Cardiac Association guidelines recommend that paediatric cardiac catheterisations should be performed with surgical back-up on site (Pepine et al. 1991; Qureshi et al. 2000).

Collating comprehensive information about the patient and the individual procedural risks prior to the intervention enhances our ability to prevent or effectively manage complications and the pre-procedure briefing can have a critical role. Real-time imaging techniques, such as point-of-care ultrasound, fluoroscopy and transthoracic or transoesophageal echocardiography aid in accurate catheter placement and reduce the risk of vascular or cardiac injuries. Complication prevention encompasses careful preparation, meticulous procedural technique and adherence to established protocols. It is crucial to maintain situational awareness at all times for potential complications and endeavour to recognise them early, ensuring timely intervention before the problem escalates. Collaborative team working including the rapid availability of surgical, intensive care and anaesthesia support are fundamental to prompt assessment and treatment of any complication and key to successful rescue of the patients to achieve a safe outcome (Jayaram et al. 2017). Surgical involvement in patients following paediatric or adult congenital percutaneous intervention can vary from surgical procedures in the catheter laboratory, emergent institution of extracorporeal membrane oxygenation (ECMO) or transfer to the operating theatre for emergency cardiac surgery.

2 Risk Scores

In order to assess the differing risks of such a diverse spectrum of procedures, several risk factor scores have been created in the last decade (Table 1). The Congenital Cardiac Catheterization Project on Outcomes (C3PO) registry prospectively collected data on all catheterisation cases performed at eight paediatric institutions since 2007. Procedure types were classified into six categories using consensus methods based on expert opinion regarding the anticipated risk of an adverse event (Bergersen et al. 2011a). Subsequently, the CHARM (Catheterization for Congenital Heart Disease Adjustment for Risk Method) was developed, using the data of C3PO registry to allow comparisons of adverse events amongst institutions performing catheterisation for congenital heart disease (Bergersen et al. 2011b). The C3PO registry showed that patients weighing less than 2 kg and less operator experience were associated with adverse events (Backes et al. 2013; Holzer et al. 2013). The IMproving Pediatric and Adult Congenital Treatment Registry (IMPACT), applying some aspects of CHARM, was directly applied to data from IMPACT and a robust risk-standardisation methodology was developed, but does not adequately factor in the combined risk of multiple concurrent interventions (Jayaram et al. 2017). The Catheterisation RISk score for Paediatrics (CRISP score) uses a ten component scoring system, based on the existing literature and expert consensus that has been prospectively validated (Hill et al. 2019). CRISP categorises procedures into three risk levels, with most cases falling into a single category, but limited risk

Table 1 Risks scores used in congenital percutaneous intervention

CHARM	IMPACT	CRISP	PREDIC3T
Based on the C3PO registry	Registry part of the NCDR	Data from the CCISC (2015)	Based on the C3PO (2014–2018)
C3PO: six categories of risk based on expert opinion	Data of 58 US centres, from 2011	11 component risk score	Includes new techniques/ procedures
Data of 8 paediatric centres (2007)	Risk predictors: baseline characteristics, comorbidities, single-ventricle physiology, haemodynamic vulnerability	The incidence of serious adverse event can be categorised into 5 risk categories based on the CRISP score	Consider the haemodynamic vulnerability score (categories: 0,1,2>+ 3)
Composite risk score categorising cases into 4 procedure-type risk categories			Procedures are categorised into 5 groups (biopsy group 0)

C3PO The Congenital Cardiac Catheterization Project on Outcomes, *CHARM* Catheterization for Congenital Heart Disease Adjustment for Risk Method, *IMPACT* IMproving Pediatric and Adult Congenital Treatment Registry, *NCDR* National Cardiovascular Data Registry, *CRISP score* Catheterisation RISk score for Paediatrics, *CCISC* Congenital Cardiac Interventional Study Consortium, *PREDIC3T* Procedural Risk in Congenital Cardiac Catheterization differentiation and nuanced differences in individual patient risk can be overlooked. Most recently, the PREDIC3T scoring system incorporates contemporary data to address some of the shortcomings of other risk scores. By considering the different haemodynamic vulnerabilities and intrinsic characteristics of a wide range of procedures. PREDIC3T aims to provide a more accurate and individualised risk assessment.

These risk scores have been used to identify risk factors associated with failure to rescue, which is critical for improving patient outcomes by enabling timely and appropriate responses to complications during and after procedures. This comprehensive approach aims to enhance patient safety and optimise procedural outcomes by providing a more detailed and accurate risk stratification (Quinn et al. 2022). Table 1 summarises the risk scores.

3 Vascular Complications

The most frequent complications after percutaneous interventions are injuries to the peripheral vascular structures, most commonly related to access site to the venous or arterial system. The majority of these injuries are minor and the compromise to the peripheral vessel is self-limiting. In minor peripheral vascular injuries, a short period of anticoagulation is frequently recommended. Occasionally, more severe issues at the access site can necessitate open surgical repair of the vessel but major vascular surgery to reconstruct the vessel and relieve ischaemia is unusual (Mullins 2006).

Vascular complications of a more central venous or larger systemic arteries can occur during interventions and are mainly caused by perforations during wire or catheter manipulation. This is more common in venous structures, which have thinner walls and where inadvertent breaches can often occur. Frequently, the injury is recognised early, after only minimal trauma and by avoiding further manipulation, any vessel injury or haemorrhage sustained is self-limiting and further injury is avoided. Inferior vena cava dissection or total disruption can occur during a wide range of procedures including PDA closure or stenting, right ventricular outflow tract stenting, atrial septostomy or during extraction of an embolised device (Figure 1). The patient can often remain haemodynamically stable if the renal veins are not involved, but in cases where reconstruction is required, mortality rates can be high. Although perforation of an artery with wires or catheters is uncommon during cardiac catheterisations in neonates, limited arterial dissections or perforations can occur in infants and small children, but surgical management is usually not required. In older children and adults, central systemic arterial injury can occur after balloon angioplasty or stenting and perforations with pleural or retroperitoneal haemorrhage may require surgical drainage. Dissections of the aorta beyond the left subclavian are usually treated with medical stabilisation and emergency surgery is almost never required. More proximal injuries to the root, ascending aorta, and arch

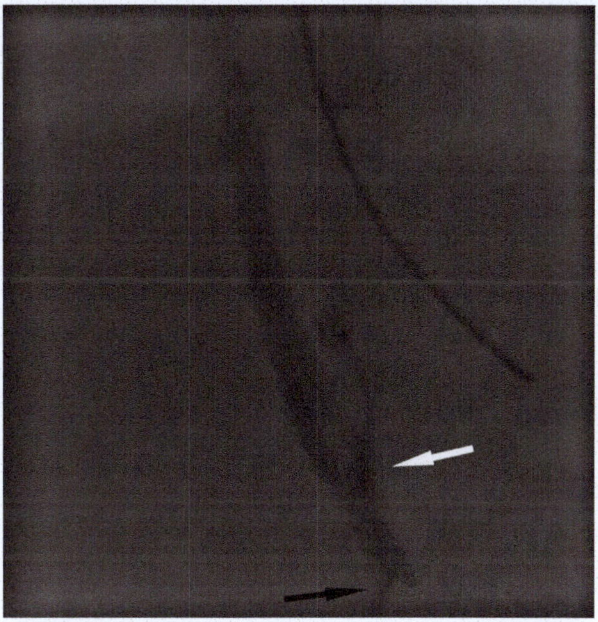

Fig. 1 Angiography showing an inferior vena cava dissection (white arrow) caused by traumatic injury of the tip of an introducer sheath on the wall of the vessel (black arrow)

are managed on an individual basis and often involve collaboration with aortic surgeons to delineate the best and safest management in the immediate aftermath.

Younger age and smaller size of the patient are independent risk factors for both minor and major vascular complications. Additional patient factors associated with arterial injuries include connective tissue disorders, high atherosclerotic burden and the presence of very tight lesions. Procedures that require stiffer wires or larger calibre introducers, catheters or wires also carry a higher risk of perforation or vessel tear.

Several well-known, protocolised techniques are used in the catheterisation laboratory to manage those complications such as major vascular injuries that carry a high mortality rate (Brotschi et al. 2015). When a systemic artery tear occurs during or after balloon dilation, if the balloon is still in place, it is reinflated at low pressure to occlude the tear without further dilation. If the balloon is removed, a larger balloon is used to occlude the tear and a bare-metal or covered stent may be required for definitive repair of an acute aortic or large vessel rupture. The patient should be prepared for transfusion, heparin reversed, thoracocentesis performed as appropriate and, if necessary, preparation for emergency surgery. Specific procedures can also add to the risk of arterial perforation such as coarctation ballooning/stenting and coronary artery intervention where intimal injury can cause occlusion or dissection by wires and catheters can occur. Major aortic injuries through perforation or dissection can be immediately life threatening due to hypovolaemia, tamponade or end-organ compromise.

Injury to the pulmonary arteries during angioplasty, stenting or deployment of a pulmonary valve is more common in congenital heart disease interventions than injury to the systemic arteries. When a perforation of a distal pulmonary artery or rupture of a capillary bed occurs, the immediate management depends upon the underlying pathology, the size of the perforation, the size of the pulmonary artery and the pulmonary artery pressure in the vessel proximal to the injury. The majority of perforations or tears are small and self-resolving and can be adequately managed in the catheter laboratory by leaving the balloon inflated for some time or using occluding devices or stents to occlude the arterial breach (Baker et al. 2000). In larger or more proximal injuries, the management is similar, but it can be important that the surgical team be prepared for the need for emergency surgery to control bleeding with repair of the tear or even lung resection in extreme cases.

4 Cardiac Perforation and Tamponade

Guidewire or catheter perforation of a vessel wall within the pericardium or of a cardiac chamber is rare, but can be seen in more complex procedures where extensive guidewire looping is required. This can occur when the tip of a guide wire is advanced through a catheter tip that has become trapped with consequent perforating the vessel or cardiac chamber. This is more common in the atria, particularly when the catheter tip is adjacent to the appendage. This risk of this major complication is reduced, but not abolished, by echocardiographic or fluoroscopic guidance. Amongst the highest risk procedures for cardiac perforation is during atrial septostomy when imaging guidance is essential to avoid accidental perforation of the atrial wall. Ventricular perforation can occur in procedures when the catheters or guidewires become embedded in the myocardium, entangled in the sub-valvar apparatus or during endomyocardial biopsy. The risk of cardiac perforation is reduced in the latter by avoiding areas of thinned out myocardium or the valvar tissue. During selective high-pressure ventriculography, 'myocardial staining' can occur when a catheter tip is wedged deep in the myocardium leading to contrast accumulation and in extreme cases can cause scars, aneurysm formation or even perforations and tamponade. Other potential perforations can occur during atrioventricular or semi-lunar valve interventions caused by the wires or the balloon. Early recognition is an important component of managing cardiac perforation or tamponade as dealing with this problem whilst still in the catheter laboratory with or without transfer to the operating theatre is preferable than returning to either after delayed recognition. Regardless of the cause or site of cardiac or intra-pericardial vessel injury, the initial management is often similar to those required to solve a vascular injury, with preparation for transfusion, heparin reversal and, if necessary, preparation for emergency surgery. Whilst in the catheter laboratory or after return, it is common practice to image the pericardial and pleural cavities and drain any collections. It is not uncommon to be able to reduce any pericardial collection, particularly if recent, with percutaneous pericardial drainage, thereby relieving any cardiac compromise by tamponade. The rate of reaccumulation and haemodynamic stability will often decide if further treatment is required, often necessitating transfer to the operating theatre or if these measures alone have stabilised the situation while the perforation seals without the need for further treatment. In general, ventricular perforation drainage alone often suffices, whereas atrial perforations often have recurrent effusions with drainage alone and so frequently require surgical drainage and repair. Should surgery be required, this is usually via primary sternotomy or repeat sternotomy for those that have had prior surgery. An experienced team is essential in these circumstances as haemodynamic instability is frequent whilst exposing the area of the perforation for repair. Cardiopulmonary bypass may be required because of haemodynamic instability or the location of the defect is not readily accessible with the heart contracting with normal pre-load. Occasionally, peripheral cardiopulmonary bypass is initiated prior to sternotomy, particularly if there has been prior cardiac surgery or the haemodynamics are particularly unstable even before incision.

5 Valvular Lesions

Puncture or tears of the valvular leaflet can also occur when crossing of the valve with guide wires, during the creation of an A-V loop or when inflation of the balloon occurs within the valve orrifice or within the leaflet tisse. Sub-valvar apparatus rupture or damage to the atrioventricular valves can occur in procedures where the equipment can be trapped and damage the papillary muscles or chordae tissue. The majority of this lesions result in haemodynamic lesions that are well tolerated, but emergency surgery is required in cases where the valvar lesion results in significant compromise.

Perforation of the valve annulus or the outflow tract related to balloon angio- or valvulo-plasty is an infrequent but reported complication. This is generally seen with oversized balloons and can be associated with tears of the valve leaflets that can manifest as valvar regurgitation. If the annular or outflow tract injury is severe or the degree of regurgitation is significant, surgical repair of the annular or outflow tract defect is required and valve repair or even replacement may be necessary.

During procedures that involve guidewires going through the tricuspid valve such as PDA device closure or right ventricular outflow tract stenting, the tricuspid valve is at risk of injury where damage to the leaflets, chordal tissue or papillary muscles can manifest as important degrees of tricuspid regurgitation. Several techniques have been developed to protect the valve and sub-valvar apparatus during these procedures (Baruteau et al. 2023).

Fig. 2 Transoesophageal image showing an atrial septal defect device (white arrow) embolised into the tricuspid valve

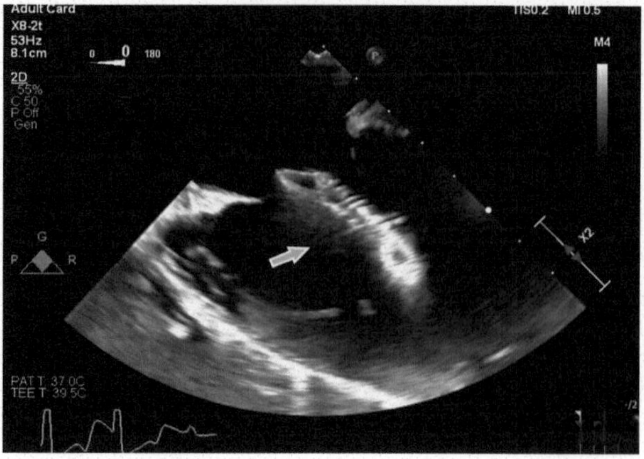

6 Device Malposition and Embolisation

Device malposition and embolisation can occur with any type of implantable device, though rates differ depending on the device used, with some devices associated with lower complication rates than others (El-Said et al. 2015).Frequently, device retrieval can be performed percutaneously, but surgical recovery may be necessary in a minority of cases. The risk–benefit of device retrieval can be challenging, particularly in complex patients with multiple prior procedures. Entanglement of the device within the sub-valvar apparatus of the atrioventricular valve can make retrieval more challenging and, in some cases, valve repair or even replacement may be required. Data from the IMPACT registry reported an embolisation rate of 2.3% of ASD devices (Figure 2), with four requiring surgical retrieval and 1.3% of PDA devices, with one requiring surgery (Moore et al. 2013).

7 Complications During Percutaneous Pulmonary Valve Implantation

Percutaneous pulmonary valve implantation is increasingly performed as a less invasive procedure to establish a competent valve in the right ventricular outflow tract and is usually deployed in the native right ventricular outflow tract or within a right ventricular to pulmonary artery conduit. During transcatheter pulmonary valve insertion, rupture of a homograft right ventricle to pulmonary artery conduit has thankfully become less frequent, principally due to decreasing the radial force exerted on the conduit through the use of progressive dilatations and smaller balloons. In most cases, conduit rupture can be managed in the catheter lab by using a covered stent, but emergency surgery may be required in cases where the rupture site cannot be sealed or haemodynamic compromise occurs. Another potential complication seen in percutaneous pulmonary valve implantation is coronary artery compression after balloon expansion of the stent or valve. This complication can be avoided by careful review of imaging and can be managed interventionally by leaving a guidewire in the coronary to allow for placement of a stent if needed (Goldstein et al. 2020). Stent and transcatheter pulmonary valve-related malposition and embolisation have a higher incidence in native right ventricular outflow tracts than those deployed within a conduit. Although the urgent need for cardiac surgery after percutaneous pulmonary valve implantation has decreased with greater experience, the mortality rate in these cases remains high (Hascoët et al. 2024).

8 Pulmonary Complications

Thrombotic or air emboli caused by catheter manipulation can cause pulmonary embolism, presenting with sudden respiratory distress that is often treated with supportive therapy in the catheter laboratory or intensive care with or without fibrinolysis and a period of anticoagulation. In severe situations, where the cardiorespiratory compromise is not well tolerated, institution of ECMO or, in some cases, thrombectomy, may be required.

The lung parenchyma can be inadvertently punctured while accessing the jugular vein or during a pericardiocentesis. Depending on the degree of respiratory compromise, drainage of the pleural cavity may be required, but surgery on the affected lung is not usually required.

9 Summary

While percutaneous interventions are an essential component of the contemporary management of congenital heart disease, they carry with them the risks that can range from minor issues to severe life-threatening complications. Awareness, early detection and collaboration between the catheter laboratory and surgical teams, as well as the timely and appropriate management, are crucial to deliver the best possible outcomes.

References

Backes CH, Cua C, Kreutzer J, Armsby L, El-Said H, Moore JW, Gauvreau K, Bergersen L, Holzer RJ (2013) Low weight as an independent risk factor for adverse events during cardiac catheterization of infants. Catheter Cardiovasc Interv 82(5):786–794. https://doi.org/10.1002/ccd.24726. Epub 2013 Mar 2. PMID: 23436647

Baker CM, McGowan FX Jr, Keane JF, Lock JE (2000) Pulmonary artery trauma due to balloon dilation: recognition, avoidance and management. J Am Coll Cardiol 36(5):1684–1690. https://doi.org/10.1016/s0735-1097(00)00904-9

Baruteau AE, Fraisse A, Butera G, Bautista-Rodriguez C (2023) The transcatheter closure of patent ductus arteriosus in extremely low-birth-weight infants: technique and results. J Cardiovasc Dev Dis 10(12):476. https://doi.org/10.3390/jcdd10120476. PMID: 38132644; PMCID: PMC10744056

Bergersen L, Gauvreau K, Marshall A, Kreutzer J, Beekman R, Hirsch R, Foerster S, Balzer D, Vincent J, Hellenbrand W, Holzer R, Cheatham J, Moore J, Lock J, Jenkins K (2011a) Procedure-type risk categories for pediatric and congenital cardiac catheterization. Circ Cardiovasc Interv 4(2):188–194. https://doi.org/10.1161/CIRCINTERVENTIONS.110.959262. Epub 2011 Mar 8. PMID: 21386090

Bergersen L, Gauvreau K, Foerster SR et al (2011b) Catheterization for congenital heart disease adjustment for risk method (CHARM). JACC Cardiovasc Interv 4:1037–1046

Brotschi B, Hug MI, Kretschmar O, Rizzi M, Albisetti M (2015) Incidence and predictors of cardiac catheterisation-related arterial thrombosis in children. Heart 101:948–953

Cassidy SC, Schmidt KG, Van Hare GF, Stanger P, Teitel DF (1992) Complications of pediatric cardiac catheterization: a 3-year study. J Am Coll Cardiol 19(6):1285–1293. https://doi.org/10.1016/0735-1097(92)90336-l. PMID: 1564229

El-Said H, Hegde S, Foerster S, Hellenbrand W, Kreutzer J, Trucco SM, Holzer R, Burch G, Mirani A, Nicolas R, Porras D, Bergersen L, Moore J (2015) Device therapy for atrial septal defects in a multicenter cohort: acute outcomes and adverse events. Catheter Cardiovasc Interv 85(2):227–233. https://doi.org/10.1002/ccd.25684. Epub 2014 Oct 13. PMID: 25257700

Goldstein BH, Bergersen L, Armstrong AK, Boe BA, El-Said H, Porras D, Shahanavaz S, Leahy RA, Kreutzer J, Zampi JD, Hainstock MR, Gudausky TM, Nicholson GT, Gauvreau K, Goodman A, Petit CJ (2020) Adverse events, radiation exposure, and reinterventions following transcatheter pulmonary valve replacement. J Am Coll Cardiol 75(4):363–376. https://doi.org/10.1016/j.jacc.2019.11.042. PMID: 32000947

Hascoët S, Bentham JR, Giugno L, Betrián-Blasco P, Kempny A, Houeijeh A, Baho H, Sharma SR, Jones MI, Biernacka EK, Combes N, Georgiev S, Bouvaist H, Martins JD, Kantzis M, Turner M, Schubert S, Jalal Z, Butera G, Malekzadeh-Milani S, Valdeolmillos E, Karsenty C, Ödemiş E, Aldebert P, Haas NA, Khatib I, Wåhlander H, Gaio G, Mendoza A, Arif S, Castaldi B, Dohlen G, Carere RG, Del Cerro-Marin MJ, Kitzmüller E, Hermuzi A, Carminati M, Guérin P, Tengler A, Fraisse A, EUROPULMS3 investigators (2024) Outcomes of transcatheter pulmonary SAPIEN 3 valve implantation: an international registry. Eur Heart J 45(3):198–210. https://doi.org/10.1093/eurheartj/ehad663

Hill KD, Du W, Fleming GA, Forbes TJ, Nykanen DG, Reeves J, Du Y, Kobayashi D (2019) Validation and refinement of the catheterization RISk score for pediatrics (CRISP score): an analysis from the congenital cardiac interventional study consortium. Catheter Cardiovasc Interv 93(1):97–104. https://doi.org/10.1002/ccd.27837. Epub 2018 Sep 9.PMID: 30196566

Holzer RJ, Gauvreau K, Kreutzer J, Moore JW, McElhinney DB, Bergersen L (2013) Relationship between procedural adverse events associated with cardiac catheterization for congenital heart disease and operator factors: results of a multi-institutional registry (C3PO). Catheter Cardiovasc Interv 82(3):463–473. https://doi.org/10.1002/ccd.24866. Epub 2013 Apr 9. PMID: 23413194

Jayaram N, Spertus JA, Kennedy KF et al (2017) Modeling major adverse outcomes of pediatric and adult patients with congenital heart disease undergoing cardiac catheterization: observations from the NCDR IMPACT Registry (National Cardiovascular Data Registry Improving Pediatric and Adult Congenital Treatment). Circulation 136(21):2009–2019

Mehta R, Lee KJ, Chaturvedi R et al (2008) Complications of pediatric cardiac catheterization: a review in the current era. Catheter Cardiovasc Interv 72:278–285

Moore J, Vincent R, Beekman R et al (2013) Impact registry: first review of community practice with respect to device closure of ASD and PDA. JACC 61(10_Supplement):E448. https://doi.org/10.1016/S0735-1097(13)60448-9

Mullins CE (2006) Cardiac catheterization in congenital heart disease: pediatric and adult. Blackwell Publishing, Oxford

Pepine CJ, Allen HD, Bashore TM, Brinker JA, Cohn LH, Dillon JC, Hillis LD, Klocke FJ, Parmley WW, Ports TA et al (1991) ACC/AHA guidelines for cardiac catheterization and cardiac catheterization laboratories. American College of Cardiology/American Heart Association Ad Hoc Task Force on Cardiac Catheterization. Circulation 84(5):2213–2247. https://doi.org/10.1161/01.cir.84.5.2213. PMID: 1934395

Quinn BP, Yeh M, Gauvreau K, Ali F, Balzer D, Barry O, Batlivala S, Berman D, Foerster S, Goldstein B, Hainstock M, Holzer R, Janssen D, O'Byrne ML, Shirley L, Trucco S, Whiteside W, Bergersen L (2022) Procedural Risk in Congenital Cardiac Catheterization (PREDIC3T). J Am Heart Assoc 11(1):e022832. https://doi.org/10.1161/JAHA.121.022832. Epub 2021 Dec 22. PMID: 34935425; PMCID: PMC9075192

Qureshi SA, Redington AN, Wren C, Ostman-Smith I, Patel R, Gibbs JL, de Giovanni J (2000) Recommendations of the British Paediatric Cardiac Association for therapeutic cardiac catheterisation in congenital cardiac disease. Cardiol Young 10(6):649–667. https://doi.org/10.1017/s1047951100008982. PMID: 11117403

Vitiello R, McCrindle BW, Nykanen D et al (1998) Complications associated with pediatric cardiac catheterization. J Am Coll Cardiol 32:1433–1440

Yilmazer MM, Ustyol A, Güven B et al (2012) Complications of cardiac catheterization in pediatric patients: a single centre experience. Turk J Pediatr 54:478–485

Penetrating Injury to Heart: Pre-hospital and Emergency Department Management

Tom Hurst, Zane Perkins, and David Lockey

Abstract Penetrating cardiac injury is a highly mortal condition, with overall mortality rates approaching 90%. However, survival rates can be dramatically improved with timely operative intervention. Prompt resuscitative thoracotomy in selected patients can achieve overall survival rates exceeding 50%. Therefore, the effective provision of resuscitative thoracotomy should be considered in all trauma systems, which deliver care for penetrating trauma.

This chapter describes the epidemiology of penetrating cardiac injury, the factors associated with survival, and reviews current guidelines governing clinical practice. The technique for resuscitative thoracotomy is described, along with a discussion of the reception and management of patients undergoing this procedure. Notably, while the majority of emergency department and pre-hospital resuscitative thoracotomies are performed by non-surgeons, it is important for surgeons to understand the circumstances and techniques used by non-surgeons to perform the technique to optimise patient outcomes following admission. Resuscitative thoracotomy also has a role in managing traumatic cardiac arrest not associated with cardiac injury. This is summarised, but is not the main focus of the chapter.

Keywords Traumatic cardiac arrest · Penetrating cardiac injury · Cardiac tamponade · Resuscitative thoracotomy · Pre-hospital resuscitative thoracotomy · Emergency department resuscitative thoracotomy (EDRT) · Bilateral finger thoracostomies · Clamshell thoracotomy · Internal cardiac massage · Aortic occlusion

T. Hurst (✉) · Z. Perkins · D. Lockey
Barts Health NHS, London, UK
e-mail: tom.hurst@nhs.net; d.lockey@nhs.net

A. Kourliouros (ed.), *Emergency Cardiac Surgery*,
https://doi.org/10.1007/978-3-032-15787-4_24

1 Introduction

Penetrating cardiac injury is a highly mortal condition, with overall mortality rates approaching 90%. However, survival rates can be dramatically improved with timely operative intervention. Prompt resuscitative thoracotomy in selected patients can achieve overall survival rates exceeding 50%. Therefore, the effective provision of resuscitative thoracotomy should be considered in all trauma systems which deliver care for penetrating trauma.

This chapter describes the epidemiology of penetrating cardiac injury, the factors associated with survival, and reviews current guidelines governing clinical practice. The technique for resuscitative thoracotomy is described, along with a discussion of the reception and management of patients undergoing this procedure. Notably, while the majority of emergency department and pre-hospital resuscitative thoracotomies are performed by non-surgeons, it is important for surgeons to understand the circumstances and techniques used by non-surgeons to perform the technique to optimise patient outcomes following admission.

Resuscitative thoracotomy also has a role in managing traumatic cardiac arrest not associated with cardiac injury. This is summarised, but is not the main focus of the chapter.

2 Epidemiology

Penetrating cardiac injuries present a formidable challenge in trauma care due to their rapid lethality and high mortality rates, with overall survival rates of 10–15% (McNicoll et al. 2023). Approximately 85% of these injuries result in pre-hospital deaths, introducing a significant survival bias in the trauma literature, as most studies report only the outcomes of patients who reach hospital. The limited population-based studies that include pre-hospital deaths reveal that the overall survival rate for patients with penetrating cardiac injury has remained stagnant at 10–15% over the past six decades, despite considerable advances in in-hospital trauma care (Demetriades and van der Veen 1983).

A substantial proportion of these pre-hospital fatalities are from potentially survivable injuries, such as single cardiac stab wounds with tamponade, if timely care had been available (Campbell et al. 1997). The incidence of penetrating cardiac injuries and the mechanisms behind them—ranging from high-energy ballistic trauma to lower energy knife wounds—vary significantly across different regions and countries. This variation influences both the clinical approach and outcomes, necessitating tailored strategies that are informed by local epidemiological data. For example, while the prevalence of penetrating trauma is reportedly increasing in the United Kingdom (Ajayi et al. 2021) and other European countries (Störmann et al. 2016), the nature of these injuries often differs from those observed in regions with higher incidences of firearm-related violence, such as in South Africa and the United

States. Despite these regional variations, the demographic profile remains remarkably consistent worldwide. These injuries predominantly affect young adults, with the vast majority (>85%) being male.

3 Traumatic Cardiac Arrest Process and Definitions

In patients who suffer cardiac arrest from non-traumatic causes (such as arrhythmia secondary to myocardial infarction), the onset is usually sudden and straightforward to diagnose. Conversely, in patients with injuries causing hypovolaemia or cardiac tamponade, the transition to cardiac arrest is often less abrupt and usually preceded by a state of low cardiac output. The criteria for diagnosing traumatic cardiac arrest are not universally standard. In some studies, patients without palpable pulses but with cardiac electrical activity are considered to have 'signs of life'. Other suggested signs of life include any recordable blood pressure, reactive pupils, spontaneous ventilation and extremity movement.

A pragmatic approach in emergency trauma care might involve determining the optimal timing for initiating interventions such as resuscitative thoracotomy. In the pre-hospital or emergency department setting, particularly with non-surgical operators, a patient should be in cardiac arrest before being considered for this procedure. This is most simply defined as being unresponsive, apnoeic (or with agonal breathing) and without palpable central pulses. Decisions on the appropriateness of resuscitative thoracotomy should also consider the likely underlying cause and the duration of cardiac arrest.

Resuscitative thoracotomy is a technique also deployed to manage potentially salvageable patients who are in cardiac arrest following trauma, irrespective of the presence of a cardiac injury. It allows for internal cardiac massage, descending aortic compression and direct treatment of cardiac injury. In mature systems, overall survival is around 7%, with appropriate patient selection being essential (Joseph et al. 2018). This role extends to patients with sub-diaphragmatic haemorrhage, although alternative techniques including resuscitative balloon occlusion of the aorta (REBOA) may also be used (ter Avest et al. 2022).

4 Outcomes and Factors Associated with Survival

4.1 Location of Intervention

Although overall survival is reported as 10–15% (Demetriades and van der Veen 1983; Kulshrestha et al. 1990), sub-group survival is variable and is determined by the mechanism of injury, the timeliness of treatment and the injury pattern. An understanding of these factors is important in considering any potential operative intervention.

Patients who survive to have operative intervention in hospital have a better outcome than those who suffer a cardiac arrest pre-hospital, with the best outcomes being in those patients who undergo surgery in an operating theatre without loss of cardiac output.

Patients who arrive without signs of life and undergo resuscitative thoracotomy in the Emergency Department have a survival of around 4%. Patients who arrive in the ED with signs of life and subsequently undergo EDRT have a survival of 15.5–21.1% (Seamon et al. 2015). In some systems, physician led pre-hospital care teams deliver resuscitative thoracotomy at scene with survival ranging from 7% to 50%, depending on duration of arrest and whether the dominant pathology is tamponade or exsanguination (Greenhalgh et al. 2023).

4.2 Duration of Cardiac Arrest

The duration of cardiac arrest is strongly correlated with mortality. Patients who undergo immediate thoracotomy, i.e. at the point of cardiac arrest, have a survival of up to 50% where tamponade is the cause and 10% where exsanguination is the cause. Survival falls rapidly to almost zero by 15 min in patients with tamponade and by 5 min in patients with exsanguination (Greenhalgh et al. 2023).

Estimating the duration of cardiac arrest is challenging in the acute situation and in exsanguination, the ECG rhythm is a valuable aid to decision making. Anything other than a narrow complex ECG is strongly associated with death in this group of patients. In patients with suspected tamponade, although the presence of a narrow complex ECG is associated with survival, survival is possible with other rhythms provided timelines are appropriate.

4.3 Mechanism of Injury

The majority of data on cardiac injuries are from penetrating injury datasets, but blunt trauma can also cause direct cardiac injury and a small number of these patients can develop tamponade from their injuries.

Penetrating cardiac injury due to knife wounds has a lower mortality than from gunshot wound (GSW) due to the higher energy transfer and greater propensity for multi-chamber and great vessel injury. Cardiac injury from firearms carries a mortality close to 100% in the demographic studies referenced.

4.4 *Structures Injured*

Injury to more than one cardiac chamber is associated with mortality rates of 95–100%, and left ventricular injury is 3–4 times more lethal than right ventricular injury. Patients with additional non-cardiac injuries also had markedly higher mortality (Sugg et al. 1968; Campbell et al. 1997)

5 Existing Guidelines

Resuscitative thoracotomy is endorsed in a number of guidelines. The European Resuscitation Council (ERC) guideline on traumatic cardiac arrest suggests that for 'penetrating chest injury', thoracotomy should be considered up to 15 min following cardiac arrest, if expertise, equipment and an appropriate environment permit (Deakin et al. 2021).

The Eastern Association for the Surgery of Trauma (EAST) strongly recommends EDRT for patients with penetrating thoracic injury who are pulseless but with signs of life (Seamon et al. 2015). The guidelines make a conditional recommendation in favour of EDRT for patients who are

- pulseless without signs of life after penetrating thoracic trauma
- pulseless with or without signs of life after penetrating extrathoracic trauma
- pulseless with signs of life after blunt trauma

They conditionally recommend against EDRT in patients who are pulseless without signs of life after blunt trauma. As described above, pulseless with signs of life encompasses those patients who despite a lack of a pulse have at least one of a range of features suggesting either a recent loss of cardiac output or some ongoing but low-volume cardiac output.

The Western Trauma Association guideline also distinguishes between patient in cardiac arrest with electrical cardiac activity or other 'signs of life' and those without. They recommend resuscitative thoracotomy for both blunt and penetrating trauma patients, with maximum CPR times of 10 and 15 min respectively. In keeping with the literature on factors associated with survival, the guidelines recommend termination of resuscitation attempts in patients with no (mechanical) cardiac activity found at operation, unless tamponade is present (Burlew et al. 2012).

6 Suggested Criteria

Based on the above, our service's criteria for pre-hospital resuscitative thoracotomy are shown herein. These criteria are also reasonable for consideration by non-surgeons for emergency department resuscitation thoracotomy. In patients arriving alive at a centre with appropriately trained and experienced surgeons, emergency thoracotomy should also be considered in patients with severe refractory shock, especially in the context of penetrating thoracic trauma.

London's Air Ambulance indications for resuscitative thoracotomy:

- Patients in cardiac arrest following trauma, diagnosed by:
  - Absent central pulse
  - Unconscious—unresponsive to stimulation
  - Apnoea or agonal respiration
  - Irrespective of ECG or ETCO2
- Suspected cardiac tamponade
  - Penetrating trauma to thorax or epigastrium (no further assessment needed)
  - Blunt trauma with ultrasound evidence of pericardial tamponade
  - Organised (narrow complex) ECG irrespective of time *or*
  - Any ECG (including asystole) if cardiac arrest duration <15 min
- Suspected exsanguination
  - Any mechanism of injury where the dominant pathology is felt to be exsanguination
  - Organised (narrow complex) ECG irrespective of time

Suspected Pathology	Cardiac Activity	
	Organised	Unorganised
Cardiac Tamponade	☑	< 15 minutes
Exsanguination	☑	☒

7 Technique

Patients in cardiac arrest or an agonal state, who meet criteria for resuscitative thoracotomy should usually undergo a clamshell incision. The incision provides rapid access to all structures in the chest to allow rapid evacuation of cardiac tamponade, ability to perform internal cardiac massage and to perform aortic compression. This technique also obviates the need for a sternal saw and has been successfully taught to non-surgeons.

The pre-hospital management approach for penetrating trauma emphasises minimising on-scene time and interventions, prioritising rapid transfer to the nearest major trauma centre. Resuscitative thoracotomy is only performed for patients with out-of-hospital TCA when clinically indicated. The operative technique employs a rapid, stepwise process with simple equipment:

Step 1: Bilateral Finger Thoracostomies

- *Identify Landmarks*: Locate the 4th intercostal space, anterior to the mid-axillary line. This can be done by counting rib spaces from the manubriosternal angle or using the 'triangle of safety' defined by the lateral borders of the pectoralis major and latissimus dorsi muscles, and a horizontal line at the level of the male nipple or 5th rib.
- *Perform Bilateral Finger Thoracostomies*: Make a 4-cm incision with a scalpel parallel to the ribs and centred over the 4th intercostal space, anterior to the mid-axillary line. Bluntly dissect through the intercostal space over the upper edge of the 5th rib using Spencer–Wells forceps or similar instruments, then open the parietal pleura. Confirm pleural entry with a finger sweep.

Bilateral finger thoracostomies are performed to rapidly exclude or treat tension pneumothorax, a reversible cause of traumatic cardiac arrest (TCA) that may coexist with cardiac tamponade or thoracic haemorrhage. In addition, starting with a familiar procedure using standard equipment helps ease the process for clinicians less accustomed to performing resuscitative thoracotomies.

Step 2: Perform a Clamshell Thoracotomy

- *Skin Incision*: Make a bold incision through the skin and subcutaneous tissues along the 4th intercostal space. From mid-sternum, the incision should skirt just below the male nipples, and then extend in a slightly upward curve to the midaxillary line to join the thoracostomy incisions.
- *Open the Chest Wall*: Identify the 4th intercostal space. Enter the space using blunt dissection directly over the upper border of the 5th rib. Using scissors, divide the intercostal muscles of the 4th intercostal space at their attachment to the 5th rib, extending the incision from the sternal edge to the mid-axillary line on each side. Using shears or a Gigli saw, divide the sternum between the thoracotomy incisions. Insert a Finochietto retractor between the cut ends of the sternum and open the chest fully.

A clamshell thoracotomy is preferred in traumatic cardiac arrest, as it provides superior exposure of thoracic contents, improved lighting into the operative field and facilitates more effective intervention, including internal cardiac massage. In female patients, retract the breasts cranially and make the skin incision in the inframammary fold. Identify the 4th intercostal space, then proceed as with male patients.

Step 3: Open the Pericardium

- *Open the Pericardium*: Lift ('tent') the pericardium in the midline with your fingers or a clamp and make a nick with scissors, then insert the scissors and widely open the pericardium with a longitudinal incision. Convert to an inverted 'T' with two small lateral incisions in the pericardium just above the diaphragm attachment, with care not to injure the phrenic nerves.

- *Evacuate Blood and Clots*: Evacuate all blood and clot present, then inspect the heart rapidly but systematically for the site of bleeding.
- *Assess Cardiac Function*: Assess if the heart begins to beat spontaneously with return of cardiac output, or if it remains agonal/asystolic. Subsequent management will be based on this evaluation.

Opening the pericardium to treat or exclude cardiac tamponade is the most important step of pre-hospital Resuscitative Thoracotomy. Pitfalls of this step include: (a) leaving the pericardium unopened because it looks 'normal', as a normal looking pericardial sac can easily hide a tamponade and (b) making the pericardial incision too short, as it can restrict access to the heart and potentially obstruct the cardiac outflow tract during internal cardiac massage.

Step 4: Dealing with Cardiac Wounds

- *Control Bleeding*: Use direct finger pressure to temporarily control bleeding. If the heart remains agonal/asystolic, then wounds should be closed quickly, followed by good-quality cardiac massage (step 5). Ventricle wounds can be closed using a skin stapler or suture. Wounds to thin-walled structures (atria, great vessels) can be closed with a Satinsky clamp or suture. In the spontaneously beating heart, small wounds can often simply be managed by direct finger pressure.

Cardiac wounds need to be closed before effective internal massage can be performed.

Step 5: Cardiac Resuscitation

- *Internal Cardiac Massage:* Good- quality bi-manual cardiac massage is required unless there is effective spontaneous activity. The rate of cardiac massage should be adjusted to allow adequate filling and may need to be relatively slow initially. It is important to ensure the heart is not lifted out of the pericardium, as this will kink venous inflow.
- *Aortic Occlusion:* This has the benefit of diverting blood flow to the brain and heart during periods of very low cardiac output, at the expense of significant visceral and lower body ischaemia. A short period of aortic occlusion can be very beneficial in protecting the brain and promoting ROSC, but longer periods are usually associated with unsurvivable multi-organ failure. Aortic control can be achieved by manually compressing the descending thoracic aorta against the vertebral bodies. Alternatively, the more complex procedure of aortic clamp application can be performed, following dissection of the pleura to allow access to the aorta.
- *Volume Resuscitation:* In almost all cases, volume resuscitation will be required and, where possible, this should utilise a balanced blood product transfusion approach.

Good-quality cardiac resuscitation requires attention to all 3 components. ROSC is directly dependant on generating adequate coronary blood flow during diastole. Aortic occlusion should not be maintained for longer than 10 min post ROSC.

8 Reception of Patients

Depending on the healthcare system, geography and timelines, there will be variation as to whether patients present to ED having undergone a pre-hospital resuscitative thoracotomy or present to the ED in extremis or cardiac arrest. In either scenario, time for preparation is likely to be very limited and so planning for this event is important.

8.1 *In Extremis*

Patients who present in, or close to, cardiac arrest with a chest wound should have a primary survey focussed on assessing and resuscitating their circulation. Rapid identification of the likelihood of cardiac tamponade is essential, with strong consideration given to point-of-care ultrasound. Vascular access should be gained and a major haemorrhage protocol activated. If the patient meets the criteria for a resuscitative thoracotomy, this should be commenced without delay, while further surgical support is being sought.

8.2 *After Thoracotomy*

Patients who have undergone RT in the pre-hospital environment will usually only be transported to hospital if a ROSC has been achieved. The reception of these patients requires a well-organised and -led trauma team, able to seamlessly continue resuscitation. Further blood product resuscitation is usually required, but care should be exercised not to overfill the heart. Aortic control should be removed as rapidly as possible if it is still being performed. Any significant bleeding that has not been identified or addressed should be controlled, but time in the ED should be kept short if possible. Drug therapy may be required to support the patient as follows:

- Inotropes: Low-dose adrenaline initially if contractility is poor.
- Sodium Bicarbonate may be required for profound acidosis or hyperkalaemia.
- Calcium should be given to maintain $iCa2+ > 1.1$ mmol/litre during ongoing transfusion.

8.3 *Transfer to Theatre*

If stability can be achieved, the patient should be transferred to the operating theatre. Any wounds not adequately treated should closed and a thorough examination of the thoracic cavity and mediastinum should be performed. The chest should be washed out and drains placed in both pleural spaces and the pericardial space. The divided internal thoracic arteries should be ligated and any bleeding controlled before the chest wall is closed.

8.4 Critical Care

A detailed description of the critical care of these patients is outside the scope of this chapter, but the following should be considered. The majority of patients will require exacting support of their cardiovascular system, as they manifest elements of cardiogenic, hypovolaemic and redistributive shock. Early advanced cardiac output monitoring should be strongly considered and a careful approach that balances the need for volume resuscitation, inotropic support and vasoconstriction instituted. A balance also needs to be struck between ensuring sufficient cerebral perfusion pressure, given the likelihood that cerebral autoregulation will be impaired, and avoiding too great a demand on the recovering heart. In patients where control of haemorrhage has been achieved but cardiogenic shock is developing, some centres are exploring the use of extracorporeal membrane oxygenation.

References

Ajayi B, Guthrie H, Trompeter A, Tennent D, Lui DF (2021) The rising burden of penetrating knife injuries. Injury Prevent 27(5):467–471. https://doi.org/10.1136/injuryprev-2020-044016

Avest ET, Carenzo L, Lendrum RA, Christian MD, Lyon RM, Coniglio C, Rehn M, Lockey DJ, Perkins ZB (2022) Advanced interventions in the pre-hospital resuscitation of patients with non-compressible haemorrhage after penetrating injuries. Crit Care 26(1):1–11. https://doi.org/10.1186/s13054-022-04052-7

Burlew CC, Moore EE, Moore FA, Coimbra R, McIntyre RC, Davis JW, Sperry J, Biffl WL (2012) Western trauma association critical decisions in trauma: resuscitative thoracotomy. J Trauma Acute Care Surg 73(6):1359–1363. https://doi.org/10.1097/TA.0b013e318270d2df

Campbell NC, Thomson SR, Muckart DJJ, Meumann CM, Van Middelkoop I, Botha JBC (1997) Review of 1198 cases of penetrating cardiac trauma. Br J Surg 84(12):1737–1740. https://doi.org/10.1002/bjs.1800841225

Deakin CD, Jasmeet S, Davies R, Patterson T, Lyon R, Nolan JP, Gabbott D et al (2021) Special circumstances guidelines

Demetriades D, van der Veen BW (1983) Penetrating injuries of the heart: experience over two years in South Africa. J Trauma Injury Infect Crit Care 23(12):1034–1041. https://doi.org/10.1016/0736-4679(84)90028-3

Greenhalgh RG, Aziz S, Whitehouse A, Read S, Foster E, Henry CL, Marsden M et al (2023) Prehospital resuscitative thoracotomy for traumatic cardiac arrest: outcomes of 601 cases at London's Air Ambulance. Scand J Trauma Resuscit Emerg Med 31(S1):54

Joseph B, Khan M, Jehan F, Latifi R, Rhee P (2018) Improving survival after an emergency resuscitative thoracotomy: a 5-year review of the trauma quality improvement program, pp 1–6. https://doi.org/10.1136/tsaco-2018-000201

Kulshrestha P, Iyer KS, Sampath KA, Sharma ML, Rao IM, Venugopal P (1990) Cardiac injuries—a clinical and autopsy profile. J Trauma Injury Infect Crit Care 30(2):203–207. https://doi.org/10.1097/00005373-199002000-00012

McNicoll CF, McNickle AG, Vanderet D, Patel PP, Souchon P, Kuhls DA (2023) Shot through the heart: a 17-year analysis of pre-hospital and hospital deaths from penetrating cardiac injuries. Injury 54(5):1349–1355

Seamon MJ, Haut ER, Van Arendonk K, Barbosa RR, Chiu WC, Dente CJ, Fox N et al (2015) An evidence-based approach to patient selection for emergency department thoracotomy: a practice management guideline from the Eastern Association for the Surgery of Trauma. J Trauma Acute Care Surg 79(1):159–173. https://doi.org/10.1097/TA.0000000000000648

Störmann P, Gartner K, Wyen H, Lustenberger T, Marzi I, Wutzler S (2016) Epidemiology and outcome of penetrating injuries in a western European urban region. Eur J Trauma Emerg Surg 42(6):663–669. https://doi.org/10.1007/s00068-016-0630-4

Sugg WL, Rea WJ, Ecker RR, Webb WR, Rose EF, Shaw RR (1968) Penetrating wounds of the heart. An analysis of 459 cases. J Thorac Cardiovasc Surg 56(4):531–545. https://doi.org/10.1016/s0022-5223(19)42812-2

Penetrating Injuries to the Heart: Emergency Definitive Treatment

Duncan Bew and Donald Whitaker

Abstract Penetrating injuries to the heart, whether iatrogenic or caused by assault, require rapid diagnosis and treatment. Preparation, training and standard operating protocols are key. This chapter describes the types of traumatic (non-iatrogenic) injuries likely to be seen, diagnosis, routes to surgical access, stabilising measures and techniques for definitive surgical repair.

Keywords Assault · Penetrating chest trauma · Penetrating cardiac injury · FAST scan · Cardiac box · Cardiac tamponade · Clamshell thoracotomy · Resuscitative thoracotomy

1 Introduction

Penetrating injuries to the heart can be divided into traumatic injuries, usually the result of assault and iatrogenic injuries during interventional cardiology or other procedures such as Swan Ganz catheterisation or even acupuncture. Iatrogenic injuries to the heart and of the major intrathoracic vessels are covered extensively in other chapters of this book, and we will therefore concentrate on the traumatic ones.

D. Bew
Consultant Trauma and Acute Care Surgeon, King's College Hospital, London, UK
e-mail: duncanbew@nhs.net

D. Whitaker (✉)
Consultant Cardiothoracic Surgeon, King's College Hospital, London, UK
e-mail: donaldwhitaker@nhs.net

A. Kourliouros (ed.), *Emergency Cardiac Surgery*,
https://doi.org/10.1007/978-3-032-15787-4_25

2 Traumatic Injuries

For the purposes of this chapter, it is assumed that no incisions have been made in the out-of-hospital setting. However, it is relatively common for the first responder team to perform resuscitative manoeuvres at the scene. Thus, patients are often brought to the emergency department having already received an anterior thoracotomy or clamshell incision.

Penetrating injuries to the heart are the most critical of surgical emergencies as the brain will die within a few minutes once cardiac output stops. When a patient arrives with a suspected penetrating cardiac injury, rapid assessment and possible intervention may both be required within minutes.

Initial management does not require advanced technology or particularly specialised surgical skills. In the authors' opinion, the most significant determinant of patient outcomes will be the prior preparation and training of the receiving medical staff. All major trauma units must therefore ensure that there is a resident team of trained medical staff who can rapidly perform the necessary resuscitative manoeuvres described in this chapter. Even if these resident staff are unable to definitively stop the bleeding, their intervention will allow time for more specialised, possibly non-resident, surgical staff to attend and to perform definitive surgical management.

3 Traumatic Injuries: Background

In our institution, Chacko et al (2019) have described that the vast majority of penetrating cardiac injuries requiring surgery over an 8-year period were caused by knives (75 out of 79—95%) compared to gunshot wounds (4 out of 79—5%). Gunshot wounds have a far higher mortality compared to knife wounds and in our experience, those that penetrate the heart rarely survive to hospital.

Trauma to the anatomic area of the anterior chest shown in all textbooks as the 'Cardiac Box' should always cause particular suspicion for a cardiac injury. This box has as its boundaries the clavicles superiorly, the costal margins inferiorly and the mid-clavicular lines laterally. It is important to appreciate that in reality, any anterior, lateral or posterior penetrating injury with a sufficiently long weapon can potentially cause cardiac injury. High-velocity blunt injuries such as fall from height or road traffic incidents may also, rarely, cause rib fractures that can penetrate the heart as well as other internal organs.

Posterior chest wounds can easily reach the heart and so a full examination of the back of the patient as recommended by ATLS protocol is essential. Also, epigastric wounds caused by a superiorly directed weapon can breach the diaphragm to injure the inferior surface of the right or left ventricles.

Injuries to the heart may be simple and only involve a single chamber or complex and include injuries beyond the myocardium. Other structures that may be injured include the coronary arteries, the valves and the septae between the atria or ventricles.

The right ventricle is the cardiac chamber with the largest area exposed anteriorly and is thus most likely to be injured from penetrating trauma. Studies (Makhadi et al. 2022) describing the incidence of injuries to the cardiac chambers from penetrating trauma consistently confirm that this holds true in practice. The right ventricle (RV) is the commonest, comprising 37–67% of all cardiac injuries, followed by the left ventricle (LV): 19–40%, right atrium (RA): 5–20% and left atrium (LA): 2–12%.

The left anterior descending coronary artery located anteriorly between the right and left ventricles for much of its course is so the commonest coronary artery to be injured. The right coronary artery also passes anteriorly in the right atrioventricular groove so may be injured. The circumflex artery is posterior and rarely injured.

4 Tamponade

Moreno in 1986, in a retrospective study that looked at 100 patients with penetrating cardiac injuries, reported higher survival (77% vs. 11%) in patients who present with tamponade. Tamponade, although clearly dangerous, may therefore also be viewed as a protective mechanism that prevents immediate exsanguination and allows time for resuscitation and repair.

Interestingly, Moreno et al. (1986) also showed that right-sided chamber injuries are associated with a higher survival of 79% compared to left-sided chamber injuries, which have a 28% survival.

5 Initial Assessment

Beck's triad of muffled heart sounds, jugular venous distension and hypotension and Kussmaul's sign of paradoxical rise in jugular venous pressure on inspiration are of limited use in the emergency setting. A rapid assessment of the patient's vital signs together with a FAST (focused assessment with sonography for trauma) scan will determine whether the patient needs an emergency room thoracotomy, direct transfer to theatre or, in the most stable, a CT scan.

If a patient is stable enough for transfer to theatre, we recommend that induction of anaesthesia, intubation and ventilation are performed in theatre. Intubation may be mistakenly considered a stabilising adjunct before transfer from the ER to the operating theatre. However, the combination of anaesthetic vasodilatation and reduced venous return with positive pressure ventilation often has a destabilising effect and leads to cardiac arrest. Cardiac arrest is more easily dealt with in the operating theatre than the ED.

The medical literature describes the subxiphoid pericardial window as a diagnostic procedure in cases of suspected tamponade. In the authors' opinion, median sternotomy is a safer approach when there is sufficient suspicion of a pericardial collection. A subxiphoid incision has no place in our practice, although some surgeons do clearly find it useful.

At our institution, median sternotomy is only performed in the operating theatre and so a thoracotomy is performed if the patient is not stable enough for transfer to theatre.

6 FAST Scan

Governatori in 2015 performed a review of multiple studies that show echocardiography has a high accuracy of up to 96–97% with sensitivity and specificity reaching near 100%. Focused Assessment with Sonography for Trauma (FAST) scanning is clearly operator-dependent, but if there is clinical suspicion of cardiac injury and pericardial fluid on the FAST scan, then rapid transfer to theatre and median sternotomy are indicated. If the FAST scan is inconclusive and the patient is stable, then CT scan with contrast is the best test.

7 Surgery

Surgery may have a resuscitative element prior to definitive repair of the injury. The principles of these overlapping components are:

1. Rapid surgical exposure
2. Simultaneous maintenance of tissue perfusion by release of tamponade, replacement of intravascular volume and with cardiopulmonary bypass as necessary
3. Temporary haemorrhage control
4. Definitive haemorrhage control

The first rule of trauma, generally known to medical students and television viewers, is that if the patient presents with the knife or other instrument in situ, this should be left in place at least until the patient is in the operating theatre and preferably until the chest has been opened and the likely injured structures fully exposed. This reduces the risk of exsanguination when the knife is removed. Again, a CT may be useful in this situation to acutely identify the path of the weapon and the anatomic structures at risk, if the patient is stable enough.

8 Left Anterior Thoracotomy

With the patient supine and the left arm abducted to 90°, incision is made with a 10-blade scalpel. The incision starts medially at left the border of the sternum and extends laterally along the 4th or 5th intercostal space to the left posterior axillary line. The subcutaneous tissues and muscle layers may be divided with a knife or scissors taking care to enter the chest over the superior surface of a rib. The ribs are then spread with whatever retractor is available. The pericardium can then be incised with scissors to release tamponade and inspect for any myocardial injury.

A left anterior thoracotomy is an excellent incision for quickly and safely relieving cardiac tamponade. However, it provides limited exposure of the ventricles and although identification and finger control of a bleeding point may be possible, definitive repair through this incision is unlikely to be possible.

If after relief of tamponade there is uncontrollable bleeding, then conversion of the left anterior thoracotomy to a clamshell incision is the next logical step. A clamshell incision will allow a midline vertical pericardial incision and maximum exposure of the anterior surface of the heart.

If after relief of tamponade the bleeding can be controlled and haemodynamic stability achieved, a decision can then be made whether to extend to a clamshell incision for definitive repair or transfer the patient to the operating theatre for either clamshell incision or a median sternotomy.

9 Clamshell Incision

This starts with the same steps as a left anterior thoracotomy and then the lower sternum is divided with strong shears, heavy scissors or a Gigli saw, followed by a right anterior thoracotomy through the same right intercostal space as the left thoracotomy. The lower parts of the internal mammary (aka thoracic) arteries will inevitably be divided. These arteries have little capacity for spasm and can cause considerable ongoing blood loss so must be ligated or clipped.

Retractors are placed in the right and left intercostal spaces, exposing the heart and both thoracic cavities.

In our experience, placing patients on central right atrial to aorta cardiopulmonary bypass is extremely difficult through a clamshell incision because exposure of the ascending aorta is limited. If bypass is required at this stage, then the options are to perform a median sternotomy in addition to the clamshell or access the femoral vessels for peripheral cardiopulmonary bypass.

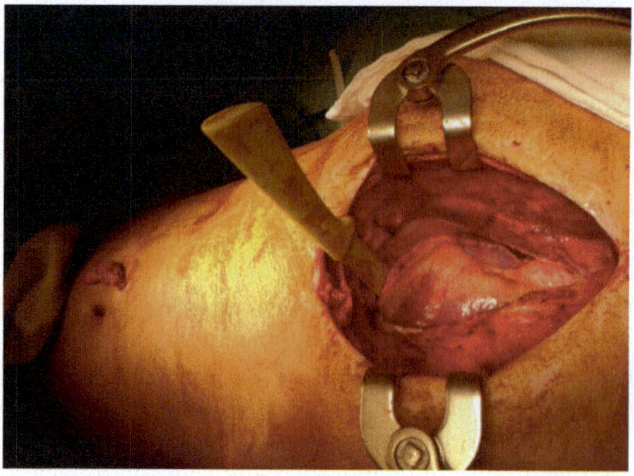

Fig. 1 Median sternotomy

10 Median Sternotomy

The technique of median sternotomy needs no description as it will be familiar to all trained cardiothoracic surgeons. In our institution, the necessary sternal saw is not available in the ED so median sternotomies will only be performed in the operating theatre or if a cardiothoracic surgeon takes a battery-operated saw to the ED. In our experience, non-cardiothoracic-trained staff can adequately resuscitate patients with the anterior thoracotomy or clamshell incision and the median sternotomy can be reserved for definitive treatment (Fig. 1).

11 Temporary Control of Bleeding

Fairly light pressure with one or several fingers, depending on the size of the defect, is usually sufficient to adequately control bleeding from the right or left ventricle. The use of skin staples or a Foley catheter are also described as temporising measures. Countertraction of a filled Foley catheter inserted into the ventricle can in theory stop bleeding but also risks worsening the defect. Rapid transfusion through a Foley catheter is also, in theory, possible, but the authors have rarely experienced this to be useful in practice. The authors have seen ventricular laceration adequately controlled with skin staples, which can then be reinforced with sutures.

As the atrial walls are much thinner, atrial lacerations can be temporarily controlled with clamps such as a Satinsky atraumatic vascular clamp or even with forceps such as Alliss forceps.

12 Definitive Control of Bleeding

12.1 Ventricular Lacerations

The two mistakes often made by inexperienced surgeons faced with a bleeding ventricular laceration are to use too small a needle on the suture and to take too small bites of the myocardium. These two errors can worsen bleeding rather than controlling it. As a general principle, it is safer to use as large a needle as possible and take deep bites in the myocardium. A 2-0 prolene suture is best for the ventricular myocardium.

A large needle allows entry to the myocardium at right angles and a full thickness or close to full thickness bite of the myocardium. This is far more secure. A deeper bite of the myocardium can also be achieved by placing the suture in two stages. The first stage puts the needle from outside the myocardium in to the defect. The needle is then repositioned and placed from the defect to the opposite side myocardium.

The right ventricle myocardium is considerably thinner than that of the left ventricle (3 mm compared to 9 mm) and thus more prone to full thickness tearing if too small bites of muscle are taken in the suture.

A median sternotomy gives excellent exposure of the right ventricle. However, the left ventricle may be obscured as it has a small anterior component and a much larger lateral surface area. Simple manoeuvres such as elevation of the left hemipericardial cradle with stay sutures or large wet packs placed behind the heart may be required to improve left ventricular exposure. Such manoeuvres are often well tolerated if performed in a step wise incremental fashion, allowing the heart to adjust. If not tolerated and unacceptable, haemodynamic compromise results, then, institution of cardiopulmonary bypass will be required.

Unless the laceration is large or complex, the heart can often be lifted manually and sutures rapidly placed during a brief period of low cardiac output. In this situation, the surgeon can lift the heart with one hand and place the sutures with the other. An assistant will be required to tie the suture with two hands.

Longer lacerations requiring more than two interrupted sutures will likely require CPB and multiple sutures buttressed on either side by a long strip of Teflon felt.

The use of Teflon pledgets is always advisable if they are available. The Teflon pledgets should ideally be large and hand fashioned from a sheet of Teflon felt. It is easier and quicker under stress to place needles through a larger pledget. Larger pledgets do not look neat and tidy (Fig. 2), but this should not be of any concern. The pledgets will spread the tension of the sutures and will allow a tighter knotting of the suture without cutting through the myocardium. When tying the prolene sutures, minimum tension to achieve haemostasis should be used. Even less tension should be used if teflon pledgets are not available. The patient's own pericardium can be fashioned into pledgets, although this is technically more difficult to handle than Teflon felt. When autologous pericardium is being used, it is easier to place the

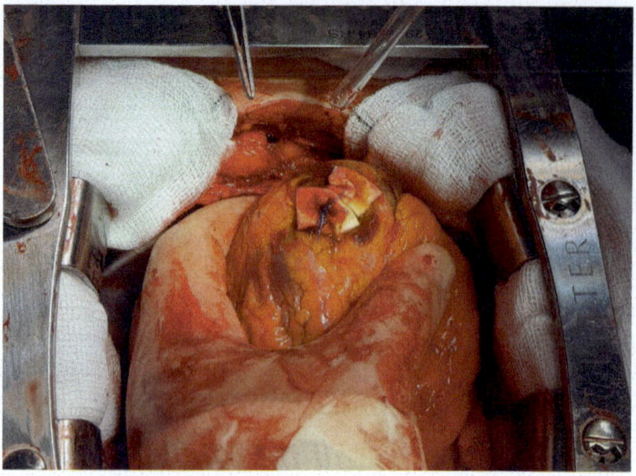

Fig. 2 Pledgetted sutures

sutures through the pericardium with the pericardium in situ and then cut out the pericardial pledget.

If a laceration lies in close proximity to a coronary artery, typically the anteriorly running left anterior descending (LAD) artery, care must be taken to not compromise the artery in the repair stitch. The recommended technique is to place the sutures deep and well beyond the coronary artery so that the suture runs below the artery and then up into the laceration. When gently tying these sutures, the surgeon should be alert to ECG changes or visible anterior wall motion reduction signifying ischaemia.

Haemostatic reinforcement adjuncts such as Bioglue may be applied once the sutures are in place and haemostasis has been achieved. Their effectiveness is unproven, and their main benefit may be to reassure the surgeon.

12.2 Atrial Lacerations

Whereas 2-0 prolene is preferred for ventricular lacerations, 3-0 or 4-0 prolene may be used for the thinner atrial tissue. Pledgets are usually not required, but may be used if the tissue is particularly fragile. Care must be taken to avoid compromising the right coronary artery if the laceration is close to the atrioventricular groove.

12.3 Coronary Artery Lacerations

Distal coronary artery lacerations can usually be tied off without consequence. Bleeding from more proximal sites will likely require cardiopulmonary bypass and grafting of the injured vessel with a length of saphenous vein to maintain perfusion and cardiac function. Coronary artery lacerations are ideally controlled with intra-coronary shunts, but these are unlikely to be available outside a cardiac surgical operating theatre and will require cardiac surgeons with 'off-pump' skills to insert them.

12.4 Internal Cardiac Injuries

In the excitement of dealing with the associated external cardiac injures, internal cardiac injuries may well be missed. A high index of clinical suspicion and a transoesophageal echocardiogram are required to identify such injuries. Some injuries such as small inter-atrial defect or a tricuspid valve injury may be well tolerated and the risk of the additional cardiopulmonary bypass that would be required to repair them not worth the benefit. Mitral valve injuries causing severe regurgitation or ventricular septal defects with significant shunt will likely need addressing if the patient is to survive.

13 Conclusions

Penetrating injuries to the heart can rapidly cause death and so rapid emergency management is essential. This chapter has described a two-stage process of initial examination and resuscitation, which may involve emergency surgical access followed by definitive management. We recommend a well-prepared resident team of ED and trauma staff as part of a trauma network who can perform the first resuscitative stage. Preparation with both wet lab training in surgical access and non-surgical human factors may aid efficient teamwork. Non-resident specialist staff can then attend for definitive surgical management.

In our experience and in the medical literature, the commonest injury requiring definitive repair is right ventricular laceration. We recommend repair with Teflon pledgetted 2.0 prolene with as large a needle as possible. We emphasise that deep, full thickness bites are safest as long as coronary arteries can be avoided. Other injuries may need more complex surgery. If haemostasis can be rapidly achieved, with or without the adjunct of cardiopulmonary bypass, patients with penetrating cardiac injury, who are usually young, can be expected to make an excellent recovery.

References

Chacko J, Whitaker D et al (2019) 8 year audit of cardiothoracic trauma at a major trauma centre. In: Presented at the Annual Meeting of the Society for Cardiothoracic Surgery (SCTS) in Great Britain & Ireland

Governatori NJ, Saul T, Siadecki SD et al (2015) Ultrasound in the evaluation of penetrating thoraco-abdominal trauma: a review of the literature. Med Ultrason 17:528–534

Makhadi S, Moeng MS, Ede C et al (2022) Penetrating cardiac injuries: outcome of treatment from a level 1 trauma centre in South Africa. Trauma Care 2:251–259

Moreno C, Moore EE, Majure JA et al (1986) Peircardial tamponade, a critical determinant for survival following penetrating cardiac wounds. J Trauma 26:821–825

Pericardial Pathologies Requiring Emergency Surgery

Andreas Gkikas and David Lawrence

Abstract The focus of this chapter is emergency surgery for pericardial conditions ranging from the rarer urgent/emergency pericardiectomy for very severe constriction, infection, and autoimmune conditions, to the more common pericardial windows for different types of effusions with tamponade physiology. The chapter is succinct, mainly addressing the surgical aspects and techniques for managing these conditions, but also aiming to evaluate outcomes and controversies in literature.

Keywords Cardiac tamponade · Pericardial effusion · Pericardiectomy · Pericardial window (subxiphoid/VATS) · Constrictive pericarditis · Purulent pericarditis · Malignant pericardial effusion · Pericardial cyst · Pericardiocentesis · Pericardial decompression syndrome

1 Introduction

1.1 Normal Pericardial Physiology

The pericardium is a fibrous sac that encloses the heart, providing a protective layer and maintaining the heart's position within the thorax. It contains a small amount of serous fluid (typically 15–50 mL), which serves as a lubricant, allowing smooth movement of the heart during the cardiac cycle (Spodick 2003). The pericardium is relatively inelastic, meaning that any significant increase in pericardial volume can lead to a rapid rise in intrapericardial pressure.

A. Gkikas
University College Hospital, London, UK
e-mail: andreas.gkikas@nhs.net

D. Lawrence (✉)
St Bartholomew's Hospital, London, UK
e-mail: david.lawrence3@nhs.net

A. Kourliouros (ed.), *Emergency Cardiac Surgery*,
https://doi.org/10.1007/978-3-032-15787-4_26

1.2 Pathophysiology of Cardiac Tamponade

1.2.1 Accumulation of Pericardial Fluid

Cardiac tamponade is a life-threatening condition resulting from the accumulation of fluid, blood, or gas within the pericardial sac, leading to increased intrapericardial pressure that compromises cardiac function. Cardiac tamponade occurs when fluid accumulates in the pericardial space faster than the pericardium can stretch to accommodate it. This fluid collection can result from various causes, including malignancy, trauma, infection, autoimmune diseases, and uraemia. The speed of accumulation plays a crucial role in determining the onset and severity of tamponade. Rapid accumulation of even a small volume of fluid (100–200 mL) can cause tamponade, while slow accumulation of larger volumes (up to 1–2 l) may be tolerated better due to the pericardium's ability to gradually stretch (Reddy and Curtiss 2017).

1.2.2 Increased Intrapericardial Pressure

As fluid accumulates in the pericardial sac, the intrapericardial pressure rises. This increased pressure compresses the heart, particularly the thin-walled atria and right ventricle, which are more susceptible to external compression compared to the thicker walled left ventricle. When the intrapericardial pressure exceeds the intracardiac pressures, the heart's ability to fill with blood during diastole is compromised, leading to a decrease in stroke volume and cardiac output (Mehta and Sloane 2020).

1.2.3 Impaired Diastolic Filling

In cardiac tamponade, the rising intrapericardial pressure creates a fixed diastolic volume within the heart chambers, primarily affecting the right atrium and right ventricle. As these chambers become compressed, venous return to the heart decreases, leading to a reduction in right ventricular preload. Consequently, there is a reduction in left ventricular filling as well, resulting in decreased stroke volume and cardiac output (Fowler 1997).

1.3 Clinical Signs of Cardiac Tamponade

1.3.1 Pulsus Paradoxus

Pulsus paradoxus is a hallmark clinical feature of cardiac tamponade, characterised by an exaggerated decrease in systolic blood pressure (>10 mmHg) during inspiration. Under normal conditions, inspiration increases venous return to the right heart, slightly reducing left ventricular stroke volume due to ventricular interdependence. In tamponade, the right ventricle's inability to expand due to pericardial compression causes further leftward displacement of the interventricular septum during inspiration, significantly reducing left ventricular filling and output. This phenomenon leads to the pronounced drop in systolic blood pressure observed in pulsus paradoxus (Nishimura and Tajik 2014).

1.3.2 Haemodynamic Consequences

The haemodynamic consequences of cardiac tamponade are profound and include the following:

- *Increased Central Venous Pressure (CVP):* As venous return to the right heart is impeded, central venous pressure rises, leading to jugular venous distension and peripheral oedema.
- *Reduced Cardiac Output:* The reduction in stroke volume directly decreases cardiac output, leading to hypotension and shock.
- *Tachycardia:* As a compensatory mechanism, the heart rate increases in an attempt to maintain cardiac output despite reduced stroke volume.

1.3.3 The Beck Triad

The classic Beck triad, although not always present, consists of hypotension, muffled heart sounds, and elevated jugular venous pressure. These clinical signs reflect the underlying pathophysiology of reduced cardiac output, pericardial fluid accumulation, and impaired venous return respectively (Beck 1935).

2 Indications for Emergency Surgery

Pericardial pathologies requiring emergency surgical intervention are relatively rare, but critically important to recognise and treat due to their life-threatening nature. These conditions range from severe pericardial constriction and infection to pericardial effusions and pericardial cysts causing tamponade physiology. This chapter provides an overview of the surgical techniques used to manage these conditions, including emergency pericardiectomy for severe constriction and infection, as well as pericardial window procedures for effusions with tamponade. Additionally, the chapter discusses outcomes and controversies in the current literature.

2.1 Pericardial Syndromes

The term pericardial syndromes is adopted from the European Society of Cardiology (ESC) guidelines that include different pathologies of the pericardium that may require surgical intervention. They comprise pericarditis, pericardial effusion, cardiac tamponade and constrictive pericarditis (Adler et al. 2015). Each of these pathologies will be addressed from the scope of emergent surgical intervention.

2.1.1 Pericardial Effusion

Increased pericardial effusion occurs either from a pathological process that leads to overproduction, decreased reabsorption of pericardial fluid or both. The pericardial effusion can be classified according to its onset (acute or chronic when lasting more or less than 3 months), composition (exudate, transudate, purulent, and blood), distribution (circumferential or loculated), and the most frequent categorisation is its size (Small : <10 mm, Mild: 10–20 mm, Large: >20 mm).

The main treatment strategy in pericardial effusion management is to diagnose and identify the underlying pathology. Pericardiocentesis with pericardial drainage is frequently the first line of treatment that allows to collect sample from the pericardial effusion and also promotes adherence of the visceral to the parietal layer of the pericardium by keeping the pericardial drain until drainage drops below 30 ml/24 h. Expeditious surgery should be considered in recurrent pericardial effusions, when the effusion becomes loculated or when tissue biopsy is required.

2.1.2 Pericardial Effusion with Tamponade

Pericardial effusion leading to cardiac tamponade is one of the most frequent indications for emergency pericardial surgery. As described previously in this chapter, tamponade occurs when fluid accumulation in the pericardial sac exerts pressure on the heart, impairing diastolic filling and reducing cardiac output, which can be rapidly fatal without intervention. The possibility of a pericardial effusion to result in cardiac tamponade depends on the size of the effusion (Large: >20 mm), the rate of the accumulation, the rigidity of the pericardial sac, as well as the filling pressures and the compliance of the heart chambers.

In cases of cardiac tamponade, it is essential to decompress the pericardial sac that will allow for venous return to the right heart. This is achieved with a needle pericardiocentesis as a first line of treatment. Emergency surgical intervention should be sought even as a first step, if tamponade occurs in the immediate postoperative period after cardiothoracic surgery, in cases of bleeding in the pericardium where haemostasis needs to be achieved, in patients with cardiac tamponade due to malignancy, trauma, or infection. The final decision between emergent needle pericardiocentesis or emergent surgical intervention needs to be tailored according to the unit's expertise and specialist's availability with main goal being the fast decompression of the pericardium.

2.1.3 Causes of Pericardial Effusion with Tamponade

- *Malignancy:* The most common cause of pericardial effusion, especially originating from lung, breast, and haematologic cancers.
- *Infection:* Particularly bacterial (e.g. tuberculosis), viral, and fungal infections.
- *Trauma:* Blunt or penetrating trauma to the chest can result in haemorrhagic effusion.
- *Autoimmune Disorders:* Conditions such as systemic lupus erythematosus and rheumatoid arthritis.
- *Post-Cardiac Surgery:* A known complication that can result in effusion and tamponade (see Chapter 'Emergency Re-exploration for Bleeding After Cardiac Surgery').

2.1.4 Constrictive Pericarditis

Constrictive pericarditis is a less common but serious condition that can occasionally present as an emergency, especially when there is rapid deterioration. It results from chronic inflammation leading to pericardial thickening and calcification, which restricts diastolic filling of the heart. Common causes include tuberculosis, post-radiation therapy, and idiopathic inflammation.

2.1.5 Infectious and Autoimmune Pericarditis

Emergency surgical intervention may be required in cases of severe infectious pericarditis (e.g. purulent pericarditis) and fulminant autoimmune pericarditis when conservative management fails, or the patient rapidly deteriorates. These conditions can lead to large effusions with tamponade or progress to constrictive pericarditis if untreated.

2.1.6 Pericardial Cysts

Pericardial cysts are rare, benign congenital anomalies that are typically asymptomatic and discovered incidentally. These cysts originate from abnormal development of the pericardium and usually remain asymptomatic throughout a patient's life. However, in rare cases, pericardial cysts can present acutely due to rupture, infection, or compression of adjacent structures, necessitating emergency surgical intervention.

Pericardial cysts are usually found in the right cardiophrenic angle, although they can appear anywhere along the pericardium. These cysts result from incomplete coalescence of mesothelial lacunae during embryologic development. Pericardial cysts are typically fluid-filled and surrounded by a thin epithelial lining. They range in size from 1 to 5 cm, though larger cysts may develop over time.

While the majority of pericardial cysts are asymptomatic, symptoms arise when the cysts compress adjacent structures such as the heart, lungs, or major blood vessels, or in cases of rupture. In rare instances, a cyst can cause cardiac tamponade or compress the bronchial tree, leading to respiratory distress (Mendes et al. 2015).

2.2 *Surgical Techniques*

2.2.1 Pericardial Window

Indications

A pericardial window is typically indicated in patients with pericardial effusion causing tamponade where percutaneous drainage is not possible, unsuccessful, or when recurrent effusions are expected, such as in malignancy.

Surgical Procedure

- *Approach:* The subxiphoid approach is most commonly used, especially for emergency cases due to its simplicity and safety, but a thoracoscopic approach video-assisted thoracoscopic surgery (VATS) or limited thoracotomy can also be utilised.
- *Technique:* After the patient receives general anaesthesia and they are positioned supine, a small vertical incision is made in the midline, below the xiphoid process to access the pericardium below the diaphragm. The xiphoid process can be resected at this stage of the operation to allow for better exposure of the pericardium. After opening of the peritoneum, the diaphragm is opened at its central tendon, which exposes the anterior mediastinum. The pericardial sac is then aspirated with sample sent for relevant tests according to the underlying pathology. A window of 4 cm is created in the pericardium, allowing the effusion to drain into the peritoneal cavity. This window can be created and remain open with the use of stapling devices placed between the parietal layer of the pericardium and the central tendon of the diaphragm. This allows for the creation of long-lasting pericardial window that will drain into the abdomen and prevent further episodes of tamponade.

- *Postoperative Care:* A chest tube in the mediastinum through the window to facilitate continuous drainage and prevent reaccumulation of fluid was advocated in the past. However, the creation of a patent window has shown to be adequate to prevent pericardial fluid reaccumulation even without a chest drain. The decision for drain insertion should, of course, remain at the discretion of the operating team.

Advantages and Outcomes

The pericardial window procedure offers immediate relief from tamponade and can be life-saving, especially in patients with malignant effusions. The procedure has a low complication rate and is associated with excellent short-term outcomes (Mercier et al. 2015). A serious but rare complication associated with this operation is the pericardial decompression syndrome. This is a paradoxical cardiovascular collapse that results from left or right ventricular failure and it is related to a high mortality of 30% (Amro et al. 2021, Kapoor et al. 2022).

2.2.2 Pericardiectomy

Indications

Pericardiectomy is the definitive treatment for constrictive pericarditis and is indicated in cases of intractable or recurrent pericardial effusion, particularly when caused by infection or autoimmune disease. Diagnosis of constrictive pericarditis that arises from clinical symptoms is considered indication to proceed with surgical intervention. The aetiology of the constrictive pericarditis, which varies from idiopathic to infectious, autoimmune, post-radiation, and post-cardiac surgery, correlates to the overall outcome of these patients.

Surgical Procedure

- *Approach:* The procedure can be performed via a median sternotomy or left anterolateral thoracotomy. The approach is chosen based on the extent of disease and surgeon's preference.
- *Technique:* The pericardium is carefully dissected from the epicardium. In a total pericardiectomy, the entire pericardium is removed, though in some cases, a partial pericardiectomy may be performed if the disease is localised. Partial pericardiectomy involves the excision of the pericardium from the left to the right phrenic nerve and avoiding only the posterior aspect of the left atrium and pulmonary veins (Nataf et al. 1993). In either total or partial peri-

cardiectomy, releasing the pericardium from the left ventricle first and then moving towards the right ventricle and atrium is advised. This reduces the chances of left ventricular failure from pericardial decompression syndrome occurring from non-compliance of the left ventricle from fluid overload when the right chambers are released first while the left ventricle remains constricted from the thickened pericardium.
- *Intraoperative Considerations:* Special care is required to avoid injury to the myocardium and the phrenic nerves, particularly in cases with extensive calcification. Bleeding control and careful dissection are paramount to prevent complications. In cases of emergency pericardiectomy, haemodynamic stability has to be maintained throughout with careful cardiovascular monitoring and cardiopulmonary bypass availability.

Outcomes and Risks

Pericardiectomy significantly improves symptoms and haemodynamic function in patients with constrictive pericarditis, but the procedure carries a notable risk, with reported mortality rates of 5–10% in experienced centres (Bertog et al. 2014). The risk is higher in patients with severe calcification or poor preoperative status.

2.2.3 Drainage of Purulent Pericarditis

Indications

Purulent pericarditis, which can rapidly progress to constrictive pericarditis, requires prompt surgical drainage to control the infection and prevent further complications.

Surgical Procedure

- *Approach:* The subxiphoid approach is most commonly used, but a thoracotomy may be required for more extensive infections.
- *Technique:* The pericardium is accessed, and the purulent material is evacuated. The pericardial sac is then irrigated with saline or antibiotic solutions, and a drainage catheter is left in place to allow for continuous drainage.

Outcomes

Timely surgical drainage combined with appropriate antibiotic therapy can lead to resolution of the infection and prevent the development of constrictive pericarditis (Spodick 2003).

2.2.4 Pericardial Cysts

Indications

Cyst Rupture

Rupture of a pericardial cyst, though uncommon, can lead to life-threatening complications such as pericardial effusion and tamponade. Cyst rupture may occur spontaneously or secondary to trauma or infection. When a cyst ruptures, it releases its contents into the pericardial space, which can cause acute pericardial effusion, leading to increased intrapericardial pressure and the development of cardiac tamponade (Roberts et al. 2012). This is an emergency that requires prompt surgical intervention.

Compression of Adjacent Structures

Large pericardial cysts can compress nearby structures, leading to symptoms such as chest pain, dyspnoea, or dysphagia. Compression of the right atrium, pulmonary artery, or superior vena cava can lead to haemodynamic compromise, while compression of the bronchial tree can result in respiratory distress. In these cases, surgical decompression is necessary to relieve the pressure on vital structures and restore normal function (Hsu et al. 2022).

Infection and Haemorrhage

Infection of a pericardial cyst, although rare, can lead to purulent pericarditis or sepsis. Haemorrhage within a pericardial cyst, either spontaneous or post-traumatic, may result in acute symptoms due to increased cyst size and the development of pericardial effusion. Both infection and haemorrhage are indications for emergency surgery to prevent further complications.

Surgical Procedure

- *Approach:* VATS is considered the preferable approach for cysts located in the anterior or lateral pericardium. This offers great visualisation of the pericardium, surrounding structures, and reduces postoperative pain and hospitalisation. Thoracotomy or median sternotomy are used in larger cysts with extensive adhesions, in cases of ruptured, infected, or actively bleeding cysts with symptoms of tamponade. Thoracotomy also offers good exposure for pericardial cysts protruding towards the posterior mediastinum with robotic-assisted approach also demonstrating great access for surgical excision for these cysts.
- *Technique:* In VATS surgery, a 3-port access along the mid- and anterior axillary line with CO_2 insufflation provides excellent exposure of the mediastinum. The pericar-

dial cyst is identified, and either decompression or complete resection is performed. If there is concern about rupture or infection, thorough irrigation of the pericardial cavity is carried out. Postoperative drainage is maintained via a chest tube to allow for fluid drainage and to prevent reaccumulation (Greig et al. 2007). For large cysts with associated infection or rupture, careful dissection is required to avoid injury to adjacent structures, and pericardial irrigation is performed.

- *Intraoperative Considerations:* In cases of VATS excision of large pericardial cysts, intraoperative needle decompression and aspiration should be performed first. This allows for easier tissue manipulation and dissection around the cyst. Even in experienced centres with thoracoscopic and robotic-assisted operations, an open approach should always be considered if intraoperative complications occur or if the surgical planes for dissection are not clear.

2.2.5 Outcomes

The prognosis following surgical intervention for pericardial cysts is generally excellent, particularly when surgery is performed before the development of severe complications. For patients with ruptured cysts and tamponade, timely surgical intervention is crucial to prevent haemodynamic collapse. Infected or haemorrhagic cysts can also be successfully treated with surgery, with a low risk of recurrence when the cyst is completely excised.

2.3 Controversies and Outcomes

2.3.1 Subxiphoid Window vs. VATS

The choice between a subxiphoid pericardial window and VATS remains a topic of debate. The subxiphoid approach is more common in emergencies in cases of tamponade from effusions and trauma. VATS approach offers superior visualisation and may be more effective for diagnostic purposes, especially for loculated effusions in the posterior pericardium where the subxiphoid approach may be difficult to reach. However, VATS is more technically demanding and requires general anaesthesia with double-lumen endotracheal tube, which may not be suitable for unstable patients who cannot tolerate single-lung ventilation (Tsang et al. 2011).

2.3.2 Timing and Extent of Pericardiectomy

There is ongoing debate regarding the optimal timing for pericardiectomy in constrictive pericarditis. While early intervention is recommended to prevent irreversible myocardial damage, the high-risk nature of the procedure necessitates careful patient selection. The extent of pericardiectomy, whether total or partial, also remains controversial, with some studies suggesting that total pericardiectomy offers better outcomes at the cost of higher surgical risk (Bertog et al. 2014).

2.3.3 Percutaneous Drainage of Pericardial Cysts

The role of percutaneous aspiration in the management of pericardial cysts remains controversial. While aspiration is minimally invasive, it is associated with a higher recurrence rate compared to surgical excision. Additionally, aspiration is not recommended for infected or haemorrhagic cysts, and its use is limited to symptomatic cysts in stable patients.

2.3.4 Prognosis and Long-Term Outcomes

The prognosis following emergency pericardial surgery largely depends on the underlying pathology. Pericardial window creation typically results in excellent immediate outcomes, with most patients experiencing significant relief from tamponade. However, the long-term prognosis is poorer in patients with malignant effusions due to the underlying advanced disease.

Pericardiectomy for constrictive pericarditis offers significant improvements in quality of life and survival, but the procedure's inherent risks necessitate thorough preoperative evaluation and careful surgical technique. Infectious pericarditis, particularly when managed early with surgical drainage and antibiotics, generally has a good prognosis, though delays in treatment can lead to complications like constriction and increased mortality (Tsang et al. 2011).

2.4 Conclusion

Emergency surgical management of pericardial pathologies is essential to prevent life-threatening complications. Procedures such as pericardial window creation and pericardiectomy provide effective relief from pericardial effusion and constrictive pericarditis respectively. However, these surgeries are not without risk, and careful consideration of patient selection, timing, and surgical technique is crucial. Ongoing research and debate continue to refine the best practices for managing these complex conditions.

References

Adler Y, Charron P, Imazio M et al (2015) ESC Scientific Document Group, 2015 ESC Guidelines for the diagnosis and management of pericardial diseases: The Task Force for the Diagnosis and Management of Pericardial Diseases of the European Society of Cardiology (ESC) Endorsed by: The European Association for Cardio-Thoracic Surgery (EACTS). Eur Heart J 36(42):2921–2964

Amro A, Mansoor K, Amro M, Sobeih A, Suliman M, Okoro K, El-Hamdani R, Vilchez D, El-Hamdani M, Shweihat YR (2021) A comprehensive systemic literature review of pericardial decompression syndrome: often unrecognized and potentially fatal syndrome. Curr Cardiol Rev 17(1):101–110

Beck CS (1935) Two cardiac compression triads. JAMA 104:714–716

Bertog SC, Thambidorai SK, Parakh K et al (2014) Constrictive pericarditis: etiology and cause-specific survival after pericardiectomy. J Am Coll Cardiol 43(8):1445–1452

Fowler NO (1997) Cardiac tamponade: a clinical or an echocardiographic diagnosis? Circulation 96(11):3163–3165

Greig JD, Ferreira HP, Roche EM et al (2007) Video-assisted thoracoscopic surgery for pericardial cysts. Ann Thorac Surg 83(1):180–182

Hsu DS, Banks KC, Velotta JB (2022) Surgical approaches to mediastinal cysts: clinical practice review. Mediastinum 6:32

Kapoor A, McWhorter Y, Polce DR (2022) Acute right ventricular failure immediately following subxiphoid pericardial window requiring temporary cardiopulmonary bypass support: a case report of pericardial decompression syndrome. Cureus 14(6):e26286

Mehta N, Sloane CM (2020) Cardiac tamponade. In: StatPearls. StatPearls Publishing, Treasure Island

Mendes RG, Costa AN, Corra RA et al (2015) Pericardial cysts: case series and review of the literature. J Clin Med Res 7(9):616–620

Mercier LA, de Guise P, Castonguay Y et al (2015) Surgical management of pericardial effusion. Ann Thorac Surg 33(1):50–53

Nataf P, Cacoub P, Dorent R, Jault F, Bors V, Pavie A, Cabrol C, Gandjbakhch I (1993) Results of subtotal pericardiectomy for constrictive pericarditis. Eur J Cardiothorac Surg 7(5):252–255;discussion 255-6

Nishimura RA, Tajik AJ (2014) The Valsalva maneuver and response revisited. Mayo Clin Proc 89(4):451–459

Reddy PS, Curtiss EI (2017) Cardiac tamponade. In: Feigenbaum's echocardiography, 7th edn. Lippincott Williams & Wilkins, Philadelphia

Roberts JT, Tiso RR, Haller JO et al (2012) Ruptured pericardial cyst presenting as hemopericardium: case report and review of the literature. Radiol Case Rep 7(2):90–93

Spodick DH (2003) Acute cardiac tamponade. N Engl J Med 349(7):684–690

Tsang TS, Oh JK, Seward JB et al (2011) Diagnostic and therapeutic approach to pericardial disease. Rev Cardiovasc Med 2(3):125–139

Emergency Cardiac Surgery for Thromboembolic Disease

Jason A. Varzaly and David P. Jenkins

Abstract Acute pulmonary embolism is a common condition that can cause shock when large volume, and emergency surgical embolectomy has a role in the treatment pathway. Guidelines for management of pulmonary embolism suggest that emergency surgery is indicated for high-risk patients that are haemodynamically unstable. Through the use of cardiopulmonary bypass, clot retrieval can be performed safely and reproducibly. The management of such patients in the modern era utilises multidisciplinary Pulmonary Embolism Response Teams (PERT) for optimal outcomes.

Keywords Acute pulmonary embolism · Pulmonary Embolism Severity Index (PESI) · Massive pulmonary embolism · Right ventricular failure · Obstructive shock · Pulmonary Embolism Response Teams (PERT) · Catheter-based pulmonary reperfusion · Surgical pulmonary embolectomy · Clot retrieval · Mechanical circulatory support

---

J. A. Varzaly (✉)
Royal Papworth Hospital, Cambridge, UK

Royal Adelaide Hospital, Adelaide, Australia
e-mail: jason.varzaly@sa.gov.au

D. P. Jenkins
Royal Papworth Hospital, Cambridge, UK
e-mail: david.jenkins1@nhs.net

A. Kourliouros (ed.), *Emergency Cardiac Surgery*,
https://doi.org/10.1007/978-3-032-15787-4_27

1 Introduction

Acute pulmonary embolism (PE) is a common medical condition in which the pulmonary arterial tree is obstructed by foreign material, usually thrombus, resulting in haemodynamic compromise proportional to the degree of occlusion. The most common source of the thrombus is the lower limb venous system. The incidence of deep venous thrombosis (DVT) in the general population is reported at between 39 and 162 per 100,000 people (Goyal 2024; Keller et al. 2020; Wendelboe and Raskob 2016).

The mortality rate associated with acute PE has historically been reported as high as 25% in patients with shock and 65% in patients who have suffered cardiac arrest as a result of the pulmonary embolism (Kasper et al. 1997).

In a recent study analysing the contemporary incidence of PE amongst patients with COVID it was identified that PE occurred in 14.7% of patients on the ward and 23.4% of patients in ICU which can represent an evolving risk factor for the acute development of this condition (Roncon et al. 2020).

Additionally, it has been identified in larger registry studies that while the overall incidence of mortality associated PE is decreasing, the overall incidence rate has been increasing across the last few decades (Sonne-Holm et al. 2022). In a broad European study this has resulted in contemporary costs ranging from 9135 to 10,620 Euros per case in the first year of follow up and a disease burden that translates to the loss of 1.2 years of health life per incident of PE case (Farmakis et al. 2022).

As such, acute PE represents a disease of significant and increasing impact on patients and healthcare systems globally.

2 Pathophysiology

The predisposing risk factors for venous thromboembolism (VTE) are extensive with the strongest risk factors including myocardial infarction in the last 3 months, hospitalisation for heart failure or atrial fibrillation/flutter, lower limb fracture, hip or knee replacement, major trauma, previous VTE and major illness such as cancer and spinal cord injury (Anderson Jr. and Spencer 2003; Rogers et al. 2012).

Once an acute PE has occurred, a well described pathophysiological spiral of events ensues that begins with right ventricle (RV) dilatation and increased wall tension, leading to RV ischaemia with decreased output that results in decreased cardiac output and ultimately obstructive shock and death (Konstantinides et al. 2020).

Care should be taken in the initial evaluation as some patients have co-existing chronic thromboembolic pulmonary hypertension (CTEPH) and present with a deterioration due to an acute chronic disease. Evidence should be looked for in the history (co-existing breathlessness), the echocardiogram (presence of RV hypertrophy and/or Pulmonary Artery (PA) systolic pressure > 60 mmHg) and CTPA (presence of typical features of CTEPH).

3 Classification

With the above outlined pathophysiological consequences of acute PE and the potentially dramatic influence it can have on a patient's haemodynamics it has become prudent to classify the severity of PE as it relates to risk of mortality, thus guiding the nature of intervention recommended (Konstantinides et al. 2020).

The most important and extensively validated risk stratification score utilised is the Pulmonary Embolism Severity Index (PESI) which has adapted to a simplified version (sPESI) and has also been validated (Konstantinides et al. 2020; Donzé et al. 2008). This score awards a single point, in patients diagnosed with PE, for each feature of age > 80 years, cancer, chronic cardiac or pulmonary disease, pulse rate > 110, systolic < 100 or arterial oxygen saturations < 90% (Table 1—adapted from ESC guidelines). If the patient has at least one of these features it increases the predicted risk of 30-day mortality to 10.9% (Konstantinides et al. 2020; Donzé et al. 2008; Righini et al. 2011).

The sPESI score can be utilised in conjunction with the patient's haemodynamic status to enable the rapid classification into low, intermediate and high risk to dictate reperfusion strategies (Table 1) (Konstantinides et al. 2020). Most useful for the surgeon is that the high risk classification dictates the need for a reperfusion strategy—either systemic thrombolysis, interventional radiological/percutaneous treatment or surgical embolectomy (in particular when thrombolysis is contraindicated, or if it has failed) (Keeling et al. 2016; Pasrija et al. 2018a; Choi et al. 2020).

Table 1 Recommendations for acute phase treatment of pulmonary embolism

	Criteria				Treatment strategy recommended	
Risk stratification	Haemodynamic instability (cardiac arrest, Systolid BP < 90 mmHg or requiring vasopressors to achieve SBP ≥ 90 mmHg)	Clinical parameters of severity (sPESI Score ≥ 1)	RV dysfunction on TTE or CTPA	Elevated cardiac troponin levels	Anticoagulation	Reperfusion
High	+	+	+	+	Unfractionated heparin + weight adjusted bolus	Surgical pulmonary embolectomy for patients whose thrombolysis has failed or is contraindicated (Class I, Level C) Percutaneous catheter-directed treatment in patients whose thrombolysis has failed or is contraindicated (Class IIa, Level C) Systemic thrombolytic therapy
Intermediate		+	+	+	Initiation of anticoagulation recommended with high probability of PE while diagnostic workup is in progress Low Molecular Weight Heparin recommended over Unfractionated Heparin	Rescue thrombolytic therapy for patients with haemodynamic deterioration on anticoagulation therapy (Class I, Level B) Surgical embolectomy or percutaneous catheter therapy can be considered with haemodynamic deterioration (Class IIa, Level C)
Low						

4 Surgical Approach

Our recommended surgical technique is through a standard median sternotomy and the utilisation of cardiopulmonary bypass. The use of inflow occlusion for clot retrieval has been described with good results, however this approach is somewhat historic as it limits the ability to retrieve clots from further distal down the pulmonary arterial tree and provides a time limit of haemodynamic stability (Clarke 1981). If CTEPH is suspected, the patient should be managed by an experienced pulmonary endarterectomy surgical service, as endarterectomy utilising Deep Hypothermic Circulatory Arrest (DHCA) will be required, which is outside the scope of this chapter.

4.1 Incision and Exposure

Midline incision, with full sternotomy. The pericardium is divided into a reverse T-shape. Pericardial stays are located from the edges of the pericardium above the superior vena cava (SVC), on either side of the aorta, at the pericardium edge over the main PA, and both sides of the inferior extent of the pericardium before the lateral extension. The critical points are good exposure over the pulmonary trunk as it continues beyond the bifurcation to the left main PA, and over the SVC with the right main PA underlying it.

4.2 Cannulation Strategy

We recommend a standard arterial inflow at the ascending aorta just proximal to the pericardial reflection. The venous cannulation is more critical—we introduce a standard two stage venous cannula from the right atrial appendage with the tip sitting in the inferior vena cava (IVC) and a separate single staged cannula (typically 30 Fr) which is then inserted through the Right Atrium free wall and up the superior vena cava (SVC) to approximately 10 cm.

This strategy is important as it enables excellent venous drainage with full decompression of the distended right heart and ensures the SVC is not compressed during dissection in the right pulmonary artery branch between the aorta and SVC.

Cardiopulmonary bypass (CPB) is then commenced, and slings are passed around the aorta, pulmonary trunk and SVC. A small PA vent can be placed to the pulmonary trunk to assist with venous drainage before the PA are opened. The typical configuration is displayed in Fig. 1.

Unlike pulmonary endarterectomy (PTE), no systemic cooling is required and normothermic CPB is standard. There is also no requirement for cardioplegic arrest, and it is actually better avoided so that there is no ischaemic insult to the right ventricle, which can be perfused throughout.

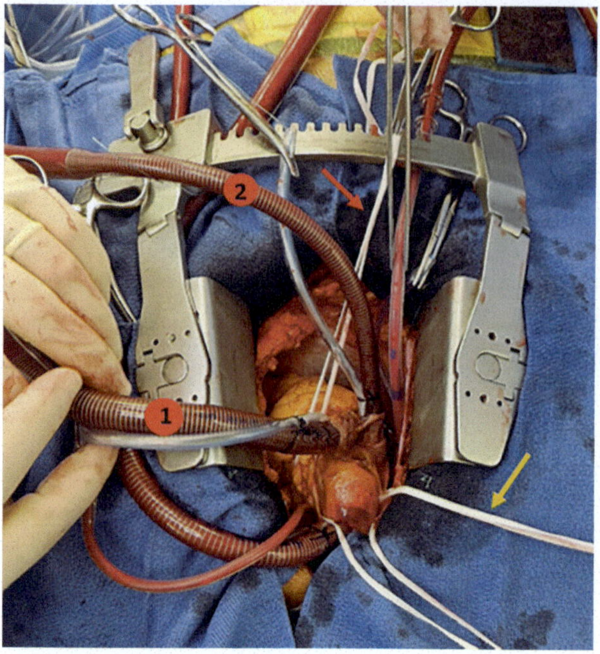

Fig. 1 Figure demonstrating cardiopulmonary bypass set up for accessing both pulmonary arteries. 1—Two staged RA to IVC venous cannula, 2—Single staged RA to SVC cannula; Red arrow demonstrates sling around PA which has been pulled tight to prevent entrainment of air through the open PA which has a vent placed; Yellow arrow demonstrates sling around the SVC which is not pulled up at this time

4.3 Clot Retrieval

4.3.1 Left Pulmonary Artery

The initial incision made in the pulmonary trunk can be extended into the left pulmonary artery by carrying it distal and gently arching to the left. We advise to stay intra-pericardial and not to go beyond the pericardial reflection as the vessel here will be more robust and the artery less likely to split distally.

The cut edges of the artery can be gently retracted using 4-0 prolene sutures on clips.

Clot retrieval can now be carried out through the utilisation of suction (we utilise a cell saver circuit) and broad forceps (DeBakey or Rampley sponge holder forceps etc.). Even without experience of PTE, it should be possible to see into the lobar and segmental divisions and retrieve all visible clot. Figure 2 demonstrates the type of acute clot specimen that can be retrieved through this method.

4.3.2 Right Pulmonary Artery

The sling passed around the SVC is pulled up and clipped to the drapes, and the aortic sling is retracted in the opposite direction and clipped to the drapes. This allows good exposure of the right main PA. Improved exposure can further be obtained through division of the pericardium between the SVC and aorta, as well as

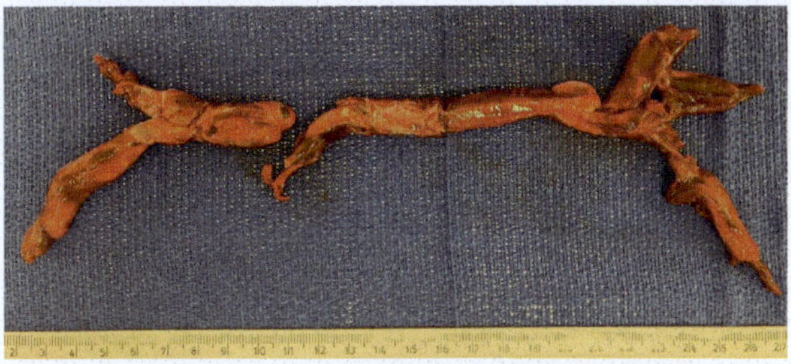

Fig. 2 Acute clot retrieved—the specimen demonstrates pulmonary arterial branching pattern down both the left and right pulmonary arteries

the use of a retractor to hold open the window being created over the right main PA. We use an Adson retractor without teeth.

Further the pulmonary trunk sling is retracted inferiorly to occlude the RV inflow.

A longitudinal incision is made in the midpoint of the right PA. The edges of the PA are retracted using half-length 4-0 prolene sutures on artery clips.

There will be collateral flow in the pulmonary artery—when in excess a small drop vent can be placed to facilitate drainage back to the pump.

Clearance of clot is as for the main PA. Once adequate clearance has been achieved, both the PA incisions can be closed using a running 5-0 prolene in two layers.

4.3.3 Special Situations

If a patent foramen ovale is present there may be clot traversing the foramen, with impending paradoxical embolism. This should be carefully removed utilising cardioplegic arrest at the start of the operation before manipulating the heart to minimise the risk of systemic embolisation.

If there is clot in the right heart, seen on CTPA or echocardiography, the right atrium should be opened with the cavae snared, and the clot should be removed, and if in the RV, through the tricuspid valve.

4.4 Weaning Strategy

Once clot retrieval has been completed and arteriotomies are closed, weaning from CPB and decannulation can take place, as for standard cardiac surgery.

While weaning greater attention must be given to the filling status of the right ventricle and care must be taken not to volume overload. A trans-oesophageal echocardiogram is useful to judge right- and left-sided filling. If anything, separating with the minimal volume able to achieve the desired haemodynamics can be beneficial, and a slow wean of 1 L at a time preferred to assess right ventricular function. If the RV function cannot sustain adequate cardiac output, temporary mechanical circulatory support may be required. We would advocate central veno-arterial ECMO (see section 6.1).

5 Outcomes

The challenge of interpreting the outcomes of surgical embolectomy in the literature is the data being captured represents both historical and contemporary outcomes as well as all-comer data that lacks the fidelity to determine the expected outcome of a well-selected modern-era patient.

One study published the results of a database query of the National Institute of Cardiovascular Outcomes Research central database in the UK retrospectively and found that from 1996 to 2018 in patients undergoing surgical pulmonary embolectomy there was an in-hospital mortality of 25% (Argyriou et al. 2024). Interestingly, they found that cardioplegic arrest was used in 53.1% and that 37.5% had pre-operative cardiogenic shock which demonstrates non-contemporary practice as well as a very sick patient population. This represents the challenges in interpreting the published literature and represents a potentially commonly held belief that the outcomes from surgical pulmonary embolectomy are generally poor.

5.1 Distilling Outcomes

In a recent scientific statement from the American Heart Association on the surgical management of pulmonary embolism, outcomes were analysed which focused on literature published from 2008 to 2020 that adjusted for acuity and patient selection (Goldberg et al. 2023). This found that mortality of surgical embolectomy ranged from 2.3 to 13.2% (with worse outcomes generally driven by the pre-operative CPR cohort) with postoperative RV failure rarely being the cause for mortality, but anoxic brain injury from CPR, or specific patient factors such as advanced cancer or infection (Goldberg et al. 2023; Neely et al. 2015; QiMin et al. 2020).

5.2 Predictors of Poor Outcome

The strongest predictor of poor outcome is pre-operative CPR (Keeling et al. 2016; Goldberg et al. 2023). While it is difficult to determine the mortality associated with pre-operative CPR, the reported mortality in patients who did not require pre-operative CPR is 2.9% (Goldberg et al. 2023). This suggests that most of the drivers for high mortality rates reported being derived from this variable.

Further, the need for postoperative ECMO increases markedly with pre-operative CPR (Goldberg et al. 2020; Pasrija et al. 2018b). This is likely driven by RV dysfunction—which all represents the acuity and fulminant state of the patient (Goldberg et al. 2023).

Failed systemic thrombolysis also impacts the morbidity and mortality associated with surgical embolectomy (Goldberg et al. 2023; Aymard et al. 2013; Azari et al. 2015). This may represent a combination of the results of antecedent thrombolytic therapy effecting surgery directly, delayed time to operation resulting in a declining patient state by the time surgery is undertaken or the severity of clot burden for it not to respond to thrombolytic therapy.

6 Team-Based Approaches and Alternative Strategies

As the management of acute pulmonary embolism progresses into the modern era, the concept of Pulmonary Embolism Response Teams (PERT) has developed (Konstantinides et al. 2020; Dudzinski and Piazza 2016). The core is to have essentially a rapid multidisciplinary meeting of specialists which may encompass any discipline that would provide input to the management of the patient—such as cardiology, pulmonology, intensive care medicine, anaesthesia, radiology and cardiothoracic surgery. Meta-analysis of the implementation of these teams, as compared to control groups, have already demonstrated increased utilisation of systemic thrombolysis, catheter-based therapies and surgical embolectomy, with a reduction in the placement of IVC filters (Fleitas Sosa et al. 2022). Further analysis have also demonstrated a reduction in mortality in addition to shorter time to initiation of therapy, reduced hospital stay and increased utilisation of advanced therapies (Gardner et al. 2024; Porres-Aguilar et al. 2022).

6.1 Mechanical Circulatory Support

The temporary use of mechanical circulatory support—typically veno-arterial extra corporeal membrane oxygenator (VA-ECMO) has been described and utilised as an adjunct in the treatment of high risk patients with high risk PE including those in a critically ill state including circulatory collapse, cardiac arrest and CPR (Konstantinides et al. 2020; Goldberg et al. 2023). The benefit from VA-ECMO is derived through offloading the right ventricle, restoring perfusion to the body and improving oxygenation while the underlying thrombus is treated. The literature on this topic is largely in the form of cohort studies that are generally retrospective, and this likely represents the use of this in an emergent situation. In general, the use of VA-ECMO offers the ability to stabilise the critically ill patient and when utilised as either stand-alone or an adjunct to a reperfusion strategy, it may offer a survival advantage (Giraud et al. 2021; Guliani et al. 2021; Hobohm et al. 2022).

The Impella RP device has also been utilised in a small number of patients with encouraging results to stabilise patients in shock and improve survival (Elder et al. 2018). These results will still need to be ratified by further studies, but may represent an additional treatment modality for such patients.

6.2 Catheter-Based Therapies

Catheter devices utilise various technologies to achieve pulmonary arterial reperfusion through mechanical fragmentation, thrombus aspiration or fragmentation/aspiration combined with locally administered thrombolysis (Konstantinides et al. 2020; Skaf et al. 2007). The results reported are generally from small trials and registries with a systematic review in 2016 summarising 35 trials demonstrating in hospital mortality rates for unstable haemodynamic status approaching 18.1% (Bajaj et al. 2016). With a more recent systematic review published in the Cochrane database finding multiple retrospective studies, prospective registries and single-arm registries suggesting the benefit of catheter-based therapies for the treatment of acute PE; however, they felt there was insufficient data to support the widespread use (Harvey et al. 2022). Another recent meta-analysis involving patients in the intermediate to high-risk PE suggested reduced mortality compared to other therapies (Ishisaka et al. 2023).

As this area continues to evolve data will become more clear as to the optimal use of catheter-based interventions which will form a treatment arm in the management of acute PE.

7 Conclusion

Acute pulmonary embolism represents a common medical condition that is potentially fatal when it causes shock. This high-risk subgroup population requires a reperfusion strategy, and surgical intervention with emergency embolectomy as an option, especially if thrombolysis is contraindicated. Patient selection and identification prior to circulatory collapse requiring CPR will optimise surgical outcomes and greatly reduce mortality rates. Regardless, the operative approach can be approached systematically and reproducibly using cardiopulmonary bypass without cardioplegic arrest. The use of PERT can optimise patient outcomes and streamline patients to those requiring mechanical circulatory support, catheter-based interventions or surgical embolectomy to achieve the best results.

References

Anderson FA Jr, Spencer FA (2003) Risk factors for venous thromboembolism. Circulation 107(23 Suppl 1):19–16. https://doi.org/10.1161/01.cir.0000078469.07362.e6

Argyriou A, Vohra H, Chan J, Ahmed EM, Rajakaruna C, Angelini GD et al (2024) Incidence and outcomes of surgical pulmonary embolectomy in the UK. Br J Surg 111(1). https://doi.org/10.1093/bjs/znae003

Aymard T, Kadner A, Widmer A, Basciani R, Tevaearai H, Weber A et al (2013) Massive pulmonary embolism: surgical embolectomy versus thrombolytic therapy—should surgical

indications be revisited? Eur J Cardio-Thoracic Surg 43(1):90–94; discussion 4. https://doi.org/10.1093/ejcts/ezs123
Azari A, Beheshti AT, Moravvej Z, Bigdelu L, Salehi M (2015) Surgical embolectomy versus thrombolytic therapy in the management of acute massive pulmonary embolism: short and long-term prognosis. Heart Lung 44(4):335–339. https://doi.org/10.1016/j.hrtlng.2015.04.008
Bajaj NS, Kalra R, Arora P, Ather S, Guichard JL, Lancaster WJ et al (2016) Catheter-directed treatment for acute pulmonary embolism: systematic review and single-arm meta-analyses. Int J Cardiol 225:128–139. https://doi.org/10.1016/j.ijcard.2016.09.036
Choi JH, O'Malley TJ, Maynes EJ, Weber MP, D'Antonio ND, Mellado M et al (2020) Surgical pulmonary embolectomy outcomes for acute pulmonary embolism. Ann Thorac Surg 110(3):1072–1080. https://doi.org/10.1016/j.athoracsur.2020.01.075
Clarke DB (1981) Pulmonary embolectomy re-evaluated. Ann R Coll Surg Engl 63(1):18–24
Donzé J, Le Gal G, Fine MJ, Roy PM, Sanchez O, Verschuren F et al (2008) Prospective validation of the Pulmonary Embolism Severity Index. A clinical prognostic model for pulmonary embolism. Thromb Haemost 100(5):943–948. https://doi.org/10.1160/th08-05-0285
Dudzinski DM, Piazza G (2016) Multidisciplinary pulmonary embolism response teams. Circulation 133(1):98–103. https://doi.org/10.1161/circulationaha.115.015086
Elder M, Blank N, Kaki A, Alraies MC, Grines CL, Kajy M et al (2018) Mechanical circulatory support for acute right ventricular failure in the setting of pulmonary embolism. J Interv Cardiol 31(4):518–524. https://doi.org/10.1111/joic.12503
Farmakis IT, Barco S, Mavromanoli AC, Agnelli G, Cohen AT, Giannakoulas G et al (2022) Cost-of-illness analysis of long-term health care resource use and disease burden in patients with pulmonary embolism: insights from the PREFER in VTE registry. J Am Heart Assoc 11(20):e027514. https://doi.org/10.1161/JAHA.122.027514
Fleitas Sosa D, Lehr AL, Zhao H, Roth S, Lakhther V, Bashir R et al (2022) Impact of pulmonary embolism response teams on acute pulmonary embolism: a systematic review and meta-analysis. Eur Resp Rev 31(165). https://doi.org/10.1183/16000617.0023-2022
Gardner TA, Fuher A, Longino A, Sink EM, Jurica J, Park B et al (2024) Reduced mortality associated with pulmonary embolism response team consultation for intermediate and high-risk pulmonary embolism: a retrospective cohort study. Thromb J 22(1):38. https://doi.org/10.1186/s12959-024-00605-8
Giraud R, Laurencet M, Assouline B, De Charrière A, Banfi C, Bendjelid K (2021) Can VA-ECMO be used as an adequate treatment in massive pulmonary embolism? J Clin Med 10(15). https://doi.org/10.3390/jcm10153376
Goldberg JB, Spevack DM, Ahsan S, Rochlani Y, Dutta T, Ohira S et al (2020) Survival and right ventricular function after surgical management of acute pulmonary embolism. J Am Coll Cardiol 76(8):903–911. https://doi.org/10.1016/j.jacc.2020.06.065
Goldberg JB, Giri J, Kobayashi T, Ruel M, Mittnacht AJC, Rivera-Lebron B et al (2023) Surgical management and mechanical circulatory support in high-risk pulmonary embolisms: historical context, current status, and future directions: a scientific statement from the American Heart Association. Circulation 147(9):e628–ee47. https://doi.org/10.1161/CIR.0000000000001117
Goyal VVASA (2024) Acute pulmonary embolism. StatPearls Publishing, Treasure Island
Guliani S, Das Gupta J, Osofsky R, Kraai EP, Mitchell JA, Dettmer TS et al (2021) Venoarterial extracorporeal membrane oxygenation is an effective management strategy for massive pulmonary embolism patients. J Vasc Surg Venous Lymphat Disord 9(2):307–314. https://doi.org/10.1016/j.jvsv.2020.04.033
Harvey JJ, Huang S, Uberoi R (2022) Catheter-directed therapies for the treatment of high risk (massive) and intermediate risk (submassive) acute pulmonary embolism. Cochr Datab Syst Rev (Online) 8(8):Cd013083. https://doi.org/10.1002/14651858.CD013083.pub2
Hobohm L, Sagoschen I, Habertheuer A, Barco S, Valerio L, Wild J et al (2022) Clinical use and outcome of extracorporeal membrane oxygenation in patients with pulmonary embolism. Resuscitation 170:285–292. https://doi.org/10.1016/j.resuscitation.2021.10.007

Ishisaka Y, Watanabe A, Fujisaki T, Iwagami M, So M, Steiger D et al (2023) Comparison of interventions for intermediate to high-risk pulmonary embolism: a network meta-analysis. Catheteriz Cardiovasc Intervent 102(2):249–265. https://doi.org/10.1002/ccd.30745

Kasper W, Konstantinides S, Geibel A, Olschewski M, Heinrich F, Grosser KD et al (1997) Management strategies and determinants of outcome in acute major pulmonary embolism: results of a multicenter registry. J Am Coll Cardiol 30(5):1165–1171. https://doi.org/10.1016/s0735-1097(97)00319-7

Keeling WB, Sundt T, Leacche M, Okita Y, Binongo J, Lasajanak Y et al (2016) Outcomes after surgical pulmonary embolectomy for acute pulmonary embolus: a multi-institutional study. Ann Thorac Surg 102(5):1498–1502. https://doi.org/10.1016/j.athoracsur.2016.05.004

Keller K, Hobohm L, Ebner M, Kresoja KP, Münzel T, Konstantinides SV et al (2020) Trends in thrombolytic treatment and outcomes of acute pulmonary embolism in Germany. Eur Heart J 41(4):522–529. https://doi.org/10.1093/eurheartj/ehz236

Konstantinides SV, Meyer G, Becattini C, Bueno H, Geersing GJ, Harjola VP et al (2020) 2019 ESC Guidelines for the diagnosis and management of acute pulmonary embolism developed in collaboration with the European Respiratory Society (ERS). Eur Heart J 41(4):543–603. https://doi.org/10.1093/eurheartj/ehz405

Neely RC, Byrne JG, Gosev I, Cohn LH, Javed Q, Rawn JD et al (2015) Surgical embolectomy for acute massive and submassive pulmonary embolism in a series of 115 patients. Ann Thoracic Surg 100(4):1245–1251; discussion 51–2. https://doi.org/10.1016/j.athoracsur.2015.03.111

Pasrija C, Kronfli A, Rouse M, Raithel M, Bittle GJ, Pousatis S et al (2018a) Outcomes after surgical pulmonary embolectomy for acute submassive and massive pulmonary embolism: a single-center experience. J Thorac Cardiovasc Surg 155(3):1095–106.e2. https://doi.org/10.1016/j.jtcvs.2017.10.139

Pasrija C, Kronfli A, George P, Raithel M, Boulos F, Herr DL et al (2018b) Utilization of veno-arterial extracorporeal membrane oxygenation for massive pulmonary embolism. Ann Thorac Surg 105(2):498–504. https://doi.org/10.1016/j.athoracsur.2017.08.033

Porres-Aguilar M, Rosovsky RP, Rivera-Lebron BN, Kaatz S, Mukherjee D, Anaya-Ayala JE et al (2022) Pulmonary embolism response teams: changing the paradigm in the care for acute pulmonary embolism. J Thrombosis Haemostasis JTH 20(11):2457–2464. https://doi.org/10.1111/jth.15832

QiMin W, LiangWan C, DaoZhong C, HanFan Q, ZhongYao H, XiaoFu D et al (2020) Clinical outcomes of acute pulmonary embolectomy as the first-line treatment for massive and submassive pulmonary embolism: a single-centre study in China. J Cardiothorac Surg 15(1):321. https://doi.org/10.1186/s13019-020-01364-z

Righini M, Roy PM, Meyer G, Verschuren F, Aujesky D, Le Gal G (2011) The Simplified Pulmonary Embolism Severity Index (PESI): validation of a clinical prognostic model for pulmonary embolism. J Thrombosis Haemostasis JTH 9(10):2115–2117. https://doi.org/10.1111/j.1538-7836.2011.04469.x

Rogers MA, Levine DA, Blumberg N, Flanders SA, Chopra V, Langa KM (2012) Triggers of hospitalization for venous thromboembolism. Circulation 125(17):2092–2099. https://doi.org/10.1161/circulationaha.111.084467

Roncon L, Zuin M, Barco S, Valerio L, Zuliani G, Zonzin P et al (2020) Incidence of acute pulmonary embolism in COVID-19 patients: systematic review and meta-analysis. Eur J Intern Med 82:29–37. https://doi.org/10.1016/j.ejim.2020.09.006

Skaf E, Beemath A, Siddiqui T, Janjua M, Patel NR, Stein PD (2007) Catheter-tip embolectomy in the management of acute massive pulmonary embolism. Am J Cardiol 99(3):415–420. https://doi.org/10.1016/j.amjcard.2006.08.052

Sonne-Holm E, Kjærgaard J, Bang LE, Fosbøl E, Carlsen J, Winther-Jensen M (2022) Pulmonary embolism: age specific temporal trends in incidence and mortality in Denmark 1999-2018. Thromb Res 210:12–19. https://doi.org/10.1016/j.thromres.2021.12.011

Wendelboe AM, Raskob GE (2016) Global burden of thrombosis: epidemiologic aspects. Circ Res 118(9):1340–1347. https://doi.org/10.1161/circresaha.115.306841

Emergency Cardiac Surgery for Complex Thoracic Resections

Marinos Koulouroudias and Apostolos Nakas

Abstract Resection of locally advanced thoracic malignancies that require unplanned use of cardiopulmonary bypass, and injuries to the origins of major vessels or other intrapericardial structures could necessitate emergency cardiac surgical management. Thoracic surgeons without cardiac surgical training or recent practice involving use of cardiopulmonary bypass could need support from a cardiac surgeon in the emergency setting. In this chapter we will identify the pathologies and circumstances that may require cardiac surgical input, review the cardiopulmonary bypass (CPB)/extracorporeal membrane oxygenation (ECMO) and repair techniques utilised and describe mitigating mechanisms and practices for optimal outcomes.

We will not cover the use of planned CPB/ECMO nor their role in lung transplantation.

Keywords Complex thoracic resection · Central airway surgery · Major vascular injury · Superior vena cava repair · Unplanned extracorporeal circulation · Emergency cardiopulmonary bypass · Extracorporeal membrane oxygenation (ECMO) · Cannulation—central and peripheral · Rapid transfusion/cell salvage · Outcomes after unplanned extracorporeal circulation

M. Koulouroudias (✉)
Department of Cardiothoracic Surgery, John Radcliffe Hospital, Oxford University Hospitals NHS Foundation Trust, Oxford, UK
e-mail: marinosk@doctors.org.uk

A. Nakas
Department of Thoracic surgery, University Hospitals of Leicester NHS Trust, Leicester, UK
e-mail: apostolos.nakas@uhl-tr.nhs.uk

A. Kourliouros (ed.), *Emergency Cardiac Surgery*,
https://doi.org/10.1007/978-3-032-15787-4_28

1 Introduction

Resection of locally advanced thoracic malignancies that require unplanned use of cardiopulmonary bypass, and injuries to the origins of major vessels or other intra-pericardial structures could necessitate emergency cardiac surgical management. Thoracic surgeons without cardiac surgical training or recent practice involving use of cardiopulmonary bypass could need support from a cardiac surgeon in the emergency setting. In this chapter we will identify the pathologies and circumstances that may require cardiac surgical input, review the cardiopulmonary bypass (CPB)/extracorporeal membrane oxygenation (ECMO) and repair techniques utilised, and describe mitigating mechanisms and practices for optimal outcomes.

We will not cover the use of planned CPB/ECMO nor their role in lung transplantation.

2 Unplanned Use of Extracorporeal Circulation for Thoracic Resections

The incidence of unplanned extracorporeal circulation (ECC) to provide stability or a bail out option in thoracic resections is, by its nature, difficult to quantify. In the largest review on this topic, unplanned circulatory support was used in 23% of all resections using CPB (Muralidaran et al. 2011). As such, this is a rare emergency in a small subset of patients with very poor prognosis if not planned for appropriately (Muralidaran et al. 2011; Machuca et al. 2015). However, appropriate planning and multidisciplinary involvement can make a significant difference in the consequences of these very challenging resections.

We propose that a clear understanding of the rationale in choosing modalities of ECC, the understanding of risk factors for potential need for ECC and meticulous multidisciplinary planning for complex resections can improve outcomes.

3 Pathologies

We suggest considering four scenarios that might necessitate use of CPB or ECMO:

(a) To *salvage* catastrophic bleeding: for example, massive pulmonary artery bleeding, aortic injury, cardiomediastinal injury without possibility for safe proximal control.
(b) To *support* respiratory instability: in the event of severe pulmonary oedema, pulmonary haemorrhage, loss of airway.

(c) To *support* cardiovascular instability: in the event of severe RV dysfunction/failure after pneumonectomy or during complex resections requiring prolonged main pulmonary artery (PA) clamping.
(d) To *facilitate* a complete resection: where the need for, e.g. superior vena cava (SVC) or left atrial or aortic resection was not anticipated on pre-operative imaging but becomes apparent on exploring the chest.

4 Intraoperative Management

1. *Modalities of Extracorporeal Support*

Briefly, the main methods available to support a complex thoracic resection with ECC are: CPB, venovenous ECMO (VV-ECMO) and venoarterial ECMO (VA-ECMO).

Cardiopulmonary bypass (CPB) has the possibility to provide full cardiac and respiratory support, can allow for shed blood salvage and autotransfusion in true exsanguinating haemorrhage and offers the possibility for any extent of mediastinal/aortic reconstruction with the possibility for deep hypothermic circulatory arrest and the use of cardioplegic cardiac arrest (Machuca et al. 2015; Fuentes-Gago et al. 2017; Salter and Burt 2019).

Venoarterial ECMO (VA-ECMO) can be helpful in situations where opening the cardiac chambers or the aorta is not necessary (c.f. CPB) and where the bleeding is more easily brought under control (no possibility for autotransfusion). If these requirements are met, patients can be supported on VA-ECMO for longer periods of time with lower ensuing coagulopathy or systemic inflammatory response (due to lower Activated Clotting Time (ACT) needs and a closed circuit with no air-blood interface etc.) (Machuca et al. 2015).

VV-ECMO can be used to provide isolated respiratory support, where right ventricular function is adequate and where no major bleeding is encountered. VV-ECMO has even lower anticoagulation requirements and is the modality with the lowest thromboembolic risk, and the use of single-site cannulation access has revolutionised its ease of institution (Rinieri et al. 2015).

2. *Access for Cannulation*

Thoracic surgery poses specific challenges in cannulation: The patient is most frequently in a lateral decubitus position compromising peripheral access and central access will also be challenging in a left posterolateral thoracotomy.

Central Cannulation One needs to be aware of the options of where to cannulate with different incisions: A right thoracotomy gives access to both the ascending aorta and the right atrium, a left thoracotomy provides more access to the descending aorta, the left atrium/pulmonary veins, LV apex and the pulmonary artery. Access to the ascending aorta and the right atrium is difficult and impossible, respectively, from the left chest.

If access is difficult and the personnel is not familiar with 'non-standard' cannulation sites, then due consideration should be given to turning the patient supine and performing either a hemi-clamshell and joining both incisions, performing a separate sternotomy incision leaving the posterolateral thoracotomy site separate or performing a full clamshell.

If the patient is too unstable for a change in position, if the exposure offered via a thoracotomy is essential in completing the resection or if the intended mode of support is better suited to a peripheral approach (i.e. VV-ECMO), then peripheral access needs to be considered.

The significant technical difficulties in controlling bleeding and performing sternotomy and central cannulation at the same time might necessitate peripheral cannulation.

Peripheral Cannulation Femoral arterial and venous access and jugular venous access are the mainstay of peripheral cannulation for ECC. Jugular venous access can be easily accomplished on the ipsilateral side of the neck outside the surgical field, and occasionally might be the only access site needed (some iterations of VV-ECMO). Femoral cut down and arterial/venous cannulation, although part of the skillset of any cardiothoracic surgeon, can be particularly challenging with the patient in the lateral decubitus position, especially with the hypovolemic peripherally shut-down patient.

If one anticipates the need for cannulation, the groins should be prepped appropriately and a guidewire can be introduced percutaneously to aid emergency exposure of the vessels. A slight tilt at the hips can be introduced at around 30° from the horizontal (similar to the 'cork screw' positioning for thoracoabdominal aortic surgery).

3. *Reference to Resection and Reconstruction Techniques for Common Lesions*

Superior Vena Cava (SVC) A lot of SVC resection/reconstruction can be performed off-pump (Lee and Flores 2017). However, good planning can anticipate the potential for haemodynamic collapse/ inadvertent injury and need for ECC. Consider venous cannulation and the risk of air locks if the cava is opened without good control of the SVC. Innominate or jugular venous cannulation supplemented by femoral venous cannulation can provide a safe exposure in the most complex on-pump resections (Lee and Flores 2017).

- When the SVC is found to be involved only tangentially by a tumour, then a Satinsky type side-clamp can be used to allow en bloc resection of the lesion with subsequent primary suture repair without causing distortion in the SVC. This can be done off-pump.
- If more extensive resection is needed (but < 30–50% of the SVC is affected) and it cannot be performed on a side-biting clamp, then proximal and distal control of the SVC-Azygos system is obtained (Lee and Flores 2017; Venuta and Rendina 2012). Occluding all SVC inflow might cause circulatory compromise and a

period of CPB or VA-ECMO support might become necessary. Then a wide autologous pericardial or prosthetic patch is anastomosed to the defect.
- If > 30–50% of the SVC is affected then the SVC needs to be completely resected and replaced with an interposition tube graft. Important considerations are, where possible to clamp above the azygous to allow for some venous return to the heart. If this is not possible then again pump support might be needed or an in situ shunt might be employed (Sekine et al. 2010).
- For very proximal SVC-innominate involvement, resection and extra-anatomical bypass from the left innominate to the right atrium can be considered (Lee and Flores 2017).

Both tube graft replacement and extra-anatomical bypass are fraught with medium- to long-term graft occlusion as this is a low pressure system (Spaggiari et al. 2002).

Key considerations also include:

1. Sound oncological staging, very poor outcomes if embarking for T4 resections with N2 disease (Spaggiari et al. 2002).
2. Left phrenic nerve function needs to be intact, the right phrenic will very commonly be sacrificed or injured (as opposed to extended thymic resections where the left phrenic might need to be sacrificed).
3. Post-operative anticoagulation is paramount, where the SVC is replaced by a graft both early (due to technical reasons) and late (due to both technical reasons and competitive flow), and is very well documented and common. Most authorities advise at least 3–6 months and up to a year of therapeutic anticoagulation (Krutman et al. 2022).

Cardiac and Aortic Involvement

In the majority of instances cardiac involvement/injury will need CPB or VA-ECMO to be addressed. Strategy for cannulation and potential need for cardioplegic or deep hypothermic arrest depends on the length of involvement, the depth of invasion and the site (cardiac chamber and ascending/arch/descending aorta) (D'Andrilli et al. 2024).

Limited left atrial resection can be done on a side-biting clamp with primary repair. Any larger resections might need prosthetic reconstruction under CPB, although there is paucity in the literature (Dawson et al. 2021).

Descending thoracic aortic invasion/injury can be approached without bypass either with partial occlusion or endovascular stent grafting. If circulatory support is required, a left heart bypass can be employed with inflow from the left atrium and outflow to the distal uninvolved aorta to preserve distal perfusion (De Perrot and Perentes 2017).

Involvement of the aortic arch or the ascending aorta will need to be most safely addressed with CPB and Deep Hypothermic Circulatory Arrest (DHCA) (for arch) and by either patch plasty of the resected portion of the aorta or conventional aortic replacement.

These are very invasive procedures, with questionable oncological outcomes (Muralidaran et al. 2011) as such planned resection is rarely undertaken, but one needs to be aware of how to deal with these entities in the emergency setting (i.e. inadvertent injury during resection of a T4 stage tumour that was underappreciated preoperatively).

Airway Surgery

Most central airway surgery can be safely and reproducibly completed with either isolated or combined use of jet ventilation, cross-field ventilation and intermittent apnoea.

In large central airway, carinal tumours involving both mainstem bronchi or large mediastinal tumours airway loss might occur during induction of general anaesthesia or during the operation. In major carinal/trachea-bronchial resections in a patient with limited cardiorespiratory reserve, adequate ventilation might not be achieved with conventional ventilation methods and urgent institution of ECMO might become necessary to complete the operation safely (Li et al. 2016; Bozer et al. 2023).

Venoarterial ECMO (VV-ECMO) needs to be considered in a proactive manner with peripheral wiring/cannulation performed awake under local anaesthesia in an optimally positioned patient rather than having to crash onto ECMO after loss of airway control.

5 Pre- and Intraoperative Steps to Optimise Outcomes

Unplanned CPB leads to worse 5-year post-operative survival for obvious reasons. In the largest relevant meta-analysis (Muralidaran et al. 2011) the only multivariate predictor of poor survival is unplanned institution of bypass. The mediastinal organ resected, or the extent of the resection do not appear to affect outcomes in these settings.

As such, prevention and controlled transition, only when absolutely necessary to extracorporeal support, are paramount in optimising outcomes.

1. Systematic examination of cross sectional imaging. We suggest that should be less than four weeks old.
2. Risk stratification for cardiac complications that can exhibit intraoperatively (Salter and Burt 2019). These patients need extensive work-up and optimisation (Echocardiography, CPET, cardiology consult for pre-optimisation)
3. In-depth MDT discussion is paramount.
   (a) In the post-PACIFIC immunotherapy era (Antonia et al. 2017), patients with likely major mediastinal structure involvement might be better treated for surgically unresectable disease and better served with radical chemoradiotherapy and immunotherapy. Similarly this needs to be considered for patients who might need a pneumonectomy but will not be fit for it.
   (b) Patients with large tumours that are likely to be resectable should be considered for neoadjuvant immunotherapy to downstage tumours and minimise possibility of unplanned need for ECC (Forde et al. 2022).

4. Plan on the day to optimise a potential unplanned transition to ECC:
   (a) Adequate briefing of the theatre team with prescribed roles in case ECMO/CPB is needed, including liaison with perfusion scientists and cardiac surgeons. Ensure all relevant equipment and cannulas on stand-by.
   (b) If need for peripheral cannulation is anticipated, consider pre-emptive awake wiring or cannulation after induction but whilst still supine, otherwise keep the groins exposed and with a lateral tilt into the field.
   (c) Early proximal and distal control of the pulmonary arteries and veins in large tumours when planes are obscured to facilitate control of major PA bleeding; early control of the SVC-innominate-azygos system if thought to be involved.
   (d) Avoid taking on a case where there is potential for major mediastinal structure involvement/risk of bleeding/risk of airway loss if in a unit with no immediate ECC support.

6 Oncological Effects of CPB/ECMO

There are some theoretical risks from in vitro studies and case series that CPB can accentuate malignant disease invasiveness and portent poorer prognosis (Lorusso et al. 2018; Pinto et al. 2013). There is no definitive literature on the effects of CPB on cancer progression. The largest review on the subject (Lorusso et al. 2018) did not find any evidence that CPB worsens outcomes (progression of disease, cardiac and non-cardiac mortality) in cancer patients.

Vignette

You are embarking on resecting a right upper lobe adenocarcinoma post-neoadjuvant immunochemotherapy (ycT3ycN0) in a 68-year-old man with Chronic Obstructive Pulmonary Disease (COPD) and previous Non-ST Elevation Myocardial Infarction (NSTEMI). His Forced expiratory volume in 1 second (FEV1) is 49% predicted and Transfer factor of the lung for Carbon Monoxide (TLCO) is 46% predicted. You start off with a standard three-port VATS approach but realise that there is extensive fibrosis and dense adhesions in the hilum so elect to convert to a posterolateral thoracotomy.

You electively sling the main right PA as it exits the pericardium in anticipation of potential difficulties, as you know how hostile the hilum and lymph nodes adhering on the PA can be post immunotherapy. You hope this will not end up needing a vascular sleeve and appreciate that this patient will not tolerate anything more than a lobectomy, but you know better than being underprepared.

After dividing the right upper lobe pulmonary vein, you turn your attention to the truncus anterior (TA) branch. You are attempting to gain better access to the right upper vessels and start dissecting off some lymph nodes around the truncus. The lymph nodes are quite adherent to the base of the truncus and are matted all the way to the ongoing interlobar PA. You suddenly find the chest filling up with dark blood and realise that there must be an injury to the PA. You alert anaesthetist to bring blood to the room and to set up cell salvage. They swiftly ensure large bore access and bring in the rapid infuser. You release traction on the lobe and place pressure on the area you think the bleeding is coming from. This buys you some time to start the major transfusion protocol and get the cell saver in the field. However, under your finger you find yourself feeling the hole enlarging and blood again floods the field. Your astute assistant snugs the umbilical tape on the right main PA. Unfortunately, you are still getting brisk back bleeding from the distal stump of the interlobar PA. You ask your assistant to take over putting pressure, and you quickly encircle and snug the middle and lower lobe veins as well, achieving full vascular control of the lung and bleeding slows down, and finally in control. You are now staring down the endothelium through a serpiginous crack extending from the TA to the interlobar PA and thinking about how to solve the problem without performing a pneumonectomy. The patient is really not tolerating the main PA being snugged and is starting to drop his blood pressure. You appreciate that the only way out of this situation is to try and fix the injury on CPB, offering cell salvage and autotransfusion, whilst supporting the circulation that is struggling with the PA snugged.

Whilst your anaesthetist is starting inopressor support, your cardiac surgery colleagues and the perfusionist swiftly arrive and they cannulate the femoral vessels after full heparinisation. You are able to perform a direct suture repair of the extension of the tear in the interlobar PA, and continue to complete the right upper lobectomy. The patient is discharged home 10 days later.

7 Conclusions

The use of CPB/ECMO can be life-saving during complex thoracic resection, but carries a substantial mortality and morbidity risk.

Planning is key in anticipation for the potential need for ECC. The main non-oncological predictor of long-term outcomes for extended resection with ECC is its emergency/unplanned use. As such every attempt should be made to employ CPB or ECMO in an as much as possible controlled manner.

References

Antonia SJ, Villegas A, Daniel D et al (2017) Durvalumab after chemoradiotherapy in stage III non–small-cell lung cancer. N Engl J Med 377(20):1919–1929. https://doi.org/10.1056/NEJMoa1709937

Bozer J, Vess A, Pineda P et al (2023) Venovenous extracorporeal membrane oxygenation for a difficult airway situation—a recommendation for updating The American Society of Anesthesiologists' 'Difficult Airway Algorithm'. J Cardiothorac Vasc Anesth 37(12):2646–2656. https://doi.org/10.1053/j.jvca.2023.04.027

D'Andrilli A, Maurizi G, Ciccone AM et al (2024) Reconstruction of the heart and the aorta for radical resection of lung cancer. J Thorac Cardiovasc Surg 167(4):1481–1489. https://doi.org/10.1016/j.jtcvs.2023.07.041

Dawson AG, Richards CJ, Hadjinikolaou L, Nakas A (2021) Metastatic renal cell carcinoma extending to the left atrium through the inferior pulmonary vein. Interact Cardiovasc Thorac Surg 32(6):991–992. https://doi.org/10.1093/icvts/ivab018

De Perrot M, Perentes JY (2017) Resection of lung cancer involving the aorta. Oper Tech Thorac Cardiovasc Surg 22(4):235–251. https://doi.org/10.1053/j.optechstcvs.2018.06.003

Forde PM, Spicer J, Lu S et al (2022) Neoadjuvant nivolumab plus chemotherapy in resectable lung cancer. N Engl J Med 386(21):1973–1985. https://doi.org/10.1056/NEJMoa2202170

Fuentes-Gago MG, Arnaiz-Garcia E, Gonzalez-Santos JM, Varela G (2017) Cardiopulmonary bypass for extended resections. Shanghai Chest 1:9–9. https://doi.org/10.21037/shc.2017.05.12

Krutman M, Nishinari K, Pignataro BS et al (2022) Postoperative anticoagulation in vascular reconstructions associated with malignancies. Ann Vasc Surg 86:219–228. https://doi.org/10.1016/j.avsg.2022.04.015

Lee DS, Flores RM (2017) Management of NSCLC invading the superior vena cava. Oper Tech Thorac Cardiovasc Surg 22(4):224–234. https://doi.org/10.1053/j.optechstcvs.2018.06.005

Li WWL, Van Boven WJP, Annema JT, Eberl S, Klomp HM, De Mol BAJM (2016) Management of large mediastinal masses: surgical and anesthesiological considerations. J Thorac Dis 8(3):E175–E184. https://doi.org/10.21037/jtd.2016.02.55

Lorusso R, Vizzardi E, Johnson DM et al (2018) Cardiac surgery in adult patients with remitted or active malignancies: a review of preoperative screening, surgical management and short- and long-term postoperative results. Eur J Cardiothorac Surg 54(1):10–18. https://doi.org/10.1093/ejcts/ezy019

Machuca TN, Cypel M, Keshavjee S (2015) Cardiopulmonary bypass and extracorporeal life support for emergent intraoperative thoracic situations. Thorac Surg Clin 25(3):325–334. https://doi.org/10.1016/j.thorsurg.2015.04.012

Muralidaran A, Detterbeck FC, Boffa DJ, Wang Z, Kim AW (2011) Long-term survival after lung resection for non–small cell lung cancer with circulatory bypass: A systematic review. J Thorac Cardiovasc Surg 142(5):1137–1142. https://doi.org/10.1016/j.jtcvs.2011.07.042

Pinto CA, Marcella S, August DA, Holland B, Kostis JB, Demissie K (2013) Cardiopulmonary bypass has a modest association with cancer progression: a retrospective cohort study. BMC Cancer 13(1):519. https://doi.org/10.1186/1471-2407-13-519

Rinieri P, Peillon C, Bessou JP et al (2015) National review of use of extracorporeal membrane oxygenation as respiratory support in thoracic surgery excluding lung transplantation. Eur J Cardiothorac Surg 47(1):87–94. https://doi.org/10.1093/ejcts/ezu127

Salter KD, Burt BM (2019) Necessity of the heart, for lung resection. J Thorac Dis 11(S9):S1132–S1134. https://doi.org/10.21037/jtd.2019.04.72

Sekine Y, Suzuki H, Saitoh Y, Wada H, Yoshida S (2010) Prosthetic reconstruction of the superior vena cava for malignant disease: surgical techniques and outcomes. Ann Thorac Surg 90(1):223–228. https://doi.org/10.1016/j.athoracsur.2010.03.050

Spaggiari L, Thomas P, Magdeleinat P et al (2002) Superior vena cava resection with prosthetic replacement for non-small cell lung cancer: Long-term results of a multicentric study. Eur J Cardiothorac Surg 21(6):1080–1086. https://doi.org/10.1016/S1010-7940(02)00175-6

Venuta F, Rendina EA (2012) Superior vena cava resection and reconstruction. Eur J Cardiothorac Surg 41(5):1177–1178. https://doi.org/10.1093/ejcts/ezr266

Emergency Cardiac Surgery During Pregnancy

Kelly Wright, Dang Nguyen, Amer Harky, and Gopal Soppa

Abstract The incidence of undertaking emergency cardiac surgery during pregnancy remains rare, though presents a critical clinical scenario demanding rapid multidisciplinary coordination in order to safeguard both maternal and foetal outcomes. Indications for emergency surgery include aortic dissection, valvular disease, cardiac trauma and end-stage heart failure, demonstrating both the unique risks of such pathologies, and requirement for individualised care. However, the timing of such surgery relative to gestational age remains critical, with the second trimester conferring optimal haemodynamic stability and foetal viability. Considerations must also be paid to the physiological and haemodynamic adaptations experienced during pregnancy, including increased blood volume and cardiac output, altered coagulation and elevated oxygen requirements. Such changes directly influence surgical decision-making, particularly in the context of intraoperative considerations to maternal positioning, foetal monitoring and cardiopulmonary bypass management. This chapter underscores the importance of personalised care delivered by a cardio-obstetric team integrating surgical, obstetric and neonatal expertise in a time-sensitive scenario. As maternal age and cardiovascular risk factors increase globally, deciphering the complexities of emergency cardiac surgery during pregnancy becomes progressively vital in order to advance survival and long-term outcomes.

Keywords Cardiac surgery in pregnancy · Pregnancy haemodynamics · Pregnancy complications · Maternal and foetal outcomes · Cardiopulmonary bypass during pregnancy · Aortic dissection in pregnancy · Valvular heart disease

K. Wright
Sheffield Teaching Hospitals NHS Foundation Trust, Sheffield, UK

D. Nguyen
Massachusetts General Hospital, Corrigan Minehan Heart Center, Harvard Medical School, Boston, MA, USA

A. Harky · G. Soppa (✉)
Department of Cardiothoracic Surgery, Liverpool Heart and Chest Hospital, Liverpool, UK
e-mail: amer.harky@lhch.nhs.uk; gopal.soppa@lhch.nhs.uk

A. Kourliouros (ed.), *Emergency Cardiac Surgery*,
https://doi.org/10.1007/978-3-032-15787-4_29

in pregnancy · End-stage heart failure in pregnancy · Cardiac trauma in pregnancy · Gestational time and cardiac surgical timing · Perioperative management in pregnancy · Multidisciplinary cardio-obstetric care

1 Introduction

Cardiovascular disease complicates 1–4% of pregnancies and is the leading cause of mortality in pregnant women in developed countries, accounting for 16% of maternal deaths. Factors that contribute to risk include maternal age, pre-existing cardiac disease and typical cardiovascular risk factors such as hypertension, smoking, obesity and diabetes mellitus (Ramlakhan et al. 2020; You et al. 2021); these factors are becoming increasingly more common with maternal age at first child and survival of children with congenital heart disease into adulthood increasing significantly over recent decades (Office for National Statistics 2024; Dellborg et al. 2023).

There are significant haemodynamic changes that occur during pregnancy such as an increase in cardiac output and blood volume which places strain on the maternal cardiovascular system. Owing to the lack of medical knowledge and awareness, cardiac diseases in pregnant women are often not detected until decompensation occurs, by which cardiac surgical intervention is then inexorable (You et al. 2021).

Key emergency cardiac procedures that occur during pregnancy include complex aortic replacement for dissection and/or aneurysm, as well as cardiac trauma and acute cardiac decompensation, all of which confer a high degree of mortality and morbidity without intervention (Harris et al. 2022; Stephens et al. 2023). Both maternal and foetal mortality need to be considered and discussed by the larger multidisciplinary team to optimise timing of surgery and weigh-up the risk of delivery versus undertaking surgery with foetus in utero. This chapter seeks to delve into the risk factors and mortality rates of different emergency procedures; discuss the physiological changes that occur during pregnancy and how this relates to adjustments needed during cardiopulmonary bypass; highlight factors that need to be considered such as foetal viability versus maternal risk and weigh-up the decision whether to deliver baby prematurely.

2 Physiological Differences in Pregnancy and Relevance to Cardiac Surgery

Cardiopulmonary bypass use is key to undertaking most cardiac surgery, allowing the machine to take over the function of the heart and lungs and enabling bloodless surgical access to the organs. There are several major parameters which must be tightly controlled whilst a patient is on bypass including activated clotting time, perfusion pressure, body temperature and acid-base management (Sarkar and

Prabhu 2017). During a healthy pregnancy, there are significant cardiorespiratory haemodynamic and haematological changes that occur to enhance uteroplacental circulation to aid foetal growth and development; these must be taken into consideration to allow cardiac surgery to be performed whilst limiting the risk to both maternal and foetal lives.

2.1 Cardiovascular

The primary change is a significant increase in cardiac output, initially because of decrease in vascular resistance leading to an increase in stroke volume. Blood volume and heart rate gradually increase throughout pregnancy and aid to maintain cardiac output when vascular resistance starts to increase throughout the third trimester (Fig. 1) (Thornburg et al. 2000; Afari et al. 2021; Sanghavi and Rutherford 2014).

Cardiac output increases abruptly during the first trimester with continued increase into the second trimester. Overall increase in cardiac output is 56% and up to ~66% versus the non-pregnant state in singleton and twin pregnancies, respectively (Afari et al. 2021; Sanghavi and Rutherford 2014; Hall et al. 2011). For most patients undergoing cardiopulmonary bypass, mean arterial pressure (MAP) targets are typically 50–60 mmHg, likely based on the lower limit of 50 mmHg needed to

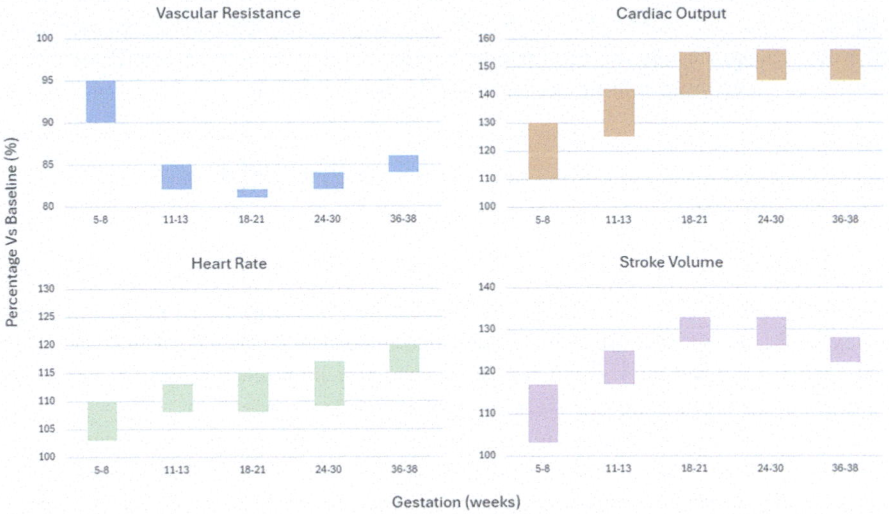

Fig. 1 Trends in vascular resistance, cardiac output, heart rate and stroke volume throughout pregnancy compared to the respective values prior to pregnancy. Vascular resistance and stroke volume are inversely proportional and trough/peak during the second trimester. Heart rate increases gradually towards the end of the pregnancy, maintaining the cardiac output when stroke volume starts to decline (Afari et al. 2021; Hall et al. 2011)

maintain cerebral autoregulation (Murphy et al. 2009). However, a MAP of > 70 mmHg is recommended in pregnancy, owing to the increased cardiac output state facilitating the maintenance of blood flow to the foetus during cardiac surgery (Stephens et al. 2023). Whilst there is ongoing debate regarding continuous versus pulsatile flow in cardiopulmonary bypass, pulsatile flow (defined as a pulse pressure > 15 mmHg) is considered to be more beneficial given it is more physiomimetic and subsequently improves microcirculation, oxygen diffusion and reduces vascular resistance (Poswal et al. 2004).

Systemic vasodilation occurs as early as week 5 of gestation, preceding the complete development of the uteroplacental circulation. Throughout the first trimester, the systemic vascular resistance decreases, reaching a minimum of around 81–85% of pre-pregnancy values around 18–21 weeks of gestation. In most uncomplicated pregnancies, the vascular resistance then plateaus, producing little haemodynamic change within the latter second trimester and early third trimester, with then a slight increase throughout the remainder of the pregnancy. This also means that peripheral systolic blood pressures follow a similar trend, decreasing by 5–10 mmHg by the second trimester, but then slowly increasing during the third trimester (Afari et al. 2021). On the contrary, heart rate gradually increases throughout pregnancy, reaching a maximum of 15–20% above baseline by delivery (Hall et al. 2011).

Moreover, the most common position used to undertake cardiac surgery is the supine position, allowing best surgical access to the thoracic cavity. Nevertheless, it is important to note that maternal positioning has a profound effect on their haemodynamic profile. The gravid uterus places pressure on the inferior vena cava in the supine position, leading to reduction in venous return and subsequent reduction in cardiac output by ~25%. However, placing a pregnant patient of greater than 20 weeks gestation into a lateral position reduces this pressure and optimises both cardiac and uteroplacental blood flow (Stephens et al. 2023).

2.2 *Respiratory*

In early pregnancy, the diameter of the chest increases by 2 cm and the subcostal angle increases by 35°, with the level of the diaphragm rising by 4 cm in later pregnancy as the uterus expands. This results in a reduction in both total lung capacity and functional residual volume but an increase in inspiratory capacity and tidal volume (up to 40%) (Ahmed 2022; Winn et al. 2021).

The increased tidal volume subsequently results in an increase in alveolar ventilation and decrease in arterial partial pressure of CO (pCO_2) from 35–40 mmHg to 27–32 mmHg in pregnancy, increasing the gradient from foetus to placenta to favour CO_2 transfer. However, renal perfusion concomitantly increases by up to 50% enhancing HCO_3^- excretion from 22–26 mmol/L to 17–19 mmol/L to maintain maternal pH (Ahmed 2022; Soma-Pillay et al. 2016). Target pCO_2 and $pHCO_3^-$ during cardiopulmonary bypass should therefore reflect these physiological changes.

On the other hand, oxygen consumption increases by up to 20% to meet increased metabolic demands and owing to the reduced functional residual volume, maternal oxygen reserve is reduced. Moreover, the oxygen-dissociation curve shifts to the right inducing a decreased affinity of haemoglobin for oxygen and therefore lower O_2 saturation for any given partial pressure of O_2 (partial pressure of oxygen) (Winn et al. 2021); women are therefore more vulnerable to hypoxemia during pregnancy and target saturations > 95% in pregnancy are recommended (Stephens et al. 2023).

2.3 Haematology

In addition to increasing blood volume, the composition of blood also changes during pregnancy. As there is a greater increase in plasma volume compared to red cell mass, physiological anaemia of pregnancy occurs with the nadir being reached between 31 and 32 weeks' gestation with an average Hb drop of 6.8 g/L (Ohuma et al. 2020).

During cardiopulmonary bypass, the addition of priming solution causes haemodilution resulting in the normal haematocrit in a healthy adult female being reduced from 37–47% to a target of 21–24%. Additional blood is added to the priming solution if the resultant haematocrit is < 24% in pregnancy (Stephens et al. 2023).

Moreover, a hypercoagulable state also occurs during pregnancy owing to an increase in several clotting factors (I, II, VII, VIII, IX and XII), a decrease in protein S, inhibition of fibrinolysis and in late pregnancy, reduced activity of activated protein C (Bremme 2003). These changes are imperative to reducing blood loss during labour but impose up to a five-fold increased risk of thromboembolism during pregnancy (Devis and Knuttinen 2017).

Activated clotting time (ACT) targets of > 480 s are typical for cardiopulmonary bypass. Typically, 300–400 U/Kg heparin is administered with further dosing required based on ACT. Nevertheless, it must be noted that given the increase in clotting factors during pregnancy, up to 30% more heparin is often required in pregnancy compared to their non-pregnant counterparts (Stephens et al. 2023; O'Carroll-Kuehn and Meeran 2007).

3 Cases Requiring Emergency Cardiac Surgery

3.1 Aortic Dissection

Aortic dissection is the most lethal of all the cardiovascular emergencies in pregnancy. The third trimester and the early postpartum period are most commonly affected (Kinney-Ham et al. 2011; Yuan 2013; Kamel et al. 2016). Aortic dissections are classified using the DeBakey or Stanford systems. Importantly, DeBakey

Type 1 dissections include the ascending aorta and the aortic root, and surgical repair must be immediate, because of the high risk of fatal complications such as cardiac tamponade and acute aortic regurgitation (Nardi et al. 2021). Delayed treatment by even an hour contributes to 1–2% higher mortality for each hour across the first 48 h for this type of critical dissection, which underscores the importance of rapid treatment (Harris et al. 2022).

In Type B dissections that just involve the descending aorta, outcomes are usually much more satisfactory, and the patient can be usually managed medically unless complications ensue (Nardi et al. 2021). Broadly, aortic surgery for Type A has a similar strategy of removing the primary intimal tear and establishing flow into the true lumen in pregnant patients, but the approach varies depending on the extent of dissection—and whether the aortic root and aortic arch are involved. If there is no dissection into the aortic root, and if the aortic valve (AV) is normal, then a supracoronary (i.e. above the origin of the coronary arteries) ascending aorta replacement might be suitable (Jormalainen et al. 2022). If the root is dilated or the aortic valve is abnormal, however, a Bentall procedure might be needed in which the aortic root, valve and ascending aorta are replaced with a composite valve-graft conduit (Shahzamani et al. 2023). There are obviously many more details to factor into decision-making, but in general terms, a valve-sparing root replacement is often used when the aortic valve leaflets are structurally normal but, nonetheless, the aortic root is dilated (Jormalainen et al. 2022). In patients whose dissection involves the arch of the aorta, what's known as a hemiarch, or total arch replacement might be needed (Coselli et al. 2024).

Special considerations in a pregnant patient include foetal monitoring, high pump flows (1.5–2.0 times body surface area) and high MAP, minimising foetal hypothermia, and duration of cardiopulmonary bypass. A simultaneous foetal delivery can be considered, if appropriate. The morbidity and mortality of repairing an aortic dissection in a pregnant female is considerably higher than in a non-pregnant patient. Maternal mortality of acute aortic dissection in pregnancy could be as high as 27% (Gurrieri et al. 2023), versus 17.3% in the non-pregnant patient population (McClure et al. 2017). Foetal mortality is 33%, and the maternal risks are preterm delivery and intrauterine growth restriction (Gurrieri et al. 2023). Reports from the literature regarding maternal and foetal mortality following cardiac surgery that include acute dissections are shown in Table 1. Long-term morbidity for the mother following dissection repair includes chronic pain, paraplegia and the need for reintervention due to false lumen expansion or aneurysm (Yuan 2013; Abo-Salem and López-Candales 2014; Price et al. 2023; Brener and Keramati 2016).

3.2 *Aortic Aneurysm*

Pregnancy is particularly risky with aortic aneurysms involving the ascending aorta, where rupture or dissection may occur due to the effects of pregnancy-induced hyperdynamic physiology and hormones, which can lead to accelerated expansion

Table 1 Maternal and foetal mortality data pooled from the literature (Strickland et al. 1991; Kapoor 2014; Yuan 2014; Schmitz et al. 2024; van Steenbergen et al. 2022; Rommens et al. 2021; Wang et al. 2023; Sepehripour et al. 2012)

Study	Procedure/Condition	Maternal mortality	Foetal mortality
Strickland et al. (1991)	Severe untreated congenital heart disease	Not reported	> 50%
	Cardiopulmonary bypass (CPB)	No increase	High (not specified)
Kapoor (2014)	CPB	3–15%	Not reported
	CPB	1.47%	16–33%
Yuan (2014)	Cardiac surgery with CPB	Not reported	18.60%
Schmitz et al. (2024)	Mechanical aortic valve thrombectomy	3%	Not reported
	Cardiac surgery with CPB (continuing pregnancy)	Not reported	29%
	Cardiac surgery after delivery	Not reported	14%
van Steenbergen et al. (2022)	Cardiac surgery (all trimesters)	7.30%	26.50%
	Cardiac surgery (third trimester)	Not reported	10.30%
Rommens et al. (2021)	Peripartum acute aortic dissection	10%	20%
Wang et al. (2023)	Aortic dissection (all types)	7.30%	Not reported
	Type A aortic dissection	4.30%	Not reported
	Type B aortic dissection	8.10%	Not reported
Sepehripour et al. (2012)	Cardiac surgery (observational study)	4.8–14.3%	14.30%
	Cardiac surgery (literature review)	2.9–5.1%	19–29%
	Cardiac surgery (observational study)	13.30%	38.50%

of an aortic aneurysm. The dimensions of the aneurysm determine the risk of adverse outcome, since the greater the aortic diameter, the more wall stress is induced (Leone et al. 2020). Areas of aortic plaque, which is common in non-Marfan aortopathies, channel blood flow and increase wall stress. Aortic repair (resection and replacement with a Dacron graft) is indicated at 5.5 cm in patients with a normal aortic valve, 5.0 cm in patients with bicuspid aortic valve and 4.5 cm in patients with Marfan syndrome (Mao et al. 2008; Gong et al. 2022; Etli et al. 2022). These size thresholds are lower during pregnancy. For ascending aortic aneurysms, aortic repair is recommended at 4.5 cm in pregnancy; for Marfan syndrome or other genetic aortopathies, it is recommended at 4.0 cm (Marfan Foundation 2022; Whelan et al. 2023; Isselbacher et al. 2022).

A major challenge in pregnant patients is additionally the timing of surgery, which aims to maximise delivering the baby at a safe gestational age and minimise aneurysm rupture risks by intervening as early as possible. If an aneurysm has a rapid expansion rate or is at high risk of rupture, there is a higher risk that ongoing expansion will cause rupture before foetal gestation is sufficiently advanced. Careful logistical coordination is required to minimise the potential delay between haemodynamic deterioration and restoration of cardiac integrity from the cardiopulmonary bypass circuit. This coordination needs attention as two operations must take place simultaneously: cardiac surgery and caesarean delivery.

3.3 *Valvular Diseases*

Pregnancy imposes a substantial haemodynamic burden, exacerbating risks for patients with pre-existing heart disease. The main valvular pathologies that have an impact in pregnancy are aortic stenosis (AS) and mitral stenosis (MS). AS in women of childbearing age is predominantly congenital, commonly bicuspid in nature, with severe cases presenting significant risks of heart failure. In symptomatic severe AS unresponsive to medical therapy, percutaneous balloon aortic valvuloplasty (PBAV) is favoured over surgical aortic valve replacement (SAVR) due to its lower maternal and foetal risk (Elkayam et al. 2022). PBAV reduces the transvalvular gradient by approximately 50%, often allowing continuation of pregnancy to term with manageable complications. Advanced imaging techniques, such as 3D echocardiography, help guide PBAV and minimise radiation exposure during pregnancy. Transcatheter aortic valve implantation, while promising, remains limited to rare cases in pregnancy due to its complexity (as the dominant pathology is bicuspid aortic valve stenosis) and potential long-term consequences.

Mitral stenosis (MS), often rheumatic in origin, poses risks such as pulmonary hypertension and thromboembolism during pregnancy. Percutaneous mitral balloon commissurotomy (PMBC) is the preferred intervention for severe symptomatic MS, especially in patients with favourable valve anatomy and minimal mitral regurgitation (Elkayam et al. 2022). When performed between 26 and 30 weeks of gestation, PMBC achieves excellent maternal and foetal outcomes, with significant symptomatic relief and minimal procedural complications. Adjunctive medical therapies, including beta-blockers and anticoagulation, are critical for optimising maternal haemodynamics and preventing thromboembolic events. Emerging transcatheter techniques for addressing failed bioprosthetic valves show promise but are currently limited to isolated cases. Both PBAV and PMBC represent valuable, minimally invasive strategies for managing critical valvular lesions during pregnancy.

3.4 *Cardiac Trauma*

Cardiac trauma during pregnancy is a rare entity but it presents some unique challenges when it occurs that demand immediate action. Motor vehicle collisions, falls and domestic violence are among the most common aetiologies (Murphy and Quinlan 2014). The gravid uterus may deflect trauma away from the heart but can also bring the heart closer to the chest wall, increasing the risk of direct injury to the heart. Pregnancy-related physiological changes such as increased blood volume may obscure the signs of hypovolaemia, which could delay the diagnosis and treatment (Hofmeyr and Mohlala 2001; Goodlin et al. 1983). The foetus may complicate imaging and surgical approaches, requiring the surgeon to balance maternal and foetal wellbeing.

It calls for coordinated care from trauma surgeons, cardiac surgeons, obstetricians and neonatologists. General initial assessment follows the standard trauma protocols with added foetal monitoring and the possibility of the perimortem caesarean section. Imaging such as chest X-ray scans to ascertain the diagnosis are often important. While the radiology examination might be warranted, adequate shielding for the foetus from the radiation must be maintained (Mattsson et al. 2021). Emergency thoracotomy might be appropriate where penetrating cardiac trauma or severe blunt-trauma cardiac rupture occur (Whang 2018; Luo et al. 2017).

The surgical interest is dictated by anatomical injury. Cardiac lacerations may be sewn directly, usually with pericardial pledgets, while larger lesions may require cardiopulmonary bypass, opening the possibility of additional surgery and risk to the maternal patient and the foetus. Injuries to coronary vessels may require direct repair, bypass grafting, or evidence of coronary occlusion may require surgery in the postpartum setting. Valvular injuries may require repair or replacement. More details on the management of cardiac trauma in the non-pregnant patients can be found in Chapters "Penetrating Injury to Heart: Pre-hospital and Emergency Department Management" and "Penetrating Injuries to the Heart: Emergency Definitive Treatment".

Outcomes are naturally dependent on the severity of injury, the gestational age of the foetus and speed of intervention. Maternal mortality for emergency cardiac surgery for trauma can exceed 37%, while foetal mortality can reach nearly 66% (Stephens et al. 2023). Foetal survivors can still experience long-term problems associated with late arrhythmias and heart failure.

3.5 *End-Stage Heart Failure*

End-stage heart failure secondary to congenital or valvular pathology complicating pregnancy poses difficult treatment choices. In states of end-stage heart failure, such as single ventricle physiology, markedly deranged right ventricular outflow tract obstruction in tetralogy of Fallot with residual right ventricular dysfunction, significant right to left shunting in Eisenmenger syndrome or accelerated disease progression of residual severe mitral or aortic stenosis, pregnancy precipitates a form of heart failure with unrelenting progressive haemodynamic compromise (Guihaire and François 2012). In previously compensated structural heart disease, normal physiological changes of pregnancy can provoke a haemodynamic event that precipitates rapid clinical decline. Management is complex and always entails weighing maternal against foetal risk invoked. When medical management such as fluid handling, diuretics or heart rhythm and rate optimisation appears insufficient, surgery may be required. Timing is critical in surgery, and when possible should ideally be deferred until foetal viability. Mechanical circulatory support may be initiated as a bridge to definitive surgery, or as terminal therapy in severe cases.

Surgery depends on the nature of the pathology; severe valvular disease can be amenable to valve repair or, if repair is not possible, then to replacement. For mechanical valve replacement, the choice of prosthesis and the post-operative anticoagulation will be unique for each case, in part determined by the need for balancing thrombosis and anticoagulation-related complications (Daughety et al. 2020). Many cases of complex congenital heart disease require more complex surgery, with next-level repair possibly including revision of previous repairs or the form of biventricular physiology from complex single ventricle physiology, and in some cases heart transplantation. Long-term maternal outcomes are often compromised by the need for repeat measures and ongoing management of heart failure. Foetal outcomes depend heavily on the timing of delivery, with prematurity and intrauterine growth restriction as major concerns. In recent decades, advancements in surgical technique, perioperative management and multidisciplinary care have helped to improve outcomes.

4 Foetal Gestation Versus Clinical Outcome

Given the haemodynamic changes that occur during pregnancy, the best outcomes for cardiac surgery occur during the late second trimester when the changes in cardiac output, stroke volume and vascular resistance are more stable. This allows surgery to occur prior to the maximal haemodynamic load that develops towards the end of pregnancy and associated increased risk of acute cardiac decompensation whilst also enabling foetal organogenesis to be completed (Stephens et al. 2023).

A meta-analysis of 386 patients undergoing cardiac surgery during pregnancy by van Steenbergen et al. (2022) demonstrated that overall maternal mortality after cardiac surgery was 7.3% (van Steenbergen et al. 2022); mortality appeared higher in the first trimester (12.1%) but with less than half of the number of patients compared to those who underwent surgery in either the second or third trimester, this risk was found not to be statistically significant. However, maternal mortality risk doubled if the patient had undergone previous cardiac surgery. On the contrary, foetal mortality was as high as 44.8% during the first trimester and significantly decreased with increasing gestational age at 34.1% and 10.3% in second and third trimester, respectively; foetal outcomes were improved where caesarean section was possible prior to undertaking cardiac surgery (van Steenbergen et al. 2022).

This may also be partially owing to the target temperatures used on cardiopulmonary bypass as emergency surgeries such as Type A aortic dissection often using deep hypothermia (20–25 °C) to offer organ protection; hypothermia has been shown to be associated with foetal bradycardia and induction of premature labour, with foetal mortality risk being highest during the cooling and warming phases.

Consequently, normothermic cardiopulmonary bypass is the preferred option during pregnancy (Stephens et al. 2023; Patel et al. 2020).

Moreover, given that prior to 22 weeks' gestation there is a consensus that there is no hope for foetal survival if delivered, then emergency surgery has no option but to take place with foetus in utero. Yates et al. (2015) demonstrated the successful delivery of 8 healthy babies in 11 patients who underwent emergency aortic surgery at 16–21 weeks' gestation, utilising pulsatile cardiopulmonary bypass with target mean arterial pressure (MAP) of 70 mmHg (Yates et al. 2015).

However, active management is usually offered to expectant mothers beyond 25 weeks' gestation, and therefore a full course of corticosteroids can be administered to reduce risk of respiratory distress syndrome of the baby; caesarean section may be considered before undertaking cardiopulmonary bypass (Patel et al. 2020; Royal College of Obstetricians and Gynaecologists 2014; Lewey et al. 2021; Kimpton et al. 2023). For those pregnancies between 22 and 25 weeks and/or where caesarean section is not undertaken, maternal corticosteroids should still be given to optimise foetal outcomes in the event of emergency delivery during or after surgery (Schmitz et al. 2024).

Despite survival rates improving for extreme preterm deliveries, the risk of developing a wide range of complications such as respiratory distress syndrome, cerebral palsy, hearing and cognitive impairment has not improved and is associated with increasing risk as gestational age decreases. For instance, a review by Crump (2020) identified that 63% of people born at full-term (> 37 weeks) have no major comorbidities at ages 18–43 years, reducing to 55% for people born prematurely (28–37 weeks) with further reductions for people born extremely premature (22–27 weeks) (Crump 2020).

5 Involvement of the Multidisciplinary Team

Given the complex nature of undertaking cardiac surgery and associated clinical decision-making during pregnancy, a wide-array of personnel are involved to ensure optimal outcome for both mother and baby. The cardio-obstetric team involves specialists such as cardiologists, cardiac surgeons, obstetricians, anaesthetists and paediatricians, with the wider multidisciplinary team including nurses, midwives, physiotherapists and pharmacists, amongst others. The team is responsible for pre-pregnancy counselling for those with pre-existing cardiac disease, pre-surgical optimisation including lifestyle modifications and medications, intraoperative maternal and foetal monitoring, post-operative maternal and foetal/neonatal care, and referral to social services including support groups and chaplaincy, where required. This means that care can be patient-centred by identifying personal needs and beliefs and offering support where required based on social circumstances (Wolfe and Yellin 2021).

Pre-pregnancy counselling involves risk-stratification. There are various models used with ZAHARA, CARPREG and modified WHO being most widely utilised for patients with known cardiovascular disease (Hagen and Roos-Hesselink 2020). These can be used by the multidisciplinary team to enable high-risk pregnancies to be identified and referred to tertiary centres for enhanced monitoring and option counselling. Likewise, the California Cardiovascular screening toolkit has been developed to identify pregnant women, without any previously known cardiovascular disease, who are at increased risk and associated complications, such as those with diabetes, chronic hypertension, obesity and/or substance misuse (Blumenthal et al. 2020).

Intraoperatively, alongside the surgical team an obstetrician and neonatal team would monitor the foetal heart rate via cardiotocography or transoesophageal echocardiography for signs of distress such as decelerations in heart rate and reduced variability and initiating delivery if survival is compromised (Ye et al. 2016; McCurdy 2020). However, some foetal heart rate changes can be anticipated depending on the anaesthetic agents used such as foetal bradycardia; this can make it challenging to interpret foetal heart rate changes and should not necessarily prompt delivery (Po' et al. 2019; Higgins et al. 2019).

The wider multidisciplinary team is a large force that comes into play post-operatively, enabling successful recovery and rehabilitation of the mother, and offering emotional, practical and social support where needed. Social support is imperative during the first 10 days post-operatively, particularly in cases where the baby was delivered prematurely, given the high risk of neonatal mortality and lengthy stay in neonatal intensive care (Seaton et al. 2019).

6 Conclusion

The incidence of emergency cardiac surgery during pregnancy is expected to increase owing to an ageing maternal population and increasing prevalence of cardiovascular risk factors. The most common and critical emergency is aortic dissection which tends to occur in the third trimester owing to the increasing cardiovascular load placed on the mother.

Whilst maternal mortality for cardiac surgery has improved and is now comparable to surgery undertaken in non-pregnant patients, risk of foetal mortality is significant and reduces with increasing gestation. Where a foetus is deemed viable, mortality reduces when caesarean section is performed prior to the patient being placed on cardiopulmonary bypass. However, where this is not possible steps can be taken to reduce risk to foetus including performing surgery during late second trimester (where possible), adjusting maternal positioning, adjusting parameters for cardiopulmonary bypass such as normothermic temperatures and increased pressure/flow rates and giving maternal corticosteroids to aid with lung development in case of emergency delivery.

Therefore, each patient should be assessed on a case-by-case basis, identifying both maternal and foetal survival chances as well as risk of future foetal comorbidities. These risks should be explained to the patient and discussed with the wider professional team to produce an optimised, personalised treatment plan.

References

Abo-Salem E, López-Candales A (2014) Diagnosis of asymptomatic aortic dissection during pregnancy using contrast echocardiography. J Cardiol Cases 9(5):200–202

Afari HA, Davis EF, Sarma AA (2021) Echocardiography for the pregnant heart. Curr Treat Options Cardiovasc Med 23(8):55

Ahmed A (2022) Fetomaternal acid–base balance and electrolytes during pregnancy. Indian J Crit Care Med 25(S3):S193–S199

Blumenthal EA, Crosland BA, Senderoff D, Santurino K, Garg N, Bernstein M et al (2020) California cardiovascular screening tool: findings from initial implementation. AJP Rep 10(4):e362–e368

Bremme KA (2003) Haemostatic changes in pregnancy. Best Pract Res Clin Haematol 16(2):153–168

Brener MI, Keramati AR (2016) Type B dissection in a pregnant woman managed with peripartum thoracic endovascular aortic repair. Circulation 133(5)

Coselli JS, Roselli EE, Preventza O, Malaisrie SC, Stewart A, Stelzer P et al (2024) Total aortic arch replacement using a frozen elephant trunk device: results of a 1-year US multicenter trial. J Thorac Cardiovasc Surg 167(5):1680–1692.e2

Crump C (2020) An overview of adult health outcomes after preterm birth. Early Hum Dev 150:105187

Daughety MM, Zilberman-Rudenko J, Shatzel JJ, McCarty OJT, Raghunathan V, DeLoughery TG (2020) Management of anticoagulation in pregnant women with mechanical heart valves. Obstet Gynecol Surv 75(3):190–198

Dellborg M, Giang KW, Eriksson P, Liden H, Fedchenko M, Ahnfelt A et al (2023) Adults with congenital heart disease: trends in event-free survival past middle age. Circulation 147(12):930–938

Devis P, Knuttinen MG (2017) Deep venous thrombosis in pregnancy: incidence, pathogenesis and endovascular management. Cardiovasc Diagn Ther 7(S3):S309–S319

Elkayam U, Bansal P, Mehra A (2022) Catheter-based interventions for the management of valvular heart disease during pregnancy. JACC Adv 1(2):100022

Etli M, Avnioglu S, Yilmaz H, Karahan O (2022) Investigation of the correlation between cardiac parameters and aortic diameter in patients with ascending aortic aneurysm. Egypt Heart J 74(1):3

Gong J, An K, Lin H, Hou J (2022) Ascending aorta diameter changes after aortic valve replacement in elderly patients with aortic valve stenosis. Cardiol Res Pract 2022:1–7

Goodlin RC, Quaife MA, Smith JJ (1983) Hypovolemic pregnant women and their risk determinants. Int J Gynecol Obstet 21(1):45–50

Guihaire J, François H (2012) The right heart in congenital heart disease, mechanisms and recent advances. J Clin Exp Cardiol 1(S8)

Gurrieri C, Manske WT, Williams C, Wildenberg JC, Keppers RJ, Tallarita T et al (2023) A 37-year-old patient presenting at 39 weeks of pregnancy with thoracic aortic dissection due to previously undiagnosed FBN1-related Marfan syndrome. Am J Case Rep 24

Hagen IMV, Roos-Hesselink JW (2020) Pregnancy in congenital heart disease: risk prediction and counselling. Heart 106(23):1853–1861

Hall ME, George EM, Granger JP (2011) El corazón durante el embarazo. Rev Esp Cardiol 64(11):1045–1050

Harris KM, Nienaber CA, Peterson MD, Woznicki EM, Braverman AC, Trimarchi S et al (2022) Early mortality in type A acute aortic dissection. JAMA Cardiol 7(10):1009

Higgins MF, Pollard L, McGuinness SK, Kingdom JC (2019) Fetal heart rate monitoring in nonobstetric surgery: a systematic review of the evidence. Am J Obstet Gynecol MFM [Internet] [cited 2024 Aug 18] 1(4). Available from: https://www.ajogmfm.org/article/S2589-9333(19)30081-3/fulltext

Hofmeyr GJ, Mohlala BKF (2001) Hypovolaemic shock. Best Pract Res Clin Obstet Gynaecol 15(4):645–662

Isselbacher EM, Preventza O, Hamilton Black J, Augoustides JG, Beck AW, Bolen MA et al (2022) 2022 ACC/AHA Guideline for the Diagnosis and Management of Aortic Disease: A Report of the American Heart Association/American College of Cardiology Joint Committee on Clinical Practice Guidelines. Circulation 146(24)

Jormalainen M, Kesävuori R, Raivio P, Vento A, Mustonen C, Honkanen HP et al (2022) Long-term outcomes after ascending aortic replacement and aortic root replacement for type A aortic dissection. Interact Cardiovasc Thorac Surg 34(3):453–461

Kamel H, Roman MJ, Pitcher A, Devereux RB (2016) Pregnancy and the risk of aortic dissection or rupture. Circulation 134(7):527–533

Kapoor M (2014) Cardiopulmonary bypass in pregnancy. Ann Card Anaesth 17(1):33

Kimpton J, Sammut A, Cox DJ (2023) Antenatal corticosteroids and longer term outcomes. BMJ 1722

Kinney-Ham L, Nguyen HB, Steele R, Walters E (2011) Acute aortic dissection in third trimester pregnancy without risk factors. West J Emerg Med 12(4):571–574

Leone O, Corsini A, Pacini D, Corti B, Lorenzini M, Laus V et al (2020) The complex interplay among atherosclerosis, inflammation, and degeneration in ascending thoracic aortic aneurysms. J Thorac Cardiovasc Surg 160(6):1434–1443.e6

Lewey J, Andrade L, Levine LD (2021) Valvular heart disease in pregnancy. Cardiol Clin 39(1):151–161

Luo L, Sun Q, Chen L, Ying D, Wu X, Chen Z (2017) Survival of the fetus during maternal thoracotomy under cardiopulmonary bypass for infective endocarditis. J Obstet Gynaecol Res 43(10):1634–1638

Mao SS, Ahmadi N, Shah B, Beckmann D, Chen A, Ngo L et al (2008) Normal thoracic aorta diameter on cardiac computed tomography in healthy asymptomatic adults. Acad Radiol 15(7):827–834

Marfan Foundation (2022) New Guidelines for the Diagnosis and Management of Aortic Disease Published by the American College of Cardiology and American Heart Association [Internet] [cited 2024 Aug 14]. Available from: https://marfan.org/2022/11/03/new-guidelines-for-the-diagnosis-and-management-of-aortic-disease-published-by-the-american-college-of-cardiology-and-american-heart-association/

Mattsson S, Leide-Svegborn S, Andersson M (2021) X-ray and molecular imaging during pregnancy and breastfeeding—when should we be worried? Radiat Prot Dosim 195(3–4):339–348

McClure RS, Ouzounian M, Boodhwani M, El-Hamamsy I, Chu M, Pozeg Z et al (2017) Cause of death following surgery for acute type A dissection. Aorta 5(2):33–41

McCurdy RJ (2020) Intraoperative fetal monitoring for nonobstetric surgery. Clin Obstet Gynecol 63(2):370

Murphy NJ, Quinlan JD (2014) Trauma in pregnancy: assessment, management, and prevention. Am Fam Physician 90(10):717–722

Murphy GS, Hessel EA, Groom RC (2009) Optimal perfusion during cardiopulmonary bypass: an evidence-based approach. Anesth Analg 108(5):1394–1417

Nardi P, Bassano C, Pisano C, Altieri C, Ferrante M, Greci M et al (2021) The effects of DeBakey type acute aortic dissection and preoperative peripheral and cardiac malperfusion on the outcomes after surgical repair. Pol J Cardio-Thorac Surg 18(1):1–7

O'Carroll-Kuehn BU, Meeran H (2007) Management of coagulation during cardiopulmonary bypass. Contin Educ Anaesth Crit Care Pain 7(6):195–198

Office for National Statistics (2024) Childbearing for women born in different years, England and Wales: 2021 and 2022 [Internet] [cited 2024 Aug 14]. Available from: https://www.ons.gov.uk/peoplepopulationandcommunity/birthsdeathsandmarriages/conceptionandfertilityrates/bulletins/childbearingforwomenbornindifferentyearsenglandandwales/2021and2022

Ohuma EO, Young MF, Martorell R, Ismail LC, Peña-Rosas JP, Purwar M et al (2020) International values for haemoglobin distributions in healthy pregnant women. EClinicalMedicine 29–30:100660

Patel C, Akhtar H, Gupta S, Harky A (2020) Pregnancy and cardiac interventions: what are the optimal management options? J Card Surg 35(7):1589–1596

Po' G, Olivieri C, Rose CH, Saccone G, McCurdy R, Berghella V (2019) Intraoperative fetal heart monitoring for non-obstetric surgery: a systematic review. Eur J Obstet Gynecol Reprod Biol 238:12–19

Poswal P, Mehta Y, Juneja R, Khanna S, Meharwal ZS, Trehan N (2004) Comparative study of pulsatile and nonpulsatile flow during cardio-pulmonary bypass. Ann Card Anaesth 7(1):44–50

Price J, Hau V, Albright CM, Buber J (2023) Successful management of pregnancies complicated by type B aortic dissections (both acute and chronic). JACC Case Rep 27:102056

Ramlakhan KP, Johnson MR, Roos-Hesselink JW (2020) Pregnancy and cardiovascular disease. Nat Rev Cardiol 17(11):718–731

Rommens KL, Sandhu HK, Miller CC, Cecchi AC, Prakash SK, Saqib NU et al (2021) In-hospital outcomes and long-term survival of women of childbearing age with aortic dissection. J Vasc Surg 74(4):1135–1142.e1

Royal College of Obstetricians & Gynaecologists (2014) Perinatal Management of Pregnant Women at the Threshold of Infant Viability (The Obstetric Perspective)

Sanghavi M, Rutherford JD (2014) Cardiovascular physiology of pregnancy. Circulation 130(12):1003–1008

Sarkar M, Prabhu V (2017) Basics of cardiopulmonary bypass. Indian J Anaesth 61(9):760

Schmitz KT, Stephens EH, Dearani JA, Patlolla SH, Rose CH, Bendel-Stenzel E et al (2024) Is cardiac surgery safe during pregnancy? A 40-year single institution experience. Ann Thorac Surg

Seaton SE, Barker L, Draper ES, Abrams KR, Modi N, Manktelow BN (2019) Estimating neonatal length of stay for babies born very preterm. Arch Dis Child Fetal Neonatal Ed 104(2):F182–F186

Sepehripour AH, Lo TT, Shipolini AR, McCormack DJ (2012) Can pregnant women be safely placed on cardiopulmonary bypass? Interact Cardiovasc Thorac Surg 15(6):1063–1070

Shahzamani M, Shirvani F, Tavakoli N, Sedighi M (2023) Bentall procedure to repair acute type A aortic dissection in pregnant Marfan syndrome woman with preservation of pregnancy. Vasc Endovasc Surg 57(7):787–790

Soma-Pillay P, Nelson-Piercy C, Tolppanen H, Mebazaa A (2016) Physiological changes in pregnancy. Cardiovasc J Afr 27(2):89–94

Stephens EH, Dearani JA, Mauermann W, Bendel-Stenzel EM, Arendt KW, Rose CH et al (2023) Cardiac surgery during pregnancy. Ann Thorac Surg Short Rep 1(1):203–205

Strickland RA, Oliver WC, Chantigian RC, Ney JA, Danielson GK (1991) Anesthesia, cardiopulmonary bypass, and the pregnant patient. Mayo Clin Proc 66(4):411–429

Thornburg KL, Jacobson SL, Giraud GD, Morton MJ (2000) Hemodynamic changes in pregnancy. Semin Perinatol 24(1):11–14

van Steenbergen GJ, Tsang QHY, van der Heijden OWH, Vart P, Rodwell L, Roos-Hesselink JW et al (2022) Timing of cardiac surgery during pregnancy: a patient-level meta-analysis. Eur Heart J 43(29):2801–2811

Wang Y, Yin K, Datar Y, Mohnot J, Nodoushani AY, Zhan Y et al (2023) Aortic dissection during pregnancy and puerperium: contemporary incidence and outcomes in the United States. J Am Heart Assoc 12(9)

Whang B (2018) Thoracic surgery in the pregnant patient. Thorac Surg Clin 28(1):1–7

Whelan AR, Ringel ME, Shalhub S, Russo ML (2023) Obstetric considerations for aortopathy in pregnancy. Ann Cardiothorac Surg 12(6):526–535

Winn HN, Chervenak FA, Romero R (2021) Clinical maternal-fetal medicine online. CRC Press, London, pp 302–303

Wolfe DS, Yellin S (2021) Maternal cardiology team: how to build and why it is necessary. Int J Cardiol Congenit Heart Dis 5:100236

Yates MT, Soppa G, Smelt J, Fletcher N, Van Besouw JP, Thilaganathan B et al (2015) Perioperative management and outcomes of aortic surgery during pregnancy. J Thorac Cardiovasc Surg 149(2):607–610

Ye X, He Y, Xia Z, Wang S (2016) Fetal descending aortic flow and heart rate monitoring with transesophageal echocardiography during maternal cardiac surgery. Can J Anesth Can Anesth 63(4):492–494

You Y, Liu S, Wu Z, Chen D, Wang G, Chen G et al (2021) Cardiac surgery under cardiopulmonary bypass in pregnancy: report of four cases. J Cardiothorac Surg 16(1):268

Yuan S (2013) Aortic dissection during pregnancy: a difficult clinical scenario. Clin Cardiol 36(10):576–584

Yuan SM (2014) Indications for cardiopulmonary bypass during pregnancy and impact on fetal outcomes. Geburtshilfe Frauenheilkd 74(1):55–62

Anaesthetic Considerations in Emergency Cardiac Surgery

James Stradling

Abstract Safe management of emergency care requires an ethos of close team-working between anaesthetists, cardiothoracic surgeons, and all members of the wider multi-disciplinary team. This chapter focuses on the key aspects of collaborative discussion which may occur throughout this challenging process, together with highlighting similarities and differences to elective patient pathways and cardiac anaesthetic principles - discussion of which is beyond the scope of this summary chapter.

Keywords Emergency cardiac anaesthesia · Emergency airway management · Damage control resuscitation · Rapid sequence intubation · Peri-arrest management · Perioperative haemodynamic monitoring and optimisation · Vasoactive agents/inotropic therapy · Ad hoc multi-disciplinary team planning · Operating theatre team briefing—WHO checklist · Emergency cardiopulmonary bypass—'crash' bypass · Emergency transoesophageal echocardiography · Post-bypass anaesthetic management

1 Introduction

Emergency anaesthesia is defined by the Royal College of Anaesthetists (UK) and NCEPOD (UK) as a requirement to proceed in immediate (within minutes) or urgent circumstances (within hours)

When applied to cardiothoracic surgery, this requirement is confined to a few pathologies which require time-critical remediation, to avoid death or severe life-altering complications.

A wide variety of presenting pathologies may be encountered including:

J. Stradling (✉)
John Radcliffe Hospital, Oxford, UK
e-mail: james.stradling@ouh.nhs.uk

A. Kourliouros (ed.), *Emergency Cardiac Surgery*,
https://doi.org/10.1007/978-3-032-15787-4_30

- Airway obstruction, tracheo-bronchial bleeding, tracheo-bronchial disruption or perforation, broncho-pleural fistula, tracheo-oesophageal fistula with gross bronchial bacterial contamination, oesophageal perforation or mediastinitis.
- Cardiac tamponade with cardiac chamber or coronary perforation: post-surgical, iatrogenic, traumatic or due to ventricular rupture following myocardial infarction.
- Acute myocardial ischaemia with risk of malignant dysrhythmia or acute ventricular dysfunction and cardiogenic shock.
- Delayed complications of previous completed myocardial infarction, causing cardiogenic shock such as ventricular septal defect, or papillary muscle rupture and severe mitral regurgitation.
- Severe primary valvular dysfunction causing cardiogenic shock.
- Acute Type A aortic dissection.
- Thoracic trauma
- Intra-cardiac masses or vegetations, with risk of systemic, coronary or pulmonary embolisation.
- Iatrogenic (vascular procedure-related) cardiac or intra-thoracic vascular injuries with hypovolaemia, haemopneumothorax or cardiac tamponade.
- Secondary post-operative cardiac arrest, bleeding, cardiac tamponade or cardiogenic shock following earlier primary cardiothoracic surgical operations.

Time-critical intervention will be required in order to prevent adverse patient outcomes, such as:

- Death, due to severe hypoxia, dysrhythmia, cardiogenic shock, hypovolaemic shock, cardiac tamponade or severe sepsis and multi-organ failure.
- Permanent end-organ dysfunction, such as renal failure.
- Long-term neurological deficit, due to stroke or hypoxic brain injury.

Or

- Permanent myocardial injury and/or valvular dysfunction with resultant long-term heart failure.

2 Patient Assessment, Optimisation and Multi-disciplinary Team Planning for Emergency Cardiac Surgical Cases

In more 'ideal' (elective) circumstances, patients presenting for cardiac surgery will undergo a thorough and stereotyped pre-operative assessment, cardiac-specific investigations and a programme of pre-operative optimisation guided by a multi-disciplinary team:

Summary of the 'ideal' pre-operative process	
Cardiothoracic investigation profile	ECG Long-term ('24-hour' tape or implantable) heart rhythm assessment Comprehensive echocardiography Invasive coronary angiography Right heart catheterisation CT coronary angiography and/or aortography CT assessment of peripheral and head/neck vasculature High resolution CT chest or CT pulmonary angiography Cardiac MRI Pulmonary function testing Diabetic control assessment and HbA1c/Glycated haemoglobin Detailed blood tests including haematology, renal, liver, and infection assessments, and transfusion screening
Screening for cardiothoracic risk factors and modifiable associated medical conditions	Obesity Obstructive sleep apnoea Smoking Chronic obstructive pulmonary disease or asthma Hypertension Anaemia Diabetes Chronic kidney disease Alcohol and/or recreational drug or steroid consumption
Pre-operative optimisation of medical conditions	Smoking cessation Weight loss, and exercise prehabilitation Treatment of sleep apnoea Optimisation of COPD, asthma or other lung conditions Antihypertensive optimisation Medical heart failure optimisation Diabetic medication optimisation Diagnosis and treatment of anaemia Alcohol moderation
Optimisation of medications (see EACTS guidelines (Jepsson et al. 2024))	Antiplatelet planning +/− pre-operative cessation Anticoagulation planning Cessation of ACE inhibitors or Angiotensin II blockers Cessation of SGLT2 inhibitors (e.g. dapagliflozin)

(continued)

Summary of the 'ideal' pre-operative process	
Multi-disciplinary team planning	Detailed case history, imaging and investigation review Organisation of further investigations or optimisation required prior to surgery Referral of complex cases to cardiothoracic anaesthetic assessment clinic Discussion of surgical, percutaneous/transcatheter, hybrid and medical treatment options—with consideration of specific patient needs and preferences Discussion of optimal timing of intervention Matching of optimal team member experience to case complexity Organisation of the perioperative and post-operative environment including specialised equipment and drugs Consideration of inter-hospital transfer where optimal needs cannot be met at a local centre

3 Considerations Prior to Urgent ('Within Hours') Surgery

Emergency cardiac surgery may occasionally be required for a small subset of the patient group described above—who have undergone thorough pre-operative assessment and optimisation but then developed unstable symptoms necessitating expedited surgery.

In contrast, however, it is common for patients requiring emergency surgery to have presented de novo with incomplete prior cardiac diagnostics and with little scope for optimisation of associated comorbidities or medication planning.

Necessary treatments (e.g. dual antiplatelet therapy for acute coronary syndromes) may be ongoing, or even acutely loaded during urgent coronary catheterisation immediately prior to surgery, with consequent impact on surgical bleeding risk. Conversely, erroneous diagnostics and treatments may have preceded referral to the cardiac surgeon: for instance, a typical and hostile scenario is the pre-treatment of aortic dissection as either acute coronary syndrome (with dual antiplatelets) or pulmonary embolism (with therapeutic anticoagulation) prior to delayed diagnosis via echocardiography or CT scanning, respectively.

When faced with a request to provide emergency care to support proposed cardiac surgery, the anaesthetist will first need to rapidly triage and identify the timeframe available for assessments and decision-making. This will be defined by the patient's current physiological status and predicted trajectory of deterioration without intervention.

At best case, where there is relative stability, and the proposed intervention is 'within hours', the anaesthetist may be able to fully assess the patient's case history, imaging and other investigations, and visit the patient for further in-person assessments, and consent.

In parallel with that urgent pre-anaesthetic assessment process, it is desirable to arrange an ad hoc emergency multi-disciplinary case discussion:

Conduct of an urgent 'ad hoc' cardiothoracic surgical multi-disciplinary meeting ('mini-MDT')	
Multi-disciplinary team members	Operating surgeon(s) Cardiothoracic anaesthetist(s) Interventional cardiologist(s) Referring team (e.g. cardiology resident/ED physician/trauma team leader) Intensivist(s) Perioperative echocardiographer Perfusionist(s) Specialist nurses (anaesthetic, ICU, operating theatre, cardiac angiography suite) ICU/cardiothoracic operating theatre coordinator
Potential locations	ED ICU Operating theatre Cardiac catheter lab Video-conferencing
Discussions	Case history and relevant investigations Any time-critical investigations which may be feasible (e.g. coronary angiography for valvular surgery, in-house CT angiography prior to aortic dissection surgery or where peripheral vascular interventions are anticipated) Specialised pre-operative optimisation strategies (e.g. pre-anaesthetic intra-aortic balloon pump, Impella or ECMO support; pre-admission to ICU for haemodynamic stabilisation or haemofiltration) Alternatives to surgery (e.g. complex percutaneous coronary revascularisation; transcatheter aortic valve intervention (TAVI); transcatheter (mitral or/and tricuspid) edge-to-edge repair; transcatheter ventriculo-septal defect closure) Appropriateness of proceeding with surgery where mortality risk or non-cardiac patient comorbidities are prohibitive Planning for salvage peri- or post-operative interventions in the event of complications (e.g. rescue percutaneous coronary intervention; intra-aortic balloon pump; advanced mechanical circulatory support such as Impella, ventricular assist device (VAD) or extracorporeal life support (ECLS/ECMO) Identification of situations where local resources are insufficient for support of complex cases, and coordination of emergency transfer to a quaternary cardiac centre (e.g. transplant centre offering mechanical circulatory support) Identification and calling of key peri-operative team members (anaesthetic team, surgical team, scrub team, perfusion/cell salvage team, echocardiographer, transfusion) Organisation of environment, equipment and drugs

Where there is consensus that emergency surgery will proceed, a WHO operating theatre team briefing should follow.

This may involve recap discussion of many of the aspects of the ad hoc multi-disciplinary discussion above, but should be attended by all members of the operating team and should include in-depth discussion of all perioperative aspect of the case such as : conduct of anaesthesia and specialised monitoring/precautions, cardiopulmonary bypass cannulation and perfusion strategy, proposed surgical technique, provisional bypass weaning plan, expectations for transfusion and haemostasis, provisional post-operative interventions expected, as well as generic safety checklists.

Aspects of emergency anaesthesia to be considered during emergency WHO team briefing and pre-operative planning:
Location of anaesthesia
Consideration of anaesthetic induction in theatre, with surgical team scrubbed and sterile precautions plus draping applied—may be necessary in some cases of cardiovascular extremis
Anaesthetic team role requirements
Lead anaesthetist
Intubator
Echocardiographer
Defibrillation and pacemaker management
Fluids and transfusion
Assistants/runners
Multiple roles may be undertaken by highly experienced anaesthetists and anaesthetic practitioners/nurses, and the minimum team number is two
However, more complex and unstable cases may benefit from the input of several anaesthetic team members, particularly where there are large or rapid transfusion requirements or a need for complex echocardiography with unstable haemodynamics as a competing demand on lead anaesthetist attention
Ideal staffing provision may be difficult to provide 'out of normal working hours' and this should be considered in the planning and governance structures of a cardiothoracic unit
Specialised monitoring
For example, cerebral oximetry for patients at high risk of neurological injury, complex cardiopulmonary bypass strategies or deep hypothermic circulatory arrest
Pulmonary artery catheter or other cardiac output monitoring according to anaesthetist's and surgeons' preference
Transoesophageal echocardiography will be required for most cases (Guidelines for the use of transoesophageal echocardiography to assist with surgical decision-making in the operating room 2020; Recommendations for transoesophageal echocardiography: update 2010 2010)
Vascular access
Anticipated rate and volume of losses, with planning for large bore venous access, fluid warming plus rapid infuser as necessary
Consideration of siting awake vascular lines in situations of anticipated cardiovascular collapse
Necessity of specialised vascular lines: additional arterial line(s) for complex cardiopulmonary bypass cannulation strategies, consideration of pulmonary artery catheterisation (after weaning from cardiopulmonary bypass), consideration of a dialysis catheter for patients with high risks of renal failure

(continued)

Aspects of emergency anaesthesia to be considered during emergency WHO team briefing and pre-operative planning:
Airway management Specific pathologies affecting the airway should be considered, these include: Surgical emphysema affecting the neck Tracheal or endo-bronchial obstructive or haemorrhagic lesion Tracheo-oesophageal fistula Upper mediastinal bleeding or mass lesion with superior vena cava compression syndrome Traumatic lung laceration or contusion with haemoptysis Broncho-pleural fistula **Pre-operative planning should include:** Discussion of specialised airway management and equipment required for non-sternotomy cases (e.g. double lumen endotracheal tube, rigid bronchoscopy, bronchial blocker) Difficult airway planning Discussion of patient fasting status Consideration of the potential necessity for rapid sequence intubation due to anticipated gastric aspiration or immediate cardiovascular collapse on anaesthetic induction Back up front-of-neck access plan for anticipated difficult airways
Respiratory management and ventilation Patients suffering from severely decompensated cardiac conditions may commonly present with secondary or coincidental respiratory conditions which affect anaesthetic management These include: Pulmonary oedema Asthma or COPD (Rarely) evolving anaphylaxis to anaesthetic agents or intravenous antibiotics Airway hyper-reactivity due to recent smoking cessation Sputum retention and bronchial obstruction Pneumonia or COVID-19 infection Septic lung emboli due to infective endocarditis Pneumothorax Haemothorax Pulmonary haemorrhage Pulmonary embolism Pre-operative planning should therefore include: Availability of bronchoscopy equipment for patients with concurrent pneumonia, or lower airway contamination (haemorrhage, broncho-pleural fistula, tracheo-oesophageal fistula). Discussion of management strategy for severely hypoxic patients—including consideration of inhaled nitric oxide or prostaglandin, intra-operative Positive End Expiratory Pressure (PEEP) strategy, potential requirement for post-operative ECMO support Consideration of use of PEEP and low tidal ventilation during cardiopulmonary bypass depending on anaesthetist's and surgeon's preferences
Pre- and post-bypass vasoactive strategy Necessity for inotrope and/or vasopressor infusions prior to induction of anaesthesia and prior to cardiopulmonary bypass Consideration of intra-aortic balloon pump prior to anaesthesia, for patients with critical ischaemia or severe ventricular failure Anticipated requirements for left and/or right ventricular support after cardiopulmonary bypass (in the event of 'plan A' surgical results or in the event of predictable complications) Epicardial pacing strategy Any potential need for mechanical circulatory support

(continued)

Aspects of emergency anaesthesia to be considered during emergency WHO team briefing and pre-operative planning:
Transfusion and haemostasis plan
Planned use of either tranexamic acid or aprotinin, as recommended in the 2017 EACTS/EACTA Guidelines (Boer et al. 2017).
Review of pre-operative haematology, including history of antiplatelet and/or anticoagulant usage, point of care tests (TEG/platelet mapping or platelet function tests, lab haematology results)
Expectations of blood loss and coagulopathy after bypass
Any prothrombotic concerns (saphenous vein grafts, known intra-cardiac, pulmonary or systematic thromboses)
Timeframe for availability of standard transfusion products (e.g. red blood cells, fresh frozen plasma, platelets or cryoprecipitate)
Availability of specialised haemostatic agents (e.g. desmopressin, prothrombin complex concentrate, fibrinogen concentrate, recombinant activated factor VIIa, andexanet alfa)
Anticipated post-operative concerns
Renal replacement therapy
Mechanical circulatory support
Advanced respiratory support, such as inhaled nitric oxide
Post-operative transfer arrangements (internal or inter-hospital)

4 The Role of the Cardiothoracic Anaesthetist in Damage Control ('Within Minutes'/Peri-arrest) Cardiac Surgery Scenarios

The above 'urgent surgery' process, where feasible, allows the cardiac anaesthetist to fully plan the location, personnel, drugs, interventions, and monitoring equipment that are necessary to provide optimised emergency anaesthesia.

In contrast, in worst case scenarios, cardiothoracic surgical emergencies frequently present with extreme cardiorespiratory instability or/and threatened exsanguination, and in some cases cardiac arrest will already have occurred by the time of arrival of the anaesthetist.

In addition, it is not infrequent for the cardiac surgical emergency team to be called to assist in the care of these severely compromised patients in 'remote anaesthesia' environments, including the emergency department, ICU, cardiac angiography or radiology suite, or even ward environments.

The anaesthetic team attending to 'in extremis' scenarios will have a very limited time for situation appraisal, and a focussed approach will be necessary (ABC assessment, resuscitation and control of time-critical pathology). Conduct of resuscitation will depend on the succinct presenting history, predicted pathology and patient location.

Summary of cardiothoracic anaesthetic considerations during damage control (incipient cardiac arrest) scenarios	
Rapid focussed anaesthetic assessment of the peri-arrest patient considered for emergency cardiac surgery	Rapid summary of clinical scenario Identification of team members; call-in and estimated time of arrival of key team members Airway planning and rapid clinical examination Fasting status/aspiration risk Vascular access Allergies, infusions and key medications Focussed investigations: Point-of-care ultrasound Echocardiography Chest X-ray or fluoroscopy Rapid review of other key imaging Blood gas, haemoglobin/platelet count Available resources: transfusion, equipment, availability of cardiopulmonary bypass or/and other mechanical circulatory support Any patient/environmental risks to staff safety
Immediate identification and treatment of immediately reversible pathologies	Obstructed airway Tension pneumothorax Immediate 'stacked' defibrillation of shockable dysrhythmias (VF/VT) Emergency pacing of severe bradycardias
Anaesthetist's/team leader's confirmation of patient-specific resuscitation pathway	Cardiothoracic ALS algorithm ('CALS') for post-operative patients with a recent sternotomy (Guideline for resuscitation in cardiac arrest after cardiac surgery 2009) ATLS algorithm for trauma patients (The ATLS Subcommittee, American College of Surgeons' Committee on Trauma, and the International ATLS working group 2013) UK REACT algorithm for patients suffering cardiac arrest during catheter-based techniques in the angiography suite (Joint British Societies Guideline on management of cardiac arrest in the cardiac catheter laboratory 2022) ALS algorithm for ward- or ICU-based pre-operative patients or patients unsuitable for immediate 'CALS' resternotomy—modified to avoid of severe post-resuscitation hypertension (Soar et al. 2021)
Damage control resuscitation interventions	Immediate CALS (minimally sterile) resternotomy ATLS resuscitative clam shell thoracotomy Completion of percutaneous coronary intervention, pacing procedure or transcatheter device deployment during mechanical CPR ('LUCAS' device) Consideration of eCPR (emergency ECMO or Impella support) where local facilities allow

(continued)

Summary of cardiothoracic anaesthetic considerations during damage control (incipient cardiac arrest) scenarios	
Definitive management strategy	Rapid stabilisation: via relief of cardiac tamponade and/or emergency haemostasis and correction of hypovolaemia with internal defibrillation, epicardial pacing, inotrope/vasopressor/mechanical circulatory support (e.g. intra-aortic balloon pump) Or Emergency cardiopulmonary bypass, including: consideration of immediate transfer to operating theatre with ongoing internal cardiac massage or severe instability versus transfer of equipment and team to remote & resource confined locations (ICU, cardiac angiography suite, ED, rarely to ward)

As such, cardiothoracic anaesthetic, cardiac catheter lab, operating theatre and ICU teams should be familiar with the above treatment guidelines, and develop staff education pathways which should ideally involve: building of familiar teams and team-based training, crisis resource management, scenario rehearsal and simulation.

Local and regional policies should include planning for provision of damage control cardiac surgical interventions, including ensuring (i) rapid availability of a mobile emergency operating and perfusion / mechanical circulatory support team to deliver care in the cardiac ICU, catheter lab, ward or emergency department (ii) immediate 24/7 access to an emergency operating theatre for definitive ongoing surgical management.

5 Practical Aspects of Modified Anaesthesia for Achieving 'Crash' Cardiopulmonary Bypass

'Time is myocardium, brain and organ function'.

Whilst urgent surgery ('within hours') may involve extreme complexity and instability, a relatively comprehensive 'ad hoc multi-disciplinary assessment' can often be arranged, and standardised pathways for conduct of anaesthesia followed (these are beyond the scope of this chapter)

In contrast, a few patients will be encountered who are suffering from one or more of the following:

(a) Coronary occlusion with evolving ventricular infarction and severe cardiogenic shock or refractory ventricular dysrhythmias
(b) A state of cardiorespiratory and metabolic extremis due to catastrophic ventricular failure and cardiac distension
(c) Exsanguination due to cardiac or major vessel perforation
(d) Incipient cardiac arrest (with ongoing resuscitation as outlined above)

In these few true emergency cases, the only feasible strategy for restoring coronary and systemic perfusion may be to establish 'crash' cardiopulmonary bypass within minutes of attendance of the operating and perfusion teams.

In such circumstances, the anaesthetist(s) will be forced to adopt a pared-down approach to all aspects of care to expedite immediate salvage cardiopulmonary bypass.

A process of minimised 'crash' cardiac anaesthesia (for a conscious, spontaneously ventilating patient but severely shocked patient) would involve the following steps:

(i) Establishment of peripheral large bore intravenous (or even intra-osseous) access, AAGBI monitoring and application of external defibrillation pads.

Whilst central venous access and arterial blood pressure monitoring are desirable—in exceptional, time-critical circumstances, these can occasionally be deferred and achieved via surgical access (e.g. temporary, direct superior vena cava line and direct aortic pressure measurement) or after stabilising the patient on cardiopulmonary bypass.

(ii) Pre-oxygenation (including consideration of apnoeic high flow nasal oxygen for patients with severe respiratory distress) followed by rapid sequence intubation (or even supraglottic airway insertion in a fasted, slim patient), invasive ventilation and maintenance of anaesthesia with volatile agent or total intravenous anaesthesia.

(iii) Immediate surgical 'knife-to-skin' after aseptic preparations and surgical draping (the surgical preparation process should however be already ongoing by the time of rapid sequence anaesthesia induction)

(iv) Surgical emergency sternotomy (for most cases) or rarely femoral vascular cut down for peripheral bypass or ECMO cannulation.

(v) Expectation of administration of bolus peripheral intravenous vasoactives (e.g. adrenaline, metaraminol, calcium) during external and then internal cardiac massage.

(vi) Supra-maximal heparinisation (at least 400 units/kg in emergency. circumstances) and testing of activated clotting time (ACT) according to local policy targets (480 s in the author's institution).

(vii) Surgical large bore ascending aortic (or occasionally, femoral) cannulation.

(viii) Restoration of circulating volume via perfusionist administration of fluid and blood products into the arterial cannula—potentially invoking the hospital 'major haemorrhage' protocol in the process.

(ix) Surgical large bore right atrial (or femoral venous) cannulation.

(x) Establishment of cardiopulmonary bypass, with potential ongoing large volume transfusion via perfusionist and anaesthetic routes.

(xi) Definitive intervention—such as arrythmia control, repair of cardiac lacerations or perforations, emergency coronary revascularisation, emergency valve intervention or simple myocardial reperfusion, metabolic optimisation and inotropic or mechanical circulatory support.

6 Post-Bypass Management After 'Crash' Emergency Anaesthesia

Following control of time-critical pathology, as above, a significant period of myocardial reperfusion, core and peripheral rewarming should follow during which surgical, anaesthetic and perfusionist team discussions can occur, with the added thinking time allowed by the stability of cardiopulmonary bypass.

Strategy discussion of the process of cardiopulmonary bypass should systemically include the following:

Priorities for discussion of cardiopulmonary bypass weaning
Intra-operative and post-operative respiratory management
Detailed assessment of tracheal tube positioning, lower airway patency and potential reversible pathologies prior to attempting weaning
Consideration of use of inhaled nitric oxide
Acknowledgement of potential deleterious effects of PEEP or lung hyper-expansion on surgical access sites, plus potential deleterious effects of hypercapnoea/acidosis on cardiac performance
Consideration of elective open chest management in cases of severe oedema of the heart-lung block
Consideration of peripheral VV or Central VA-ECMO as a planned or rescue strategy
Vasoactive management
Epicardial pacing strategy, including haemodynamic benefits of atrial or atrioventricular pacing, weighted against increased bleeding risk of atrial epicardial pacing wires
Consensus planned inotropic support, acknowledging potential deleterious effects of team's preferred agents
Consideration of intra-aortic balloon pump, Impella, LVAD or RVAD, or ECMO support as a primary or salvage vasoactive strategy
Consideration of elective or rescue open chest management, acknowledging benefits for right ventricular and lung performance, weighted against bleeding and infection concerns engendered
Planning of key diagnostics and monitoring metrics from transoesophageal echocardiography
Haemostasis strategy
Further planned transfusion requirements and strategy for haemostatic agents
Consideration of reduced volume interventions for patients with severe lung and/or right heart oedema
Consideration of on bypass haemofiltration to allow for further transfusion requirements and coagulopathy correction
Predicted ongoing support requirements post-operatively in intensive care
Pre-discussion and/or second opinion input from ICU medical staff may be beneficial even prior to cardiopulmonary bypass weaning , in order to facilitate a smooth and safe handover and consensus agreed management strategy

7 Conclusions

When faced with a necessity for time-critical salvage intervention, due to severely decompensated cardiovascular physiology, it is essential that the emergency cardiothoracic surgical team maintains a culture of streamlined, focussed decision-making and cohesive team working. This process should be underpinned by closed-loop communications, particularly between the anaesthetic, surgical and perfusion roles.

Pre-rehearsal of agreed team strategies for all phases of care is essential, ideally via a comprehensive team briefing process, where time allows. However, on those occasions where a crisis scenario dictates that split-second decision-making is necessary, then familiar teams will be able to resort to pre-practised stereotyped drills of each care phase, steered by expert cardiothoracic anaesthetic and surgical team co-leaders.

Acquisition of requisite skills for effective team working in emergency care will be enhanced by familiarity of team members who work together regularly, and an education framework that includes regular multi-disciplinary training, ideally with scenario practice and simulation, plus a programme of regular case review and team debriefing, again, led by expert anaesthetic and surgical leaders.

References

Boer C et al (2017) EACTS/EACTA Guidelines on patient blood management for adult cardiac surgery. Journal of Cardiothoracic and Vascular Anesthesia 32(1):88–120

Guideline for resuscitation in cardiac arrest after cardiac surgery (2009) Eur J Cardio-Thoracic Surg 36(1):3–28

Guidelines for the use of transesophageal echocardiography to assist with surgical decision-making in the operating room: a surgery-based approach from the American Society of Echocardiography in Collaboration with the Society of Cardiovascular Anesthesiologists and the Society of Thoracic Surgeons (2020) J Am Soc Echocardiograph 33:692–734

Jepsson et al (2024) 2024 EACTS Guidelines on perioperative medication in adult cardiac surgery. Eur J Cardio-Thoracic Surg. https://academic.oup.com/ejcts/advance-article/doi/10.1093/ejcts/ezae355/7815986

Joint British Societies Guideline on management of cardiac arrest in the cardiac catheter laboratory (2022) Heart 108(12). https://heart.bmj.com/content/108/12/e1

Recommendations for transoesophageal echocardiography: update 2010 (2010) Eur J Echocardiograph 11:557–576

Royal College of Anaesthetists: Guidelines for the Provision of Anaesthetic Services, Chapter 5, Guidelines for the Provision of Emergency Anaesthesia

Soar J, Deakin CD, Nolan JP, Perkins GD, Yeung J, Couper K, Hall M, Thorne C, Price S, Lockey A, Wyllie J, Hampshire S (2021) Adult advanced life support guidelines. Resuscitation Council UK. https://www.resus.org.uk/library/2021-resuscitation-guidelines/adult-advanced-life-support-guidelines

The ATLS Subcommittee, American College of Surgeons' Committee on Trauma, and the International ATLS working group (2013) Advanced trauma life support (ATLS®): the ninth edition. J Trauma Acute Care Surg 74(5):1363–1366

Perfusion Considerations in Emergency Cardiac Surgery

Lydia Wilkinson

Abstract The use of cardiopulmonary bypass during cardiothoracic emergencies is often dependent upon the requirement to provide end-organ perfusion during periods of reduced cardiac output or wherein a surgical repair is indicated. Such eventualities pose various considerations for the perfusionist and conduct of cardiopulmonary bypass; primarily determined by the degree of notice presented by the surgical emergency. This falls into three distinct categories; 'elective' emergencies wherein an emergency can be anticipated and planned for, semi-planned emergencies in which surgery is required within a defined timeframe and true emergencies which cannot be anticipated. Considerations predominantly vary across cardiopulmonary bypass circuit adaptations, cannulation strategy and ability to induce systemic anticoagulation. Though cardiopulmonary bypass conduct including rapid cooling, haemofiltration and oxygenated arterial flow rates must also be considered.

Keywords Cardiopulmonary bypass (CPB) · Emergency cardiac surgery · Perfusion strategies · Cannulation techniques · Deep hypothermic circulatory arrest · Aortic dissection · Cardiac tamponade · Oxygen delivery · CPB circuit adaptation · Haemodilution management · Rapid initiation of CPB · Anticoagulation during emergency CPB

1 Introduction

'Emergency' cardiac surgery is generally defined as a time-critical event requiring urgent surgical intervention; the nature of which directly determines whether cardiopulmonary bypass (CPB) is required. CPB is often utilised in instances of inadequate end-organ perfusion during a period of reduced, or absent, cardiac

L. Wilkinson (✉)
Department of Clinical Perfusion, John Radcliffe Hospital, Oxford University Hospitals NHS Foundation Trust, Oxford, UK
e-mail: Lydia.Wilkinson@ouh.nhs.uk

A. Kourliouros (ed.), *Emergency Cardiac Surgery*,
https://doi.org/10.1007/978-3-032-15787-4_31

output and wherein a bloodless surgical field to facilitate a surgical repair is necessary. Perfusion considerations in such emergencies, for example circuit adaptation, prime composition and cannula selection, are predominantly determined by the degree of notice presented by an emergency with three defined periods identified. (1) 'Elective' emergencies in which a potential emergency scenario is anticipated such as 'high risk' pacemaker and implantable cardioverter-defibrillator lead extractions, (2) semi-planned emergencies wherein cardiac surgery is required within four hours and (3) unplanned or 'salvage' emergencies, occurring commonly as a result of cardiac arrest, in which CPB is required to provide cardiac output. Whilst the perfusion techniques executed at each stage differ the common denominator, providing adequate perfusion remains the common goal and will therefore be elucidated at each differentiated emergency timeframe, respectively.

2 'Elective' Emergencies

The juxtaposing term 'elective emergency' is herein defined as a planned procedure within which an emergency situation requiring CPB support is anticipated and can be planned for. The nature of the elective procedure enables prior planning via multidisciplinary team (MDT) discussion, and also ensures wider MDT availability in the event of an emergency due to compliance with $n + 1$ staffing during working hours. Such procedures include the explant of permanent pacemaker or implantable cardiac defibrillator leads, with risk stratified according to duration of implantation, and on the basis of patient factors including low body mass index, extremes of age and reduced left ventricular ejection fraction. For example, the extraction of indwelling permanent pacemaker leads > 20 years is likely to be deemed high risk due to the formation of severe lead adhesions which, upon removal, may induce cardiac or vascular perforation and rapid onset of circulatory decompensation (Kancharla et al. 2019). In such instances, emergency sternotomy and the immediate evacuation of any pericardial collection is required, with time to intervention being the single most important factor in preventing a major complication leading to death (Boarescu et al. 2022). It is assumed that such interventions must occur no longer than 10 min post vascular collapse, after which the risk of severe neurological injury and death increases dramatically (Tułecki et al. 2022). Due to this, it is commonplace for a full cardiothoracic surgical team to be present in the cardiac catheterisation lab for the duration of 'high risk' lead extractions, to promptly attend to the potential emergency.

Perfusion techniques in this context relate primarily to the execution of CPB itself rather than preoperative CPB considerations as, due to the elective nature of the emergency, time is allocated for circuit priming, completion of a pre-bypass safety checklist and addressing patient-specific requirements including cannula choice and comorbidity consideration. Once an emergency has been established, likely due to a pericardial collection leading to tamponade physiology and circulatory decompensation, the CPB run is anticipated to share many similarities to salvage emergencies as the direct cause of the emergency cannot be anticipated. Therefore, standard aortic arterial cannulation and two-stage venous cannulation may not be possible due to the potential for right atrial wall damage and superior vena cava (SVC) perforation. However, in order to rapidly establish CPB a dual-stage venous cannula will often be utilised to obtain venous drainage, though the potential for modification to this cannulation strategy must be considered. For example, to obtain access to the SVC to facilitate a surgical repair, the dual-stage venous cannula may be inserted into the right atrium and deployed further into the inferior vena cava (IVC), whilst a bullet tipped sucker may be inserted into the SVC to provide cerebral venous drainage and improve visibility, therefore reinforcing the importance of the presence of an emergency trolley, containing CPB cannula, connectors and commonly prescribed drugs and fluids, to accommodate such adaptations to cannulation.

The rapid establishment of CPB induces widespread haemodilution due to the inability to perform blood-conserving techniques such as retrograde autologous priming (RAP), removing the CPB prime solution by displacement with autologous blood, and is exacerbated further by volume resuscitation with crystalloid and colloid fluids. Therefore, it is common to encounter a reduced rate of oxygen delivery (DO_2i), indexed to body surface area (BSA), due to diminished haemoglobin values as the delivery of oxygen relies upon arterial pump flow rate and the oxygen content of arterial blood (CaO_2). CaO_2 is determined by the sum of oxygen dissolved in the plasma and oxygen bound to haemoglobin, the formula for which is presented below (Baker 2017):

$$DO_2i\left(\text{mL}/\text{min}/\text{m}^2\right) = DO_2 / \text{Body surface area}\left(\text{m}^2\right)$$

$$DO_2\left(\text{mL}/\text{min}\right) = Q \times CaO_2 \times 10$$

$$CaO_2 = \left(\text{Hb}[\text{g}/\text{L}] \times 1.34 \times SaO_2[\%]\right) + \left(PaO_2[\text{mmHg}] \times 0.003\right)$$

DO_2—delivery of oxygen, Q—arterial pump flow (litres per minute), CaO_2—total arterial oxygen content, Hb—haemoglobin, SaO_2—arterial oxygen saturation, PaO_2—partial pressure of oxygen in arterial blood.

A DO_2i below 260 mL/min/m^2 is associated with organ dysoxia, increased peak lactate and CO_2 production (VCO_2) during CPB, and subsequent tissue acidosis (Ranucci et al. 2006). This in turn may be a determinant of impaired post-operative organ function, specifically contributing to acute kidney injury (Newland and Baker 2017). Hence, it is pertinent to restore the DO_2i rapidly by elevating the haemoglobin via packed red blood cell transfusions and incorporating a haemofilter into the CPB circuit to remove excess fluid, haemoconcentrate plasma factors and elevate haemoglobin values. It should be considered that restoring a reduced intravascular volume requires a holistic approach, by transfusing fresh frozen plasma, platelets and cryoprecipitate collectively alongside packed red blood cells to replicate the intravascular volume lost during haemorrhage.

3 Semi-planned Emergencies

A semi-planned emergency procedure refers to the urgent nature of a condition requiring emergency cardiac surgery within four hours. Examples exist across the adult and paediatric setting including Stanford type A aortic dissections (STAAD) and presentations of total anomalous pulmonary venous drainage, respectively, though CPB considerations in the adult patient population will be focused upon.

Depending on clinical urgency a team brief is usually able to be undertaken during which the surgical plan and cannulation strategy is discussed, whilst time is also allocated for CPB circuit modifications as with aforementioned 'elective' emergencies. Therefore, when considering such modifications and perfusion techniques for a STAAD, a highly optimised CPB circuit is required to facilitate antegrade cerebral perfusion during deep hypothermic circulatory arrest (DHCA). This often requires the addition of a bifurcated arterial line, a preconstructed example of which is displayed in Fig. 1, which allows for simultaneous arterial cannulation sites, commonly the axillary or subclavian arteries to enable cerebral perfusion. Furthermore, Fig. 1 also demonstrates a recirculation line with three Luer locks, allowing for the addition of isolated perfusion lines which are routinely deployed for cerebral perfusion during DHCA, and myocardial perfusion in instances of beating heart circulatory arrest. Such a feature also negates the need to directly cut into the arterial line to incorporate a bifurcation and, thus, reduces the risk of desterilisation and potential introduction of bacteria.

A further consideration during STAAD's is the potential for a prolonged CPB run due to the complexity of surgical repair, and the subsequent impact upon oxygenator performance. Many commonly utilised oxygenators, such as the Sorin Inspire 8F, are rated for up to 6 hours or less clinical use at a maximum arterial pump flow rate defined by individual oxygenator specifications. Post 6 hours clinical use this rate of oxygenation is not guaranteed and thus must be considered during CPB circuit adaptation prior to an anticipated prolonged surgical case. The incorporation of a 'parallel replacement of oxygenator not transferring oxygen' or 'PRONTO' loop into the CPB circuit, between the arterial pump outlet and oxygenator inlet, provides the ability to exchange and prime an oxygenator without terminating CPB (Groom et al. 2002). The

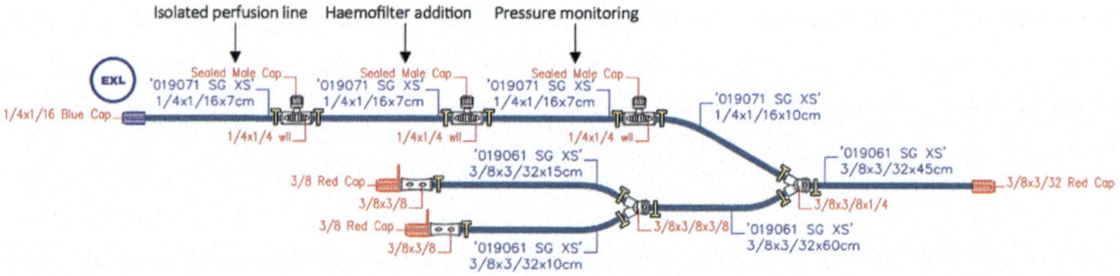

Fig. 1 CPB circuit diagram of a pre-constructed bifurcated arterial line utilised at the John Radcliffe Hospital, Oxford, during instances of multiple CPB arterial cannulation sites, manufactured by Liva Nova

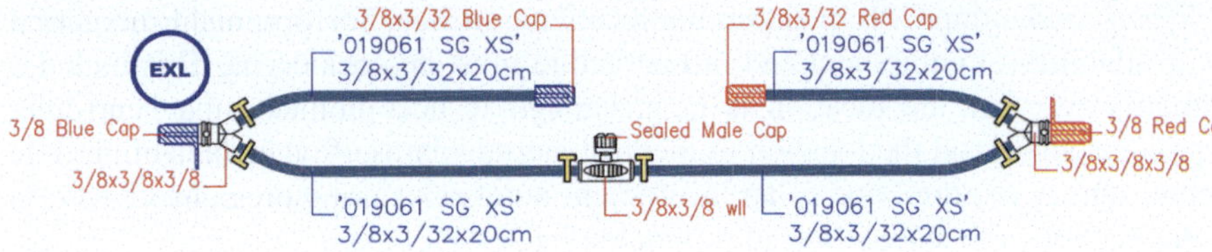

Fig. 2 CPB circuit diagram of a parallel replacement of oxygenator not transferring oxygen (PRONTO) loop in use at the John Radcliffe Hospital, Oxford, manufactured by Liva Nova

CPB circuit diagram of a PRONTO loop is displayed in Fig. 2. Such a feature therefore provides an element of safety against progressive oxygenator function decline post 6 hours clinical use, and is frequently employed outside of STAAD procedures at the John Radcliffe Hospital, Oxford, wherein a prolonged CPB run is anticipated.

Furthermore, STAADs are often misdiagnosed as an acute coronary syndrome with adenosine diphosphate (ADP) receptor inhibitors, such as clopidogrel and ticagrelor, immediately prescribed as monotherapy or as part of dual antiplatelet therapy (Xue et al. 2019). However, patients receiving such therapy and subsequently requiring emergent cardiac surgery upon STAAD diagnosis are at an increased risk of post-operative bleeding, hospital stay and morbidity, impairing outcomes post surgery. However, the inclusion of a CytoSorb® device (CytoSorbents Inc, Monmouth Junction, NJ), a blood purification filter containing adsorbent polymer beads, into the CPB circuit has been demonstrated to intraoperatively reduce circulating plasma ticagrelor concentrations during CPB by 67.1% (Hassan et al. 2023). This in turn has been associated with significantly reduced bleeding complications in non-deferrable cardiac surgery, and subsequently patients received fewer transfusions of blood products and experienced a shorter intensive care stay (Hassan et al. 2019). Therefore, recent evidence proposes the benefit of such a device in this context, and may also impart a cost benefit due to reduced blood product administration.

4 Unplanned 'Salvage' Emergencies

In true or 'salvage' emergencies, CPB is often utilised to assist in recovering patients with total, near-total or expectant imminent cardiovascular collapse. This requires initiating treatment where presented, such as in Accident and Emergency or Intensive Care Departments, during which establishing CPB in a timely manner is of utmost importance to limit mal-perfusion duration and the secondary sequelae of hypoxia-induced morbidity. Therefore, there is by nature, no prior warning of the event, and thus no time allocated preceding a CPB run to create a surgical plan or execute CPB circuit modifications. However, it must be considered that the end point of such interventions is not CPB, but rather the resolution of structural or physiological disturbances which preceded and initiated the event requiring CPB support.

When conducting CPB in unfamiliar locations, such as Accident and Emergency, the availability of equipment and infrastructure must be considered. This includes primarily whether the location is large enough to accommodate the heart-lung bypass machine, and the location of medical gas supply as often a pendant gas line splitter unit is required due to an insufficient number of gas outlets. Moreover, in such situations the availability of a portable bag containing a variety of CPB cannula and essential fluids and drugs, such as compound sodium lactate (Hartmann's) solution and unfractionated heparin, is useful during hours of reduced staffing when transportation of larger equipment is unachievable.

The timing and nature of a true emergency cannot be anticipated; the priority in these cases is likely to establish oxygenated arterial flow. Therefore, a standby CPB circuit must be available at all times to immediately support as wide a range of adult patients as possible. In such cases, the use of highly optimised or miniaturised circuits as emergency pumps may be counterproductive as they may not suit the oxygenated arterial flow requirements of the patient. Rather, a 'standard' adult circuit which can generate a minimum of 6 L/min arterial flow should be available to account for a broad spectrum of scenarios encountered in the adult patient population. This approach is more difficult in paediatric centres due to the variation in patient BSA and thus arterial flow requirements, and as such a 'one size fits all' approach to circuit configuration cannot be undertaken. It also varies across perfusion departments as to whether a primed CPB pump is available at all times, which is more common in high-throughput centres, though it is recommended that a dry-build CPB circuit is continually available to be rapidly primed in case of adult emergencies. The approach to emergency priming at the John Radcliffe Hospital, Oxford, is to administer 2 L of Plasma-Lyte148 into the reservoir via the rapid prime line, ensuring that oxygenated arterial flow can be established quickly. There may not be time to complete a comprehensive pre-bypass safety checklist, in which situation the circuit must be free of air, and the reservoir level, bubble detection and arterial circuit pressure alarms engaged and functionality checked as minimum. Should there also be insufficient time to prime the cardioplegia circuit, the cardioplegia blood line may be clamped off at the outlet of the oxygenator to prevent air entrainment during any period of negative arterial circuit pressures.

The administration of systemic anticoagulation preceding CPB is also of paramount importance to prevent activation of the coagulation system, and subsequent global clot formation, resulting from contact between blood and the artificial surface of the CPB circuit (Sniecinski and Chandler 2011). Heparin sodium is the common anticoagulant of choice administered prior to CPB, of which an empirical dose of 300–500 IU/kg is used to achieve an activated clotting time above 400 s (Young et al. 1978). By potentiating the action of antithrombin III 1000-fold heparin inhibits both thrombin and factor Xa formation and their pro-coagulant activity, though the response is naturally heterogenous across patients. However, in the context of total cardiovascular collapse, systemic heparin administered will unlikely be effective solely through intravenous administration due to the absence of cardiac output, thus anticoagulation may be inadequate upon CPB initiation. In order to mitigate against this, heparin is often an additive to CPB priming solutions and administered either as a fixed dose ranging from 2500 to 10,000 IU in adult circuits, or based on patient weight. A further consideration is that should the emergency be due to tamponade, the CPB suckers will often be placed directly in the chest upon sternotomy and opening of the pericardial sac in order to improve visibility of the surgical field. However, blood aspirated via such means is often shed prior to systemic heparinisation and as such, will not be anticoagulated. Additionally blood stasis within the pericardium also propagates Virchow's triad of thrombosis, resulting in hypercoagulable blood aspirated into the CPB circuit. To mitigate against this, 2500 IU of heparin may be added directly to the tubing of each sucker by removing the tubing prior to the one-way valve connection, if present, and introducing heparin. Alternatively a sterile needle may be used to inject heparin into the sucker tubing lumen at the level of the roller pump inlet; however, the resulting puncture must be sealed with a sterile, non-absorbable product such as surgical-use bone wax to prevent blood loss.

Cannulation strategy must also be considered as the urgency of the situation will take priority over complex cannulation techniques; thus, central or femoral cannulation will often be utilised to achieve a rudimentary 'one pipe in, one pipe out' approach to CPB. In cases presenting in intensive care units secondary to cardiac surgery, Cardiac Advanced Life Support treatment encourages reopening of the previous sternotomy and as such, central cannulation will likely be the fastest way to initiate CPB with full flow immediately achievable (Brand et al. 2018). However, femoral cannulation via a cut-down approach may be required in a primary presentation, examples of this potentially include hypothermic arrest in colder climates and cardiac arrest due to drug toxicity. Such incidences may also call for extracorporeal membrane oxygenation (ECMO) support, though this should only be deployed if ECMO availability is equal to, or faster than, initiating CPB as time to establishing extracorporeal support is a direct predictor of end-organ viability (Debaty et al. 2017).

With the arterial cannula in place, CPB can be rapidly initiated provided a degree of venous return is obtained. It must be considered that this may employ 'sucker bypass' which entails delivering a degree of arterial flow which matches the rate of aspirated blood returned to the CPB circuit from the surgical field via the suckers, until venous access is confirmed by the surgeon and visualised by the perfusionist. However, in such situations, a single-stage cannula or a Ross Atrial Basket, may be introduced into the right atrium to provide basic venous drainage. During such periods a more modest flow target should be accepted with adequate perfusion pressures and oxygenation prioritised. However, it can also be mentioned that the suture lines for venous cannulation may not be robust due to the clinical urgency to establish a form of CPB. Therefore, the perfusionist may keep a partial clamp on the venous line to prevent air entrainment through loose purse strings, avoiding a venous 'air-lock', whilst simultaneously allowing for full venous drainage. In addition, little is often known about the patient's physiology, therefore a target arterial flow must be estimated, with 4 L/min and 5 L/min generally accepted as sufficient for adult females and males, respectively.

If full flow is not achievable or reduced on grounds of surgical need, aggressive cooling of the patient is strongly indicated. Cooling reduces basal metabolic rate by

7% for every 1 °C reduction in core temperature from 37 °C, which enables low flow states to be well tolerated as oxygen requirements are reduced (Bjertnæs et al. 2022). In the extreme this can permit deep hypothermic circulatory arrest with no arterial CPB flow required. Whilst there is a general trend to perform circulatory arrest at warmer temperatures up to 24 °C, 18 °C remains the useful target threshold from which mortality data is available, with 40- and 60-min markers for adverse neurological morbidity and mortality indices, respectively (Salehi Ravesh et al. 2022).

Upon obtaining vascular access and stability on CPB, the conduct of CPB concerning biochemical and metabolic disturbances must be addressed. Should hypotension and hypoperfusion have preceded CPB support, consideration must be paid to the resulting hypoxia and oxygen debt which will likely result in profound metabolic and lactic acidaemia. The establishment of CPB may result in reperfusion washout of such metabolites into the circulation that will likely necessitate the employment of techniques including zero-balance ultrafiltration and the addition of buffering solutions.

5 Conclusions

The utilisation of CPB during emergency cardiac surgery is dependent upon the clinical presentation and subsequent requirement for either cardiorespiratory support, bloodless surgical field or both. Perfusion considerations inevitably vary depending upon the time available to conduct circuit modifications and establish CPB; however, further considerations include the conduction of a pre-bypass safety checklist, cannulation strategy and CPB conduct. Regardless of clinical urgency, the requirement to provide an adequate amount of oxygenated arterial flow on CPB to prevent end-organ mal-perfusion remains the goal.

References

Baker RA (2017) Variation in measurement and reporting of goal directed perfusion parameters. J Extra Corpor Technol 49:P2–P7

Bjertnæs LJ, Næsheim TO, Reierth E et al (2022) Physiological changes in subjects exposed to accidental hypothermia: an update. Front Med (Lausanne) 9:824395. https://doi.org/10.3389/fmed.2022.824395

Boarescu P-M, Popa ID, Trifan CA et al (2022) Practical approaches to transvenous lead extraction procedures—clinical case series. Int J Environ Res Public Health 20:379. https://doi.org/10.3390/ijerph20010379

Brand J, McDonald A, Dunning J (2018) Management of cardiac arrest following cardiac surgery. BJA Educ 18:16–22. https://doi.org/10.1016/j.bjae.2017.11.002

Debaty G, Babaz V, Durand M et al (2017) Prognostic factors for extracorporeal cardiopulmonary resuscitation recipients following out-of-hospital refractory cardiac arrest. A systematic review and meta-analysis. Resuscitation 112:1–10. https://doi.org/10.1016/j.resuscitation.2016.12.011

Groom RC, Forest RJ, Cormack JE et al (2002) Parallel replacement of the oxygenator that is not transferring oxygen: the PRONTO procedure. Perfusion 17:447–450. https://doi.org/10.1191/0267659102pf606oa

Hassan K, Kannmacher J, Wohlmuth P et al (2019) Cytosorb adsorption during emergency cardiac operations in patients at high risk of bleeding. Ann Thorac Surg 108:45–51. https://doi.org/10.1016/j.athoracsur.2018.12.032

Hassan K, Geidel S, Zamvar V et al (2023) Intraoperative ticagrelor removal via hemoadsorption during on-pump coronary artery bypass grafting. JTCVS Open 15:190–196. https://doi.org/10.1016/j.xjon.2023.04.013

Kancharla K, Acker NG, Li Z et al (2019) Efficacy and safety of transvenous lead extraction in the device laboratory and operating room guided by a novel risk stratification scheme. JACC Clin Electrophysiol 5:174–182. https://doi.org/10.1016/j.jacep.2019.01.001

Newland RF, Baker RA (2017) Low oxygen delivery as a predictor of acute kidney injury during cardiopulmonary bypass. J Extra Corpor Technol 49:224–230

Ranucci M, De Toffol B, Isgrò G et al (2006) Hyperlactatemia during cardiopulmonary bypass: determinants and impact on postoperative outcome. Crit Care 10:R167. https://doi.org/10.1186/cc5113

Salehi Ravesh M, Friedrich C, Schoettler J et al (2022) Association between duration of deep hypothermic circulatory arrest and surgical outcome in patients with acute type A aortic dissection: a large retrospective cohort study. J Clin Med 11:644. https://doi.org/10.3390/jcm11030644

Sniecinski RM, Chandler WL (2011) Activation of the hemostatic system during cardiopulmonary bypass. Anesth Analg 113:1319–1333. https://doi.org/10.1213/ANE.0b013e3182354b7e

Tułecki Ł, Czajkowski M, Targońska S et al (2022) The role of cardiac surgery in transvenous lead extraction. A high-volume center experience with 3207 procedures. Kardiochir Torakochirurgia Pol 19:122–129. https://doi.org/10.5114/kitp.2022.119759

Xue Y, Chong H, Zhu X et al (2019) Aortic dissection patients mimic acute coronary syndrome with preoperative antiplatelet therapy. J Thorac Dis 11:3385–3390. https://doi.org/10.21037/jtd.2019.08.02

Young JA, Kisker CT, Doty DB (1978) Adequate anticoagulation during cardiopulmonary bypass determined by activated clotting time and the appearance of fibrin monomer. Ann Thorac Surg 26(3):231–240

Emergency Re-exploration for Bleeding After Cardiac Surgery

Metesh Acharya and Giovanni Mariscalco

Abstract Bleeding is a common post-operative phenomenon after cardiac surgery and in some circumstances can be severe enough to warrant emergency re-exploration. This is a high-risk intervention owing to the haemodynamic instability of the patient, ischaemic injury from end-organ hypoperfusion and deleterious effects of excessive blood product transfusion. This chapter aims to provide a comprehensive overview of the predictors and causes of bleeding after cardiac surgery, potential bleeding sources at re-exploration, indications and optimal timing for re-exploration, surgical technique for re-sternotomy, prognostic and economic implication of re-exploration and strategies to minimise excessive bleeding and re-exploration.

Keywords Post-operative bleeding · Emergency re-exploration · Emergency re-sternotomy · Cardiac tamponade · Impact of re-exploration · Measures to minimise post-operative bleeding

Abbreviations

BARC	Bleeding Academic Research Consortium
CABG	Coronary artery bypass graft
CALS	Cardiac Advanced Life Support
CPB	Cardiopulmonary bypass
ICU	Intensive care unit
PRBC	Packed red blood cells
UDPB	Universal definition for perioperative bleeding

M. Acharya (✉) · G. Mariscalco
Department of Cardiac Surgery, Glenfield Hospital, Leicester, UK
e-mail: metesh.acharya@doctors.org.uk; giovanni.mariscalco@uhl-tr.nhs.uk

A. Kourliouros (ed.), *Emergency Cardiac Surgery*,
https://doi.org/10.1007/978-3-032-15787-4_32

1 Introduction

The advent of cardiopulmonary bypass (CPB) has since led to the worldwide adoption of open-heart cardiac surgical procedures and their development into mainstream therapeutic modalities for cardiovascular disease. Despite refinements in surgical techniques and advances in perioperative care and diagnostics, the early post-operative period may be complicated by excessive bleeding, haemodynamic instability and cardiac arrest, which may necessitate re-exploration for resolution. The incidence of re-exploration in cardiac surgical patients is estimated at between 2 and 6% (Dacey et al. 1998; Unsworth-White et al. 1995; Sellman et al. 1997; Choong et al. 2007; Karthik et al. 2004; Moulton et al. 1996). Re-exploration is particularly important considering that most underlying causes will be reversible, with survival being significantly greater following cardiac arrest after cardiac surgery than any other aetiology (Dunning et al. 2009).

Re-exploration refers to the systematic process whereby the thoracic cavity of a post-operative cardiac surgical patient is re-entered, usually in an operating room setting, but also within intensive care unit (ICU) or ward environments, to determine the cause of, and address, specific complications where conservative measures have failed. The principal indications for emergency re-exploration after cardiac surgery include excessive bleeding, cardiac tamponade and bypass graft failure. Non-emergency re-exploration may be necessary for infective complications, such as mediastinitis but will not be discussed further here.

The generalised attitude maintained throughout the cardiac surgical community is that re-exploration should be performed following cardiac arrest in post-operative cardiac surgical patients on the ICU should initial resuscitation measures prove unsuccessful (Dunning et al. 2009; Society of Thoracic Surgeons Task Force on Resuscitation After Cardiac Surgery 2017). This is usually executed emergently to prevent life-threatening deterioration of a patient's clinical status and to afford them the best opportunity for survival. Decision-making for re-exploration involves rapid yet accurate clinical assessment, the timely performance and careful interpretation of diagnostic investigations and a collaborative approach comprising cardiac surgeons, intensivists, anaesthetists and nursing staff, often during stressful situations. The optimal timing and strategy for re-exploration demand special consideration, since delays in intervention may be associated with prolonged periods of haemodynamic instability, excessive blood product utilisation and detrimental physiological and metabolic sequelae, with resultant significant morbidity and mortality.

This chapter aims to provide a comprehensive overview on the predictors and causes of bleeding after cardiac surgery and potential sources of bleeding at re-exploration. The indications and optimal timing for emergency re-exploration specifically relating to bleeding are reviewed. The technique for emergency re-sternotomy, prognostic and economic implications of re-exploration and strategies to minimise bleeding and re-exploration are also discussed.

2 Predictors of Bleeding After Cardiac Surgery

Bleeding after cardiac surgery has a multi-factorial aetiology comprising patient-related factors, procedure-related factors and impaired haemostasis from coagulopathy (Moulton et al. 1996; Biancari et al. 2012; Vivacqua et al. 2011). Several patient-related risk factors for re-exploration have been identified, including advanced age, male gender, poorly controlled diabetes mellitus, renal and hepatic dysfunction, peripheral vascular disease, connective tissue disorders such as Ehlers-Danlos syndrome, impaired left ventricular ejection fraction, increased EuroSCORE, low pre-operative haematocrit, and pre-operative exposure to aspirin or warfarin (Moulton et al. 1996; Biancari et al. 2012; Ranucci et al. 2008; Despotis et al. 1994, 2008, 2009; Kristensen et al. 2012; Petrou et al. 2016; Ruel et al. 2017). Hereditary or acquired defects affecting platelets or coagulation factors, such as von Willebrand disease or haemophilia, negatively impact the haemostatic system and may also cause excessive bleeding.

Cardiac surgical patients undergoing urgent or emergency surgery, redo sternotomy, more complex procedures other than coronary artery bypass graft (CABG) surgery and procedures requiring deep hypothermic circulatory arrest or prolonged durations of CPB are more susceptible to bleeding complications and therefore re-exploration (Moulton et al. 1996; Biancari et al. 2012; Ranucci et al. 2008; Vivacqua et al. 2011). The incidence of re-exploration following CABG has been reported at 4.5%, 5.5% for isolated valve procedures, 9.6% for combined procedures and 15% for emergency operations (Fröjd and Jeppsson 2016). Advanced age, reduced body mass index, congestive heart failure or shock, severe angina, chronic steroid use, greater number of distal anastomoses and internal mammary artery use have been associated with a greater risk of bleeding, and therefore re-exploration (Dacey et al. 1998; Sellman et al. 1997; Moulton et al. 1996; Fröjd and Jeppsson 2016; Despotis et al. 1994; Kristensen et al. 2012). Patients receiving clopidogrel within five days of surgery, ticagrelor within three days of surgery, heparin, warfarin or novel oral anticoagulants are at increased susceptibility to bleeding complications (Ul Islam et al. 2021). The effects of residual heparin resulting from incomplete reversal or heparin rebound also play an important role in post-operative bleeding.

Cardiac surgery procedures under CPB are associated with increased bleeding risk for several reasons. Firstly, extracorporeal circulation induces a haemodilution effect from fluid administration into the circuit to compensate for bleeding or cell salvage losses, whilst the specific type of fluid used for intravascular replacement may itself cause specific abnormalities in coagulation factor or platelet function or adhesion. Secondly, hypothermia exerts an inhibitory effect on coagulation factor and platelet function. Autotransfusion of shed mediastinal blood in conjunction with tissue injury and contact activation may result in a consumptive state comparable to disseminated intravascular coagulation. Similarly, excessive thrombin generation and fibrinolysis can result from activation of both intrinsic and extrinsic pathways, and lead to platelet and coagulation factor depletion.

Finally, an understanding of the clinical variables linked to post-operative bleeding can be used to develop simple yet effective risk estimation tools. As an example, the Bedside Risk Score has been validated as a predictive model to estimate patient-specific risk for re-exploration for bleeding after CABG (Mehta et al. 2009).

3 Medical Versus Surgical Causes for Bleeding After Cardiac Surgery

Prior to any decision for re-exploration, it is essential to differentiate between the so-called medical and surgical causes of bleeding, acknowledging that both can occur simultaneously.

"Medical" bleeding is a term ascribed to the coagulopathy arising from the patient- and procedure-related factors previously alluded to, including residual heparin effects, deficiencies in platelet number and function, coagulation factor depletion and hyperfibrinolysis (Brand et al. 2018; Besser et al. 2015). "Medical" bleeding is usually correctable and point-of-care evaluation of platelet, coagulation factor and fibrinogen levels and function can facilitate the diagnosis of haematological abnormalities. Furthermore, "medical" bleeding is generally responsive to the judicious administration of haemostatic blood components and adjunctive pharmacological therapies, for example protamine, desmopressin, anti-fibrinolytics and factor concentrates (Despotis et al. 2009). Uncorrected coagulopathy will exacerbate coexisting surgical causes of bleeding. Post-operative bleeding in the presence of a confirmed coagulopathy in a haemodynamically stable patient is therefore initially managed medically. Such a coagulopathy usually manifests as a diffuse bleeding or oozing which can be distinguished intra-operatively by experienced surgeons. In contrast, persistent bleeding despite normalisation of coagulation parameters in suspected "medical" bleeding may imply "surgical" bleeding and should prompt consideration of re-exploration.

"Surgical" bleeding refers to surgically induced injury to blood vessels which can be localised intra-operatively and controlled by surgical intervention. Active "surgical" bleeding will generate greater volumes of blood loss over a shorter time period and thus predispose to haemodynamic instability and the accompanying metabolic derangements. Common causes of "surgical" bleeding early after cardiac surgery include anastomotic suture lines and cannulation sites, side branches of arterial and venous bypass conduits, sternal sites including periosteum, bone marrow and wire holes, and dissected surfaces such as the internal mammary artery bed, pericardium and thymus (Moorjani et al. 2013).

4 Sources of Surgical Bleeding at Re-exploration

In one study by Hall and colleagues in 2001 with 82 patients undergoing re-exploration for post-operative haemorrhage out of 2263 cardiac cases, a surgical cause of bleeding was found in 66%, with the most common sites for bleeding consisting of the side branches of bypass conduits and the chest wall (Hall et al. 2001). Karthik and co-workers in 2004 identified a surgical source of bleeding in 67% of their re-explored patient cohort of 89 patients out of 2898 patients undergoing CABG, with the foremost bleeding sites being the conduit or anastomosis (57.5%), sternum or internal mammary bed (31.5%), extra-pericardial bleeding vessels (8.2%) and from cannulation and cardiotomy sites (2.8%) (Karthik et al. 2004). Out of 18,892 patients undergoing primary and repeat CABG, valve or combined operations, Vivacqua and associates in 2011 demonstrated the major sites of bleeding related to the sternum (30%), mediastinum (24%), internal mammary artery bed (16%) and coronary anastomosis (11%) (Vivacqua et al. 2011). Surgical causes of bleeding were identified in a considerable 76.9% of patients undergoing re-exploration in the analysis by Ali and co-workers, attributable to conduit side branches in 35.9%, sternal wire holes (17.9%), cannulation sites (15.4%) and epicardial pacing wire sites (7.7%) (Ali et al. 2019). A large meta-analysis encompassing 51,497 patients by Biancari and associates in 2018 evaluated bleeding sources in 2455 patients, out of which surgical bleeding points were identified in 65.7%, with the principal bleeding sites comprising bypass grafts (20.2%), the sternum (17.0%), vascular sutures (12.5%), the internal mammary artery harvest site (13.0%) and anastomoses (9.9%) (Biancari et al. 2018). Amongst the 127 cases of active bleeding at the time of re-exploration in 229 patients in the analysis by Tirilomis and co-workers in 2020, the principal sources of bleeding were anastomoses (26.0%), internal mammary artery or venous graft side branches (17.3%) and epi-/myocardial harvesting sites (11.8%) (Tirilomis et al. 2020). Most recently in 2023, Shou and colleagues discovered that amongst 251 patients undergoing re-exploration for post-cardiac surgery bleeding, the primary bleeding site was a suture line (28%), the chest wall (19%), mediastinum (15%) and multiple sites (8%) (Shou et al. 2023). Knowledge of these more frequent bleeding sources is valuable in directing surgeons during re-exploration and informing intra-operative decision-making processes.

5 Indications for Emergency Re-exploration for Bleeding

The general indications for emergency re-exploration comprise excessive bleeding, as evidenced by a greater volume of haemorrhagic drainage via the chest tubes, cardiac arrest due to severe bleeding and impending or established cardiac tamponade where an abrupt reduction in chest tube drainage from obstruction by clot may precede circulatory collapse. The common pathway is of haemorrhagic shock resulting in reduced effective circulating volume, tissue hypoperfusion, increased anaerobic metabolism, lactic acidosis, reperfusion injury, endotoxin translocation and eventual multi-organ dysfunction (Cecconi et al. 2014). However, there remains significant variation in the absolute volumes of intra- and post-operative bleeding in patients who eventually undergo re-exploration (Fröjd and Jeppsson 2016; Dyke et al. 2014).

The severity of bleeding in adult cardiac surgery has been categorised from 0 (insignificant bleeding) to 4 (massive bleeding) according to the universal definition for perioperative bleeding (UDPB) (Dyke et al. 2014). Re-exploration is indicated for Class 3 (severe) bleeding, associated with a post-operative chest tube blood loss of 1001–2000 mL over a 12-h period and transfusion of 5–10 units each of packed red blood cells (PRBC) and fresh frozen plasma. By incorporating multiple easily measurable criteria such as the volume of chest tube loss and units of PRBC and blood components transfused, the UDPB facilitates the assessment of bleeding severity when it occurs, but perhaps is not employed as often as it should be in clinical practice.

Significant bleeding warranting re-exploration after cardiac surgery has also been detailed by the Bleeding Academic Research Consortium (BARC) (Mehran et al. 2011). BARC type 3b bleeding includes that associated with a haemoglobin drop $\geq$ 5 g/dL, culminating in cardiac tamponade and requiring intravenous vasoactive drugs for surgical intervention for control. Specific to CABG, BARC type 4 bleeding implies that which mandates re-operation after sternal closure, transfusion of $\geq$ 5 PRBC within 48 h or that has chest tube drainage $\geq$ 2 L within 24 h.

Most institutions adhere to the criteria for early re-exploration proposed by Kirklin and Barratt-Boyes based on the magnitude of blood loss, comprising drainage of > 500 mL during the first hour, drainage of > 400 mL during each of the first 2 h, drainage of > 300 mL during each of the first 3 h or > 1000 mL in total during the first 4 h. However, widespread consensus is lacking on clear-cut thresholds for the absolute volumes of chest drainage above which re-exploration should be performed, and in most cases, this is left to the discretion of the supervising surgeon.

Additional reported indications for re-exploration due to bleeding are persistent bleeding over 12 h not meeting the Kirklin and Barratt-Boyes criteria but amounting to a total drainage rate exceeding 100 mL/h, sudden massive bleeding, persistent bleeding despite correction of any co-existing coagulopathy and cardiac arrest in the context of persistent bleeding (Ranucci et al. 2008). Should bleeding persist after normalisation within four post-operative hours of deranged coagulation indices, re-exploration should be performed to exclude a surgical bleeding source. Haemodynamic instability in combination with low cardiac output states despite adequate filling pressures with volume resuscitation, escalating inotropic/vasopressor requirements and a downwards trend in haemoglobin levels regardless of PRBC transfusion is concerning, and most units would advocate early re-exploration in such circumstances (Ranucci et al. 2008). On balance, a more conservative approach avoiding urgent re-exploration may suffice when stable haemodynamic parameters and haemoglobin levels are maintained independent of PRBC transfusion.

Re-exploration itself carries a mortality risk surpassing 3% even without PRBC transfusion (Ranucci et al. 2008).

Whilst the above represents a generalised guide to facilitate decision-making, submitting a patient to re-exploration is a complex and dynamic undertaking which ultimately remains at the judgement of the responsible clinician. A multitude of factors influence the decision, including the haemodynamic stability and metabolic profile of the patient, the individual surgeon's threshold for excessive bleeding, information discerned from point-of-care coagulation studies and echocardiography, and the availability of operating room resources and supporting personnel.

6 Timing of Re-exploration for Bleeding

The timing of re-exploration is of paramount importance with most groups advocating earlier re-exploration (Choong et al. 2007; Karthik et al. 2004; Ranucci et al. 2008; Kristensen et al. 2012; Ul Islam et al. 2021; Ali et al. 2019; Canádyová et al. 2012; Pasrija et al. 2020; Haneya et al. 2015; Soletti Jr et al. 2024). Increasing time to re-exploration has been independently associated with worse mortality and morbidity (Shou et al. 2023). Unnecessary delay in re-exploration whilst modifiable causes of bleeding such as hypothermia, acidosis and coagulopathy are addressed can subject patients to a continued low cardiac output state, the attendant end-organ malperfusion, deleterious effects of higher-dose inotropes and vasopressors, and the not insignificant risks relating to blood product transfusion (Fröjd and Jeppsson 2016; Ul Islam et al. 2021; Hall et al. 2001; Koch et al. 2006a, b, 2009). Another perhaps intentional reason in delaying for re-exploration is that the operating surgeon may perceive a theatre return as a personal failure. This, particularly in the current era when re-exploration is scrutinised as a quality performance metric, may incline the surgeon to pursue medical management of bleeding for as long as is feasible. Delaying re-exploration only translates into amplified risk by way of increased allogenic blood product utilisation, with the number of PRBC transfused being an independent risk factor for morbidity and mortality (Ranucci et al. 2008). Bleeding patients who do not undergo re-exploration and instead receive massive PRBC transfusion have a greater mortality risk (Ranucci et al. 2008). Even with negative intra-operative findings, retained clot evacuation and subsequent reduction in mediastinal fibrinolytic activity is therapeutic in itself (Pelletier et al. 1998) and reduce infection rates by removing clots as a culture medium for bacterial proliferation.

There is now significant evidence that deferring re-exploration for > 12 h post-operatively despite an unacceptable haemoglobin level leads to greater morbidity, such as an extended ICU stay, renal failure, prolonged mechanical ventilation beyond 24 h and greater requirement for intra-aortic balloon pump support, and mortality, in the face of continued hypovolaemia and tissue hypoxia (Choong et al. 2007; Karthik et al. 2004). The time until re-exploration is often significantly prolonged in patients who die following re-exploration (Canádyová et al. 2012). A recent analysis which stratified mortality according to time to re-exploration revealed significantly increased mortality with re-exploration at 0–4 h post-operatively (12.3%), compared to 25–48 h (37.5%) (Shou et al. 2023). For example, re-exploration after the day of surgery has been associated with a 6.4-fold increase in mortality risk presumably due to the consequences of prolonged haemodynamic instability and uncorrected bleeding (Ruel et al. 2017). Results from a large meta-analysis have suggested that re-exploration be performed as soon as excessive bleeding, as defined above, and/or cardiac tamponade become evident (Biancari et al. 2012). Importantly, within the first 12 h of the index cardiac operation, there does not appear to be any adverse impact of time delays to surgical re-exploration on clinical outcomes (Ranucci et al. 2008). In fact, a reduction in stroke and renal failure may be achieved with early re-exploration at < 5 h, perhaps due to less time spent in an ischaemic state (Ohmes et al. 2017).

Since most bleeding in cardiac surgical patients, in some reports up to 82% (Karthik et al. 2004), originates from a surgical source and more favourable outcomes are achievable by expedited re-exploration, most institutions in the reported literature therefore adopt an aggressive approach with an earlier re-exploration policy in the presence of haemodynamic instability and low haemoglobin (Choong et al. 2007; Karthik et al. 2004; Ranucci et al. 2008; Vivacqua et al. 2011). Such patients with suspected surgical bleeding should be re-explored promptly. Nevertheless, there is no universal time cut-off within which re-exploration should be performed, although post-operative time, volume of blood loss and patient's haemodynamic condition must be carefully considered.

7 Technique of Emergency Re-sternotomy

This section will provide a practical overview of emergency re-sternotomy performed at the patient's bedside for cardiac arrest, and can be performed for all cardiac surgical patients within 10 days of their last operation in accordance with standardised Cardiac Advanced Life Support (CALS) protocols (Dunning et al. 2009; Society of Thoracic Surgeons Task Force on Resuscitation After Cardiac Surgery 2017). CALS protocol emergency re-sternotomy is performed immediately for post-cardiotomy cardiac arrest at the patient's bedside, when haemodynamic instability precludes patient's transfer. However, it is certainly preferable to transfer a bleeding yet non-arrested patient manifesting haemodynamic deterioration, albeit with a degree to responsiveness to fluid resuscitation and vasoconstrictor therapy, to a more controlled operating theatre environment for definitive intervention.

Whilst non-sterile staff perform external cardiac massage as part of CALS, a gown and gloves are donned in a sterile fashion using a closed glove technique by two to three staff members, with one acting as the primary operator, one as an assistant and one as a scrub nurse. Skin preparation with antiseptic solution and hand-washing are not necessary. Non-sterile external cardiac massage continues until a sterile "all-in-one" thoracic drape is applied to cover the whole bed with the clear and adhesive plastic window section applied over the sternal region, after which the scrubbed staff resume sterile external cardiac massage and the re-sternotomy kit is opened on the sterile drape. The simplified re-sternotomy kit comprises a scalpel, wire cutter, heavy needle holder, suction and single-piece sternal retractor.

The scalpel is used to open the sternotomy incision all the way down to the sternal wires. If skin clips have been used for skin closure, these are not removed but instead a new skin incision is made adjacent and parallel to the existing one. The primary operator then pulls the sternal wires using the heavy needle holder to expose a free section which can be cut by the assistant using wire cutters. The sternal wires are then pulled out by the primary operator, causing the sternal edges to separate and relieve cardiac tamponade if present. Suction is used to carefully evacuate blood or clot before the sternal retractor is inserted to spread the sternal edges. Chest re-entry should be accomplished within 5 min from cardiac arrest.

Clots overlying the heart are then removed whilst paying special attention to important structures that may be obscured from view, such as internal mammary and other bypass grafts, and chest tubes are repositioned outside the surgical field. Internal cardiac massage using single- or two-handed techniques based on the primary operator's experience can now be performed if there is no cardiac output, at a rate of 100 compressions per minute to achieve a systolic blood pressure of 60 mmHg, alongside internal defibrillation if appropriate. The apex of the heart should not be lifted for internal cardiac massage following mitral valve repair or replacement to avoid posterior ventricular rupture. Cardiopulmonary bypass or extra-corporeal membrane oxygenation may be instituted according to the clinical status of the patient, to ensure systemic perfusion whilst resting the heart.

All surgical sites are systematically examined for active bleeding, which may be addressed by diathermy, application of stainless-steel clips or active topical haemostatic materials, or suturing. The sternal wound is irrigated with saline or antibiotic solution, residual blood in the pericardial and pleural cavities is evacuated and chest tubes are replaced. The sternum may be closed primarily if haemostasis is secured, otherwise with ongoing coagulopathy, areas of concern are packed with sterile gauze without causing a compressive effect and a sterile transparent adhesive drape is applied over an open sternal wound. Further re-exploration is then scheduled once permitted by haemodynamic stability and resolution of clotting derangements.

8 Re-exploration in Operating Theatre

There will be circumstances where the surgical team will still elect to transfer the patient to the operating theatre for further management after achievement of haemodynamic stability with bedside CALS re-exploration. The following practical steps are applicable to the post-arrest patient who was successfully resuscitated with CALS and then returned to the operating theatre, but also for emergency re-explorations where relative haemodynamic stability allows transfer to operating theatre as the most appropriate environment. Anaesthetic and perfusion principles of emergency re-opening and salvage scenarios are presented in detail in Chapters "Anaesthetic Considerations in Emergency Cardiac Surgery" and "Perfusion Considerations in Emergency Cardiac Surgery".

Following return to the operating theatre, CPB lines can be prepared and brought to the operating table in anticipation of potentially complex reparative procedures necessitating CPB. On re-opening, saline washout of the pericardial cavity may not be performed immediately as clots may conveniently denote the location of an underlying active bleeding point. For inspection of distal coronary anastomoses, the sternal retractor should be opened widely to permit excellent exposure and a deep Trendelenburg position can counterbalance haemodynamic fluctuations. Ventilation can be temporarily discontinued to facilitate exposure. Cardiac tissue stabilisers and/or positioning devices provide enhanced retraction capabilities and, coupled with expert anaesthetic management, may avoid the need for re-institution of CPB for repair of bleeding coronary anastomoses. As previously mentioned in the internal massage scenario, lifting of the heart should be avoided in the presence of mitral prostheses, including annuloplasty rings. If performed, it should be done gently and with minimal displacement only when there is high level of suspicion and by someone who can deal with the complications, occasionally catastrophic, of such a manoeuvre. When emergency CPB cannot be circumvented in an arrest scenario, cannulae may be introduced into the aorta and right atrium without prior placement of purse-string sutures, and held in position by assistants until controlled purse-string suture application on CPB. Notably, the ascending aorta may be flaccid with systemic hypotension and/or severe hypovolaemia and arterial blood may not rise to the top of the inserted aortic cannula, mandating careful wet connection to the arterial return of the CPB circuit. Similarly, connection of the venous cannula to the CPB circuit can mitigate blood loss during its insertion into a tense right atrium associated with significantly higher chamber pressures than those observed on routine cannulation.

9 Prognostic and Financial Impact of Emergency Re-exploration for Bleeding

Despite the best efforts of the clinical team to save life during highly stressful bleeding scenarios, re-exploration is a hazardous affair with potential implications for longer-term outcomes. Patients undergoing re-exploration experience significant deteriorations in their post-operative outcomes as consistently corroborated by numerous studies demonstrating up to fourfold increases in mortality, renal failure, sepsis, atrial arrhythmias, prolonged mechanical ventilation, requirement for circulatory support and longer length of hospital and ICU stay (Karthik et al. 2004; Moulton et al. 1996; Biancari et al. 2012; Ranucci et al. 2008; Vivacqua et al. 2011; Fröjd and Jeppsson 2016; Ruel et al. 2017; Hall et al. 2001; Shou et al. 2023; Haneya et al. 2015; Ohmes et al. 2017; Heimisdottir et al. 2022; Affronti et al. 2021; Unsworth-White et al. 1995).

Patients undergoing re-exploration > 24 h after their index operation suffered 3-fold greater morbidity and 15-fold greater mortality than their counterparts undergoing re-exploration within the first 4 h post-operatively (Shou et al. 2023). At a tertiary Canadian centre, re-exploration after the day of surgery was associated with a 6.4-fold increase in mortality risk (Ruel et al. 2017). From their meta-analysis, Biancari and co-workers indicate that re-exploration for bleeding represents an independent predictor of immediate post-operative mortality (Biancari et al. 2012). Fröjd and colleagues showed that cardiac surgical patients undergoing re-exploration had approximately double the odds of mortality not only in the early post-operative period, but extending up to 90 days from re-exploration (Fröjd and Jeppsson 2016), although survival seems comparable to patients without re-exploration in those surviving beyond 90 days from their index operation (Heimisdottir et al. 2022).

The concomitant requirement for blood product transfusion in this population predisposes them to ischaemic injury from micro-emboli and micro-thrombi, and more intense inflammatory responses, whilst potentially conferring increased stroke and short- and long-term mortality risks above those for re-exploration alone (Vivacqua et al. 2011; Despotis et al. 2008). Indeed, the number of PRBC transfused is itself an independent risk factor for low cardiac output, renal failure, sepsis and mortality, with each PRBC unit administered in this setting imparting an approximate 0.25% increase in mortality (Ranucci et al. 2008). Besides multi-organ failure, sepsis and increased blood product utilisation as the principal determinants of mortality in patients undergoing re-exploration, the more complex pre-operative risk profile in this group might explain their globally poorer outcomes (Spadaccio et al. 2023).

There are substantial economic implications for resource utilisation and expenditure amongst patients undergoing re-exploration, not limited to extended ICU and hospital stay (Spadaccio et al. 2023; Alström et al. 2012; Herwaldt et al. 2003). In their study assessing the costs associated with re-exploration compared with prophylactic haemostatic agents in patients undergoing re-exploration after isolated CABG in Sweden, Alström and associates calculated a mean incremental cost of € 6290 per re-explored patient, with 48% (€ 3001) due to prolonged ICU and hospital stay, 31% (€ 1928) due to surgical/anaesthetic costs, 20% (€ 1261) due to increased blood product transfusion and < 2% (€ 100) due to the cost of haemostatic drugs (Alström et al. 2012). Herwaldt and colleagues determined that the cost attributed to re-exploration following CABG in the USA was US$ 9912, compared to US$ 3312 for medically managed bleeding (Herwaldt et al. 2003). The adjusted incremental cost of excessive bleeding in a German cardiac surgical cohort was € 6251, although costs relating specifically to re-exploration (3%) and blood transfusion (4%) contributed only minimally to overall hospital expenditure (Christensen et al. 2009).

These adverse clinical and economic consequences of re-exploration for bleeding highlight the need for prophylactic strategies to diminish the requirement for re-exploration.

10 Intra-operative Surgical Measures to Minimise Post-operative Bleeding

In CABG operations, the in situ internal mammary artery graft should be examined for bleeding points before being stowed in a papaverine-soaked gauze for later use and the internal mammary artery bed and distal stump should be checked before proceeding with cannulation. Intended coronary targets should be identified before cross-clamp application and excellent visualisation of coronary targets is mandatory to ensure technical excellence with anastomotic technique. Each distal coronary anastomosis must be inspected and repaired, as necessary, before embarking on the next step of the operation, and reassessed again whilst on CPB. Accumulated pleural blood should be drained before closure.

In aortic valve replacement operations, the requirement for a right superior pulmonary vein vent and retrograde cardioplegia cannula should be carefully considered, since inadvertent injury to the pulmonary vein or coronary sinus, respectively, on insertion may be troublesome to repair. Each of these should be oversewn at the end. Aortic tissue quality should be assessed and the level and length of the aortotomy precisely determined, to avoid calcification in the aortic wall which can complicate closure whilst being cognisant of thinner aortic walls in patients with a bicuspid aortic valve and/or connective tissue disease. Aortic annular breaches occurring during valve excision should be repaired, and the aortotomy closed with either a single- or double-layered closure, depending on tissue quality. There should be a low threshold for patch augmentation of the aortotomy to relieve excess tension and reduce the risk of aortic rupture. Additional interrupted sutures, with or without Teflon pledget reinforcement, may be placed to control aortotomy bleeding points during low-flow states on CPB. Less severe and non-surgical bleeding from the aortotomy following termination of CPB may be better addressed by packing using gauze swabs, or topical haemostatic agents.

Special considerations to minimise bleeding after mitral valve surgery are avoidance of lifting the heart after implantation of a mitral annuloplasty ring or prosthetic valve, and not oversizing the valve prosthesis, both of which may cause atrio-ventricular disruption. This feared complication, which may manifest as haematoma formation over the posterior cardiac surface rather than frank bleeding, is best managed with resumption of cardiopulmonary bypass, prosthetic valve or annuloplasty ring explantation and patch repair. Atrio-ventricular rupture may also result following excessive decalcification of the posterior mitral valve annulus, when pre-emptive patch insertion is prudent. Finally, a satisfactory technique for left atriotomy closure is mandatory, since bleeding from this posterior incision usually necessitates return to CPB with cross-clamping for control.

Several intra-operative steps may be performed to reduce the higher bleeding risks associated with complex aortic surgery involving the aortic root, ascending aorta and arch. Aortic tissue quality is again an essential consideration. It is advisable to mobilise soft tissue off the aortic root, ascending aorta, arch and neck vessels prior to heparin administration. Size mismatch of valved conduits and prosthetic grafts should be avoided to minimise problematic bleeding from anastomotic discrepancies. When performing a closed distal aortic anastomosis, an adequate portion of aorta should be ensured beyond the cross-clamp and the vascular graft can be invaginated into the aorta. For root replacement surgery, competence of the graft prosthesis, native aortic root and coronary buttons can be tested by the administration of pressurised cardioplegia. It is vital to interrogate all completed anastomoses carefully, especially the posterior aortic root, left coronary button and distal arch, which may be less accessible afterwards.

Prior to closure, the pleurae are drained and all surgical sites are re-examined for haemostasis. Adjunctive techniques to promote haemostasis in cases of mild non-surgical bleeding range from warm saline irrigation of the pericardial cavity to application of topical haemostatic materials. Additional protamine may be necessary if the activated clotting time has not returned to baseline levels. Chest tubes are placed into any opened thoracic cavity, usually the pericardium, pleura(e) and retrosternal space and placed on suction whilst the sternum is being closed. An additional Redivac negative pressure suction drain can be placed in the posterior pericardium and left clamped until chest tube or temporary pacing wire removal. It may be unclamped beforehand to relieve suspected pericardial blood accumulation. However, if drain output is unacceptably high, further evaluation is needed and the chest should not be closed immediately.

11 Minimising Re-exploration for Bleeding

Greater awareness of the predictors and sources of bleeding should emphasise the fundamental importance of meticulous surgical technique with attainment of haemostasis from the outset, to reduce the prevalence of bleeding and re-exploration (Biancari et al. 2018). Careful haemostasis should be observed in the preliminary set-up of the operation up to and including cannulation for CPB, and all surgical sites should be inspected before termination of CPB and re-inspected before protamine administration.

Further intra-operative measures which may help to prevent re-exploration include acute normovolaemic haemodilution, maintenance of haematocrit $\geq 24\%$ during CPB, cell salvage, ultrafiltration and pharmacological agents (Ruel et al. 2017; Shah et al. 2020). The anticipated introduction of more potent antiplatelets and anticoagulants will provide a unique opportunity for further research into the development of novel haemostatic technologies.

Effective application of dedicated haemostasis checklists covering both surgical and coagulopathy components of intra-operative bleeding, and mandating surgical and anaesthetic team cooperation have already demonstrated significant benefit in clinical practice by reducing early post-operative blood loss and re-exploration rates, whilst generating meaningful cost savings (Ali et al. 2019; Elassal et al. 2021; Loor et al. 2013).

Bleeding that may be anticipated in specific patient populations, such as the elderly, those with multiple systemic comorbidities or bleeding diatheses and those receiving antiplatelet or anticoagulant medications with sub-optimal pre-operative cessation, should serve as a focus for pre-emptive intervention. Predictive models, such as the bedside risk score (Mehta et al. 2009), can be used to characterise those populations at elevated bleeding risk, thus permitting pre-emptive optimisation to minimise excessive bleeding and re-exploration. The judicious empirical administration of blood products and procoagulant agents following termination of CPB and prior to chest closure, as guided by clinical experience and point-of-care diagnostic testing, can augment early post-operative haemostasis (Hall et al. 2001). Delayed sternal closure may be more appropriate in the presence of obvious intrinsic coagulopathy, when overlying skin can be closed over a stented sternum.

The universal adoption of standardised definitions of severe post-operative bleeding (Dyke et al. 2014) can increase staff vigilance towards unfavourable trends associated with bleeding and thereby encourage the timely implementation of established departmental protocols. This can steer individual and unit practices towards a multidisciplinary and collaborative routine aimed at reducing re-exploration rates, whilst also homogenising indications for re-exploration when necessary.

As a final consideration, cardiac surgical institutions should embrace the opportunity for reflection and learning when re-explorations occur. This will enable the multidisciplinary team caring for post-operative cardiac surgical patients to gain insight into the underlying causes through institutional governance processes and establish management frameworks to mitigate future occurrences.

12 Conclusions

Excessive bleeding that demands emergency re-exploration is an infrequent yet potentially catastrophic event after cardiac surgery. A thorough appreciation of the inherent risk factors, aetiology and potential intra-operative sources for bleeding can facilitate the pre-emptive recognition of populations vulnerable to post-operative bleeding. Familiarity with the indications, optimal timing and conduct of re-exploration are paramount to achieve the best possible outcomes for patients in such adverse circumstances.

References

Affronti A, Sandoval E, Muro A, Hernández-Campo J, Quintana E, Pereda D, Alcocer J, Pruna-Guillen R, Castellà M (2021) Impact of bedside re-explorations in a cardiovascular surgery intensive care unit led by surgeons. J Clin Med 10:4288

Ali JM, Gerrard C, Clayton J, Moorjani N (2019) Reduced re-exploration and blood product transfusion after the introduction of the Papworth haemostasis checklist. Eur J Cardiothorac Surg 55:729–736

Alström U, Levin LÅ, Ståhle E, Svedjeholm R, Friberg O (2012) Cost analysis of re-exploration for bleeding after coronary artery bypass graft surgery. Br J Anaesth 108:216–222

Besser MW, Ortmann E, Klein AA (2015) Haemostatic management of cardiac surgical haemorrhage. Anaesthesia 70(Suppl 1):87–95

Biancari F, Mikkola R, Heikkinen J, Lahtinen J, Airaksinen KE, Juvonen T (2012) Estimating the risk of complications related to re-exploration for bleeding after adult cardiac surgery: a systematic review and meta-analysis. Eur J Cardiothorac Surg 41:50–55

Biancari F, Kinnunen EM, Kiviniemi T, Tauriainen T, Anttila V, Airaksinen JKE, Brascia D, Vasques F (2018) Meta-analysis of the sources of bleeding after adult cardiac surgery. J Cardiothorac Vasc Anesth 32:1618–1624

Brand J, McDonald A, Dunning J (2018) Management of cardiac arrest following cardiac surgery. BJA Educ 18:16–22

Canádyová J, Zmeko D, Mokrácek A (2012) Re-exploration for bleeding or tamponade after cardiac operation. Interact Cardiovasc Thorac Surg 14:704–708

Cecconi M, De Backer D, Antonelli M, Beale R, Bakker J, Hofer C, Jaeschke R, Mebazaa A, Pinsky MR, Teboul JL, Vincent JL, Rhodes A (2014) Consensus on circulatory shock and hemodynamic monitoring. Task force of the European Society of Intensive Care Medicine. Intensive Care Med 40:1795–1815

Choong CK, Gerrard C, Goldsmith KA, Dunningham H, Vuylsteke A (2007) Delayed re-exploration for bleeding after coronary artery bypass surgery results in adverse outcomes. Eur J Cardiothorac Surg 31:834–838

Christensen MC, Krapf S, Kempel A, von Heymann C (2009) Costs of excessive postoperative hemorrhage in cardiac surgery. J Thorac Cardiovasc Surg 138:687–693

Dacey LJ, Munoz JJ, Baribeau YR, Johnson ER, Lahey SJ, Leavitt BJ, Quinn RD, Nugent WC, Birkmeyer JD, O'Connor GT (1998) Re-exploration for haemorrhage following coronary artery bypass grafting. Incidence and risk factors. Arch Surg 133:442–447

Despotis GJ, Santoro SA, Spitznagel E, Kater KM, Cox JL, Barnes P, Lappas DG (1994) Prospective evaluation and clinical utility of on-site monitoring of coagulation in patients undergoing cardiac operation. J Thorac Cardiovasc Surg 107:271–279

Despotis G, Eby C, Lublin DM (2008) A review of transfusion risks and optimal management of perioperative bleeding with cardiac surgery. Transfusion 48:2S–30S

Despotis G, Avidan M, Eby C (2009) Prediction and management of bleeding in cardiac surgery. J Thromb Haemost 7(Suppl 1):111–117

Dunning J, Fabbri A, Kolh PH, Levine A, Lockowandt U, Mackay J, Pavie AJ, Strang T, Versteegh MI, Nashef SA (2009) EACTS Clinical Guidelines Committee. Guideline for resuscitation in cardiac arrest after cardiac surgery. Eur J Cardiothorac Surg 36:3–28

Dyke C, Aronson S, Dietrich W, Hofmann A, Karkouti K, Levi M, Murphy GJ, Sellke FW, Shore-Lesserson L, von Heymann C, Ranucci M (2014) Universal definition of perioperative bleeding in adult cardiac surgery. J Thorac Cardiovasc Surg 147:1458–1463.e1

Elassal AA, Al-Ebrahim KE, Debis RS, Ragab ES, Faden MS, Fatani MA, Allam AR, Abdulla AH, Bukhary AM, Noaman NA, Eldib OS (2021) Re-exploration for bleeding after cardiac surgery: revaluation of urgency and factors promoting low rate. J Cardiothorac Surg 16:166

Fröjd V, Jeppsson A (2016) Reexploration for bleeding and its association with mortality after cardiac surgery. Ann Thorac Surg 102:109–117

Hall TS, Brevetti GR, Skoultchi AJ, Sines JC, Gregory P, Spotnitz AJ (2001) Reexploration for hemorrhage following open heart surgery differentiation on the causes of bleeding and the impact on patient outcomes. Ann Thorac Cardiovasc Surg 7:352–357

Haneya A, Diez C, Kolat P, Suesskind-Schwendi M, Ried M, Schmid C, Hirt SW (2015) Re-exploration for bleeding or tamponade after cardiac surgery: impact of timing and indication on outcome. Thorac Cardiovasc Surg 63:51–57

Heimisdottir AA, Nielsen SJ, Karlsson M, Jeppsson A, Gudbjartsson T (2022) Long-term outcome of patients undergoing re-exploration for bleeding following cardiac surgery: a SWEDEHEART study. Eur J Cardiothorac Surg 62:ezac208

Herwaldt LA, Swartzendruber SK, Zimmerman MB, Scholz DA, Franklin JA, Caldarone CA (2003) Hemorrhage after coronary artery bypass graft procedures. Infect Control Hosp Epidemiol 24:44–50

Karthik S, Grayson AD, McCarron EE, Pullan DM, Desmond MJ (2004) Reexploration for bleeding after coronary artery bypass surgery: risk factors, outcomes, and the effects of time delay. Ann Thorac Surg 78:527–534

Koch CG, Li L, Duncan AI, Mihaljevic T, Cosgrove DM, Loop FD, Starr NJ, Blackstone EH (2006a) Morbidity and mortality risk associated with red blood cell and blood-component transfusion in isolated coronary artery bypass grafting. Crit Care Med 34:1608–1616

Koch CG, Li L, Duncan AI, Mihaljevic T, Loop FD, Starr NJ, Blackstone EH (2006b) Transfusion in coronary artery bypass grafting is associated with reduced long-term survival. Ann Thorac Surg 81:1650–1657

Koch C, Li L, Figueroa P, Mihaljevic T, Svensson L, Blackstone EH (2009) Transfusion and pulmonary morbidity after cardiac surgery. Ann Thorac Surg 88:1410–1418

Kristensen K, Rauer L, Mortensen P, Kjeldsen B (2012) Reoperation for bleeding in cardiac surgery. Interact Cardiovasc Thorac Surg 14:709–713

Loor G, Vivacqua A, Sabik JF 3rd, Li L, Hixson ED, Blackstone EH, Koch CG (2013) Process improvement in cardiac surgery: development and implementation of a reoperation for bleeding checklist. J Thorac Cardiovasc Surg 146:1028–1032

Mehran R, Rao SV, Bhatt DL, Gibson CM, Caixeta A, Eikelboom J, Kaul S, Wiviott SD, Menon V, Nikolsky E, Serebruany V, Valgimigli M, Vranckx P, Taggart D, Sabik JF, Cutlip DE, Krucoff MW, Ohman EM, Steg PG, White H (2011) Standardized bleeding definitions for cardiovascular clinical trials: a consensus report from the Bleeding Academic Research Consortium. Circulation 123:2736–2747

Mehta RH, Sheng S, O'Brien SM, Grover FL, Gammie JS, Ferguson TB, Peterson ED (2009) Society of Thoracic Surgeons National Cardiac Surgery Database Investigators. Reoperation for bleeding in patients undergoing coronary artery bypass surgery: incidence, risk factors, time trends, and outcomes. Circ Cardiovasc Qual Outcomes 2:583–590

Moorjani N, Viola N, Ohri SK (2013) Key questions in cardiac surgery. TFM Publishing Ltd, Harley

Moulton MJ, Creswell LL, Mackey ME, Cox JL, Rosenbloom M (1996) Re-exploration for bleeding is a risk factor for adverse outcomes after cardiac operations. J Thorac Cardiovasc Surg 111:1037–1046

Ohmes LB, Di Franco A, Guy TS, Lau C, Munjal M, Debois W, Li Z, Krieger KH, Schwann AN, Leonard JR, Girardi LN, Gaudino M (2017) Incidence, risk factors, and prognostic impact of re-exploration for bleeding after cardiac surgery: a retrospective cohort study. Int J Surg 48:166–173

Pasrija C, Ghoreishi M, Whitman G, Ad N, Alejo DE, Holmes SD, Schena S, Salenger R, Mazzeffi MA, Fonner CE, Taylor B (2020) Investigators for the Maryland Cardiac Surgery Quality Initiative. Mitigating the risk: transfusion or reoperation for bleeding after cardiac surgery. Ann Thorac Surg 110:457–463

Pelletier MP, Solymoss S, Lee A, Chiu RC (1998) Negative reexploration for cardiac postoperative bleeding: can it be therapeutic? Ann Thorac Surg 65:999–1002

Petrou A, Tzimas P, Siminelakis S (2016) Massive bleeding in cardiac surgery. Definitions, predictors and challenges. Hippokratia 20:179–186

Ranucci M, Bozzetti G, Ditta A, Cotza M, Carboni G, Ballotta A (2008) Surgical reexploration after cardiac operations: why a worse outcome? Ann Thorac Surg 86:1557–1562

Ruel M, Chan V, Boodhwani M, McDonald B, Ni X, Gill G, Lam K, Hendry P, Masters R, Mesana T (2017) How detrimental is reexploration for bleeding after cardiac surgery? J Thorac Cardiovasc Surg 154:927–935

Sellman M, Intonti MA, Ivert T (1997) Reoperations for bleeding after coronary artery bypass procedures during 25 years. Eur J Cardiothorac Surg 11:521–527

Shah A, Palmer AJR, Klein AA (2020) Strategies to minimize intraoperative blood loss during major surgery. Br J Surg 107:e26–e38

Shou BL, Aravind P, Ong CS, Alejo D, Canner JK, Etchill EW, DiNatale J, Prokupets R, Esfandiary T, Lawton JS, Schena S (2023) Early reexploration for bleeding is associated with improved outcome in cardiac surgery. Ann Thorac Surg 115:232–239

Society of Thoracic Surgeons Task Force on Resuscitation After Cardiac Surgery (2017) The Society of Thoracic Surgeons Expert consensus for the resuscitation of patients who arrest after cardiac surgery. Ann Thorac Surg 103:1005–1020

Soletti G Jr, Cancelli G, Dell'Aquila M, Caldonazo T, Harik L, Rossi C, Tasoudis P, Leith J, An KR, Dimagli A, Demetres M, Gaudino M (2024) Re-exploration for bleeding and long-term survival after adult cardiac surgery: a meta-analysis of reconstructed time-to-event data. Int J Surg 110:5795–5801

Spadaccio C, Rose D, Nenna A, Taylor R, Bittar MN (2023) Early re-exploration versus conservative management for postoperative bleeding in stable patients after coronary artery bypass grafting: a propensity matched study. J Clin Med 12:3327

Tirilomis T, Bougioukas IG, Friedrich MG, Danner BC, Schoendube FA (2020) Re-exploration early after cardiac surgery in adults: the importance of bleeding-related complications. Heart Surg Forum 23:E174–E177

Ul Islam M, Ahmad I, Khan B, Jan A, Ali N, Hassan Khan W, Farooq O, Khan H, Ahmad Ali F, Shahid M (2021) Early chest re-exploration for excessive bleeding in post cardiac surgery patients: does it matter? Cureus 13:e15091

Unsworth-White MJ, Herriot A, Valencia O, Poloniecki J, Smith EE, Murday AJ, Parker DJ, Treasure T (1995) Resternotomy for bleeding after cardiac operation: a marker for increased morbidity and mortality. Ann Thorac Surg 59:664–667

Vivacqua A, Koch CG, Yousuf AM, Nowicki ER, Houghtaling PL, Blackstone EH, Sabik JF 3rd. (2011) Morbidity of bleeding after cardiac surgery: is it blood transfusion, reoperation for bleeding, or both? Ann Thorac Surg 91:1780–1790

Risk Stratification and Outcome Reporting in Emergency Cardiac Surgery

Rana Sayeed

Abstract Accurate risk stratification is essential to guide clinical decision-making and enable comparison between surgeons and institutions. Current risk prediction models based on logistic regression show good discrimination but are poorly calibrated for emergency and other high-risk cardiac surgery. Better risk prediction may be achieved by combining risk models into a two-stage approach, modifying existing risk models with additional variables to create disease-specific tools, e.g. for acute aortic dissection, or novel machine learning models. Current machine learning models offer a slight improvement in performance over established logistic regression models, but further improvements and refinements are likely to achieve even better reliability.

Keywords Emergency cardiac surgery · Risk stratification · Risk prediction · Machine learning · Artificial intelligence

1 Risk Stratification in Cardiac Surgery

Successful clinical outcomes in cardiac surgery depend upon careful patient selection and meticulous operative technique in the undertaking of the correct operative procedure; these factors attain greater significance in emergency surgery. The technical aspects of emergency operative procedures are described in other chapters. This chapter focuses on risk stratification in emergency cardiac surgery to guide clinical decision-making and compare clinical outcomes between surgeons and surgical centres.

The principles of risk stratification for risk-benefit analysis and patient selection are well described. In combination with careful clinical assessment, risk-scoring

R. Sayeed (✉)
Consultant Cardiac Surgeon, Oxford Heart Centre, John Radcliffe Hospital, Oxford University Hospitals NHS Foundation Trust, Oxford, UK
e-mail: rana.sayeed@ouh.nhs.uk

A. Kourliouros (ed.), *Emergency Cardiac Surgery*,
https://doi.org/10.1007/978-3-032-15787-4_33

systems help guide complex decision-making in the emergency setting. The most widely used risk-scoring systems are the European System for Cardiac Operative Risk Evaluation (EuroSCORE), currently EuroSCORE II, and the Society of Thoracic Surgeons (STS) score (Pittams et al. 2021).

1.1 EuroSCORE

The EuroSCORE was first developed in 1999 to predict the risk of in-hospital mortality after cardiac surgery (Roques et al. 1999). The current iteration, EuroSCORE II, based on newer outcome data and a revised model, was released in 2012 (Nashef et al. 2012). It is the most well-known risk stratification system in cardiac surgery worldwide. The original EuroSCORE comprised 17 pre-operative variables, divided into patient-related, cardiac-related, and surgical-related factors, and was developed by multivariate logistic analysis of a European multinational database of more than 19,000 patients in 128 European centres. EuroSCORE II updated the EuroSCORE risk model based on the outcomes of more than 22,000 patients from 154 centres across 43 countries in Europe, North America, Asia, and Africa to achieve a better predictive model than logistic EuroSCORE. Notably, less than 5% of cases were emergency (4.3%) or salvage (0.5%) procedures.

1.2 STS Score

The STS score is a risk stratification model based on 30 variables to predict short- and long-term mortality *and* morbidity after cardiac surgery.[1] In addition to patient demographic and cardiac factors, the STS score includes a broader range of pre-operative comorbidities, such as an immunocompromised state and dialysis, which are poor prognostic indicators. There are separate online tools to determine the risk of mortality after isolated coronary artery bypass graft (CABG) surgery, isolated valve procedures, or combined CABG and valve procedures. The STS score was first developed in 1999 and updated regularly according to the STS National Database. The model was developed from surgeon-specific mortality and morbidity data in a bivariate random-effects model, enabling STS risk prediction scores for mortality, morbidity, and individual morbidities such as deep sternal wound infection, prolonged ventilation, renal failure, and stroke. However, the STS score underestimates the risk of mortality compared with EuroSCORE II, and the latter allows risk prediction for a wider range of procedures.

---

[1] The Society of Thoracic Surgeons. Risk calculator. Available at: https://www.sts.org/resources/risk-calculator. Accessed 16 December 2024.

2 Limitations of Risk Prediction Models in Emergency Cardiac Surgery

Risk models are assessed by two criteria: calibration (how close is the predicted outcome to the observed outcome?) and discrimination (how accurate is the model in distinguishing between a high-risk and a low-risk patient?). EuroSCORE II broadly overestimates contemporary risk in overall UK cardiac surgery, but this 'calibration drift' results from the age of the model—EuroSCORE II is based on data collected in 2010 and the use of risk modelling as a quality control measure in the UK and the consequent robust quality monitoring in UK national cardiac surgical practice have helped to identify and correct any clinical underperformance.

Furthermore, the validation and calibration of a risk prediction model depends on the original modelling data set and may vary according to procedure and location. An analysis of 3,342 emergency cardiac procedures between 2008 and 2011 in the UK National Institute for Cardiovascular Outcomes Registry (from a total of 109,988 operations, a lower proportion than the EuroSCORE II data set) found that (logistic EuroSCORE and) EuroSCORE II had poorer discrimination and calibration for emergency cardiac surgery compared with non-emergency and all cardiac procedures (Grant et al. 2013). Several risk factors were not important in determining in-hospital mortality after emergency cardiac surgery, including female sex, chronic pulmonary disease, neurological disease, active endocarditis, unstable angina, recent myocardial infarction, and pulmonary hypertension.

In summary, the most widely used risk prediction models perform poorly in emergency cardiac surgery. What are the possible solutions?

3 Improving Risk Stratification in Emergency Cardiac Surgery

Current risk prediction models are less accurate in emergency cardiac surgery because their databases contain a small proportion of these cases and because particular risk factors predictive in other settings are not valuable in emergency cardiac surgery. Strategies to improve risk prediction in emergency cardiac surgery include combining risk scores into a two-stage approach, disease-specific risk models, and machine learning to develop new predictive models.

3.1 Two-Stage Risk Prediction

The Italian Surgical and Clinical Outcome Research (SCORE) Group has developed a two-stage model to predict mortality after high-risk cardiac surgery (Ranucci et al. 2016). An analysis of 105 patients with predicted operative mortality > 25%

by either the EuroSCORE II or the ACEF (Age, creatinine, ejection fraction) score (Ranucci et al. 2009) confirmed the limitations of established risk models in a high-risk cohort. The observed mortality was 26%; expected mortality was underestimated by EuroSCORE II (16%) and overestimated by ACEF (36%), although EuroSCORE II maintained good discrimination. In this high-risk population, independent risk factors for mortality were emergency surgery, serum creatinine, pulmonary hypertension, and pre-operative anaemia. A two-stage strategy (first stage: EuroSCORE II/ACEF score risk > 25%; second stage: reclassification based on pulmonary hypertension, serum creatinine, and anaemia) accurately predicted an expected 26% mortality with good discrimination and might represent one solution to risk prediction in emergency and other high-risk settings.

3.2 Risk Prediction Models for Aortic Dissection

Aortic dissection is the most common cardiac surgical emergency, and reliable risk stratification is essential for optimal case selection. EuroSCORE II includes *thoracic aortic surgery* as an operative risk factor, but there is no distinction based on the extent of aortic surgery. Nonetheless, studies have confirmed the predictive accuracy of EuroSCORE II in elective and emergency thoracic aortic surgery in its original form (Nishida et al. 2014). A modified version, including aortic dissection and pre-operative malperfusion as additional risk factors, has improved the predictive value of EuroSCORE II for aortic surgery (Barmettler et al. 2004).

Several groups have developed risk prediction models for aortic dissection based on national or institutional outcomes registries. The International Registry of Acute Aortic Dissection (IRAD) score was created from the IRAD observational registry to create a simple risk model for in-hospital mortality based on age > 70 years; history of aortic valve replacement; presenting hypotension, shock, or tamponade; migrating chest pain; pre-operative cardiac tamponade; any pulse deficit; and ECG infarct, new Q waves, ST elevation, or ischaemia. The risk prediction tool had good discrimination and agreement between observed and predicted mortality (Rampoldi et al. 2007).

Given the critical importance of pre-operative malperfusion, the Penn Group developed its classification based on the categorisation of acute aortic dissection patients into four groups according to the presence and extent of any ischaemia and malperfusion: class A (no branch-vessel malperfusion or circulatory collapse); class B (localised branch-vessel malperfusion with ischaemia, including stroke, renal failure, paraplegia, limb ischaemia, and mesenteric ischaemia), class C (circulatory collapse with or without cardiac involvement); and class BC (branch-vessel malperfusion in conjunction with circulatory collapse). A systematic review found that although the Penn classification has good discrimination, with an incremental increase in mortality with the progression across Penn groups, it is poorly calibrated (Chandiramani et al. 2024). In contrast, another centre developed a novel risk model based only on serum creatinine, serum lactic acid, and liver malperfusion with good predictive ability after multivariate analysis (Ghoreishi et al. 2018).

Finally, the German Registry of Acute Aortic Dissection Type A (GERAADA) score was developed as an online risk scoring system to predict 30-day mortality after acute type A aortic dissection repair. The GERAADA score includes many factors within EuroSCORE II but does not include factors related to malperfusion. A recent comparison found that although GERAADA and EuroSCORE II had good calibration, EuroSCORE II had better discrimination (Nezic et al. 2021).

At present, there is no widely adopted risk model for elective or emergency aortic surgery, although the STS has an aortic surgery risk model and calculator under development.

3.3 Machine Learning to Predict Cardiac Surgical Mortality

EuroSCORE II was developed using logistic regression to analyse perioperative factors collected in its database. EuroSCORE II has clinical utility because the relevant risk factors needed to calculate a score are routinely available, but it tends to overestimate contemporary surgical mortality because of calibration drift and inherently weaker calibration for emergency and other high-risk procedures. Logistic regression is an established and widely used tool to create risk prediction models, but it is limited because of its key assumption of a linear relationship between variables and a need for regular time-consuming revision, such as the different iterations of EuroSCORE. Machine learning-based prediction modelling has the advantages of not assuming linearity and utilising many different self-generated algorithms to study complex variable interactions. There have been significant advances in machine learning across many disciplines, and recent studies confirm that current machine learning models showed some statistical improvements in discrimination, calibration, and clinical utility compared with EuroSCORE II (Sinha et al. 2023).

The performance of machine learning models will continue to improve because machine learning improves with additional data; it does not assume linearity when the interaction of many cardiac risk factors is not linear, and automated retraining of models will reduce calibration drift in established risk prediction models.

4 Clinical Outcome Reporting in Emergency Cardiac Surgery

Clinical outcomes after emergency cardiac surgery, e.g. death or stroke, are highly variable owing to the diverse range of presentations that need emergency surgery described elsewhere in this volume, including acute aortic dissection, post-infarction ventricular septal or papillary muscle rupture, and failed PCI. Without an established and accurate risk model, published series or regional and national registries provide the most valuable contemporary outcomes for defined conditions for patient consent and benchmarking clinical practice. For example, the UK National Consultant Information Programme portal reported a 17.8% in-hospital and 23.8% 1-year mortality after surgery for acute type A aortic dissection over 2020–2023, comparable to published series.

Surgeon-specific risk-adjusted outcomes for cardiac surgery are published in the public domain in a few countries, including the UK and USA (California, New York). The benefits of the public availability of such outcome data include an associated improvement in risk-adjusted outcomes, better quality and completeness of data collection and validation, and public reassurance about the safety and quality of services (Jenkins and Cooper 2017). However, there are potential detrimental effects of the publication of surgeon-specific data, including gaming—distorting the process of care to meet targets or manipulating data to misrepresent actual performance—and adverse selection/inequity ('risk-averse behaviour') - avoiding the most severely ill patients. In cardiac surgery, emergency cases are excluded from outcome reporting to prevent risk-averse behaviour affecting the decision to operate on emergency high-risk cases. Nonetheless, a survey of UK cardiac surgeons reported that both gaming and risk-averse behaviour were observed in clinical practice (Jarral et al. 2016).

5 Summary

Existing risk prediction models show good discrimination but need better calibration and overestimate mortality for emergency and other high-risk cardiac surgery. Better risk prediction may be achieved by combining risk models into a two-stage approach, adding variables to create disease-specific tools, e.g. for acute aortic dissection, or using machine learning models. Current machine learning models offer a slight improvement in performance over established logistic regression models, but further improvements in are likely to achieve even better reliability.

References

Barmettler H, Immer FF, Berdat PA et al (2004) Risk-stratification in thoracic aortic surgery: should the EuroSCORE be modified? Eur J Cardiothorac Surg 25:691–694

Chandiramani A, Al-Tawil M, Rajasekarz T et al (2024) Incidence rates of Penn classes and class-specific mortality in acute type A aortic dissection patients: an epidemiologic systematic review and meta-analysis. J Cardiothorac Vasc Anesth 38:1558–1568

Ghoreishi M, Wise ES, Croal-Abrahams L et al (2018) A novel risk score predicts operative mortality after acute type A aortic dissection repair. Ann Thorac Surg 106:1759–1766

Grant SW, Hickey GL, Dimarakis I et al (2013) Performance of the EuroSCORE models in emergency cardiac surgery. Circ Cardiovasc Qual Outcomes 6:178–185

Jarral O, Baig K, Pettengell C et al (2016) National survey of UK consultant surgeons' opinions on surgeon-specific mortality data in cardiothoracic surgery. Circ Cardiovasc Qual Outcomes 9:414–423

Jenkins DP, Cooper G (2017) Publicly available outcome data for individual surgeons: lessons from cardiac surgery. Eur Urol 71:309–310

Nashef SAM, Roques F, Sharples LD et al (2012) EuroSCORE II. Eur J Cardiothorac Surg 41:734–745

Nezic DG, Zivkovica IS, Milicic MD et al (2021) On-line risk prediction models for acute type A aortic dissection surgery: validation of the German Registry of Acute Aortic Dissection Type A score and the European System for Cardiac Operative Risk Evaluation II. Eur J Cardiothorac Surg 61:1068–1075

Nishida T, Sonoda H, Oishi Y et al (2014) The novel EuroSCORE II algorithm predicts the hospital mortality of thoracic aortic surgery in 461 consecutive Japanese patients better than both the original additive and logistic EuroSCORE algorithms. Interact Cardiovasc Thorac Surg 18:446–450

Pittams AP, Iddawela S, Zaidi S et al (2021) Scoring systems for risk stratification in patients undergoing cardiac surgery. J Cardiothorac Vasc Anesth 36:1148–1156

Rampoldi V, Trimarchi S, Eagle KA et al (2007) Simple risk models to predict surgical mortality in acute type A aortic dissection: The International Registry of Acute Aortic Dissection score. Ann Thorac Surg 83:55–61

Ranucci M, Castelvecchio S, Menicanti L et al (2009) Risk of assessing mortality risk in elective cardiac operations. Age, creatinine, ejection fraction, and the law of parsimony. Circulation 119:3053–3061

Ranucci M, Di Dedda U, Castelvecchio S et al (2016) In search of the ideal risk-scoring system for very high-risk cardiac surgical patients: a two-stage approach. J Cardiothorac Surg 11:13

Roques F, Nashef SAM, Michel P et al (1999) Risk factors and outcome in European cardiac surgery: analysis of the EuroSCORE multinational database of 19030 patients. Eur J Cardiothorac Surg 15:816–823

Sinha S, Dong T, Dimaglia A et al (2023) Comparison of machine learning techniques in prediction of mortality following cardiac surgery: analysis of over 220 000 patients from a large national database. Eur J Cardiothorac Surg 63(6):ezad183

Index

A. Kourliouros (ed.), *Emergency Cardiac Surgery*,
https://doi.org/10.1007/978-3-032-15787-4

R